CLINICAL DENTAL PROSTHETICS

CLINICAL DENTAL PROSTHETICS

H.R.B. Fenn

K.P. Liddelow A.P.Gimson

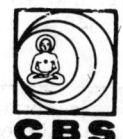

CBS Publishers & Distributors Pvt. Ltd.

New Delhi • Bengaluru • Chennai • Kochi • Kolkata • Mumbai
Hyderabad • Nagpur • Patna • Pune • Vijayawada

ISBN: 81-239-1079-7

First Indian Edition: 1986
Reprint: 1998, 2002, 2004, 2008

This edition has been published in India by arrangement with
John Wright & Sons Ltd., U.K.

Published by **Satish Kumar Jain** and produced by **Varun Jain** for
CBS Publishers & Distributors Pvt. Ltd.,
4819/XI Prahlad Street, 24 Ansari Road, Daryaganj, New Delhi - 110002
delhi@cbspd.com, cbspubs@airtelmail.in • www.cbspd.com
Ph.: 23289259, 23266861, 23266867 • Fax: 011-23243014

Corporate Office: 204 FIE, Industrial Area, Patparganj, Delhi - 110 092
Ph: 49344934 • Fax: 011-49344935
E-mail: publishing@cbspd.com • publicity@cbspd.com

Branches:
• *Bengaluru:* 2975, 17th Cross, K.R. Road, Bansankari 2nd Stage,
  Bengaluru - 70 • Ph: +91-80-26771678/79 • Fax: +91-80-26771680
  E-mail: cbsbng@gmail.com, bangalore@cbspd.com
• *Chennai:* No. 7, Subbaraya Street, Shenoy Nagar, Chennai - 600030
  Ph: +91-44-26681266, 26680620 • Fax: +91-44-42032115
  E-mail: chennai@cbspd.com
• *Kochi:* Ashana House, 39/1904, A.M. Thomas Road, Valanjambalam,
  Ernakulum, Kochi • Ph: +91-484-4059061-65
  Fax: +91-484-4059065 • E-mail: cochin@cbspd.com
• *Kolkata:* 6-B, Ground Floor, Rameshwar Shaw Road, Kolkata - 700014
  Ph: +91-33-22891126/7/8 • E-mail: kolkata@cbspd.com
• *Mumbai:* 83-C, Dr. E. Moses Road, Worli, Mumbai - 400018
  Ph: +91-9833017933, 022-24902340/41 • E-mail: mumbai@cbspd.com

Representatives:
• Hyderabad: 0-9885175004   • Nagpur: 0-9021734563
• Patna: 0-9334159340   • Pune: 0-9623451994
• Vijayawada: 0-9000660880

Printed at:
India Binding House, Noida, UP (India)

To

ALL PAST, PRESENT AND FUTURE DENTAL STUDENTS

AND TO

ALL TECHNICIANS WITHOUT WHOSE CRAFTSMANSHIP

THE CLINICIAN'S EFFORTS WOULD BE VALUELESS

CONTENTS

PREFACE TO THE FIRST EDITION

The justification for adding yet another textbook to the shelves of dental literature is to be found in the presentation of the subject matter and not in any novelty of technique. As teachers of undergraduate dental students we have become increasingly aware of the fact that the purely clinical aspect of dental prosthetics is still to quite a large extent overshadowed by dental mechanics in current textbooks. Another shortcoming which we desired to remedy is that whilst there are many books on full denture construction there are few on partial dentures and none which give adequate information on both full and partial dentures in the same volume.

An attempt has been made to explain the principles of denture construction, both full and partial, together with a detailed description of the clinical work involved and the reason for each particular operation. As this book is intended primarily for undergraduate students whose time is necessarily limited, many excellent but more complicated techniques have purposely been omitted but it is hoped that this book is sufficiently comprehensive to guide the operator in the construction of dentures for all but the most unusual cases.

The purely mechanical side of denture construction is not mentioned as it is already well catered for and the present trend in dental education is, rightly or wrongly, to increase the clinical knowledge and skill at the expense of the purely laboratory work.

It will be obvious that we have freely consulted the available dental literature and whilst we have neither quoted from it verbatim nor duplicated any illustrations we have in a few instances followed it fairly closely and where this has occurred we should like to express our appreciation to the Authors concerned.

We would like to express our indebtedness to our many colleagues whose help and encouragement has made the production of this book possible. In particular we should like to thank Mr R. D. G. Gain for the very valuable help and advice he has given in proof reading; Miss M. J. Waldren and Miss P. Carter of the Medical Illustration Department of Guy's Hospital for the illustrations; Mr A. Smith of the Photographic Department of King's College Hospital for taking many of the photographs; Miss E. Young and Mrs K. A. Short for typing the manuscript; Mr H. Bone and the technical staff of King's College Hospital for preparing the models used for the illustrations and other invaluable assistance; and finally we should like to express our thanks to the publishers for their ready co-operation and for including all the illustrations for which we asked. Especially should we like to thank in this connexion Miss E. Hewson and her staff of the Publishing Department and Mr G. Hill and his staff of the Production Department.

H. R. B. F.
K. P. L.
A. P. C.

PREFACE TO THE SECOND EDITION

The first edition of this book, while covering the basic essentials of prosthetics, gave no information in the wider fields of the subject. Also since no textbook can remain permanently up to date, it was decided to revise certain sections and make some additions.

The section on partial dentures has been largely re-written with many new illustrations. Several new chapters have been included dealing with perfecting the occlusion and articulation; obturators; appearance and overlay and implant dentures, thus presenting in one volume all the essentials which a student should know before qualification and also making the book more useful to the practitioner.

An experiment has been tried in this new edition with some trepidation – which is to drop the use of the term 'bite' taking, substituting where possible the word 'record' taking as being more in keeping with modern teaching: time will show whether this change is justified or not.

The many suggestions and criticisms which have been received have all been carefully considered and we are grateful for them, even though we have not been able to incorporate them all.

We should like to express our thanks particularly to Mr Wesley Johnson, who devoted a lot of his own time to preparing a detailed, constructive criticism of the first edition. This was of great help to us and many of his valuable amendments and suggestions have been incorporated in the second edition. We should also like to thank those who have so kindly and readily loaned us illustrations: Mr Adrian Halder, for fig. 181 (a), Mr Denis Glass for fig. 520, Professor Malcolm Gibson for fig. 514, and Mr Maurice Kettle for figs. 513, 565, 579, 580.

Some of the additional photographs have been kindly taken by Mr A. Smith of the Photographic Department of King's

College Hospital whilst Mr H. Bone, Mr T. Marshall, Mr F. Treacher, Mr G. Hough and Mr P. Nowell have produced many of the appliances and models used for illustration.

Mr Roy Honeywood and Mr A. J. Bailey are responsible for the additional line illustrations and Mrs M. Harrison and Miss S. and Miss V. Liddelow have patiently typed and re-typed the new manuscript.

To all of them we say thank you indeed for both your work and your forbearance.

We should also like to record our appreciation of both the help and courtesy which we have received from the Production Department of Staples Press, especially from Mr Derek Morrison and Mr N. J. Cowan.

Finally, but by no means least, we should like to record our gratitude to our wives for their help and forbearance during the long period of production of both the original and this second edition, without which the work could never have been completed.

H. R. B. F.
K. P. L.
A. P. G.
King's College Hospital,
Dental Department and School,
London, S.E.5.

INTRODUCTORY HISTORICAL NOTES

Dental prostheses are undoubtedly among the earliest forms of dental treatment, the oldest existing denture being one of the lower six anterior teeth bound together with gold wire and attached by the same means to the adjacent natural teeth. It was made by the Etruscans in about 300 B.C. and shows a much higher degree of skill and craftsmanship than many specimens of a considerably later date. The early Japanese, in particular, constructed very crude dentures of wood with pebbles inserted to represent the teeth.

Probably the earliest written reference to full dentures is in the preface to Blagravi's 'Mathematical Jewel' (1585) in which the author mentions his nephew 'who caused his teeth to be all drawn out and after had a sett of ivory teeth in agayne.'

Until the middle of the nineteenth century dentures were usually carved out of a solid block of ivory or bone, sometimes with natural teeth inserted in them and usually the anterior six uppers and lowers (*see* fig. 181(*a*)). The useful life of these dentures was short as the materials were of course subject to caries and the fit could never have been more than approximate. The carving was by trial and error though undoubtedly some marking medium was used in the mouth and Purman in 1684 mentions making a model of the mouth but from his description it is not clear whether his model was an impression or a cast. It was not until 1782 that impression taking is mentioned, by William Rae who describes a technique for taking an impression in wax and pouring into it a cast of plaster of Paris.

Although Philip Phaff of Prussia is usually credited with the introduction of models made of plaster of Paris.

Pierre Fauchard may truly be regarded as the 'Father of Dentistry' and his 'Chirurgien Dentiste' published in 1728 contains many detailed descriptions of various prostheses, including no fewer than five different types of obturators.

He obviously encountered some difficulty in keeping his dentures in place since he describes the use of springs for retention 'where necessary'. It is interesting to note that George Washington's dentures were retained by springs.

The disadvantages of ivory and bone were obviously serious and metal bases of swaged gold or platinum were commonly used by the beginning of the nineteenth century and Chemant of Paris tried fused porcelain for both bases and teeth but his contemporaries, among whom was John Hunter, soon abandoned it, having been unable to overcome the shrinkage when fusing. About 1774 Duchâteau, an apothecary of Paris, and Dubois de Chemant, a dentist, made a whole denture from fused porcelain, but it was not until 1808 that Fouzi of Italy started making individual porcelain teeth and later (1837) Claudius Ash of London introduced fused porcelain tube teeth for the same purpose.

The first thermoplastic denture base was probably used by Harrington of Portsmouth who in 1830 softened and moulded tortoise-shell but the introduction of vulcanized rubber by Goodyear in 1839 was really the beginning of modern dental prosthetics.

A quotation from Gutmann of Leipzig written in 1827 is interesting as showing the appreciation of the trifold functions of a denture. 'In order to render the use of artificial teeth more widespread and more serviceable to the community, I refuse to accept a fee for installing them until patients have had one, or in certain circumstances even two, months in which to convince themselves of their suitability for ornament, for clear enunciation and for mastication.'

The technique of the casting of metal has a long history and the lost wax process was probably used by the Egyptians and the goldsmiths of Solomon to produce decorations for the temple. It was Taggart, however, in 1907 who first used this process for producing gold inlays and later it was used for dentures. A lot of trouble was experienced with the contraction of the metal and it is only in recent years that really accurate metal casting has been made possible.

Chrome cobalt or an alloy of similar metals was discovered by Elwood Haynes in 1907 when experimenting to find a durable alloy for the electrodes ot sparking plugs. In 1929 R. W. Erdle and C. H. Prange of Austenal Laboratories modified this alloy for casting dentures and patented it as Vitallium. It is interesting to note that this alloy played an important part in the development of the jet engine because its ability to maint in its physical properties at high temperatures was invaluable in this field.

The acrylic resins are of comparatively recent development and were first used for denture bases in 1935.

The most recent developments in prosthetic dentistry are probably the alginate materials introduced in about 1938 and the rubber base impression materials introduced in the '50s.

CHAPTER I

INTRODUCTION TO PROSTHETICS

Definition of Prosthetics

A Prosthesis may be defined as an appliance which replaces lost or congenitally missing tissue. Some prostheses restore both the function and the appearance of the tissue they replace, others merely restore one of these factors.

Prosthetics is the art and science of designing and fitting artificial substitutes to replace lost or missing tissue. Dental Prosthetics is a subdivision which deals with its application to the mouth.

By definition dental prosthetics includes the replacement of any lost tissue and therefore embraces the filling of teeth and the fitting of artificial crowns. In actual practice, however, the term has come to mean the fitting of appliances such as artificial dentures, bridges, obturators, surgical prostheses and lip supports, and it is in this sense that the term will be used throughout this book.

WHY ARE DENTURES NECESSARY?

Before studying in detail the methods, techniques and theories employed in and relating to dental prosthetics, it is necessary to have clearly in mind the purpose which is being served. It is pertinent, therefore, to commence a book of this character by asking and answering the question – 'Why do we make dentures?'

In order to answer this question the functions of the teeth must be understood. These are threefold:

(1) To divide the food finely so that a large surface area is available for the action of the digestive juices.

(2) To assist the tongue and lips to form some of the sounds of speech.

(3) The teeth form an important feature of the face, and by supporting the lips and cheeks enable these structures to

perform their functions of manipulating the food and expressing emotion.

The teeth are also mutually interdependent; premature loss of any tooth may cause a collapse of the dental arch, and movement of individual teeth, with loss of interproximal contacts, thus giving rise to food-packing and gingival troubles. Function is necessary :

(1) To minimize the risk of caries by preventing food stagnation.

(2) To preserve the health of the soft tissues by the massaging action of the passage of food.

(3) To prevent the over-eruption which may occur if a tooth is unopposed.

Prior to the comparatively modern development of highly refined foods the loss of natural teeth often resulted in severe malnutrition but nowadays it is quite possible to live a· perfectly healthy life with no teeth at all; in spite of this complete edentation is an unpleasant state for the following reasons:

(1) It places limitations on the diet and all hard and fibrous foods require to be finely divided or else digestive troubles may result.

(2) It produces a certain sibilance in the speech because those consonant stops requiring the presence of the teeth cannot be made efficiently.

(3) It results in a prematurely aged appearance due to the loss of support and consequent falling in of the lips and cheeks, and the fact that the jaws can be overclosed produces a bunching up of the soft tissues around the mouth and close approximation of the chin and nose.

(4) It can produce loss of confidence and even psychological disturbances from the mutilated appearance.

The results of edentation so far mentioned apply generally; there are other disadvantages applying individually. For instance: wind instrument players and singers are quite unable to perform; clergymen cannot preach; actors and photographers' models cannot follow their employment; and the pipe smoker loses half the enjoyment of his pipe if he cannot hold it between his teeth.

To the majority of people, therefore, the loss of the teeth is a matter of great concern, and their replacement by artificial substitutes is vital to the continuance of normal life.

WHAT ARE THE DIFFERENCES BETWEEN NATURAL TEETH AND ARTIFICIAL DENTURES?

Having seen that the replacement of the lost natural teeth by artificial substitutes is essential to the continuance of a normal life, the questions which logically follow must be answered.

The essential difference between natural and artificial teeth is that the former are firmly rooted in the bone of the jaws, and in consequence they can incise, tear and finely grind food of any character because the lower teeth can move across the upper teeth with a powerful shearing action. Artificial dentures, on the other hand, merely rest on the gums and are held there by weak forces. In addition they are subjected to powerful displacing forces, so their efficiency as a masticating apparatus is limited. This efficiency can vary within wide limits depending on the shape and size of the edentulous jaws, the type of gum tissue covering these jaws, the mental attitude of the patient to the dentures, his ability to learn to use them, and the skill of the operator. These factors are discussed at length in Chapter II.

Aesthetically, artificial teeth can be indistinguishable from natural teeth, and in many cases they can enhance the appearance if the natural teeth were hypoplastic, grossly carious or unpleasantly irregular. The speech of artificial denture wearers should be normal once the tongue and lips have adapted themselves to the dentures. Other functions such as singing, or musical instrument playing, can be made possible by modifying the dentures in various ways.

The main limitations of artificial dentures therefore are that they lack stability, and the masticatory force which can be applied by them is limited by this fact, and also by the pressure which the gums will tolerate. In other respects they can closely rival natural teeth.

WHAT ARE THE DISPLACING FORCES CAUSING INSTABILITY?

The most powerful displacing forces are the muscles surrounding the oral cavity, and the tongue. One of the functions of the lips, cheeks and tongue is to receive and manipulate the food and pass it backwards and forwards between the teeth until it has been reduced to a sufficiently fine state for it to be formed into a bolus and swallowed. These movements are powerful, and unless the dentures are very firmly seated – which can be the case only if they have been properly designed and made by a careful and exact technique – and until the wearer has become skilful in manipulating them, they are liable to be moved about with the food. In addition, every time the mouth is opened the muscles of the cheeks tense, and if the lower denture is over-extended at the edges it will be raised. Also during speech the tongue tends to tip, and, in bad cases, eject the lower denture unless it is properly designed.

Other displacing forces requiring to be reduced by careful technique and design are:

(1) The interference and locking of the cusps of the teeth as the lower move across the upper in chewing. This interference tends to displace both dentures from their seating.

(2) Viscous and sticky foods tend to unite the dentures and displace them.

(3) Gravity will tend to unseat the upper denture.

WHAT ARE THE RETAINING FORCES AVAILABLE TO COUNTERACT DISPLACEMENT?

These can be divided into two classes:

(A) Positive physical forces.

(B) Acquired muscular control by the denture wearer.

(A) *The Physical Forces*

1. *Adhesion and Cohesion*

Adhesion is defined as the apparent force of attraction existing between dissimilar bodies in close contact. This force acts most powerfully at right angles to the surface, and is proportional to the area of the surfaces in contact. Cohesion is the apparent force of attraction existing between similar bodies in close contact.

An example of adhesion is afforded by two microscope slides with a very thin film of water between them. The force required to separate the slides, provided it is applied at right angles, will be great, but if it is applied at a lesser angle the slides immediately commence to slip over one another and separate easily. The force of adhesion acts from one surface of the film of water to one glass slide and from the other surface of the film to the other glass slide. Within the film of water the force of cohesion unites the molecules, and the thinner the film the more powerful is this force.

A denture base is made accurately to fit the mucous membrane on which it rests, and intervening between the two surfaces is saliva. The similarity to the microscope slide analogy is therefore obvious. Thus adhesion may or may not play an important part in retaining a denture in place, depending on the shape of the mouth, its surface area, the closeness of apposition of the denture to the tissues, and the direction of the displacing forces. The accompanying diagrams should make this clear (*see* figs. 1 and 2).

Adhesion is by far the greater of these two forces, as can easily be shown by placing a dry slide on a moist one and then forcibly separating them; both will be found to be wet, proving that the force holding the molecules of water together is less than that holding the water to the glass.

A lower denture covers a very small surface area compared with an upper, and its adhesion is correspondingly less.

The viscosity of the saliva is of importance in the phenomenon of cohesion. Saliva which is more viscous than normal, i.e. it contains a larger percentage of mucin, prevents the denture and tissues coming into sufficiently close contact because it increases the thickness of the saliva film and this reduces the cohesive force.

2. *Atmospheric Pressure (Suction)*

The periphery of a denture should bed slightly into the soft tissues in the sulci, and except for the back edge of the upper denture it will be covered by the lips and cheeks, wrapped up as it were in the surrounding soft tissues.

When an upper denture is inserted air is expelled from between it and the mucous membrane, and provided the fit of the periphery to the tissues is good no air can get in because this edge-fit provides an efficient seal (*see* fig. 3). This means

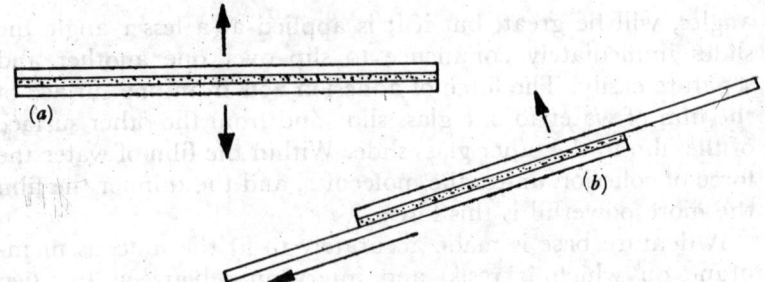

Fig. 1

(a) The large flat surface of a microscope slide provides excellent adhesion when resisting vertical separation.

(b) A sliding force allows easy separation.

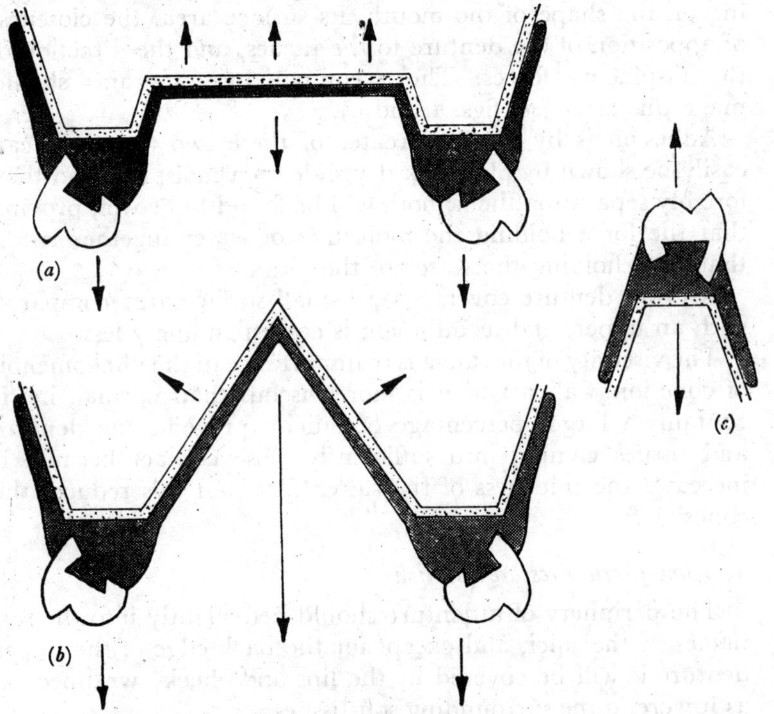

Fig. 2

(a) A flat palate will provide good surface adhesion.

(b) A V-shaped palate allows sliding and therefore retention by adhesion is reduced.

(c) A lower denture provides a very small surface for effective adhesion.

that the pressure acting on the fitting surface of the denture is less than that acting on the non-fitting surface (atmospheric pressure). The difference between these two pressures gives a positive force holding the denture in place. Furthermore, if the denture tends to move out of contact with the tissues, provided the seal at the periphery is not broken, the pressure under the denture will tend to fall still further and the atmospheric force will increase.

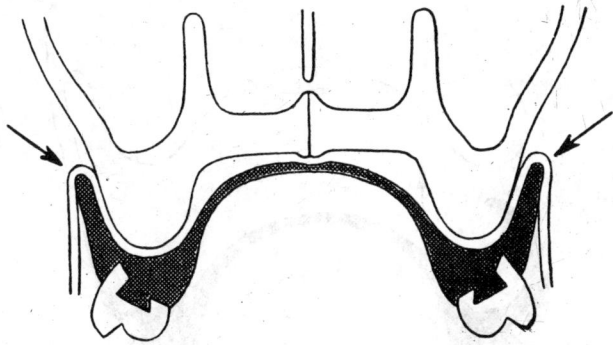

FIG. 3. – Arrows indicate tissues sealing the edges of the denture and so preventing ingress of air.

3. *Undercut Area*

It is often possible to insert a denture in one direction into what, from another direction, is an undercut area and thus obtain a purely mechanical retention (*see* fig. 4).

(B) *Acquired Muscular Control*

Dentures are always foreign bodies in the mouth and when fitted for the first time most muscular actions tend to expel them. Gradually, however, the wearer learns to differentiate between the food and the dentures and, at first consciously but later subconsciously, to control and stabilize them with the tongue and the cheeks. The tongue, by resting on top of the lower denture and pressing it downwards and forwards, can control its tendency to rise, and also counterbalance to a large degree unstabilizing masticatory forces. The tongue can also be unconsciously trained to prevent the back edge of the upper denture dropping while the front teeth are incising.

The muscular cheeks can be trained, again unconsciously, to press downwards on the buccal flanges of the lower denture, whilst still carrying out their function of placing food between the teeth.

If full use is to be made of muscular control of dentures, their design must follow certain lines which are fully explained in the following chapters.

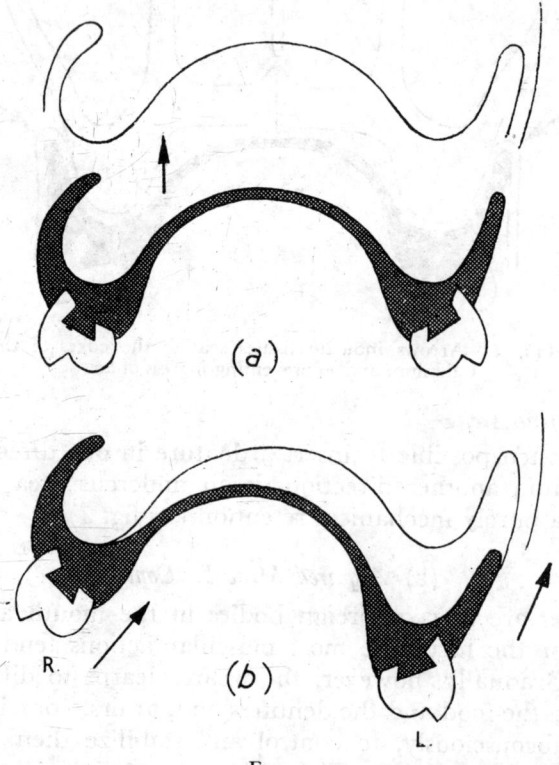

FIG. 4

(a) If the denture is inserted directly upwards it will not go into place.

(b) If the denture is inserted from the right side, the flange of the denture will go into place and the opposite side may be rotated upwards. The right side of the denture will be retained by the undercut, once in place.

WHY ARE THERE SO MANY TECHNIQUES?

The novice in prosthetics may become bewildered by the plethora of techniques which exist for achieving the same result. For example, there are at least a dozen techniques for taking an impression of the mouth, and almost as many for determining the relationship which the jaws bear to one another. There are many different types of articulator and an equal number of posterior tooth forms. This list could be greatly extended, but the examples given serve to draw attention to the fact.

Furthermore, individual operators tend to select and practise a very limited number of techniques, and regard the others with indifference or even open hostility. The explanation for this state of affairs is briefly as follows:

Prosthetics is not an exact science; it is very largely an art, and although certain aspects of it do follow rigid laws the major part of the subject follows lines laid down by practitioners who have developed their craft by their own clinical experience and research. Such practitioners have given rise to what may be termed 'schools of thought', and pupils who have learned from them have perpetuated their methods.

In addition, mouth conditions of individuals vary within wide limits; some presenting jaw formations which make the fitting and subsequent function of dentures a comparatively simple matter, while in others difficulties of retention and occlusal relationship and other factors require that special techniques be used in order to make use of every small advantage which is presented, if the dentures are to have any chance of success.

In an attempt to achieve this, many techniques with the same aim have been evolved, and no one of them has been of such outstanding merit as to displace the others entirely. Closely bound up with this is the fact that all these techniques require the development of a high degree of skill in the prosthetist who practises them, and if one technique is producing good results in the hands of one practitioner he is likely to advocate its use and continue to practise it to the exclusion of others.

Finally, in certain aspects of prosthetics, agreement has not been reached on how and why certain phenomena and functions occur and, as in other branches of science, conflicting theories exist, each with its adherents.

For example, in the field of articulation of the teeth, Gysi and Hanau have related the movements of the mandible to the guidance it receives from both the temporo-mandibular joints and the slope of the tooth surfaces in contact during movement. Monson and Boyle, on the other hand, have evolved the theory that the movements of the mandible follow the segment of a sphere, the centre of which is located near the crista galli. Articulators and posterior teeth have been designed to enable dentures to be made conforming to the principles of these theories, and as both apparently produce satisfactory results both have their adherents.

Speed and economy have also had a powerful effect on the development of techniques because the cost of artificial dentures bears a very definite relationship to the time spent on their construction, and simple quick methods have a wide appeal in spite of the fact that they frequently produce dentures which are very inferior in comparison with those which could be made by more elaborate and time-consuming techniques.

The only safe guide to be followed by the student of prosthetics is to learn to anticipate the difficulties which a given case will present, study any technique which is designed to overcome the difficulties, and select for his practice the one which appeals to him most and produces in his hands the best result.

Chapter II

APPLIED ANATOMY

This section indicates how a knowledge of the structure and function of the tissues in the immediate vicinity of the dentures can be used to determine their logical design and provides reasons for, and answers to, some of the difficulties which are encountered in full denture prosthesis.

The mouth only represents a true cavity when opened to receive food or during the formation of certain sounds of speech; at other times it is filled almost completely by the tongue and edentulous alveolar ridges.

Fig. 5 shows the appearance of an open edentulous mouth with the tongue depressed.

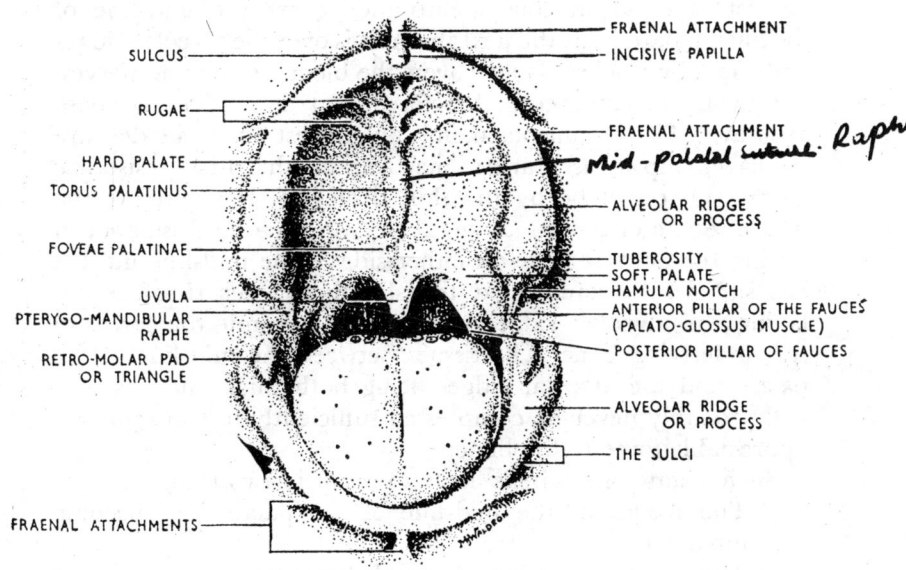

FIG. 5. – The open edentulous mouth with the tongue depressed; illustrating the structures which are visible.

The Mucous Membrane

TISSUE COMPRESSION

The varying thickness of the mucous membrane and sub-mucous tissue covering the bones forming the palate and alveolar ridges results in the forces which are applied to the denture during mastication being transmitted unevenly to these supporting structures.

In addition to this varying thickness, there is a variation in the closeness of packing of the fibrous elements of the corium.

Soft tissue is compressed when a force is applied to it due to the fact that some of the fluids (blood and lymph) which it contains, are temporarily driven out of it. The amount of fluid which a soft tissue contains is dependent both on its thickness and the density of its elements.

Reference to figs. 6 and 7 will show that the thinnest and densest layer of mucous membrane covers the mid-line of the hard palate; that the next thinnest is over the alveolar ridges and that the thickest layer covers the blood vessels and nerves.

It will be apparent, therefore, that if a denture base accurately fits the mucous membrane at rest when the denture is driven upwards during mastication the first resistance offered to it will be by the thin tissues of the centre of the palate. Some of the remaining force will then be dissipated in flexing the denture base on either side of the mid-line until it has sufficiently compressed the slightly thicker tissues over-laying the alveolar ridge; which then transmit the forces to the underlying bone. The tissues between the mid-line of the palate and the alveolar ridges being both thick and vascular will probably never be compressed sufficiently to transmit any appreciable force to the bone.

Such a state of affairs is likely to result in two things:

(1) The tissues in the mid-line of the palate will become inflamed.

(2) The constant flexing of the denture base will cause its fracture from fatigue.

Means of overcoming these results of uneven soft tissue distribution are dealt with in the chapter on impressions.

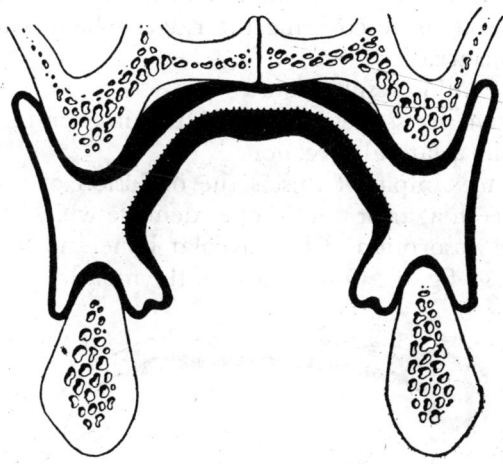

FIG. 6. – This coronal diagram through the 1st molar region illustrates the varying thickness of the mucous membrane covering the oral structures.

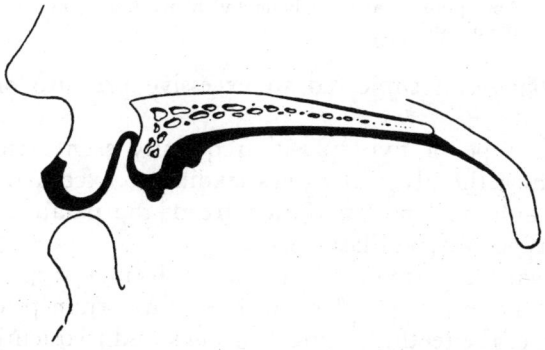

FIG. 7. – Mid-line sagittal diagram illustrating varying thickness of mucous membrane overlying hard palate.

Abnormally Thick Mucous Membrane

It is not uncommon for the fibrous tissue of the corium of the mucous membrane covering the alveolar ridges to proliferate producing a soft tissue covering the ridges which is thick and flabby in some areas.

Such proliferation results from:

(1) Excessive stress being applied to an edentulous ridge particularly in a lateral direction.

A common example of this is the occlusion of six natural lower front teeth against a full upper denture which frequently results in the absorption of the alveolar bone and hyperplasia of the gums (*see* fig. 8). Other areas of the mouth may undergo

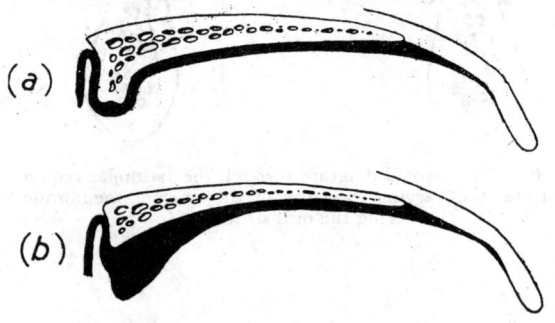

FIG. 8

(*a*) Sagittal diagram showing normal thickness of mucous membrane covering alveolar ridge and palate.

(*b*) Absorption of alveolar bone and hyperplasia of mucous membrane.

similar changes if subjected to excessive pressure or lateral stress.

Another type of hyperplasia frequently seen results from absorption of the alveolar ridges leading to excessive pressure being brought to bear on the centre of the palate causing a granular type of hyperplasia (*see* fig. 9).

(2) Advanced periodontal disease results in absorption of the alveolar bone and hyperplasia of the gum corium prior to the extraction of the teeth, leading to a thick and frequently flabby mucosal covering of the resultant edentulous ridges (*see* fig. 10).

The correct manner of dealing with these types of mucous

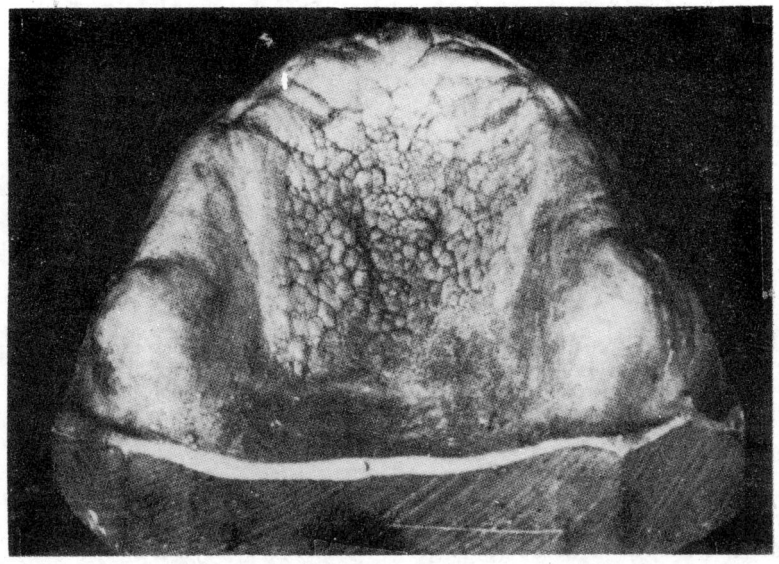

Fig. 9 – Model showing hyperplasia of the palate; note the granular appearance.

membrane is discussed in the chapters on surgical preparation and impressions of the mouth.

TISSUE COMPRESSION AND PERIPHERAL SEAL

Attention has been drawn to the fact in Chapter I that a powerful factor in the retention of full dentures is atmospheric pressure. To be effective this requires a good seal to be maintained at the periphery of the denture.

Those parts of the periphery of the denture which terminate in the sulci may be adequately sealed by virtue of the fact that the mucous membrane is reflected over them covering them completely, and so preventing the ingress of air. Posteriorly, however, the periphery lacks this natural seal and it is necessary to ensure that these edges sink slightly into the tissues. In order to achieve this, these edges must be placed over very compressible tissue. In the upper jaw such tissue is found in the region of the junction of the hard and soft palates and the correct area to place the back-edge of the upper denture is

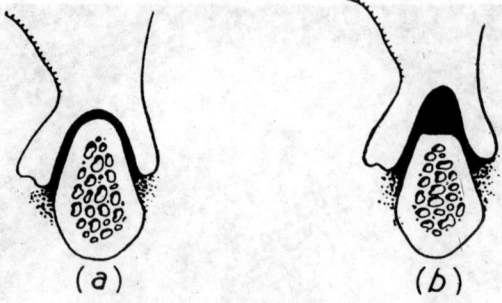

FIG. 10

(a) Coronal diagram showing normal thickness of mucous membrane covering lower alveolar ridge.

(b) Hyperplasia of mucous membrane and absorption of alveolar bone resulting from advanced periodontal disease.

just on to the soft palate but not so far back that it encroaches on the movable tissue (*see* figs. 7 and 11). The junction of the hard or soft palates is sometimes delineated by a faint transverse groove and the foveae palatinae. If the posterior edge of the upper denture is placed on the hard palate the mucous membrane covering the bone is too thin to allow the edge to sink into it sufficiently to provide an adequate seal without ulceration resulting (*see* fig. 12).

The details for placing the back edge of the upper denture correctly are dealt with in the chapter on registering the occlusion.

In the lower jaw compressible tissue is found in the retromolar pads and the posterior edges of the lower denture should be placed so as to cross these structures (*see* fig. 13). (*See* correct model preparation for the Fournet-Tuller technique, Chapter V.)

The Alveolar Ridges

It must be remembered that edentulous alveolar ridges are not natural structures – they are what is left of a bone after disease and surgery have been applied to it.

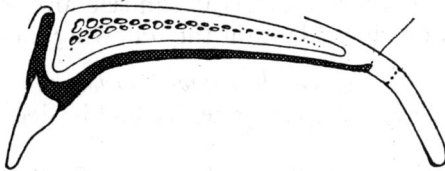

FIG. 11. – Correct placing of the posterior border of the
upper denture just on to the non-movable part of the soft
palate. The dotted line indicates the vibrating line, the point
behind which movement of the soft palate occurs.

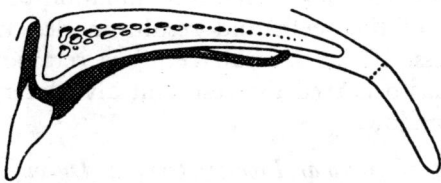

FIG. 12. – Incorrect placing of the posterior border of the
upper denture. The effect is magnified to illustrate what
occurs.

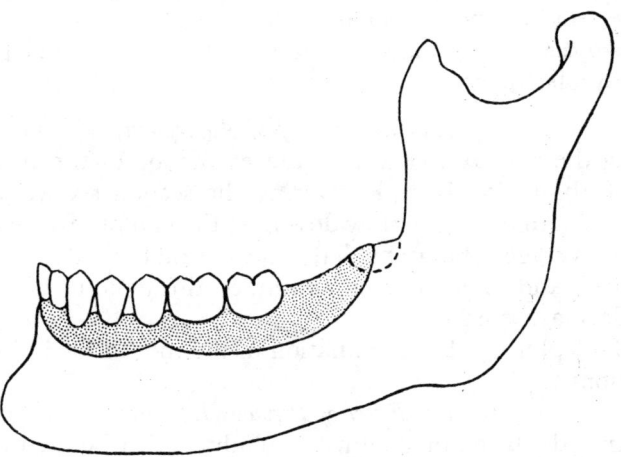

FIG. 13. – The back-edge of the lower denture should cross
the retromolar pad. The retromolar pad is indicated by
the dotted line.

The alveolar ridges vary greatly in size and shape and their ultimate form is dependent on the following factors:

1. *Developmental Structure*
The individual variation in bone size and its degree of calcification is great.

2. *The Size of the Natural Teeth*
The teeth like the bones show wide individual variation in size. Large teeth are supported by bulky ridges – small teeth by narrow ones.

3. *The Amount of Bone Lost Prior to the Extraction of the Teeth*
Periodontal disease is a chronic inflammation of the supporting structures of the teeth and results in destruction of the alveolar process. If the natural teeth are retained until gross alveolar loss has occurred the resultant alveolar ridges will be narrow and shallow.

4. *The Amount of Alveolar Process Removed During the Extraction of the Teeth*
During extraction with forceps the buccal alveolar plate is sometimes fractured and removed with the tooth. The commonest sites for this occurrence are the upper and lower canine and first molar regions.

When teeth are removed by dissection some alveolar process is always destroyed.

5. *Rate and Degree of Absorption*
During the first six weeks after the extraction of the teeth the rate of absorption is rapid. During the second six weeks it is fast but commencing to slow down. At the end of three months, on an average, the immediate post-extraction absorption is complete and thereafter it continues throughout life at an ever decreasing pace.

(*See* chapter on the examination of the mouth for individual variations.)

6. *The Effect of Previous Dentures*
Ill-fitting dentures, or dentures occluding with isolated groups of natural teeth, may cause rapid absorption of the alveolar process in the areas where they cause excessive pressure or lateral stress.

Types of Alveolar Ridges and Palate Formation and
Their Significance

Upper

1 Well developed but not labnormally thick ridges and a
  palate with a moderate vault (*see* fig. 14). This is a favourable formation because:

(*a*) The centre of the palate presents an almost flat horizontal
     area and this will aid adhesion (*see* Chapter I).

(*b*) The roomy sulcus allows for the development of a good
     peripheral seal.

(*c*) The well-developed ridges resist lateral and antero-
     posterior movement of the denture.

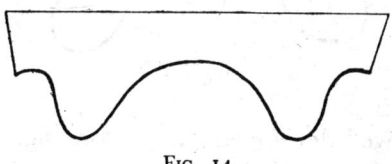

Fig. 14

2 High V-shaped palate usually associated with thick
  bulky ridges (*see* fig. 15). This is an unfavourable formation
  because the forces of adhesion and cohesion are not at
  right angles to the surface when counteracting the normal
  displacing forces of gravity.

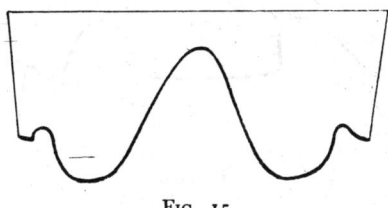

Fig. 15

3 Flat palate with small ridges and shallow sulci (*see* fig. 16)
  This is an unfavourable formation because:

(*a*) The ill-developed ridges do not resist lateral and antero
     posterior movement of the denture.

(*b*) The sulci being shallow do not form a good peripheral seal

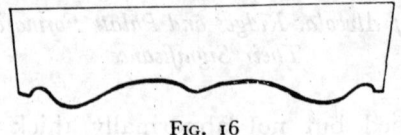

FIG. 16

4 Ridges exhibiting undercut areas (*see* fig. 17). These are unfavourable because frequently the flanges of the denture need to be trimmed in order to be able to insert it and this reduces the peripheral seal.

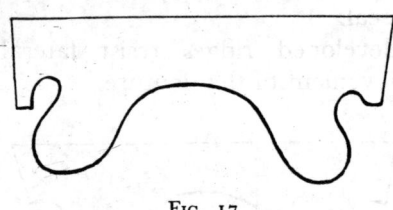

FIG. 17

Lower

1 Broad and well-developed ridges (*see* fig. 18). This is a favourable formation because:

(*a*) It provides a large area on which to rest the denture and prevents lateral and antero-posterior movement.

(*b*) The surface presented for adhesion is as large as it can ever be in a lower jaw.

(*c*) The lingual, labial and buccal sulci are satisfactory for developing a close peripheral seal.

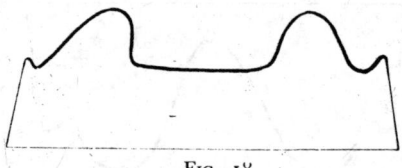

FIG. 18

2 Ridges exhibiting undercut areas (*see* fig. 19). Unfavourable because:

(*a*) If the denture is not eased away from the undercuts pain and soreness will result and, if it is eased, food will lodge under the denture.

(*b*) The easing of the periphery will spoil the peripheral seal.

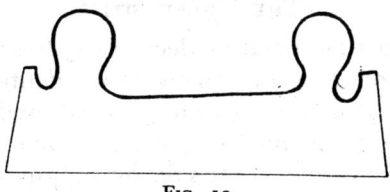

FIG. 19

3 Well developed but narrow or knife-like ridges (*see* fig. 20). These are unfavourable because:

(*a*) The pressure of the denture during mastication on the sharp ridge will cause pain.

(*b*) There is no suitable surface presented for adhesion.

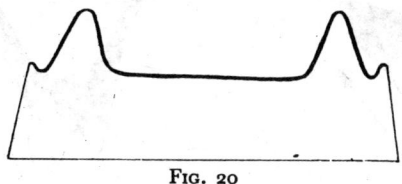

FIG. 20

4 Flat ridges (*see* fig. 21).

These are unfavourable because no resistance is offered to anteroposterior or lateral movements. In addition, such ridges are frequently found to have absorbed to the level of the attachments of the mylohyoid, genioglōssus and buccinator muscles and, if the denture base is kept sufficiently narrow not to encroach on these structures, its area is too small to be functional. If the area is increased by encroachment on the muscles they may move the denture when they contract.

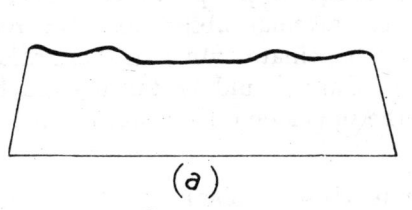

(*a*)

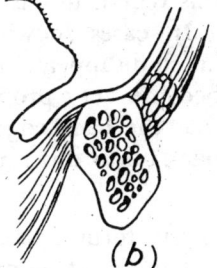

(*b*)

FIG. 21

(*a*) Illustrates a flat lower ridge in coronal section.
(*b*) Illustrates the closeness of the attachments of the buccinator and mylohyoid muscles to a flat ridge.

THE TUBEROSITIES

Large tuberosities bounded by deep sulci offer very satisfactory resistance to the lateral movement of the denture.

Tuberosities sometimes exhibit buccal undercut areas. If only one tuberosity is undercut this can sometimes be utilized to retain the denture on that side by slipping the distobuccal flange up over the bulge first and then raising the other side of the denture (*see* fig. 22).

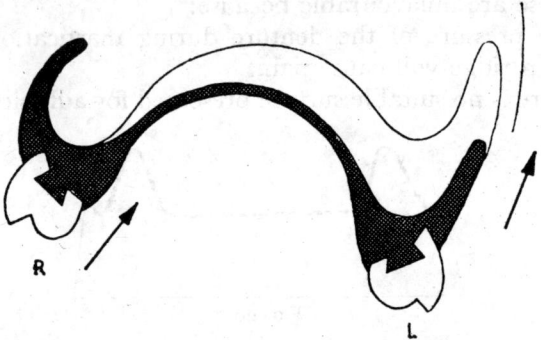

FIG. 22 – If the denture is inserted from the right side, the flange of the denture will go into place and the opposite side may be rotated upwards. The right side of the denture will be retained by the undercut, once in place.

Tuberosities exhibiting gross undercuts may require surgical treatment (*see* chapter on surgical preparation).

THE HAMULAR NOTCH

The tissues in the hamular notch are easily compressed and the post-dam line of the upper denture should be carried into this region to ensure an adequate peripheral seal (*see* fig. 23).

In cases showing gross alveolar absorption, the hamular notch disappears and the buccinator fibres in that region may become very prominent. Care should be taken in such cases that the back edge of the upper denture is not carried too far back on to this raphe.

THE HARD PALATE

If the torus palatinus is very prominent it may increase the difficulties of obtaining a stable upper denture for the reasons

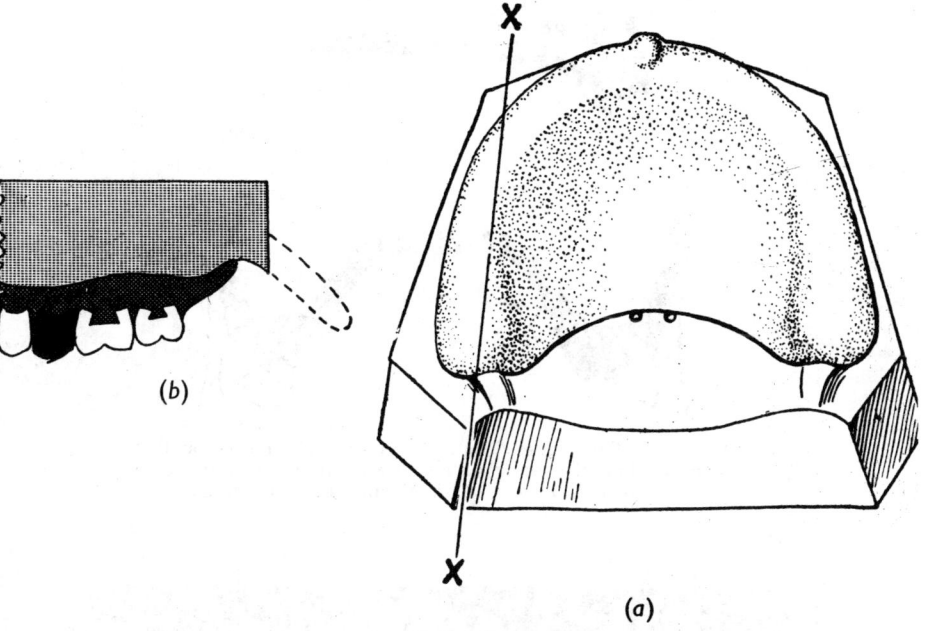

FIG. 23. – Illustrating the manner in which the posterior border of the upper denture should be carried into the hamular notch.

(a) In plan.

(b) Section through the line **XX**. Dotted line represents position of soft palate.

given in the section on mucosa compressibility. Steps must be taken to obtain adequate relief for it (*see* fig. 24), either by using special impression techniques, mechanical relief or, as a last resort, by its excision surgically.

THE RUGAE

These are said to be associated with the sense of taste and the function of speech. They ~~assist~~ the tongue to absorb via its papillae, the fluids containing the four primary flavours. They also enable the tongue to form a perfect seal when it is pressed against the palate in making the linguopalatal consonant stops of speech (*see* chapter on phonetics).

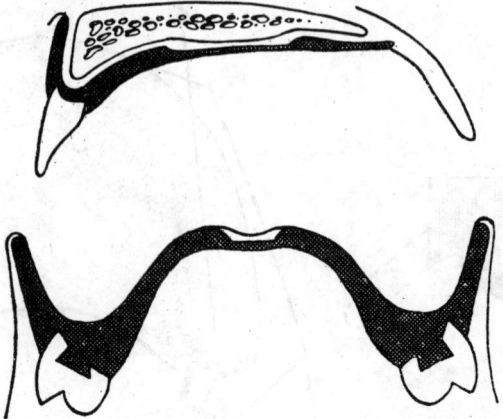

FIG. 24. – This figure illustrates in sagittal and coronal diagrams how the fitting surface of a denture is relieved to prevent it rocking on a prominent torus palatinus.

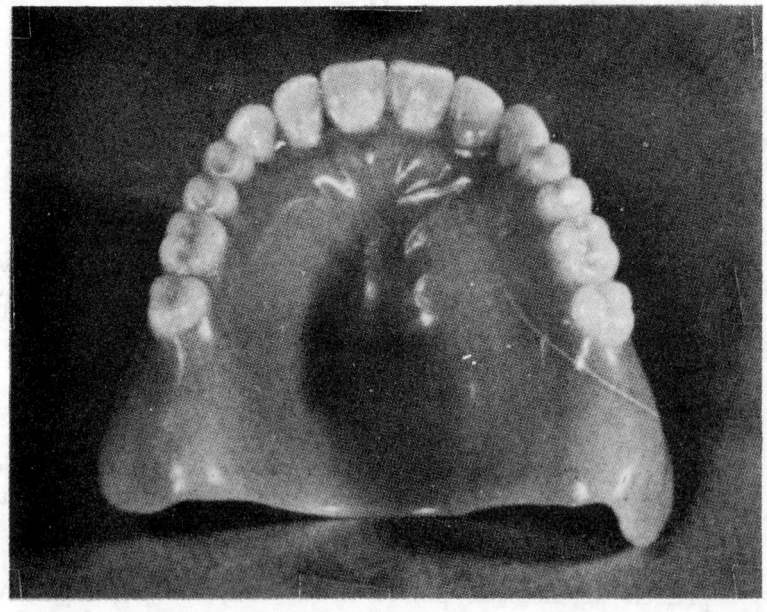

FIG. 25. – Denture with artificial rugae.

When a smooth, thick artificial denture palate covers these elevations of the mucosa, difficulty is sometimes experienced with both taste and speech. The high degree of adaptability of the normal individual usually results in rapid adjustment to these disabilities but the copying of rugae on the palatal surface of a denture or especially the corrugation of a thin metal palate helps to reduce the disability in some cases (*see* fig. 25).

THE PALATAL BLOOD VESSELS

Dentures made when using certain compression impression techniques may bring pressure to bear on the foramina through which the blood vessels pass. Relief of the anterior and posterior palatine foramina should be ensured in such cases

THE SOFT PALATE

Attention has already been drawn to the correct placing of the posterior edge of the upper denture on to the non-movable tissue of the soft palate. Patients may be broadly divided into two classes with regard to this non-mobile area:—

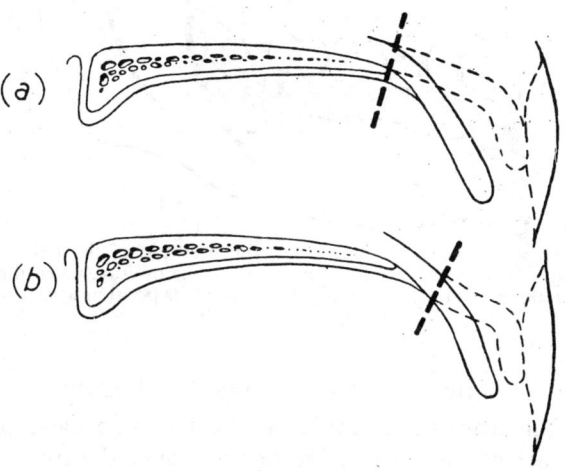

Fig. 26. – Sagittal diagram illustrating variations in the position of the vibrating line of the soft palate (marked by broken line).

(*a*) Movement occurs at the junction of the hard and soft palates.

(*b*) Movement occurs some distance behind the junction.

(1) Those whose palates exhibit movement at the junction of the hard and soft palates.

(2) Those whose soft palates move some distance behind the junction (*see* fig. 26).

The correct manner of assessing the area in which to place the back edge of the upper denture is dealt with in Chapter VI.

THE ANTERIOR PILLARS OF THE FAUCES

The palatoglossal arch follows the movements of the tongue. When the tongue is protruded or moved sideways the arch is pulled forwards. If the posterolingual edge of the lower denture is extended backwards so that it prevents this forward movement of the arch, soreness will result.

The most forward position of the palatoglossal arch, therefore, determines the position to be occupied by the posterolingual edge of the lower denture (*see* fig. 27).

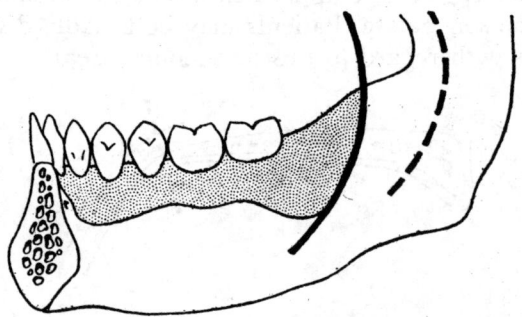

FIG. 27. – Diagram illustrating the positions of the palatoglossal arch. The dotted line indicates its position when the tongue is at rest, and the thick black line its position when the tongue is protruded.

THE PTERYGO-MANDIBULAR RAPHE

Originating from the hamular process it is in close proximity to that part of the distal edge of the upper denture resting in the hamular notch. If this edge is overextended, when the mouth is opened and the pterygo-mandibular raphe becomes tense it elevates a fold of soft tissue which will impinge on the denture either causing inflammation which is reported by the patient as soreness of the throat, or, if over-extension is gross, the back-edge of the denture will be flicked downwards each time the mouth is opened, causing the denture to drop.

THE FRAENA

These move with the muscles of the lips, cheeks, and tongue during speech and mastication. The peripheries of the dentures must be designed to allow for these movements but such allowance must not be gross enough to spoil the peripheral seal. The correct and incorrect method of allowing for fraena is illustrated in fig. 28.

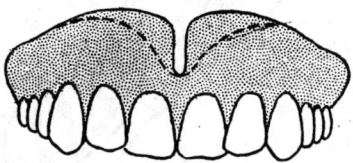

FIG. 28. – The method of shaping the periphery to allow for fraena. The continuous line illustrates the correct contour; the dotted line the incorrect, because the latter shape breaks the peripheral seal.

Overdeveloped fraena, or those which are attached too high on the alveolar ridge, may be removed surgically. In mouths exhibiting very poor retention, the removal of all the fraena materially increases the peripheral seal.

THE SULCI

The depth of the sulci is dependent on the height of the alveolar ridges and the mobility and tension of the surrounding muscles. Overextension of the denture in this area will cause instability, or soreness, or both.

THE PERIPHERAL OUTLINE AND FORM OF THE DENTURES
The Lower Denture

Tracing the periphery of the lower denture, commencing with the distobuccal aspect, the outline necessary to conform to the muscle attachment is as follows:

The periphery runs downwards and outwards from the

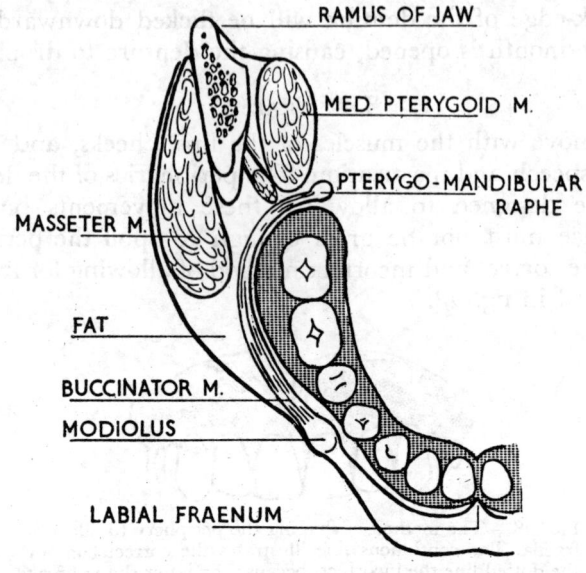

RAMUS OF JAW

MED. PTERYGOID M.

PTERYGO-MANDIBULAR
RAPHE

MASSETER M.

FAT

BUCCINATOR M.

MODIOLUS

LABIAL FRAENUM

FIG. 29

retromolar pad to the first molar region following the attachment of the buccinator muscle as it sweeps outward from its
origin along the pterygo-mandibular raphe (*see* figs. 29 and 30).

In the region of the first molar, there is no muscle attachment
to bone and the periphery curves outwards here to fill the small
pouch which is a vestigial remnant of a far better developed
structure found in some monkeys. In this region the polished
buccal surface of the denture is concave looking outwards and
upwards in order that the buccinator muscle as it contracts
and forces the cheek inwards may press the denture downwards (*see* fig. 31). From this point the periphery runs forwards
sweeping sharply in again in order that it may not encroach
on the modiolus situated in the premolar region (*see* figs. 29,
30 and 32). This tendinous band is pulled inwards and backwards and pressed hard against the teeth in order to provide a
fixed base from which the orbicularis oris can contract. The
lower denture base requires to be kept as narrow as possible in
this region in order that the pressure of the modiolus may be

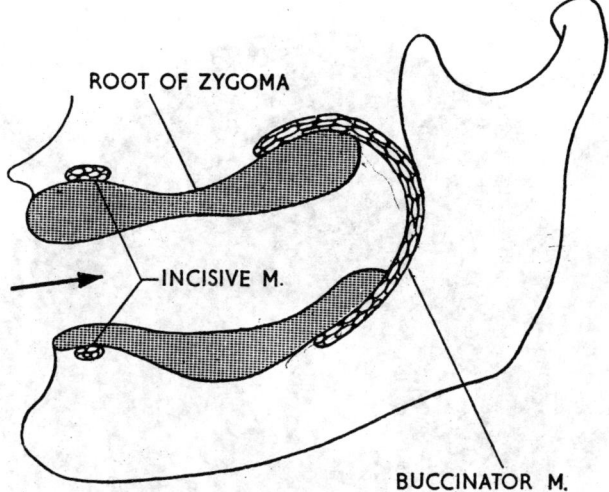

ROOT OF ZYGOMA

INCISIVE M.

BUCCINATOR M.

FIG 30. – The arrow indicates the area of action of the modiolus.

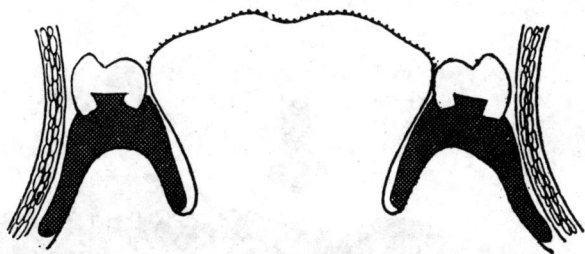

FIG. 31. – Illustrating the correct curvature of the buccal flange of a lower denture in order that the buccinator muscle may assist in the retention of the denture.

taken by the upper denture which, due to its greater stability, is far better able to withstand it.

From this point the periphery curves outwards and downwards again but it must not be carried too deeply in the canine region else the incisive muscle when contracting to assist in the fixation of the orbicularis oris will force the denture upwards (*see* fig. 30). Overextension of the periphery in the incisor region will cause lifting of the denture resulting from contraction of the mentalis muscle.

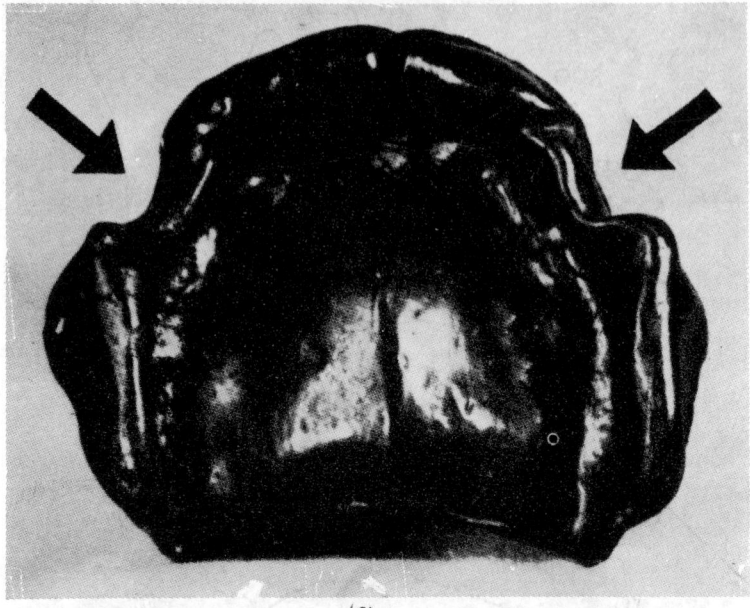

(a)

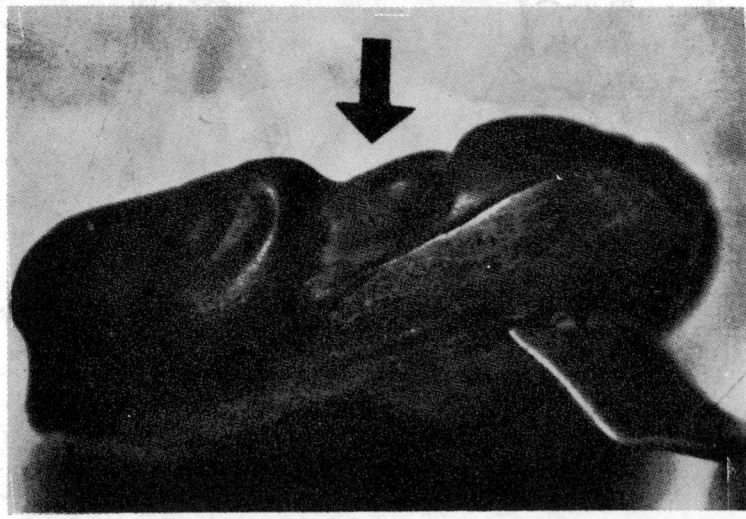

(b)

FIG. 32. – A composition impression showing the effect of the modiolus (arrowed) when the muscles inserted into it contract: (a) From above. (b) From the side. Note that the modiolus is a broad band.

In the mid-line the periphery is shaped to allow room for the labial fraenum (*see* fig. 29).

Lingually, commencing at the crest of the ridge in the retromolar area, the periphery runs as follows:

It runs downwards and slightly forwards, its direction being dictated by the most forward position assumed by the palato-glossus muscle (*see* fig. 27). The depth to which it descends depends on the degree of absorption of the alveolar ridges and the laxity of the soft tissues. If there is little alveolar ridge the lingual pouch in this region is shallow. The periphery follows the curve of the palatoglossal arch and, as it runs forwards along the floor of the mouth its depth is limited by a slip of the superior constrictor muscle crossing to be inserted into the tongue. The tissues enveloping the periphery in this region rise to their highest position during swallowing and thus limit the depth of the denture which must not interfere with this movement. This position can be ascertained by placing a finger in the lingual pouch and asking the patient to swallow.

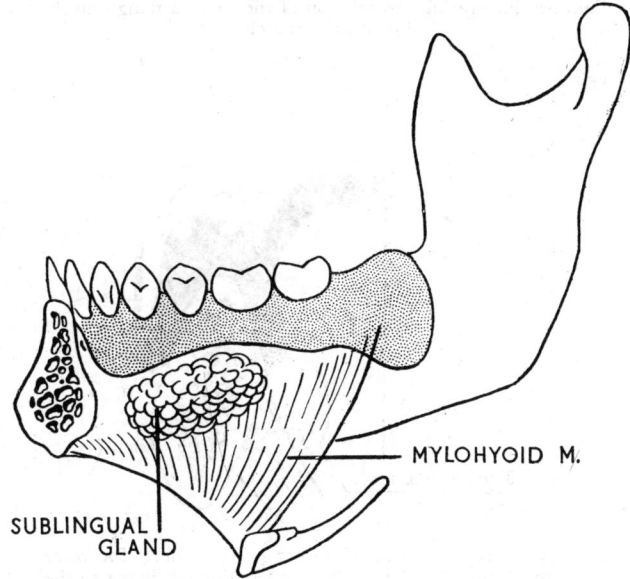

MYLOHYOID M.

SUBLINGUAL GLAND

Fig. 33. – Illustrating the outline of the lingual flange of the lower denture in relation to the structure in contact with it.

From here it rises slightly to cross the narrow posterior edge of the mylohyoid muscle which sometimes is sufficiently well defined to produce a definite notch in the periphery in this region (*see* figs. 33 and 34).

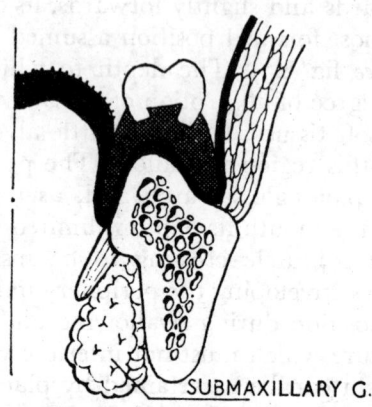

Fig. 34. – Diagram through 2nd molar region of a lower denture, illustrating the relation of the lingual flange to the mylohyoid muscle.

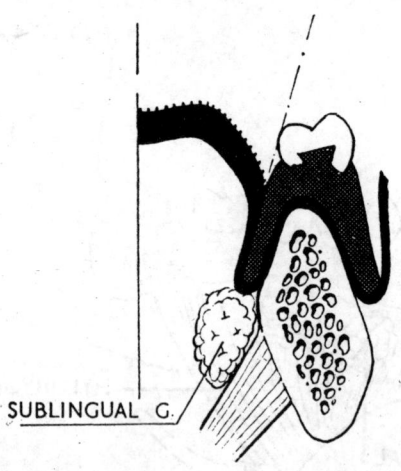

Fig. 35. – Diagram through the 1st molar region of a lower denture, illustrating the relation of the lingual flange to the tongue, the sublingual gland and the mylohyoid muscle. Dotted line indicates the slope of the lingual flange.

From this point forwards the periphery usually follows a gentle curve with the concavity looking downwards, dictated by the body of the sublingual gland which lies immediately underneath the mucous membrane forming the floor of the mouth (*see* figs. 33 and 35). When it reaches the first premolar region it descends again for a short distance and then rises to clear the lingual fraenum which sometimes presents a very broad attachment to the mandible (*see* fig. 36).

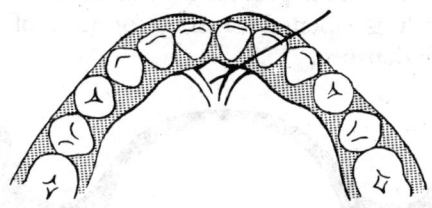

Fig. 36. – Lingual fraenum in relation to the lingual flange of the lower denture.

The polished lingual surface of the lower denture slopes downwards and inwards so as to present no area which overhangs the tongue (*see* fig. 35).

The Upper Denture

The periphery of the upper denture commencing with the posterior edge is as follows:

This edge, as already pointed out, should sink slightly into the non-movable tissues of the soft palate following a line from the hamular notch of one side to that of the other close to the foveae (*see* fig. 23). The posterior border then traverses the hamular notch and rises up into the sulcus on the buccal side of the tuberosity (*see* fig. 30). The height to which it rises is determined by the attachment of the buccinator muscle in this region. From this point it commences to descend following the buccinator attachment, the lowest point of this descent being at the root of the zygoma (*see* fig. 30). The zygoma having been cleared, the periphery rises again but the height to which it is carried should not be excessive else the upper incisive muscle, when contracting, will displace the denture. Finally the periphery is shaped to clear the labial fraenum (*see* fig. 28).

The polished buccal surface of the upper denture should be hollowed slightly with the concavity looking downwards and outwards so that the buccinator muscle when contracting may press the denture upwards (*see* fig. 37). Care should always be taken to ensure that the buccal flange in the second molar region is not excessively thick in cases with well-developed ridges since the coronoid process may strike against the flange when the mouth is opened causing soreness of the cheek or dropping of the denture.

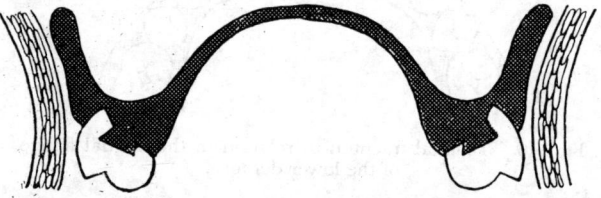

FIG. 37. -- Correct contouring of polished buccal surface upper denture.

The orbicularis oris muscle when contracting to press the lips against the teeth does not affect the upper denture as much as it does the lower because of the greater stability of the former. Therefore, the upper front teeth may be placed sufficiently far forward in most cases to suit the aesthetic requirements of the case and thickening of the labial flange to plump out the lips may be tolerated provided it is not carried to excess.

THE PERIPHERAL MUSCULATURE IN RELATION TO IMPRESSION TAKING

Trays used for impression taking should have a similar outline to that described for dentures.

The commonest fault found in stock trays is that they are overextended and especially is this the case with the disto-buccal region of lower trays.

Overextended trays lead to overextended impressions and this means that the muscles surrounding the oral cavity have been forcefully pushed out of the way and dentures made to such overextended impressions will be displaced by the muscles returning to their normal positions (*see* fig. 38).

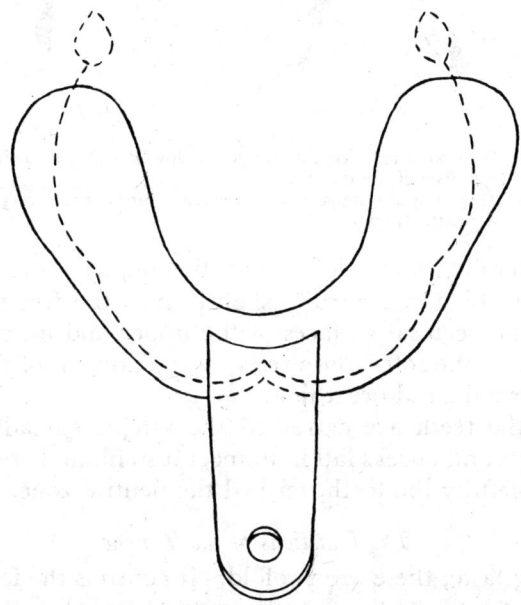

FIG. 38. – Overextended buccal flanges of a stock tray and insufficient length to include the retro-molar pads.

Particular attention should be paid to the posterolingua flanges of the lower tray because if these are overextended they will push the floor of that part of the mouth and the palatoglossus muscles downwards and backwards. On the other hand, if the flanges are short the lateral borders of the tongue will get under the tray and spoil the impression (*see* fig. 39).

THE TONGUE

The Rest Position of the Tongue

The dorsum rests against the roof of the mouth and the tip of the tongue rests in contact with the lingual surfaces of the lower incisor teeth.

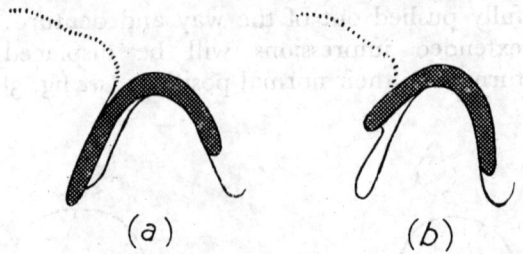

FIG. 39

(a) Overextended lingual flange of lower tray distorting
     the floor of the mouth.
(b) Short lingual flange of a lower tray trapping the tongue
     beneath its edge.

The lateral borders lie against the lingual borders of the posterior teeth and protrude slightly into the free-way space between the occlusal surfaces of the upper and lower teeth.

Posteriorly the soft palate rests on the dorsum of the tongue during normal nasal breathing.

When the teeth are extracted the tongue spreads laterally and the lips and cheeks fall in to meet it so filling between them the space left by the teeth, termed the neutral zone.

The Functions of the Tongue

Excluding taste, these are twofold. It controls the food during mastication and swallowing. It controls and directs, with the aid of the lips, teeth and palate the vibrating air stream from the larynx to form the sounds of articulate speech.

During mastication it performs as follows:

As the piece of food is being incised it controls and steadies it with its tip. In the case of food which does not require incising the tongue is protruded slightly and its centre depressed to form a shallow concavity into which the food is placed.

Next the food is quickly transferred backwards along the depressed surface of the tongue by a series of muscular waves until it has reached a level with the teeth by which it is to be chewed. Hard food is placed farther back than soft or fibrous food because the mandible is a lever of the third class and the farther back the food is placed the shorter is the arm of the lever.

The middle of the tongue now rises and forces the food laterally between the occlusal surfaces of the teeth which have parted to receive it. The lateral borders of the tongue at this time are on a level with the occlusal surfaces of the lower teeth and pressed hard against their lingual aspects so as to prevent the food passing downwards between the teeth and the tongue into the lingual sulcus.

The teeth occlude, dividing the food some of which is squeezed out, some lingually and some buccally. The tongue depresses in the centre gradually to receive the food as it is forced lingually by the occluding teeth and then returns it to them again as they separate. The cheek controls and replaces the food displaced buccally.

This cycle, smoothly continuous, proceeds until the food has been adequately divided and insalivated. The tongue then collects the food and forms it into a bolus which it holds in its central depression. A series of waves travelling posteriorly along the tongue then passes the food backwards. As the bolus reaches the back of the tongue the soft palate rises and the tongue and the palate holding the bolus between them pass it into the pharynx whence it is directed over the epiglottis into the oesophagus.

Finally the tongue scavenges the sulci with its tip to clear the mouth of fragments of food which have escaped the formation of the bolus.

From the foregoing it will be realized that the tongue is a powerful factor mitigating against the stability of the lower denture because of its power and latitude of movement. Care must be taken, therefore, to design the dentures so that they impede the movements of the tongue as little as possible and, to gain this end, attention must be paid to the following:

(1) The teeth must never be set inside the ridge or they will cramp the tongue causing movement of the dentures and irritation to the patient (*see* fig. 40).

In cases where dentures have been worn for some time the tongue space should be carefully measured from the old dentures and copied in the new ones. (*See* chapter on Setting Up and Immediate Dentures.)

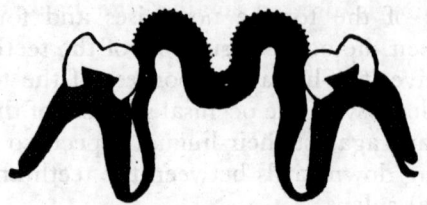

FIG. 40. – The tongue cramped.

(2) The lower denture should present lingual flanges to the tongue which slope slightly inwards from above downwards (*see* fig. 35). In no circumstances should the lingual cusps of the posterior teeth overhang the tongue (*see* fig. 41). In other words no concavities should be presented to the tongue into which its lateral borders can expand and so lift the denture.

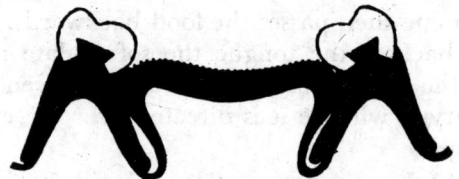

FIG. 41. – Lingual cusps overhanging the tongue.

(3) The palate of the upper denture should be as thin as is commensurate with the strength of the material used in its construction.

(4) The occlusal plane of the lower denture should be kept low, this allows the lateral borders of the tongue to rest upon the occlusal surfaces of the teeth when the mouth is opened to receive food and so prevent the lower denture from rising (*see* fig. 42).

The Tongue as a Controlling Influence

Observation of individuals who wear full dentures satisfactorily, discloses that the tongue is used very largely to control the dentures. It acts in the following ways:

(1) The dorsum is pressed against the back of the upper denture to prevent it dropping when incising (*see* fig. 43).

(2) The tip is pressed forwards and downwards against the anterior lingual surface of the lower denture when the lower lip tends to force the denture backwards (*see* fig. 43).

(3) The lateral borders of the tongue rest on the occlusal surfaces of the lower denture when opening the mouth (*see* fig. 42).

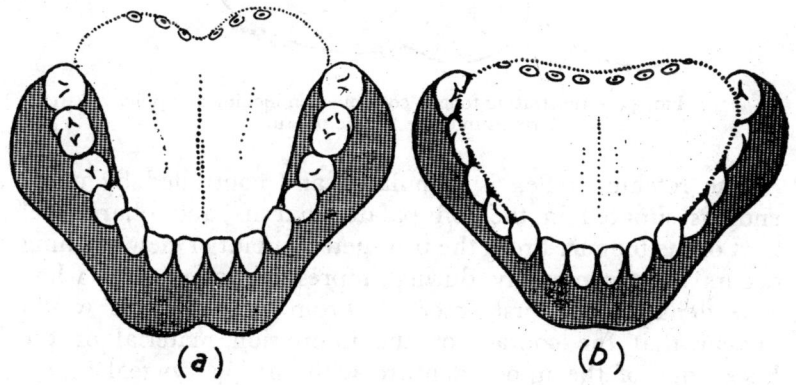

(a)   **(b)**

Fig. 42

(*a*) High occlusal plane preventing the tongue resting on the occlusal surface.

(*b*) Low occlusal plane allows the tongue to rest on the occlusal surface.

Such control takes time for wearers of new dentures to master, and a small percentage never learn at all. Attention to the design discussed earlier in this section gives patients a better chance of learning this control.

THE TONGUE IN RETCHING AND NAUSEA

Anything held on the anterior two-thirds of the tongue is under complete control and can be manipulated by the tongue at will and, if necessary, ejected from the mouth altogether. Once it has passed on to the pharyngeal part of the tongue, however, this ease of control is lost and, if it is required to eject a foreign body, an ejectory contraction of the muscles forming the pharyngeal sphincter, termed retching, must occur, and the foreign body is then forcefully expelled.

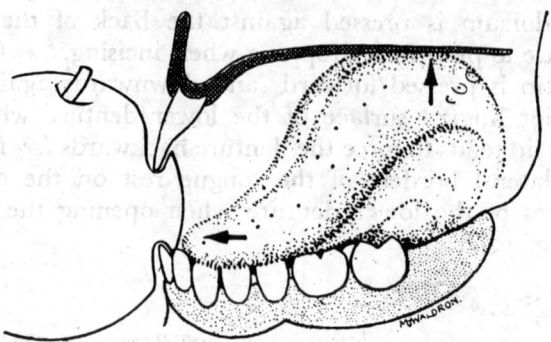

FIG. 43. – Illustrating tongue control when incising an apple.
Arrows indicate tongue pressure.

The retching reflex is stimulated and controlled by nerve endings situated in the soft palate, pharynx and pharyngeal part of the tongue. From the prosthetist's point of view retching occurs most commonly during impression taking and when new dentures are first inserted. From experience it would appear that the contact of the impression material or the back edge of the upper denture with the pharyngeal aspect of the tongue is the chief cause of the trouble. Methods of taking impressions without causing retching are dealt with in the chapter on impressions.

With regard to the back edge of the upper denture, it is its thickness more than the position it occupies which causes the retching. A thick square edge irritates the pharyngeal surface of the tongue constantly when it is in its rest position and so initiates the retching reflex. A thin back-edge properly post-dammed so as to sink into the compressible tissues of the palate will not irritate the tongue (*see* fig. 44). Light or intermittent pressure is another cause of nausea and a further reason for post-damming in this area.

The rationale of prescribing the sucking of boiled sweets for individuals showing a tendency to retch when dentures are first fitted is that the act of sucking and the swallowing induced by the increased flow of saliva keep the tongue occupied and prevent it resting against the back-edge of the new denture before it has learned to tolerate it.

Wearing dentures during sleep is to be recommended during the learning period for a very similar reason because tolerance is gained by the tongue during the night. If the dentures are removed before retiring the tolerance gained during the day is lost and the early morning is a time when many people are especially susceptible to retching.

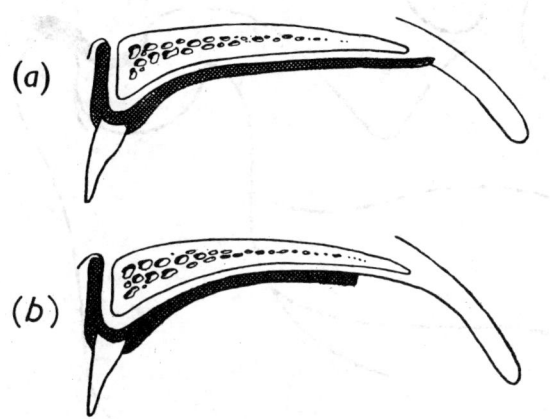

FIG. 44
(a) Showing posterior edge of upper denture correctly post-dammed.
(b) Thick square edge of upper denture incorrectly post-dammed.

THE TEMPORO-MANDIBULAR JOINT

The Normal Position of the Condyle

When the natural teeth are in centric occlusion (this term is discussed in Chapter VI), the anterosuperior aspect of the head of the condyle should articulate through the agency of the meniscus with that part of the fossa formed by the squamous temporal bone (see fig. 45). When the mouth is opened or the jaw protruded or moved laterally, the condyle should travel down the articular eminence and, in the widest position of opening, rest just short of the crest of the articular tubercle.

THE MUSCLES OF MASTICATION

The muscles of mastication when contracting are capable of applying a force of over 400 lb. between opposing molar

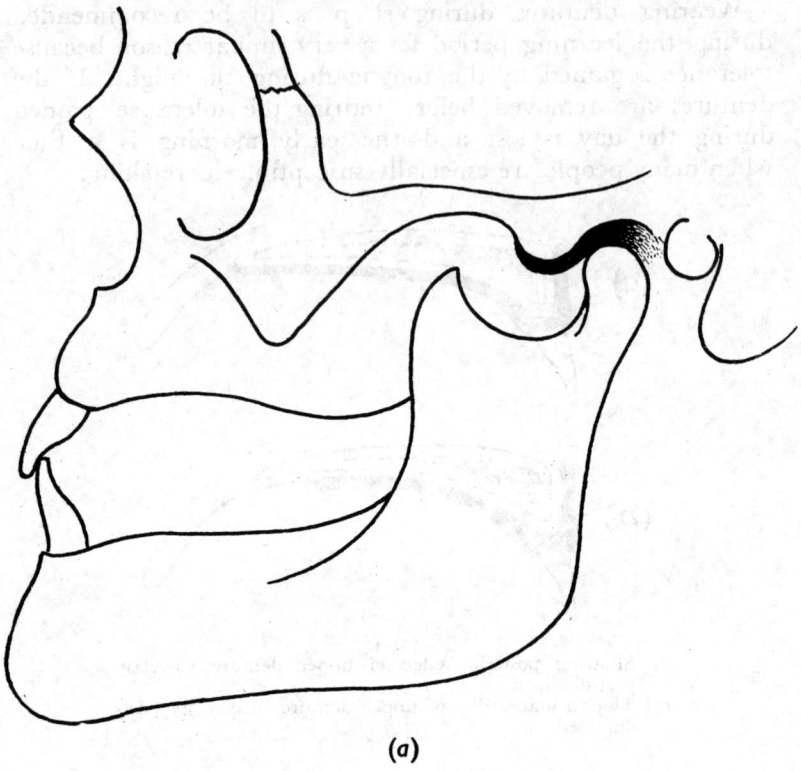

(a)

FIG. 45. – The relation of the head of the condyle to the fossa –
(a) When the mouth is closed.

teeth. This is very greatly reduced when artificial dentures are fitted because the mucous membrane cannot stand such pressure, a figure of 30 lb. never having been recorded.

The mandible, its joints and the muscles of mastication together constitute a double lever of the third class (*see* fig. 46).

The muscles which apply the powerful closing force to the mandible are the temporalis and the masseter and it is thus obvious that the farther back in the mouth (i.e. the nearer to the insertions of these muscles) a piece of food is placed the greater the power which can be brought to bear on it.

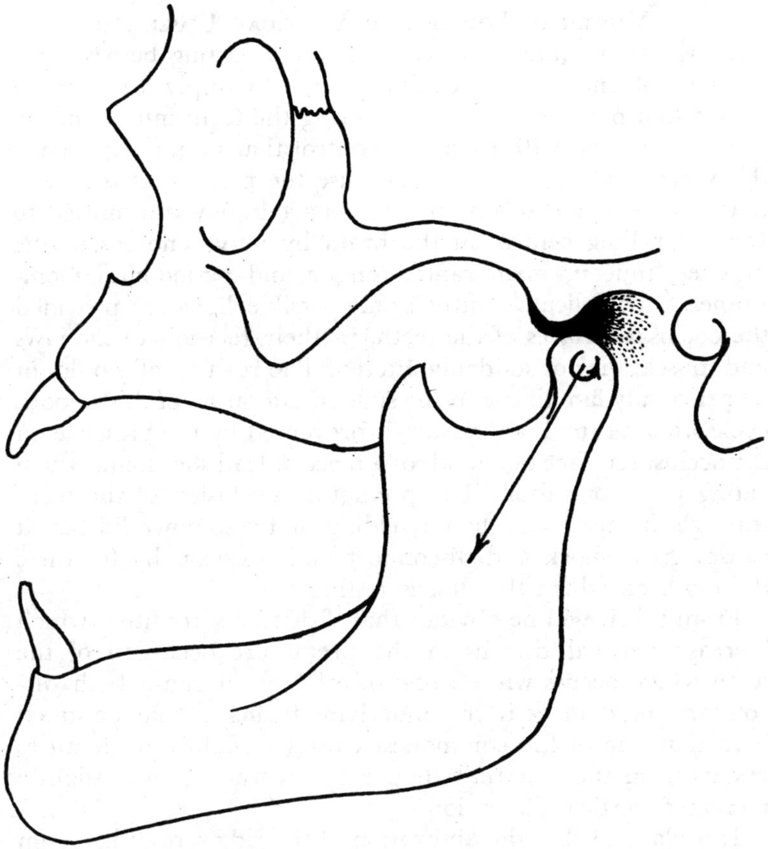

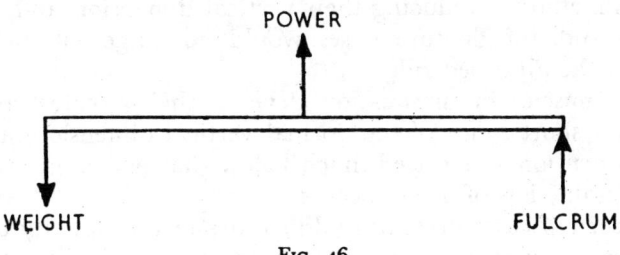

(b)

Fig. 45. – The relation of the head of the condyle to the fossa –
(b) When the mouth is open.

POWER

WEIGHT

FULCRUM

Fig. 46

MUSCULAR POWER AND VERTICAL DIMENSION

The beautiful control and co-ordination existing between the muscles of mastication enables them to apply their great power to a piece of food and yet bring the teeth into occlusion after its division with such fine control that no jarring occurs. They are enabled to do this because the position of the teeth and jaws in space at any moment is accurately transmitted to the controlling centres in the brain by nerve endings in the muscles, mucous membranes, tongue and periodontal membranes. Such delicate control is only possible, however, provided the occlusal surfaces of the teeth, in their relation to the jaws and muscles, is not suddenly altered. The reader will no doubt be personally familiar with the sudden alteration of this smooth cycle when normal jaw closure is prevented by the presence on the occlusal surface of a tooth of a piece of lead shot found when eating game or rabbit. The premature occlusion of the teeth through the agency of the unyielding shot is so powerful that it causes great shock and discomfort and occasionally fractures the tooth on which the shot is resting.

From this it will be obvious that if dentures are fitted which increase vertical dimension the premature occlusion of the teeth which occurs will be so powerful as to cause both discomfort and damage to the underlying tissues. It may be stated here that one of the commonest causes of failure of dentures results from the fact that they are constructed to a slightly increased vertical dimension.

It is claimed that the absorption of the ridges resulting from the force of occlusion occurring with an excessive vertical dimension soon reduces its height and restores equilibrium. It is doubtful, however, whether many patients would tolerate such a method of reducing their vertical dimension and, even if they did, the denture bases would no longer fit the new form of the absorbed ridges.

The muscles of mastication develop their greatest power within a short range of the normal vertical dimension, and if this dimension is reduced much below that which is normal considerable loss of power occurs.

In certain cases presenting difficulties in the stability of the dentures, advantage may be taken of this power loss associated with closure of the vertical dimension to reduce the forces applied to the dentures. Such closure of the vertical dimension, however, should be carried out with care and a full realization of the other disadvantages which may accrue; these are discussed elsewhere in the book.

Muscle Tone and Antagonism

In a normal mouth with a complete complement of natural teeth the elevator, depressor, protruder and retractor groups of muscles, or more accurately muscle fibres, balance one another and gravity and so control the movement of the mandible with great precision.

For example in protrusion the lateral pterygoid muscles draw the head of the condyle and the articular disc forwards, the medial pterygoid muscles produce a strong component force pulling the angle of the mandible forwards, the superficial fibres of the masseter muscle and to a slight extent the anterior fibres of the temporalis muscle also bring a forward traction to bear on the mandible. When posterior teeth are present the forward pull of these muscle fibres is accurately balanced by the gradual relaxation of the posterior fibres of the temporalis muscle and some of the deep fibres of the masseter.

In retrusion the reverse action occurs. When the posterior teeth are lost and mastication is performed entirely on the front teeth or when a long period of edentation precedes the fitting of full dentures, abnormal habits of chewing with the mandible forward are acquired which results in the delicate balance between the protruding and retruding groups of muscle fibres being temporarily lost, the protruding group becoming dominant due to excessive use.

In such cases difficulty may be anticipated when registering the anteroposterior bite relationship, and great insistence must be placed on complete muscular relaxation and a very gentle closing movement thus tending to eliminate the dominance of the protruding group of muscle fibres in such cases.

THE FREEWAY SPACE

When the mandible is at rest it is supported by the elevator group of muscle fibres which are not fully relaxed but are in a condition of partial contraction, termed tonus, which is sufficient to counterbalance comfortably the tonus of the depressor muscles of the mandible, and gravity.

The position which the mandible assumes when at rest is probably constant for each individual and normally when it is in this position the occlusal surfaces of the maxillary and mandibular teeth are separated by 2–4 mm ($\frac{1}{8}$ in.). This space between the occlusal surfaces of the teeth is termed the freeway space and its importance in gauging the vertical dimension is dealt with in Chapter VI.

THE LIP MUSCLES

The orbicularis oris closes the lips and when contracting, its lateral insertions into the modeoli are fixed by the contraction of the quadratus labii superioris and inferioris, zygomaticus, triangularis, and buccinator muscles. The incisal muscles also fix it to the alveoli.

During such function considerable inward pressure is brought to bear on the labial surfaces of the teeth and also the labial sulci are reduced in depth. The upper denture, due to its inherent stability, can withstand such pressure provided its labial flanges have not been overextended. The lower denture, however, in cases presenting poorly formed alveolar ridges is likely to be raised from the ridge in front and pushed backwards. Experienced denture wearers counteract this pressure of the lip by a forward pressure of the tongue but assistance can often be given to the tongue by carrying the heels of the lower denture up the ascending rami of the mandible in such cases.

The effect of the modioli on denture design has already been discussed.

The elevator and depressor muscle groups antagonize the orbicularis oris and one another thus opening the lips and producing facial expression. It must be remembered, when closing the vertical dimension, that the origins of the elevator and depressor groups of muscles will be moved closer together thus causing a bunching up of the muscles with consequent loss of tone. This causes drooping of the mouth, puckering and wrinkling of the skin of the lips and face and a flattening of the philtrum giving an aged and bad tempered appearance. Some of this damage can be mitigated by plumping the lateral labial flange of the upper denture (*see* fig. 47) thus causing the muscles of the

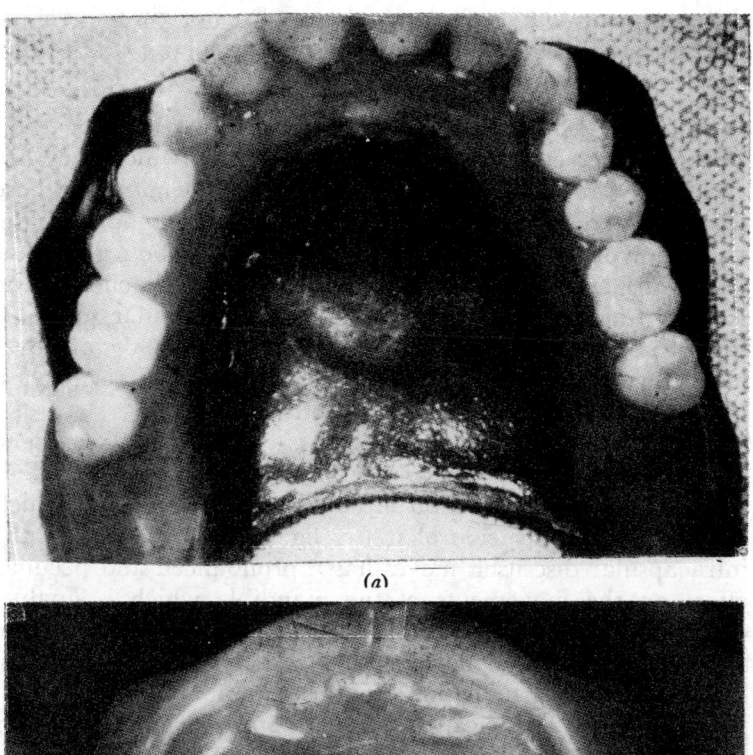

(a)

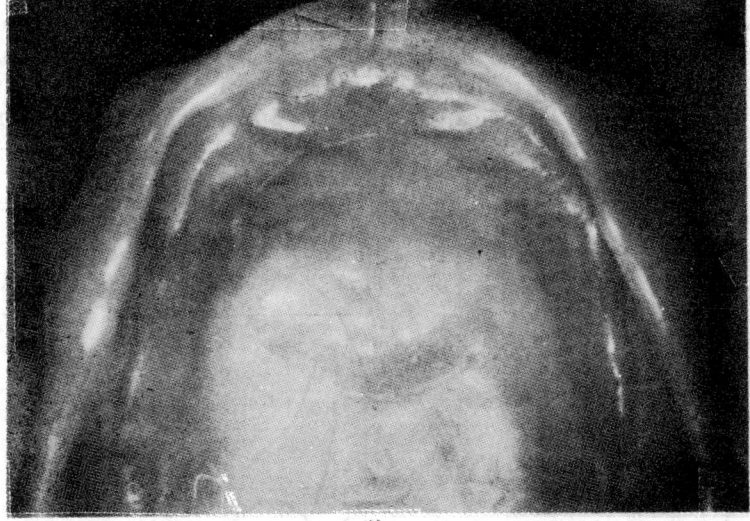

(b)

FIG. 47. – A 'plumped' denture, or one built out to support the circumoral musculature. (a) At the try in stage. (b) Finished denture. Note that the support is in the area of the modiolus and thus the attachments of all the muscles are supported; compare with fig. 32.

elevator group to follow a longer course from origin to insertion and so restoring their tone, but the only true cure is to restore the height of the bite.

The Mandibular Movements of Mastication

The natural teeth are embedded in bone to which they are attached by means of the fibrous periodontal membrane, whose resilience may here be disregarded. The bones comprising the upper jaw move only with the skull and so may be regarded as the fixed factor whilst the lower jaw, which is attached to the skull by the two very mobile temporo-mandibular joints, is capable of many complicated movements. It is these movements together with those of the surrounding muscles which are of such importance to the prosthetist.

The temporo-mandibular joint is unique because some muscle fibres are attached to the intracapsular disc which is thus moved during function in its relation to the bones which articulate on either side of it (*see* fig. 45). The fact that the intracapsular disc itself moves has a pronounced and peculiar effect on the movements of the mandible which is unable, except within very strict limits, to move with a pure hinge rotation; it is forced to move forwards when moving downwards.

The normal articulation of the anterior teeth in most Europeans and Americans is with the uppers slightly anterior

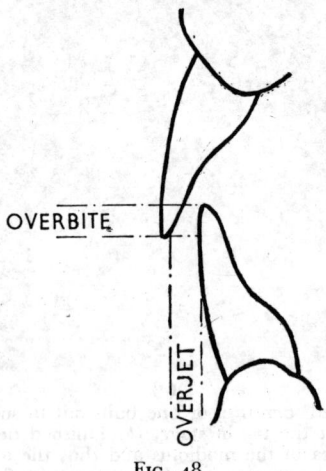

OVERBITE

OVERJET

Fig. 48

to the lowers and overlapping them by 1 mm. to 4 mm., a fact which must be borne in mind when considering normal mandibular movement. The overlap in the horizontal plane is termed the overjet and that in the vertical plane the overbite (*see* fig. 48).

Now to consider what happens when a piece of food is bitten off, chewed and swallowed (*see* fig. 49).

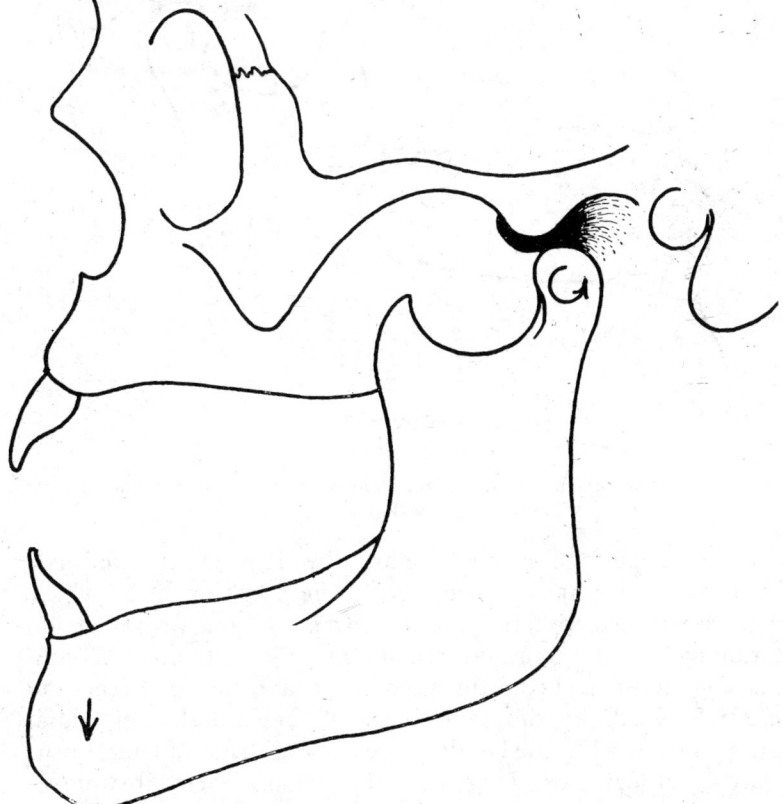

FIG. 49. – Opening and incising movements of the mandible.
(*a*) Opening movement – condyles rotate and move forwards to bring incisors into vertical relationship.

First Movement – The Opening Movement

The first movement of the mandible, which is confined to the lower articular cavity of the joint, is a pure rotation of the

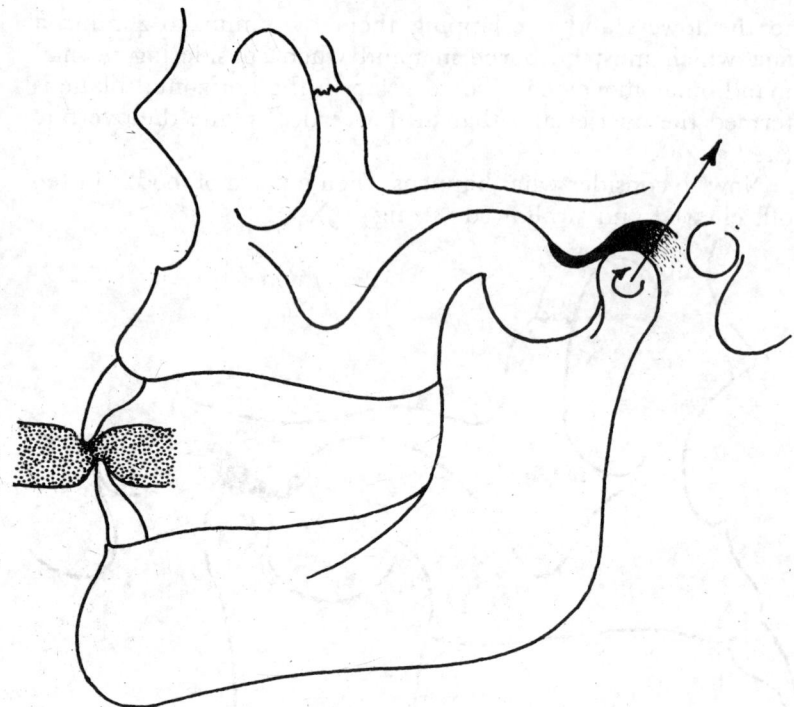

FIG. 49. – (b) Food is interposed between front teeth and condyles rotate upwards and backwards.

condylar heads against a stationary disc. It is mainly produced by gravity and the contraction of the anterior belly of the digastric muscle but the jaw is prevented from dropping too suddenly by the gradual relaxation of the temporalis and masseter muscles. From this point the mandible commences to move forwards by the contraction of the lateral and medial pterygoid muscles, the condylar heads and discs moving downwards and forwards along the articular eminences, this movement occurring in the upper joint cavity. The condyle heads are still able to rotate in relation to the discs thus controlling the vertical relationship of the teeth though not the anteroposterior

Second Movement – The Closing Movement

When the upper and lower front teeth have parted sufficiently,

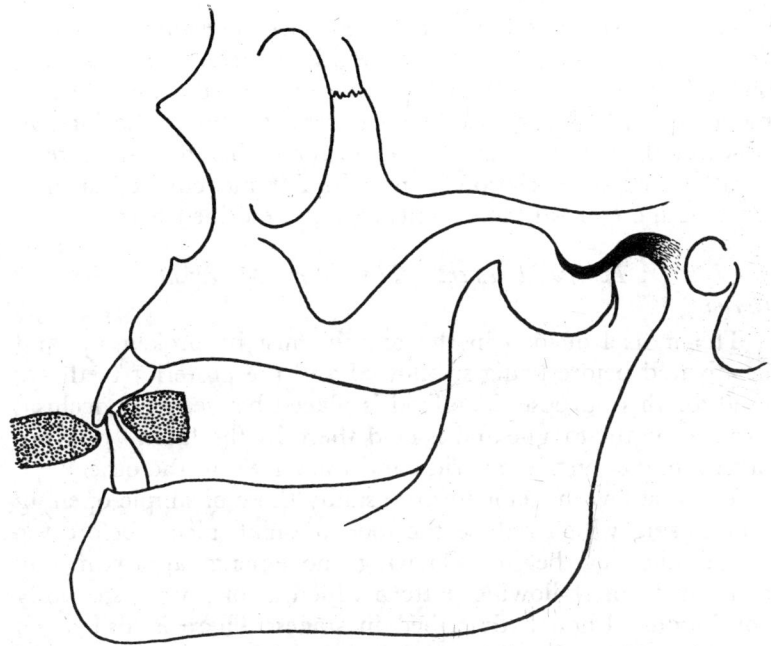

FIG. 49. – (c) Teeth meet and lower incisors slide with shearing action up palatal inclines of upper incisors until heads of condyles are physiologically retruded in glenoid fossae.

the food to be bitten off is placed between these teeth and the reverse movement back to centric occlusion takes place beginning with some degree of approximation of the incisive edges depending on the resistance offered by the food. This is brought about by the contraction of the masseter and medial pterygoid muscles and results in a crushing rather than a cutting action.

Third Movement – The Shearing Movement

The final return of the teeth to centric occlusion is the result of further contraction of these muscles and by the posterior fibres of the temporalis accompanied by gradual relaxation of the pterygoid muscles. This muscular synergy returns the condyle heads and discs to the rest position in the glenoid fossae at the same time producing a shearing action between the incisive edges of the teeth.

These movements have been described as though of equal degree on both sides, but of course this is not so and invariably one side moves more than the other thus producing a lateral movement which increases the shearing action of the incisive edges of the teeth. It must also be remembered that there is great individual variation in mandibular movement but only the average general movements can be described here.

Fourth Movement – The Lateral Movement
Chewing
The morsel of food in the mouth must be broken up and insalivated before being swallowed and the posterior teeth are used for this purpose, The food is placed between the occlusal surfaces by the tongue and is held there by the lateral pressure of the tongue on the one side and the cheek on the other.

The first few movements are usually those of simple opening and closing which reduce the food to small pieces before the actual chewing begins. Chewing movements approximately conform to the following pattern which is, of course, smoothly continuous although described in stages. There is also much greater individual variation of these lateral movements than of the incisive ones just described, owing to the prevalence of malposition of the teeth and cuspal interference found in the civilized races.

Chewing begins with a simple opening movement and the placing of the food on the occlusal surfaces of the posterior teeth on one side, called the working side. There is then a lateral rotation of the mandible towards the working side which is brought about by the condylar head and disc of the opposite side being pulled downwards and forwards on the articular eminence by the lateral pterygoid muscle. At the same time the condylar head on the working side rotates about a vertical axis and moves slightly backwards and laterally by contraction of the masseter and temporalis, thus causing a slight but definite lateral shift of the whole mandible. This movement is called the Bennet movement. The mandible now moves upwards in this lateral position until considerable resistance is encountered or until the opposing cusps, having penetrated the food, come into contact with each other. The

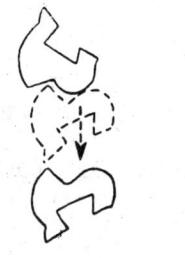 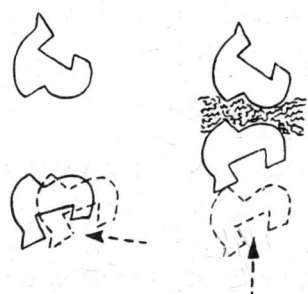 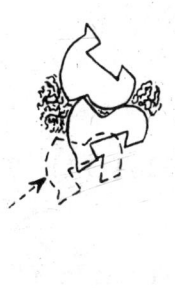

FIG. 50. – The chewing cycle.

final movement is the upward and sideways return to centric occlusion and it is during this last small movement that the cutting and tearing of tough fibres and the crushing and grinding of hard particles takes place between the approximating cusps (*see* fig. 50).

CHAPTER III

HISTORY TAKING AND EXAMINATION OF THE MOUTH

Success in full denture prosthetics depends on three factors:
  (1) The patient's attitude to dentures and his ability to learn to use them.
  (2) The condition of the mouth.
  (3) The skill of the operator who must acquire all the information he can, in order to anticipate difficulties which may arise and select the technique best suited to overcome them. He must be in a position to warn a patient of expected difficulties, not only in order to gain his co-operation and later perseverance, but also to save himself from possible recriminations when dentures, constructed for abnormal conditions, do not appear to the patient to be as comfortable or efficient as those of his relations or friends. Finally, though of the greatest importance, he should be able to recognize the oral symptoms of such general systemic diseases as syphilis, pernicious anaemia, malignant tumour and in fact any other oral manifestations since he will sometimes see these conditions before a medical practitioner has been consulted.

History taking and examination of the mouth will be described separately, but this is only for convenience and it must be realized that in practice they are inseparable. For the same reasons of convenience the patient's mental attitude will be discussed when describing history taking. The usual method, in medicine, of describing the information obtained about a patient is to say that it is made up of signs and symptoms, a sign being a fact which the investigator finds for himself, and a symptom something which is told him by the patient.

1. History Taking

This will be described under separate headings merely for convenience and frequently runs concurrently with the examination of the mouth. It should be directed towards discovering those aspects of the case which cannot be observed and augmenting, where necessary, those which can.

(a) THE PATIENT'S ATTITUDE TO DENTURES

Although it is true that nearly all edentulous people who go to consult a dental surgeon want to have dentures, it must not be assumed that they are all equally willing to play their part in making such dentures successful. An attitude of mind will have been formed by the patient's own past experience of dentures, if any, or from his observation of friends or relatives who wear dentures. If, prior to being rendered edentulous, a partial denture was worn with comfort and efficiency, the same will be expected of full dentures. It should be explained to such patients that, although partial denture experience is helpful in relation to full dentures, the latter require a considerably greater degree of control because they are not, as were the partial dentures, retained or supported by the natural teeth. If this difference in the two types of denture is not explained, the initial difficulty experienced in learning to use the full dentures compared with the partial dentures may cause the patient much disappointment, and he may condemn the dentures as being faulty, not knowing that a little perseverance is necessary.

If full dentures are already being worn and they have been comfortable and efficient, the same will be expected of the new dentures. If the old full dentures were troublesome, the attitude may be expectant of better results with the new dentures or pessimism that nothing better can be hoped for. If no previous denture experience exists, friends or relations may have coloured the patient's mind with their own attitudes.

In such cases the efficient control and use of full dentures depends to a very large extent on the formation of new habits, and a new pattern of muscular movement. This demands time and some patience on the part of the wearer. Many full denture troubles can be traced to the fact that no preparation of the patient's mind preceded the fitting of the dentures. If a leg is amputated the patient anticipates a long learning period before he can walk confidently with its artificial substitute, and he never expects to be able to walk as well with it as he did with his natural leg. In addition he is taught to use the artificial limb and this learning period may extend over several months. It is necessary, therefore, that the correct attitude to full dentures be instilled into the patient's mind. This cannot be done in a few minutes as the patient is being shown out of the surgery at the final visit; it should be a gradual process spread over all the visits necessary to complete the dentures, and should be related to the attitude already existing in the patient's mind.

The patient should be told what to expect when he commences to wear the dentures; how long the period of learning is likely to be; how considerable perseverance will be required before any degree of skill is attained in their use. This prognosis will bear a very definite relationship to what is discovered during the history taking and mouth examination.

(b) The Existence of Old Dentures

Most patients volunteer information about the existence of old dentures even if it is not already obvious, but every edentulous patient who does not mention old dentures of his own accord should be questioned concerning them. Questions are directed to elicit information regarding the length of time dentures have been worn; how many sets have been made since the teeth were extracted; the success of the existing or old dentures and the attitude of the patient to their appearance.

All this information is important because if the existing dentures have been satisfactory and only the passage of time has made them ill-fitting, any gross alteration of the new dentures will almost certainly mean their failure. A person who has worn comfortable and efficient dentures has developed a complete control of them which is entirely reflex and is dependent on a subtle appreciation by the tongue, cheeks and lips of the shape and position of the polished surfaces of the dentures, the height of the occlusal plane and exactly when the teeth will make contact. If any of these is altered grossly or suddenly the established reflexes are upset and conscious control of the dentures must again be exercised. With an experienced denture wearer such control is a thing of the past, and if it can be dispensed with by copying certain aspects of the old dentures success with the new dentures is assured. If on the other hand certain alterations in the new dentures are essential, e.g. altering the occlusal plane for reasons of appearance or restoring the correct vertical height to correct an overclosure, then this must be explained to the patient and he must be told that conscious control of the new dentures will be required until new reflex habits are formed.

(c) Information Regarding the Loss of the Natural Teeth

If the teeth were not extracted by the dental surgeon who is constructing the dentures information regarding their extraction should always be sought. A history of difficult extractions should be followed by a radiographic examination of the jaws to verify the absence of retained roots.

Questioning should be directed to eliciting the general order in which the teeth were lost. For example, if all the posterior teeth were extracted some years before the anterior ones and no partial dentures were worn in the meantime, then a habit of eating with the front teeth will have been formed which, if persisted in, will have a pronounced unstabilizing effect on full dentures.

A similar condition will exist in individuals who have been edentulous for a considerable length of time and have not worn dentures, for thus they are only able to approximate their jaws in the anterior region and consequently forward travel of the mandible is necessary all the time during eating.

When there is a history of abnormal mandibular function or movement, then difficulty can be anticipated when registering the anteroposterior occlusal relationship.

(d) The Patient's Age

In general, though there are many exceptions, increasing age decreases the readiness to form new habits and also the muscular efficiency is often impaired. Thus the elderly patient will require a longer learning period than the younger individual when dentures are fitted for the first time. Impaired muscular efficiency of old age may demand special types of posterior teeth.

(e) The Patient's Occupation

This will frequently have a relation to the design of the dentures and the technique used in impression taking, for example:

(i) With most professional men and many others whose occupation entails intimate contact with their fellows, appearance and retention are more important than efficiency.

(ii) Public speakers and singers require not only perfect retention but also particular attention to palatal shape and thickness because of the importance of these in phonation.

(iii) Wind instrument players often require a special modification of the shape and position of the anterior teeth.

(f) The 'Patient's Attitude to Appearance

This is often a matter of supreme importance to the individual and where this is the case the operator must be prepared to devote extra time and care to this part of denture construction, often to the extent of making individual teeth.

The oral examination will be described under three headings: (1) Visual examination. (2) Digital examination. (3) X-ray examination.

2. Visual Examination

(a) Colour of the Mucous Membrane

Any variation from the normal must be investigated, and though whitish patches or spots of hyperkeratinisation are not uncommon the most usual variation found is an increased redness due to the inflammation caused by irritation either mechanical, chemical or bacteriological.

Common Prosthetic Causes of Irritation

(i) *Overextension of the Periphery of the Denture.* – This is frequently seen as a bright red line which may break down to an ulceration if the irritation is continued (*see* fig. 51). It may be due to overextension of the periphery of new dentures or

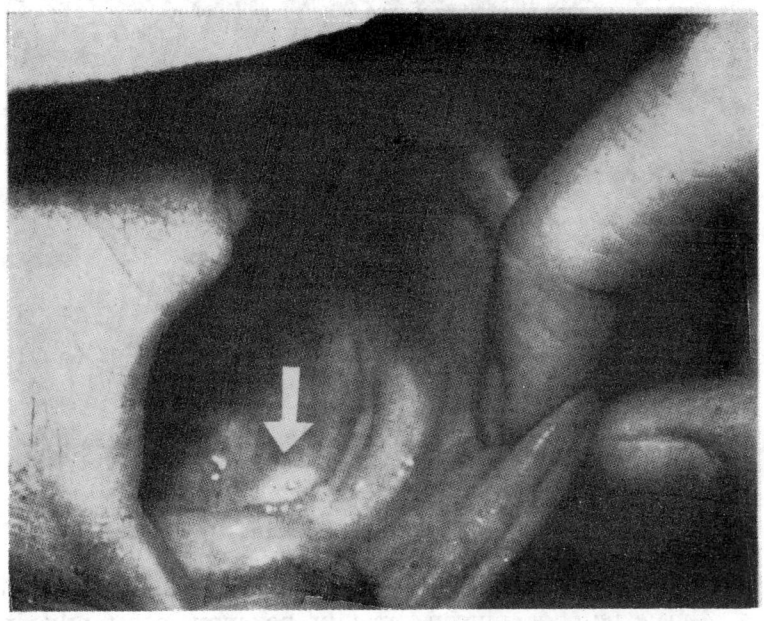

Fig. 51. – Traumatic ulcer (arrowed) caused by overextended lingual flange of denture.

to the altered position of existing dentures due to alveolar absorption, the latter being almost entirely confined to the lower as there is no appreciable absorption of the hard palate and when seen in the upper it is caused by tilting of the denture. In some cases this irritation, if continued over a long period of time, will cause a proliferation of the mucous membrane which is visible as a ridge, flap or series of flaps (*see* fig. 52).

(ii) *Dirty, Ill-fitting Dentures.* – The movement of an ill-fitting denture may of itself cause inflammation, and this is much more likely to occur if the denture is also dirty and consequently harbouring fermenting foodstuffs and bacteria or deposits of salivary calculus. The inflammation

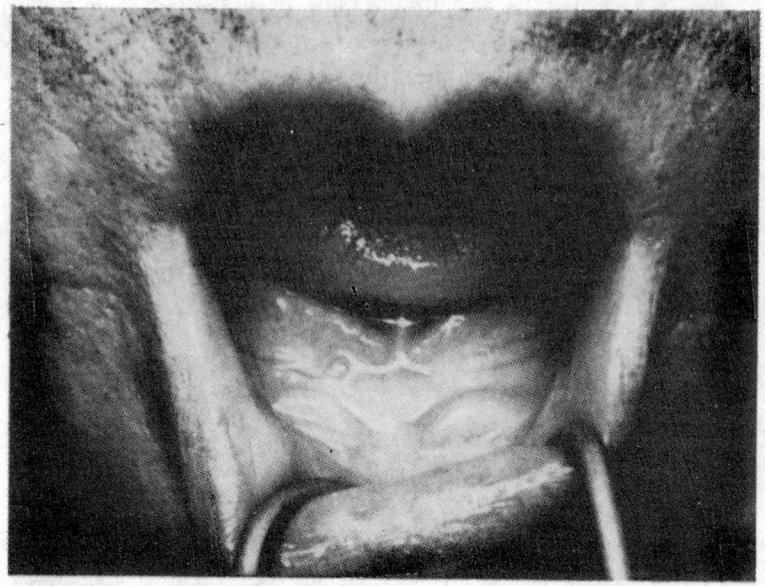

FIG. 52. – Hyperplasia or granuloma caused by long continued overextension of labial flange of lower denture.

usually appears as an ill-defined red area which varies with the extent of mucous membrane most constantly in contact with the denture.

(iii) *Continuous Wearing of a Denture.* – A denture which is worn continuously day and night may cause a chronic inflammation of the underlying mucosa. Particularly is this so if the denture is not kept clean. In the case of an upper denture a granular type of hyperplasia of the palatal mucosa may develop and this is of diagnostic value in spotting the continuous denture wearer (*see* fig. 53).

A similar condition of palatal inflammation sometimes develops in individuals whose dentures move excessively although they do not wear them at night.

(iv) *Faulty Articulation of the Teeth.* – Inflammation may be found on the crest of the alveolar ridge if the occlusion is too heavy in one particular spot, or on the sides of the ridge if there is a lateral drag caused by cuspal interference.

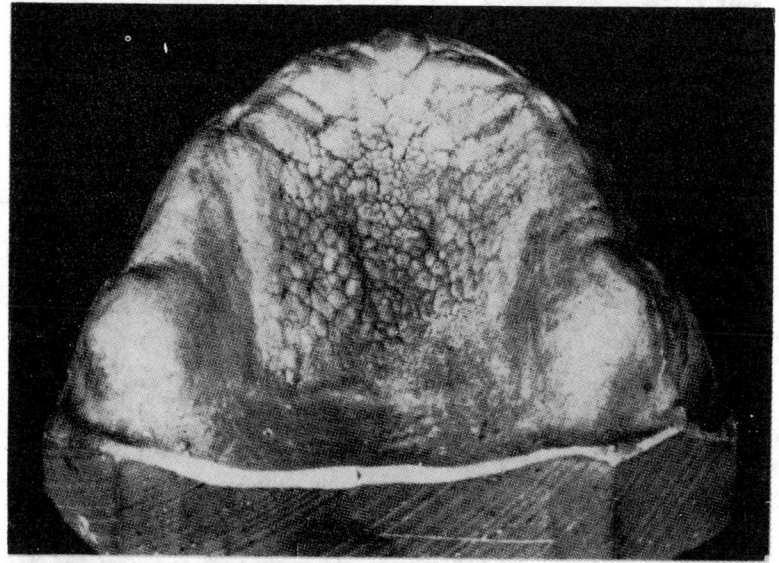

FIG. 53. – Model showing hyperplasia of the palate; note the granular appearance.

This condition is often seen in an edentulous upper in the incisor region when the natural lower anterior teeth are still standing and faulty habits of mastication on the front teeth have been acquired with resultant tipping of the upper denture and consequent trauma.

(v) *Rubber Suction Discs.* – These are removable rubber discs attached by means of a metal stud to the fitting palatal surface of an upper denture. The development of an area of decreased pressure within the disc aids in the denture retention (*see* fig. 54).

They cause chronic inflammation of the mucous membrane with resultant hyperplasia if the inflammation is continued. This is due to the softness of the rubber and the fact that it perishes rapidly, thus the area of contact with the tissues is constantly altering. A number of cases have been reported of perforation of the palate and malignant tumours, attributed directly to the use of rubber suction discs. Their use cannot be condemned too strongly.

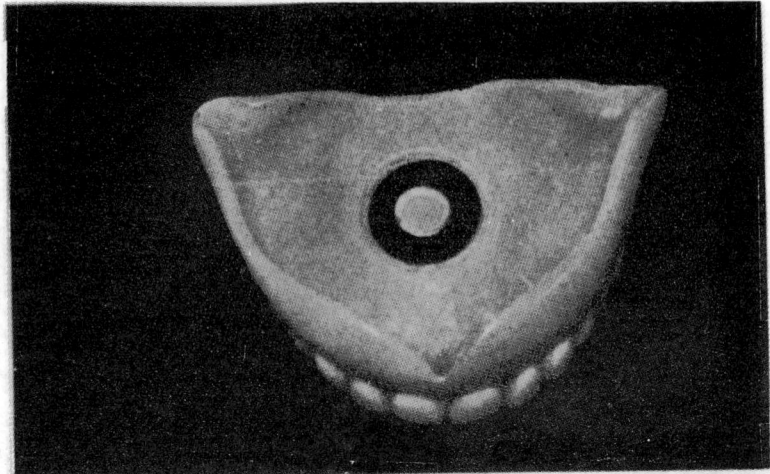

(a) The disc as fitted to the denture.

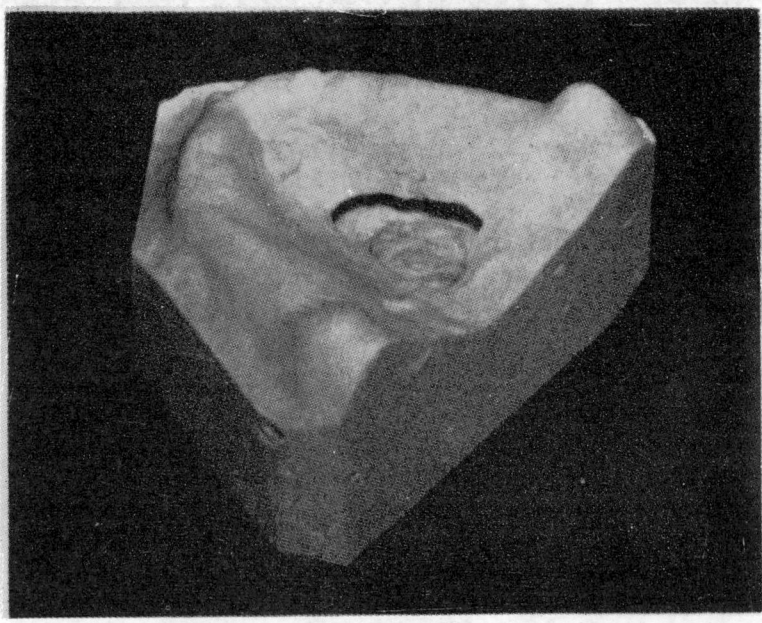

(b) Perforation of the palate resulting from the prolonged use of a disc.

FIG. 54. – Rubber suction disc

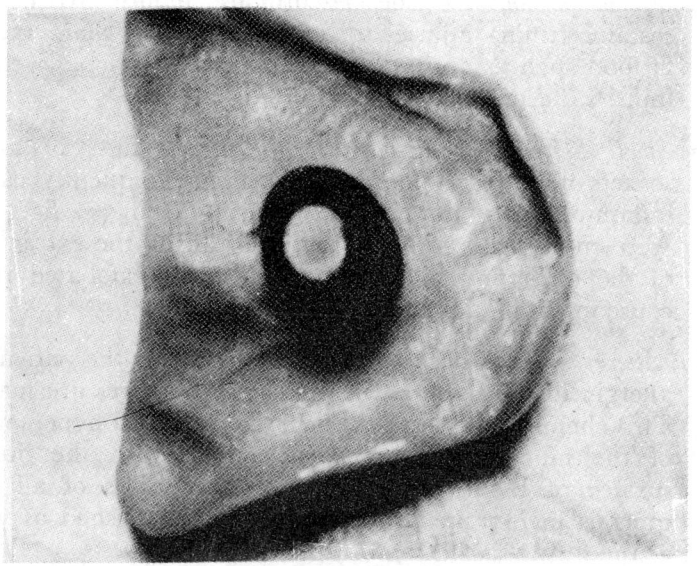

(c) Suction disc on denture.

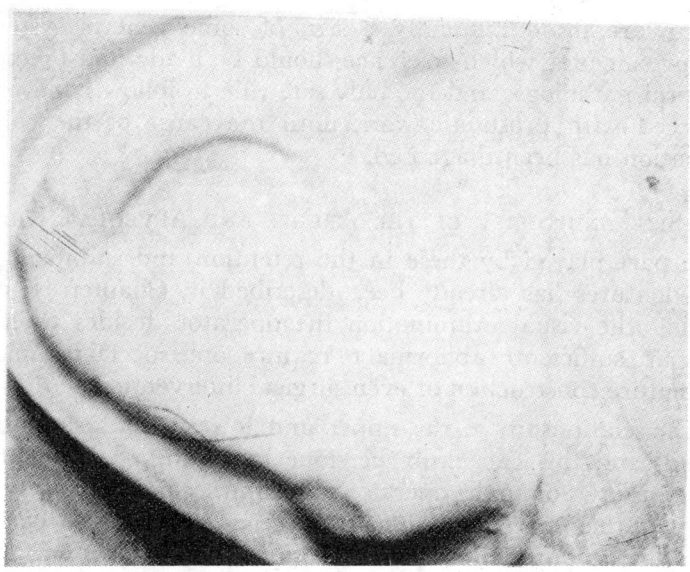

(d) Damage which it has inflicted on patient.
Fig. 54. – Rubber suction disc

(vi) *Traumatic Injury.* – The edentulous mouth frequently sustains trifling injuries to the mucosa from sharp pieces of food such as crusts or small bones. Occasionally these injuries become infected.

(vii) *Small Spicules of Alveolar Bone.* – Sharp edges of tooth sockets not yet rounded by absorption frequently cause inflammation of the mucosa overlying them (*see* fig. 55). Also small pieces of bone fractured during the extraction of the teeth and in the process of being exfoliated may cause inflammation.

(viii) *Allergy.* – Cases occasionally arise in which the patient is allergic to the material of which the dentures are made. This chemical irritation is visible as a general hyperaemia of the mucous membrane in contact with the fitting surface of the denture and in severe cases of all the mucous membrane in contact with the polished as well as the fitting surfaces.

Other Causes of Colour Variation

These are most frequently a sign of some general systemic disturbance for which reference should be made to a textbook on oral pathology, and the only safe rule to follow is never to proceed with prosthetic work until the cause of the colour variation has been diagnosed.

(*b*) SIZE AND SHAPE OF THE ARCHES AND ALVEOLAR RIDGES

The part played by these in the retention and stabilizing of the dentures has already been described in Chapter II, and during the visual examination the operator decides whether they are sufficiently abnormal to require some special technique of denture construction or even surgical intervention.

The relationship of the upper and lower arches should be noted, and this can easily be done by asking the patient to close his jaws on to the operator's first and second fingers. If the lips are then parted at the side the jaw relationship can be seen at the approximate vertical separation which will exist when dentures are fitted.

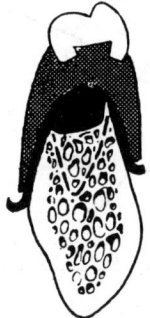

FIG. 55. – Mucous membrane pressed against sharp edge of tooth socket by the denture.

The jaw relationship in different cases will vary from normal to inferior protrusion on the one hand to inferior retrusion on the other (*see* fig. 56).

It is important to gain some knowledge of the jaw relationship at an early stage so that possible difficulties may be foreseen, the rims of the record blocks constructed in their correct positions and the set-up and occlusion of the teeth related to the individual case as discussed later in the book.

(*c*) SHAPE OF THE HARD PALATE

When considered in conjunction with the alveolar ridges, the experienced operator is able to judge with considerable accuracy any unusual difficulties the patient is likely to experience in the retention of his dentures and should inform him of them at this early stage (*see* Chapter II for details).

(*d*) DEPTH OF THE SULCI

Whenever a very shallow sulcus is encountered a special impression technique will be required in order to obtain an adequate peripheral seal and so utilize atmospheric pressure to the full as a retentive force (*see* Chapter II for details).

(*e*) INTERFERENCE FACTORS

The size of the tongue, tightness of the lips and any abnormal

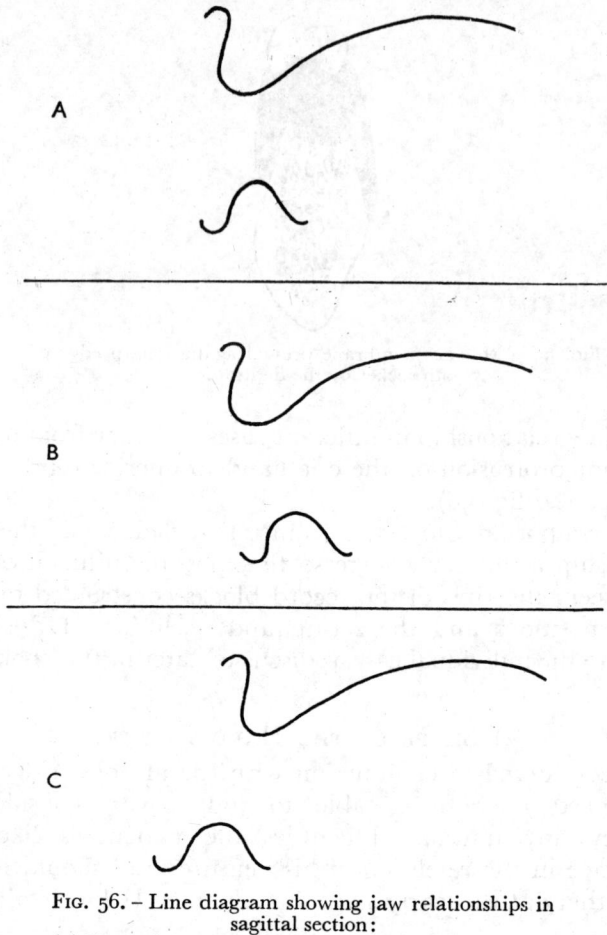

Fig. 56. – Line diagram showing jaw relationships in
sagittal section:
(A) Normal.
(B) Inferior retrusion.
(C) Inferior protrusion.

muscular or fraenal attachments must be noted as they will
influence the design of the future dentures and the type and
position of the artificial teeth used (*see* Chapter II for details).

(*f*) UNEXTRACTED ROOTS

These may be seen flush with, or protruding above, the surrounding mucous membrane (*see* fig. 57), with or without an obvious

area of inflammation round them. They may be loose or firm, and in the latter case it is always wise to take an X-ray photograph. Rarely should a denture be made covering unextracted roots, but in the very exceptional cases where it must be done, the denture should be freely relieved over them, otherwise it is likely to rock and probably fracture.

(g) Sinuses

An infected area in the bone, such as surrounds the retained broken-off apex of a tooth, usually communicates with the surface through a channel known as a sinus (*see* fig. 57).

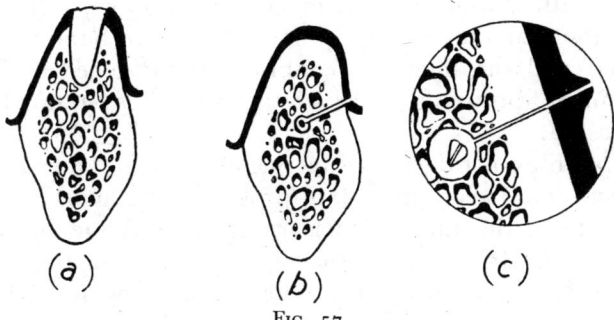

FIG. 57

(*a*) Root visible on surface.
(*b*) Buried root with sinus communicating with buccal sulcus.
(*c*) Enlarged view of sinus.

The appearance in the mouth is usually that of a very small nipple-shaped elevation with a hole in its centre, most commonly found on the sulcus side of the ridge. Pressure with the finger, above in the upper and below in the lower, directed towards the opening will cause the extrusion of a droplet of pus or serum in most cases; this is usually diagnostic and whenever seen should be followed by an X-ray photograph to locate the position and extent of the infected area.

(h) Unilateral Swellings

Any abnormal swellings in the mouth must be investigated and diagnosed, and when found only on one side they are much more likely to be pathological than when they are bilateral.

3. Digital Examination

Before starting to explore the mouth with the finger tips the patient should be asked to indicate immediately if any pain is felt and the cause of such pain must be found. Any area which is painful to the pressure of a soft finger is unlikely to tolerate the pressure of a hard denture.

(a) Firmness of the Ridges

This is most conveniently tested by placing a finger on each side of the ridge and applying alternate lateral pressure. Ridges vary in firmness; the normal is composed of bone covered with a thin layer of mucous membrane, others may appear the same but it may be found that the bone has been absorbed and the mucous membrane is thickened and contains much fibrous tissue which is displaced by the lateral pressure test.

Flabby, fibrous ridges may be encountered in all parts both of upper and lower jaws, but probably the most common position is in the upper anterior region and the history in these cases is almost invariably one of loss of all the natural teeth except the lower anteriors. Later, owing either to the failure to wear a partial lower denture or to the wearing of an inefficient denture, the patient acquires the habit of eating entirely on the anterior teeth with resultant torsion on the upper full denture which leads to rapid absorption of the anterior alveolar ridge and its replacement by fibrous tissue (*see* fig. 58).

(b) Irregularities of the Alveolar Ridge

The general size and shape of the ridges will be noted during the visual examination, but palpation will be necessary to determine irregularities of the underlying bone. The information sought is quite apart from that discussed later under the heading of 'hard and soft areas' and is directed at determining the shape and regularity of the underlying hard tissues. Alveolar absorption is never uniform and hard nodules, sharp edges, spikes and irregularities are frequently felt and pain on pressure over these areas is common (*see* figs. 59 and 60). The prosthetist must at this stage decide whether surgical

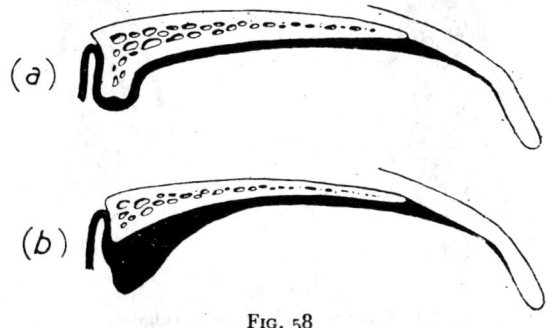

FIG. 58

(a) Sagittal diagram showing normal thickness of mucous membrane covering alveolar ridge and palate.
(b) Absorption of alveolar bone and hypertrophy of mucous membrane.

correction is needed, or whether they will remedy themselves in time in the course of normal absorption, or whether relief of the denture alone will be satisfactory.

(c) VARIATIONS OF MUCOUS MEMBRANE

The ideal mucosa on which to seat full dentures should be:

(i) *Firmly bound down* to the sub-adjacent bone by union with the periosteum which will thus prevent the denture and mucosa moving together in relation to the supporting bone.

(ii) *Slightly Compressible.* – This will allow the denture to bed comfortably into place because the mucosa will adjust itself slightly to the fitting surface of the denture: this will very materially increase the retention by adhesion and cohesion because the film of saliva between the denture and the mucous membrane will be very thin. It will also allow maximum retention from atmospheric pressure because the denture bedding slightly into the tissue will prevent air leaks. In addition such mucosa will act as a cushion to the normal stresses of mastication and prevent the development of sore spots and painful areas from pressure on the underlying bone.

(iii) *Of an Even Thickness.* – This condition is never realized because in a normal mouth the membrane on the crest of the ridges covers scar tissue resulting from the extraction of the teeth, and this varies in thickness.

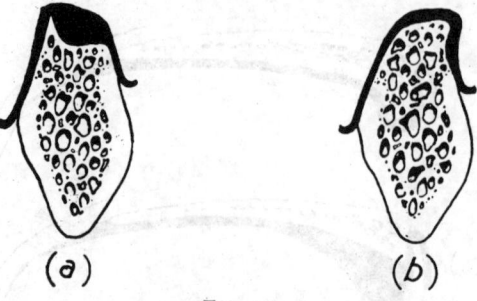

FIG. 59

(a) Sharp edge of alveolar ridge.
(b) Bony nodule.

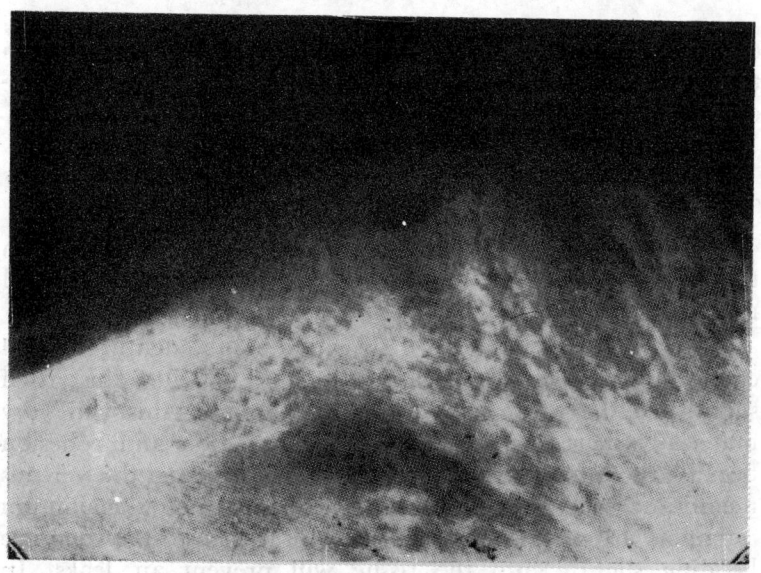

FIG. 60. — Rough irregular surface of alveolar ridge in 4321 area.

In the mid-line of the palate the membrane is thinner than elsewhere. The sides of the vault of the palate are traversed by the anterior palatine, nasopalatine and greater palatine arteries and veins and these are protected by a layer of sub-mucous connective tissue and fat (*see* fig. 61). The tissue of the retromolar pad is often much thicker than any other lower ridge tissue.

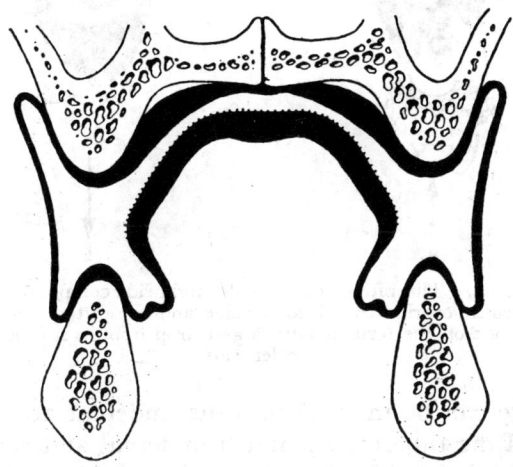

Fig. 61. – This coronal diagram through the 1st molar region illustrates the varying thickness of the mucous membrane covering the oral structures.

Where the differences in compressibility of the mucosa are not great or of large extent they will be found to be clinically unimportant, but where the reverse conditions are present the prosthetist will need to have recourse to a special impression technique or alteration in normal denture construction.

Thin mucosa covering a well-defined torus palatinus and flanked by thick, compressible membrane, will result in a denture which rocks during function, causing pain to the patient and frequently fracture of the denture due to the repeated flexure the base is required to undergo during mastication (*see* fig. 62).

(d) MAXILLARY TUBEROSITIES

These may be found on visual examination to be bulbous and to have a definite undercut area above them, but only by palpation can it be determined whether the bulbous portion is composed of hard or of soft tissue, that is, whether

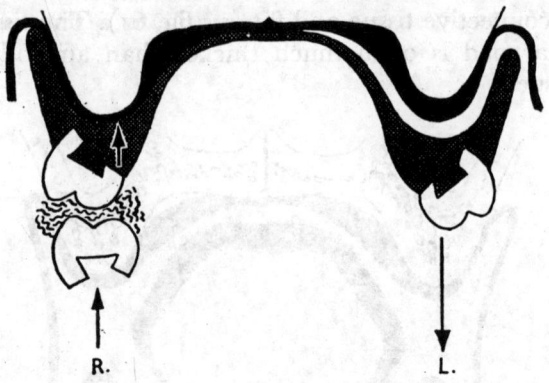

FIG. 62. – The biting force on the right side compresses the mucosa covering the alveolar ridge and causes the denture to rock on the torus palatinus and drop from its seating on the left side.

the denture can be inserted into the undercut area or not (*see* fig. 63). If the tuberosity is much undercut and covered with only a thin layer of mucous membrane, then the surgical removal of part of it may be necessary.

(e) MYLOHYOID RIDGES

It is only in the neighbourhood of the second or third molars that the mylohyoid ridges have any prosthetic significance,

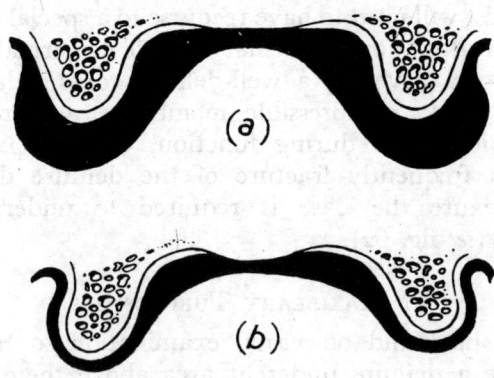

FIG. 63.
(a) A buccal undercut formed by soft tissue.
(b) A buccal undercut formed by bone.

but in this region it is sometimes possible to carry the denture into the undercut area below and behind the ridge. In the majority of cases these ridges are felt to be pronounced and sharp, which is a contra-indication for extending the denture over them, unless the denture is relieved, but where they feel ill-defined and rounded a lingual extension is usually successful (*see* fig. 64).

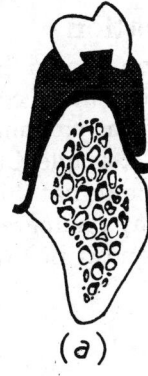 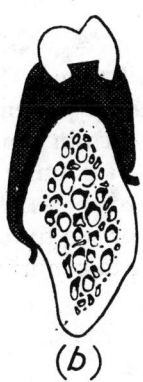

$$(a) \qquad\qquad (b)$$

Fig. 64

   (a) Sharp mylohyoid ridge with lingual flange of denture finished above the ridge.

   (b) Rounded mylohyoid ridge which may allow the lingual flange of the denture to be carried beneath the ridge.

(*f*) LINGUAL POUCH

This is the area bounded medially by the tongue, laterally by the mandible, posteriorly by the palatoglossus muscle and anteriorly by the posterior 3 mm. of the mylohyoid muscle. The extent of the pouch with the tongue at rest and with the tongue protruded sufficiently to lick the lips and also during the act of swallowing should be noted. This is most conveniently done by gently inserting the index finger into the pouch and asking the patient to perform the above actions when the alterations in the extent of the pouch can be felt. If a pouch persists during tongue movement and swallowing then the lingual flange of the denture can probably be carried into this area which will materially assist in the retention of the lower denture.

(g) Painful Areas

This is not a separate examination of itself and pressure pain may be encountered during any of the digital examinations already mentioned. The whole of the denture-bearing mucous membrane should be palpated and any painful areas must be diagnosed and treated before successful dentures can be constructed.

4. X-ray Examination

Ideally a full mouth X-ray examination should be made of every edentulous patient prior to starting denture construction, otherwise a certain number of pathological or abnormal conditions will pass unrecognized, as for example buried roots and unerupted teeth. When it is considered that this routine is uneconomic or too time-consuming, X-ray photographs should still be taken to confirm or assist in diagnosis in the following cases:

(i) Buried roots.
(ii) Sinuses.
(iii) Unilateral swellings.
(iv) Rough alveolar ridges.
(v) Areas painful to pressure.

The information which has been given in this chapter is now tabulated (*see* opposite page) for the convenience of the beginner.

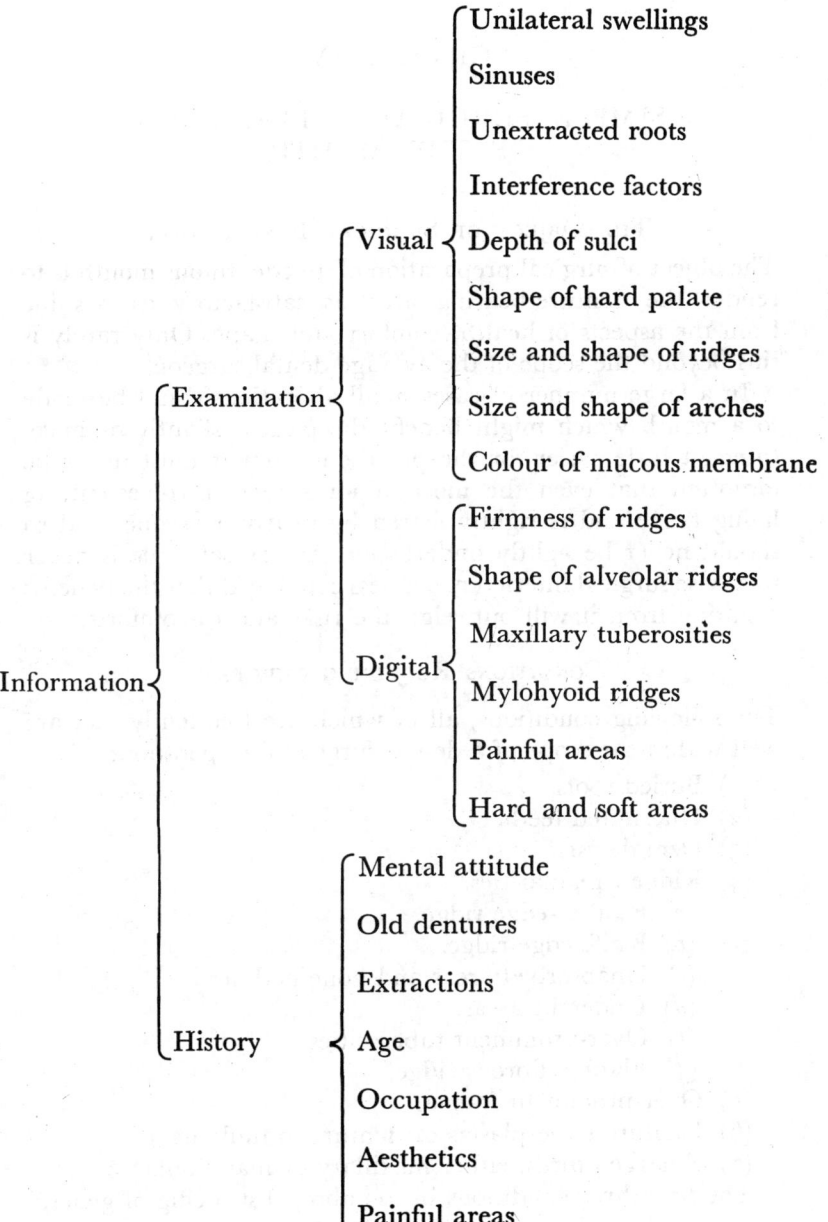

Information
- Examination
  - Visual
    - Unilateral swellings
    - Sinuses
    - Unextracted roots
    - Interference factors
    - Depth of sulci
    - Shape of hard palate
    - Size and shape of ridges
    - Size and shape of arches
    - Colour of mucous membrane
  - Digital
    - Firmness of ridges
    - Shape of alveolar ridges
    - Maxillary tuberosities
    - Mylohyoid ridges
    - Painful areas
    - Hard and soft areas
- History
  - Mental attitude
  - Old dentures
  - Extractions
  - Age
  - Occupation
  - Aesthetics
  - Painful areas

Chapter IV

SIMPLE SURGICAL PREPARATION
OF THE MOUTH

The Object of Surgical Preparation

The object of surgical preparation of an edentulous mouth is to render the denture-bearing area as satisfactory as possible from the aspects of health, comfort and shape. Only rarely is this beyond the scope of the average dental surgeon.

In a large number of cases small alterations could be made to a mouth which might benefit the patient slightly or make things a little easier for the prosthetist, but it must never be forgotten that even the most minor surgery involves cutting living tissue and is rightly feared by nearly everyone, and so should never be lightly undertaken. A very safe rule is never to advise surgical interference unless convinced that the benefits resulting from it will outweigh the risks and discomforts.

Conditions Requiring Surgery

The following conditions, all of which are frequently met are well within the scope of a dental surgeon for operation:

(1) Buried roots.
(2) Unerupted teeth.
(3) Dental cysts.
(4) Ridge irregularities.
    (a) Feather-edge ridge.
    (b) Knife-edge ridge.
    (c) Unabsorbed areas and bone nodules.
    (d) Undercut areas.
    (e) Over-prominent tuberosities.
    (f) Flabby, fibrous ridge.
(5) Over-prominent fraena.
(6) Denture hyperplasias or denture granulomata.
(7) Enlarged torus, either maxillary or mandibular.

The first three conditions in the above list, being of general dental application rather than purely prosthetic, will not be mentioned further except to stress that they should almost invariably be dealt with before denture construction is begun.

GENERAL SURGICAL PRINCIPLES

Before outlining the techniques of individual operations a few general principles are given.

(1) Asepsis must be observed. Since it is quite impossible to sterilize the oral cavity it is perhaps not immediately apparent why sterility on the part of the operator is so essential. Every healthy animal has acquired a high degree of immunity to the bacteria normally present in its mouth. If a dog injures itself it licks the wound and although its saliva is teeming with bacteria the wound rarely becomes septic, but if the same dog were to bite a man and he did nothing about cleansing the injury it would almost certainly turn septic. So although a sterile field for operations in the mouth is impossible every care must be taken to prevent the introduction of foreign bacteria.

(2) Incisions through the mucoperiosteum must be made with firmness, otherwise reflection without tearing is impossible.

(3) Incisions should err on the side of being too long rather than too short; one extra stitch is of no consequence to the patient whilst a little extra vision or space is frequently of great assistance to the operator. In addition, tissue which is well reflected is in less danger of being traumatized during the operation.

(4) When operating under local anæsthesia it should be remembered that bone cutting with a hammer and chisel causes much more jarring and discomfort to the patient than cutting with burs.

(5) Decide beforehand, as far as possible, what is to be done and be sufficiently radical; results will not be obtained by reflecting the mucous membrane and then just scratching the bone.

(6) If there is any doubt whether a flap will stay in place, suture it. A suture is painlessly inserted under anaesthesia and can be painlessly removed a few days later.

Diagnosis of Conditions Requiring Surgery

By far the largest numbers of edentulous mouths which require some surgical preparation for the reception of dentures are those in which there is an abnormal condition of the bony ridges and, whilst the general technique of operating remains the same, the surgeon should differentiate between the various conditions before starting to operate: slight variations in technique will be needed for the different conditions.

Feather-edged Ridge

This can usually be detected on palpation as a thin, irregular, sharp edge painful to pressure. It is apparently due to irregular alveolar absorption, and as it is most frequently found following the extraction of teeth for periodontal disease it is sometimes wrongly described as residual sepsis. The radiographic appearance is of a very irregular alveolar crest with no clearly defined outline, the bone appearing to fade away (*see* fig. 60).

On exposing the bone exactly the same picture is seen; it is found to be cancellous in type, uncovered by a cortical layer, the alveolar crest presenting innumerable spicules and irregularities.

Knife-edged Ridge

On palpation the ridge is felt to be thin buccolingually, sharp but smooth and, like the feather edge, painful on pressure. Found only in the mandible it appears to be due to absorption which is greater buccolingually than vertically. X-ray photographs show a thin ridge with a clearly defined outline, the cancellous bone being covered with a cortical layer. The appearance of the exposed bone confirms this (*see* fig. 65).

Unabsorbed Areas and Bone Nodules

These can usually be felt as smoothly rounded hard lumps under the mucous membrane and their cause is apparently unknown. Radiographically they show as small roundish areas of increased density.

On exposure the nodules are easily seen as raised lumps of smooth, hard, cortical bone.

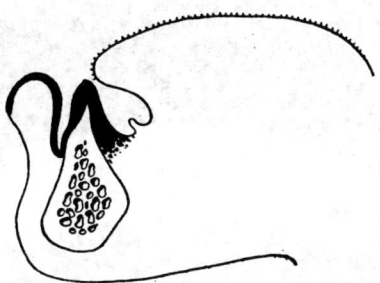

Fig. 65. – Sagittal diagram showing knife edge ridge in lower anterior region.

Alveolectomy

This is the name given to the operation for the removal of alveolar bone, and is equally applicable to the removal of one small nodule or the excision of bone from the entire alveolar ridges of both jaws.

This operation is most frequently performed under local anaesthesia as it is both more convenient to work in a dental surgery and is generally preferred by patients.

Technique of Alveolectomy

The Incision

An incision is made just below the crest of the alveolus on the buccal side, and care must be taken that all fibres of the muco-periosteum are severed. This is not always easy if the under-lying bone is rough and irregular, and a heavy scalpel is preferable to one having a light and flexible blade as the cutting edge must be pressed firmly against the bone (*see* figs. 66 and 67).

Further incisions at each end of this transverse cut will be needed on the labial or buccal surfaces, and these should be continuous with the first incision, joining it in a gentle curve and not at right angles, otherwise the small piece of muco-periosteum in the angle is difficult to retain in place during healing.

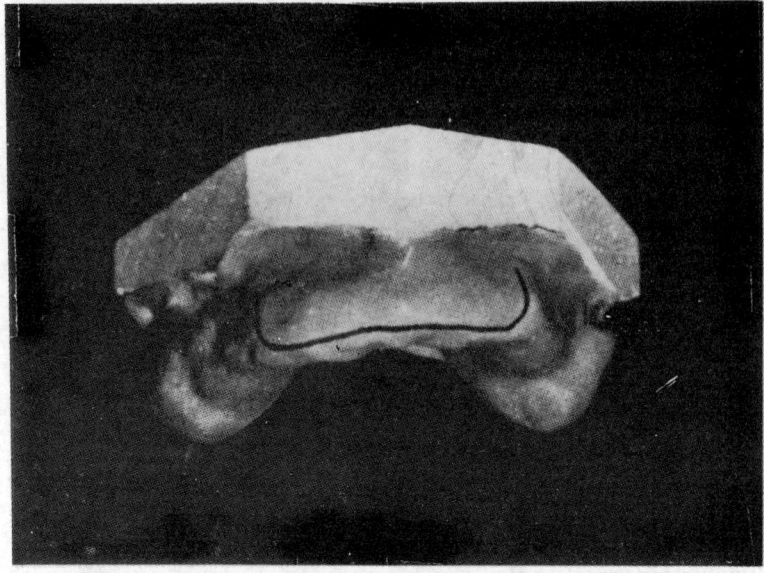

FIG. 66. – Alveolectomy of the upper anterior region.
The line of the incision.

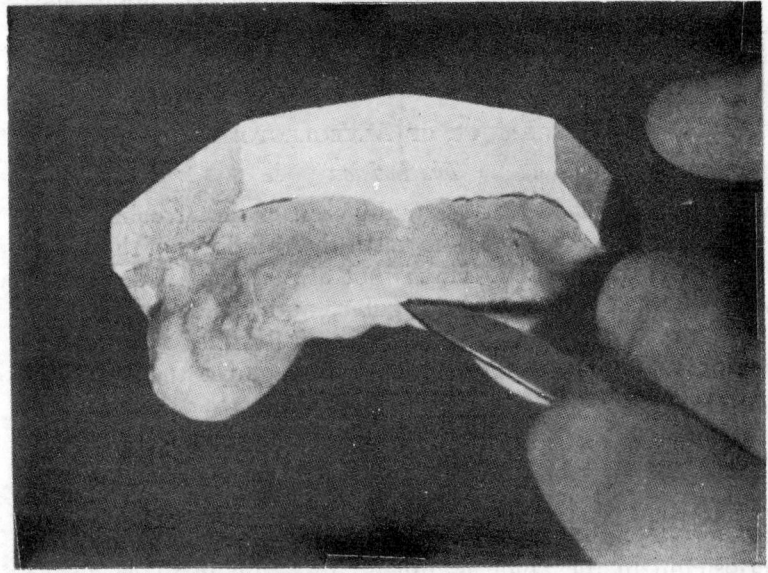

FIG. 67. – Alveolectomy of the upper anterior region.
Making the incision.

The incisions should be carried no deeper into the sulci than is absolutely necessary because the tissues in this area are looser and more vascular than elsewhere and their severance will result in greater post-operative swelling and haematomata. On the lingual or palatal surfaces further incisions are rarely necessary as the soft tissues here will be reflected towards the inner side of the arch where, instead of being stretched, they will have more room.

Reflection of Tissues

The next step is the reflection of the mucoperiosteum with a periosteal elevator, and is often the only difficult part of an otherwise simple operation. The soft tissues are very adherent to the bone and if thin, great care must be taken not to tear them; this is not easy as often considerable force is required particularly when starting to lever up this membrane. This reflection is continued until all the bone to be removed is fully exposed (see fig. 68).

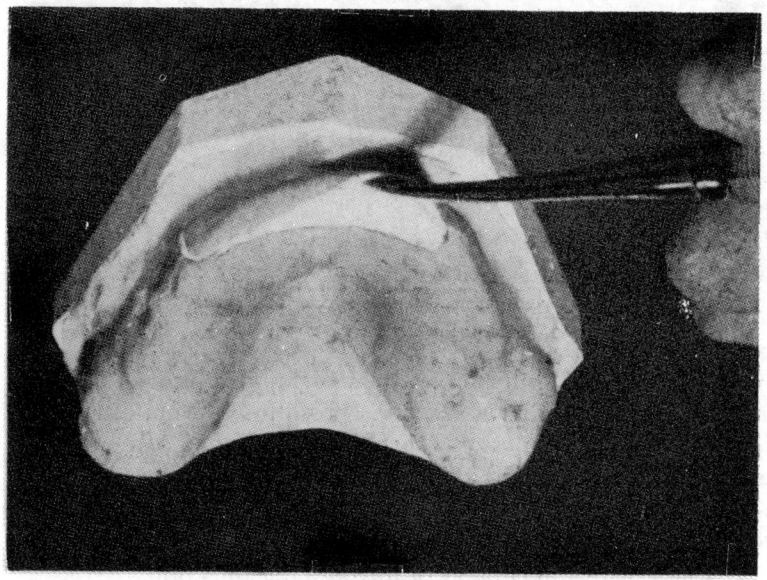

Fig. 68. – Alveolectomy of the upper anterior region. Reflection of the mucoperiosteum.

Removal of Bone

With a pair of rongeurs the alveolus is trimmed to the desired shape (*see* fig. 69). Some operators prefer to use large, bone-cutting burs for trimming the alveolar ridge, and with their use a jet of water constantly playing on the bur will be found a great help as it will keep the field clear of blood, saliva and debris. It will also keep the bur from clogging and heating, and the water is easily removed from the mouth by an efficient "sucker".

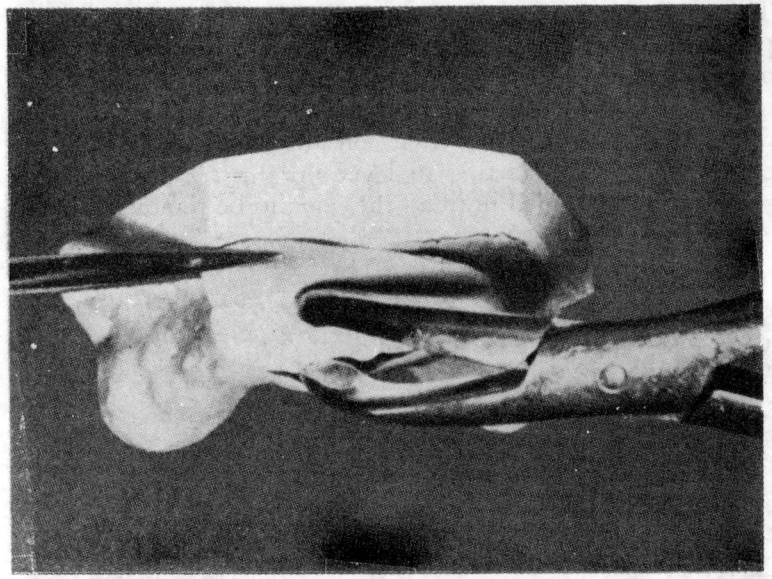

FIG. 69. – Alveolectomy of the upper anterior region.
Removal of bone with rongeurs.

Having removed the gross mass of bone it is necessary to smooth the remainder as much as possible with bone files (*see* fig. 70). The smoothness or otherwise of the bone can easily be ascertained by running the tip of the finger over the area, having first replaced the mucoperiosteum. This last point is very important for these reasons:

(1) There is less likelihood of introducing infection.

(2) Exposed cancellous bone always feels rough.

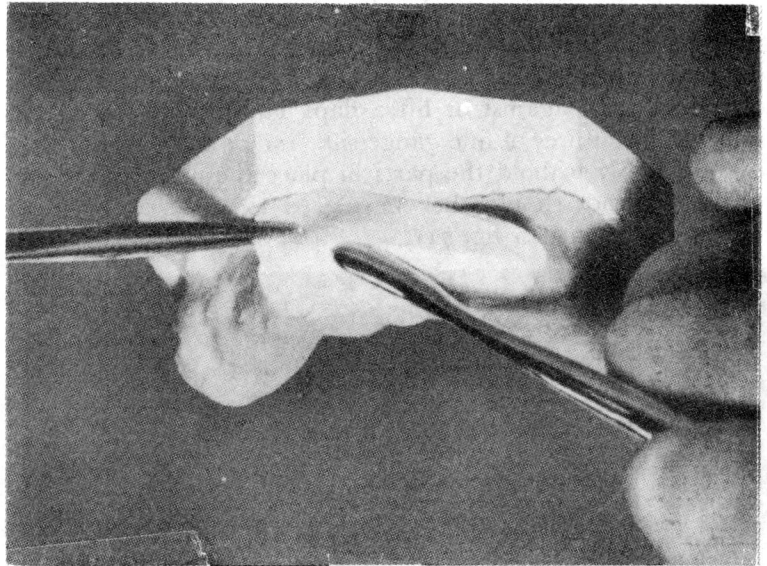

Fig. 70. – Alveolectomy of the upper anterior region.
Smoothing the bone with a bone file.

(3) Dental surgeons are accustomed to judging the shape and
smoothness of bone through an intervening layer of
mucous membrane.

When satisfied with the feel of the bone, the debris caused
by filing should be washed away by a gentle jet of warm normal
saline solution and the flaps of soft tissue replaced. These
flaps will be found now to overlap, and they must be trimmed
till their edges just approximate without tension. If too much
tissue is removed there will be a gap between the edges which
must epithelialize over and healing will be retarded, whilst if
too little is cut away a thick fibrous band will be left which
may well make the later wearing of a denture very difficult.
A pair of dissecting forceps to hold the strip being removed
and a pair of serrated-edged scissors are the best instruments
to use as the wet, fibrous tissue is rather difficult to control and
the serrations on the blades of the scissors prevent the tissue
slipping.

Suturing

The operation is completed by stitching the flaps in place, sufficient stitches being used to make it impossible for the tongue to catch against or lift a flap. The needles should be fine and the sutures of fine gauge silk, and as the object of the stitches is only to hold the parts in place they must never be pulled tight nor should they be placed too near an edge in case they pull out (*see* fig. 71).

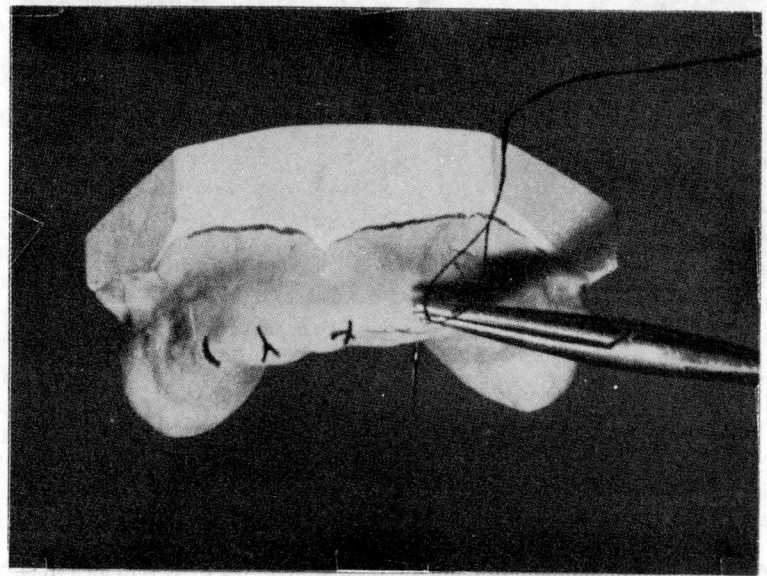

Fig. 71. – Alveolectomy of the upper anterior region. Suturing the mucoperiosteal flap back into position.

The patient may now rinse the mouth out gently, and if dentures are worn they may be inserted, as they will protect the wound from the inquisitiveness of the tongue and so allow healing in the minimum length of time. Some operators line such dentures where they cover the wound with B.I.P. paste, a paste composed of bismuth, iodoform and paraffin, whilst others use penicillin paste in the same way, but neither is usually necessary.

The patient may be given two aspirin-phenacetin-codein tablets to take, as the effect of the anæsthetic is being lost, to minimize any after-pain of the operation. Two more tablets every four hours may be prescribed if pain persists. A mouth-wash is quite unnecessary but if the patient particularly wishes, anything mild and bland such as glycerin-thymol will do no harm.

Post-operative Procedure

The patient should be seen twenty-four hours later to make sure that there is no undue swelling or pain, though both are usually absent. Three or four days later the stitches may be removed by holding them steady with a pair of tweezers and cutting with a sharp pair of fine pointed scissors or a scalpel. If pain is caused in removing these stitches it is caused by clumsiness or inefficiency on the part of the operator.

No attempt has been made to describe the quantity of bone which should be removed, and this omission is deliberate since every case differs and each must be treated according to its individual needs. The general principle is never to operate if the same results can be obtained within a reasonable time by alveolar absorption, but where an operation is necessary the object of an alveolectomy is so to shape the bone that it will form the best possible painless base to support a denture.

REMOVAL OF BONE NODULES

The commonest variation of the above technique occurs when dealing with small nodules of bone. It is often impossible to remove these nodules with nibblers which tend to slip over the hard, convex surfaces without sufficient grip to cut; when this does occur recourse must be had to a bone-cutting bur. The nodules are also very easily removed by a hammer and sharp chisel – a suitable method when operating under a general anaesthetic.

UNDERCUT AREAS

When these are too deep to permit the entry of a denture they should generally be removed or reduced, and the only guidance is the judgment of the operator as to whether retention of the denture will be satisfactory if the undercut is left and the periphery of the denture adjusted to permit its insertion. The most common positions requiring surgical interference are the

maxillary tuberosities and the lower incisor region, either
lingually, labially, or both.

OVER-PROMINENT MAXILLARY TUBEROSITIES

The operation for eliminating an undercut in the region of the
maxillary tuberosities in no way differs from other forms of
alveolectomy, except in the first incision which is best made in
the form of a semicircle extending along the alveolar crest
below the bone to be removed and sweeping mesially to it, up
to the required height in the sulcus (*see* fig. 72).

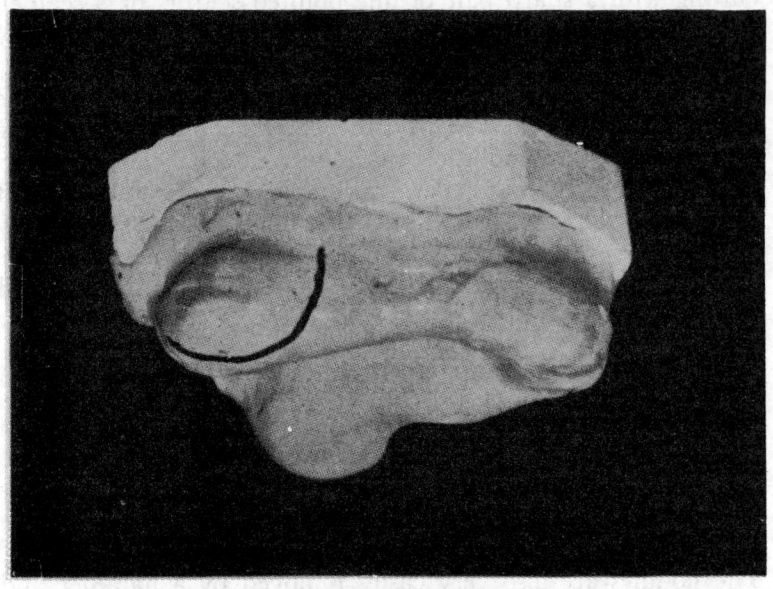

FIG. 72. – Alveolectomy of the tuberosity.
The line of the incision.

An incision of this shape will make the reflection of the mucoperiosteum considerably easier, and in cases where it is only
necessary to remove a little bone it will obviate the necessity
of stitching as the small semicircular flap will be held in place
by the pressure of the cheek. If the removal of much bone is
contemplated it is wise to X-ray the cases pre-operatively to
ascertain the size and proximity of the maxillary antrum.

INTERFERING FRAENA

Fraenal attachments rarely require excision as it is nearly always possible to design the denture to accommodate them, but cases do occur where, unless removed, they make the satisfactory wearing of a denture impossible.

The operation of fraenectomy is a simple one, the denture being used to keep the cut surfaces apart and so prevent their re-uniting. The impression, from which the denture is constructed, must be taken in an easy flowing material such as plaster of Paris so that the position of the easily displaced fraenum is accurately recorded. When the denture is ready for processing the fraenal attachment on the model is cut away and the sulcus trimmed to the desired depth, the flange of the denture is waxed into this sulcus, and the denture processed (*see* fig. 73).

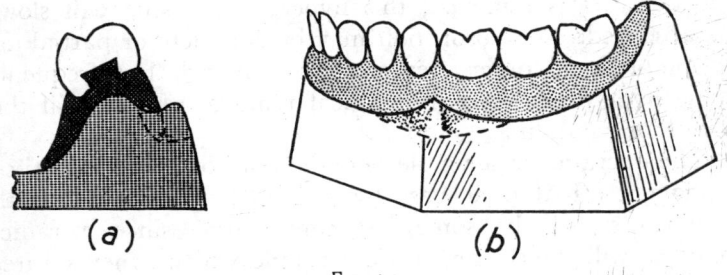

(a)   **(b)**

FIG. 73

(a) Coronal section through the buccal fraenum on the plaster model. Dotted line indicates the depth to which the model is trimmed.

(b) Side view of the fraenum showing the depth to which the model is trimmed.

TECHNIQUE OF FRAENECTOMY

The operation consists of anaesthetizing and then excising the fraenum with scalpel or scissors to the same depth as was previously done on the model. As soon as the bleeding is checked, the denture is inserted and the patient instructed that it must not be removed, except for cleaning, until the cut surfaces have completely epithelialized over. The patient should be seen occasionally during this period so that any soreness arising from the wearing of the new denture can be speedily dealt with, as under no conditions may it be left out for more than a few minutes at a time.

DENTURE HYPERPLASIA

These benign overgrowths of mucous membrane are usually associated with old dentures where alveolar absorption has resulted in settling of the denture leading to chronic irritation of the sulci from the now over-extending denture flange. These hyperplasias are often multiple, one flap having grown and then become enclosed under the denture either because of the looseness of fit or because the patient finds it more comfortable in this position. A second flap forms and is in turn enclosed, and so on until in some cases there are six or eight of these overgrowths like leaves of a book (*see* figs. 74 and 52).

If the irritation, caused by the over-extended periphery of the denture, is removed, this hyperplastic tissue will slowly be absorbed. The absorption may be complete or partial and if complete no other treatment is required, but frequently these hyperplasias require surgical removal especially if they are of long standing.

The operation is a simple one, the flaps of fibrous soft tissue being cut off at their base by a scalpel or scissors, but the removal should be somewhat conservative since a radical removal will leave a much wider wound which, when sutured, will tend to reduce the sulcus depth considerably. Where the wound is a small one it can usually quite satisfactorily be left to epithelialize over, but if there is a persistent slight haemorrhage which cannot be controlled by the application of hot saline solution the edges must be gently drawn together by one or two sutures.

FLABBY, FIBROUS RIDGES

A condition is quite frequently encountered where an alveolar ridge which appears normal is found on palpation to lack bony support and to be readily displaceable on pressure. The cause is usually over-stimulation of the alveolar ridge, often from lateral pressure, which has resulted in its excessive absorption whilst at the same time the mucous membrane has become thickened and fibrous (*see* Chapter II).

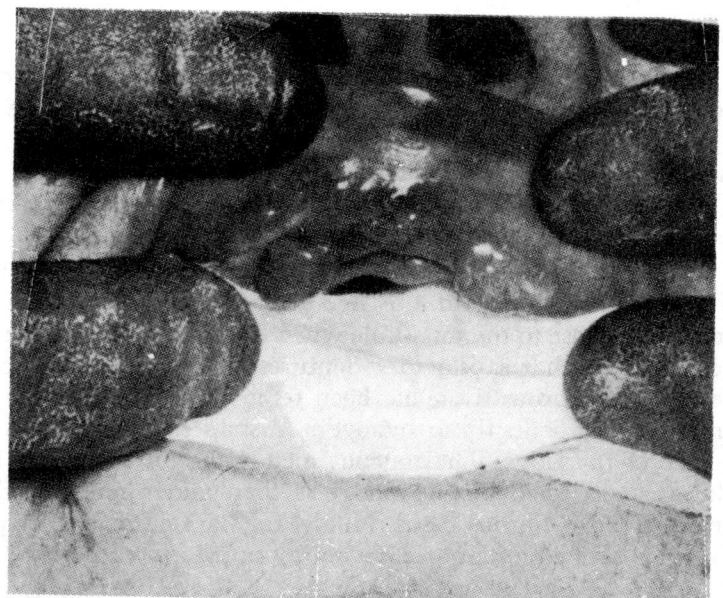

(a) Two granulomata of labial sulcus.

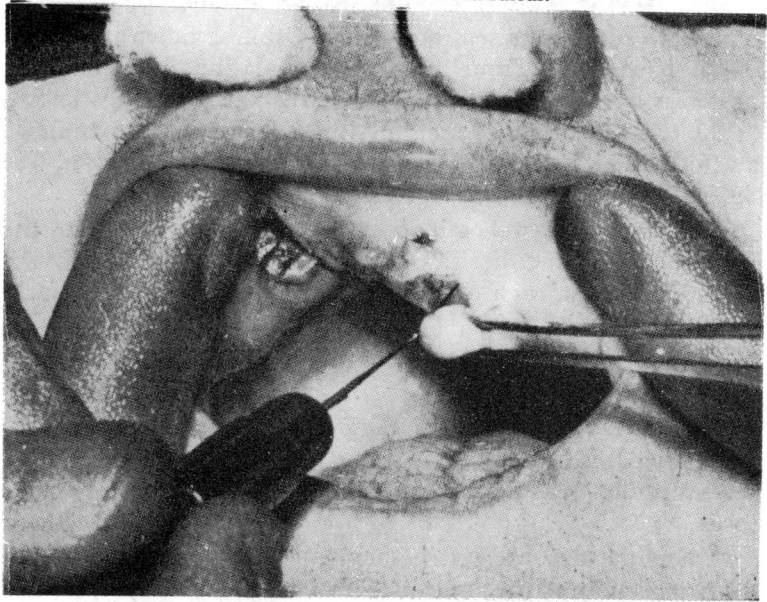

(b) Ezcision of granuloma by Mr P. A. Trotter, using monopolar electrode of M.S.5 surgical unit.

FIG. 74. – Denture granulomata.

It is rarely necessary or even desirable to remove this fibrous tissue as in most cases a flabby ridge is better than no ridge at all, and by using special techniques satisfactory dentures can usually be constructed. When, however, it is decided to operate the treatment should be as conservative as possible, the minimum amount necessary being removed.

The position where it is commonly necessary to remove fibrous tissue is around the maxillary tuberosities, where it may be so close to the mandible when the latter is in its normal rest position that satisfactory dentures cannot be made until some of the fibrous tissue has been removed. The technique of the operation is firstly to remove a V shaped wedge from the centre of the ridge. The mucous membrane on either side of the area occupied by the wedge is then undermined by the removal of the fibrous tissue. Finally the flaps of mucous membrane so formed are approximated by sutures (*see* fig. 75).

LARGE TORUS, MAXILLARY OR MANDIBULAR

There is usually a raised, bony ridge running down the centre of the hard palate from the anterior palatine foramen to the posterior border, or any part of this distance, which is known as the torus palatinus. Sometimes this ridge is very pronounced and covered with only a thin layer of mucous membrane (*see* fig. 76).

There may be two eminences on the lingual aspect of the mandible, one on either side of the mid-line and usually in the premolar region, each of which is called a torus mandibularis.

These conditions do not inconvenience the patient until he is obliged to wear dentures, when pressure may cause considerable pain.

The correct treatment for these cases, unless they are very pronounced, is to leave them alone and to relieve the dentures so that under no conditions can they exert any pressure on the torus.

If it is decided to reduce them surgically it will be found after reflection of the mucous membrane that they present a hard, smooth, cortical layer of bone which it is almost impossible to remove with nibblers. A bone-cutting bur or

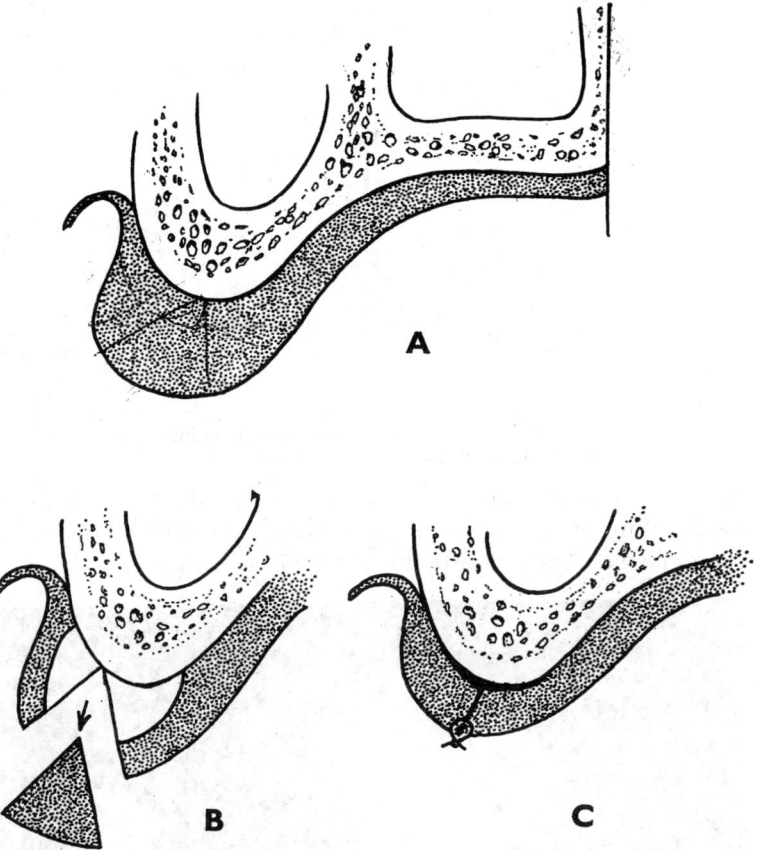

FIG. 75. – Technique of reducing a fibrous tuberosity:
(A) The bulbous tuberosity.
(B) A V-shaped section removed and the tissue remaining undermined.
(C) The undermined tissues sutured together.

hammer and chisel is the best instrument to use, followed by the usual bone-files.

It should be stressed that the genial tubercles, which lie immediately on either side of the mid-line on the lingual side of the mandible, must not be mistaken for the torus mandibularis. When there has been considerable absorption of the mandible the genial tubercles stand up prominently above the

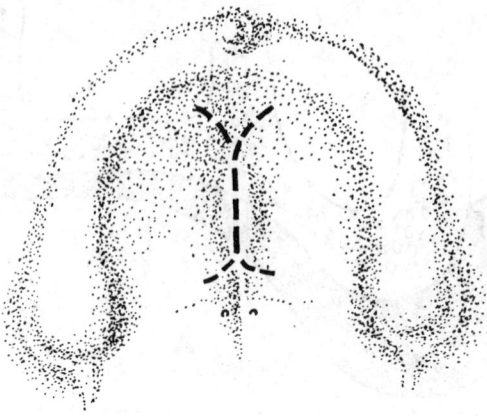

Fig. 76. – Illustrating a pronounced torus palatinus and the incision made if it is intended to reduce it surgically.

general level and are a considerable handicap to the prosthetist, but on no account may they be removed since the genioglossus muscle is attached to them (*see* fig. 77).

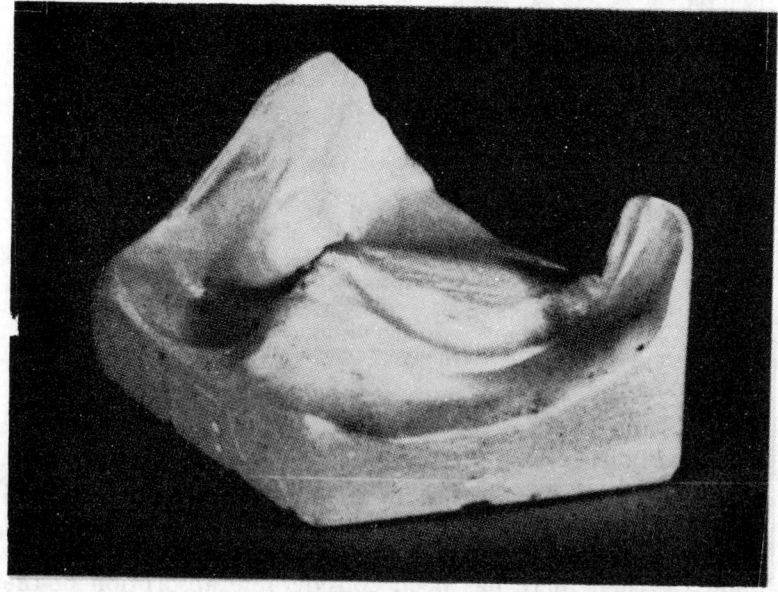

Fig. 77. – A prominent attachment of the genioglossus muscle.

DIFFICULTIES

Since there are no large blood vessels in the mucous membrane covering the alveolar processes, serious haemorrhage will not be encountered but capillary bleeding or the cutting of a small vessel may sometimes be troublesome: both may be easily controlled. For capillary oozing the application under pressure of gauze soaked in hot (120° F.) saline solution is all that is required, whilst small blood vessels may be crushed with tweezers or Spencer-Wells forceps. The application of Oxycel in cases of persistent oozing after suturing is complete usually stops the bleeding.

When operating under a general anaesthetic it may still be advisable to inject a local anaesthetic at the site of operation because of its properties of vasoconstriction. The anaesthetist should be consulted before this is done as the effect of the adrenaline on the heart of a patient under a general anaesthetic is variable.

Swelling may be controlled by the intra- or extra-oral application of ice packs, whilst haematomata and bruising, though often alarming to the patient, are usually better left alone and disappear quite rapidly.

Sepsis, though rare, will usually yield rapidly to correct antibiotic treatment.

More extensive operations such as those for bilateral mandibular resection, epithelial inlays, etc., are outside the scope of the average dental surgeon and consultation with an oral or a plastic surgeon is necessary. Any description of these more serious operations is out of place in a book of this description, but they are excellently dealt with in current surgical literature.

CHAPTER V

IMPRESSION TAKING

In order that a denture may be correctly designed and the necessary constructional work carried out accurate models of the patient's mouth are necessary and various methods by which these may be obtained will be described in this chapter.

Whilst all operators agree that the models must be an accurate reproduction of the mouth there is considerable difference of opinion over the interpretation of the word accurate. The base on which the denture will rest is covered with mucous membrane which is compressible or distortable and the shape of this base at rest differs from the shape when resisting the stresses of mastication imposed through the denture which it supports. Further, the denture will be surrounded by moving tissues and the question arises, what position should these tissues occupy when taking an impression to produce an accurate model?

Ideally one wishes to obtain from the impressions, models of those areas of the mouth which will be covered by the dentures, together with the soft tissues which will be in contact with their peripheries during any normal movements made in speech and mastication. Also the model should represent the bearing surface as it will be when the denture is functioning during mastication, i.e. transmitting pressure.

The area which should be included in the impression is frequently far greater than can be used, but it is not possible to design a denture accurately unless the whole area which it could occupy is included in the model, although, for reasons which have been discussed in Chapter II it is not always desirable to finish a denture to this outline. The extent of the impression should be as follows:

The Edentulous Upper

From the functional depth of the labial sulcus anteriorly to
2 mm. or 3 mm. beyond the posterior border of the hard
palate, as ascertained by palpation. Laterally from the functional depth of the buccal sulcus on one side to the functional
depth of the sulcus on the other (*see* fig. 78).

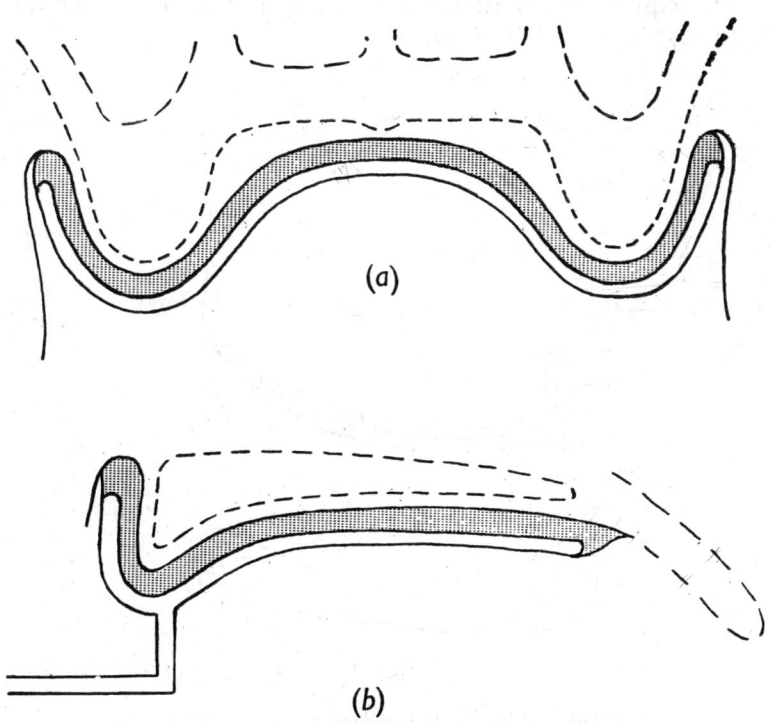

FIG. 78

(*a*) Coronal, and (*b*) Sagittal views of the correct extent of an
upper impression.

The Edentulous Lower

From the functional depth of the labial sulcus anteriorly to
2 or 3 mm. above the retromolar pad, posteriorly.

From the functional depth of the buccal sulcus to the functional position of the floor of the mouth laterally, on both sides (*see* fig. 79). The position of the floor of the mouth depends on the position of the tongue and, as overextension of the denture is apt to cause ulceration of the mucous membrane and instability of the denture, it is desirable to take the impression with the floor of the mouth raised to the functional position, which is obtained posteriorly by protruding the tongue to the extent required to moisten the lips, and anteriorly by raising its tip upwards and backwards.

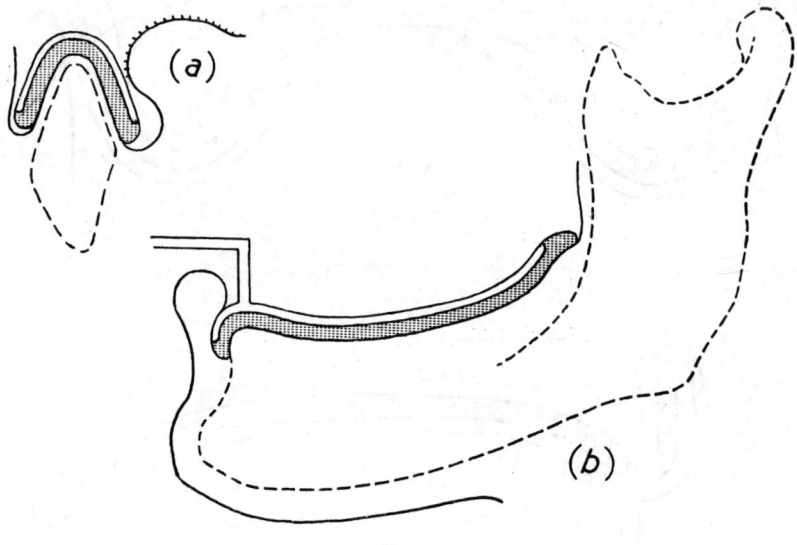

FIG. 79

(*a*) Coronal, and (*b*) Sagittal views of the correct extent of a lower impression.

THE IDEAL IMPRESSION MATERIAL

Many materials have been advocated for impression taking and whilst none is perfect each is usually superior to the others in some respect and, in order to have some means of comparison, it is useful to enumerate the properties which would be possessed by an ideal impression material.

An ideal impression material would:

(1) Be non-injurious to the tissues.
   Non-poisonous and non-irritant.

(2) Be capable of compressing the soft tissues to any desired degree without itself being distorted.
   This would enable an impression to be taken of the tissues in the position they will occupy under masticatory stresses.

(3) Be sufficiently fluid on insertion to give accurate surface detail.
   Closeness of fit is all important if the full advantages of adhesion and cohesion are to be obtained (*see* Chapter I).

(4) Be able to reproduce accurately any undercuts which are present.
   This implies that the material shall be either sufficiently elastic to spring out of the undercuts or sufficiently brittle to break easily. If brittle, the material should be capable of easy reassembly.

(5) Have a pleasant taste, smell and appearance.

(6) Have no dimensional changes either in or out of the mouth at all normal degrees of temperature and humidity.
   This is necessary in the interests of accuracy.

(7) Set, or harden, at, or near, mouth temperature.
   If this is not the case then the removal of the impression from the mouth without distorting it will be virtually impossible.

(8) Have a setting time under the control of the operator.
   This is required to allow for individual variations of skill and speed.

(9) Be capable of having additions made and of reinsertion in the mouth, without distortion.
   This will allow minor corrections to be made without having to take an entirely new impression.

(10) Have a simple technique.

(11) Be compatible with all materials in general use for model making.

      It is undesirable that the choice of the material for model making should be governed by the impression material.

(12) Be cheap enough to use once only or capable of easy sterilization if used more than once.

Before describing any actual techniques of impression taking there are a few general considerations, common to all, which must first be discussed.

The Position of the Patient and Operator

For most prosthetic operations the dental chair is set in the upright position, this being specially important during the impression taking since one of the fears existing among patients is that of being choked by the material in use. When the patient is seated the chair should be adjusted so that the head and neck are in line with the trunk (*see* fig. 80). If the head is allowed to bend backwards from the neck the supra and infrahyoid muscles will be tense and difficulty in swallowing will result, also, should a fragment of impression material break away from the main impression it can more easily fall into the throat and possibly cause obstruction in the airway. Apart from the dangers, the patient's comfort must be considered if the operator is to receive the full co-operation required to produce a satisfactory impression.

A suitable covering in the form of an apron or large towel should be provided to protect the patient's clothing and also, ready at hand, a warm, flavoured mouth-wash with which remaining fragments of impression material can be rinsed away on instruction from the operator.

The positions of the operator are shown in figs. 81 and 82.

Impression Trays

Impression trays are used as rigid containers for carrying the impression material into the mouth, for maintaining it in

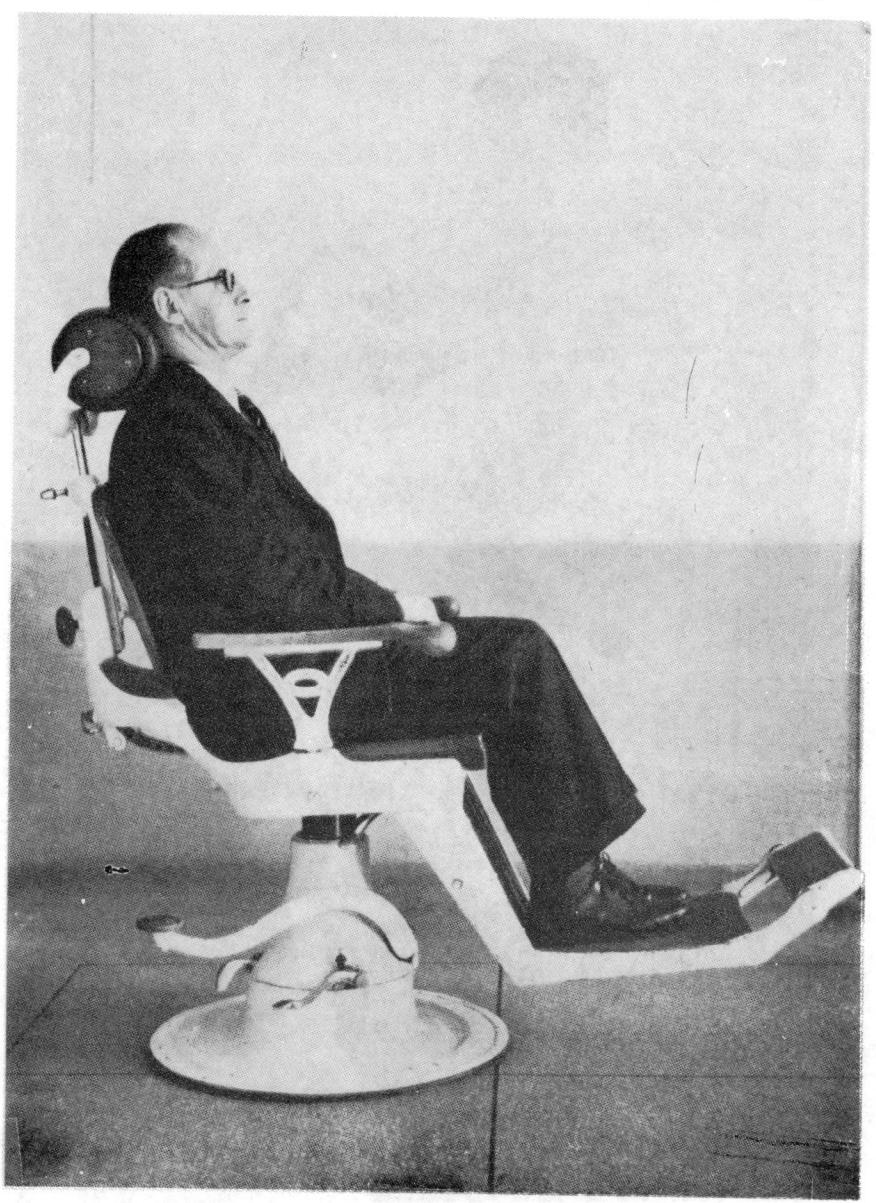

FIG. 80

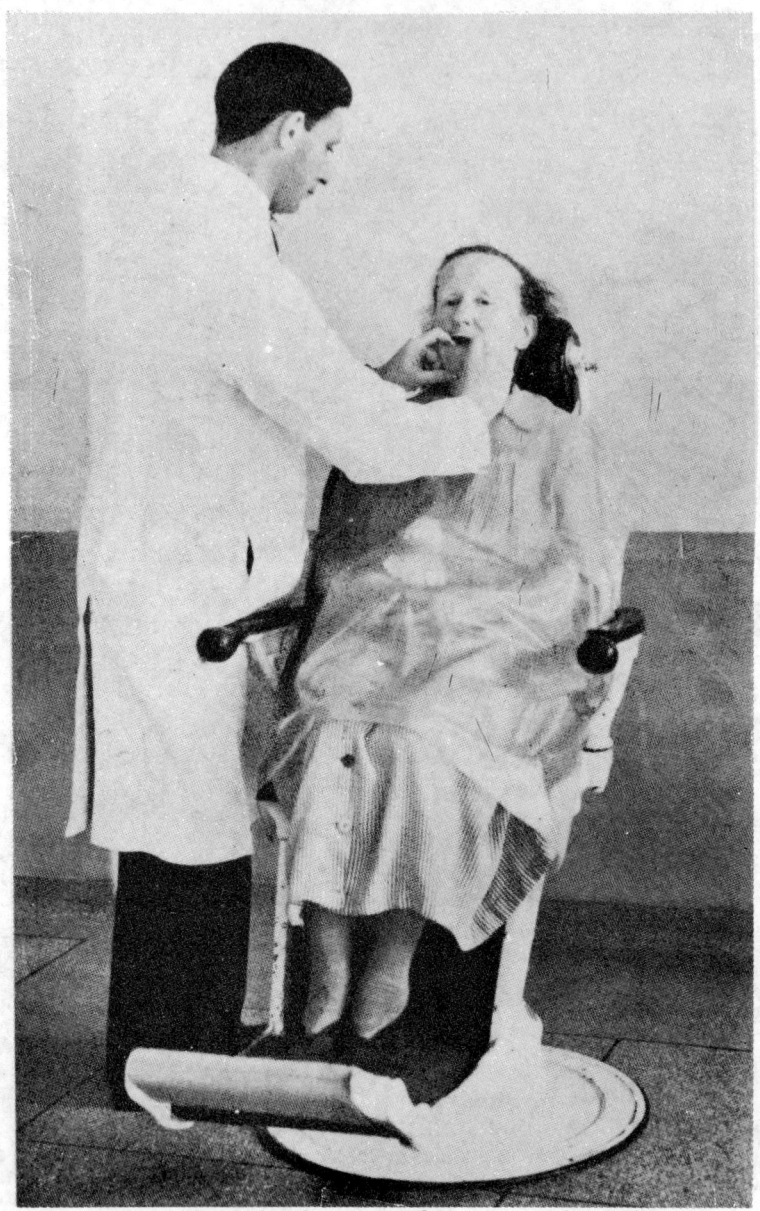

FIG. 81. – Illustrating the position of the operator when taking
a lower impression.

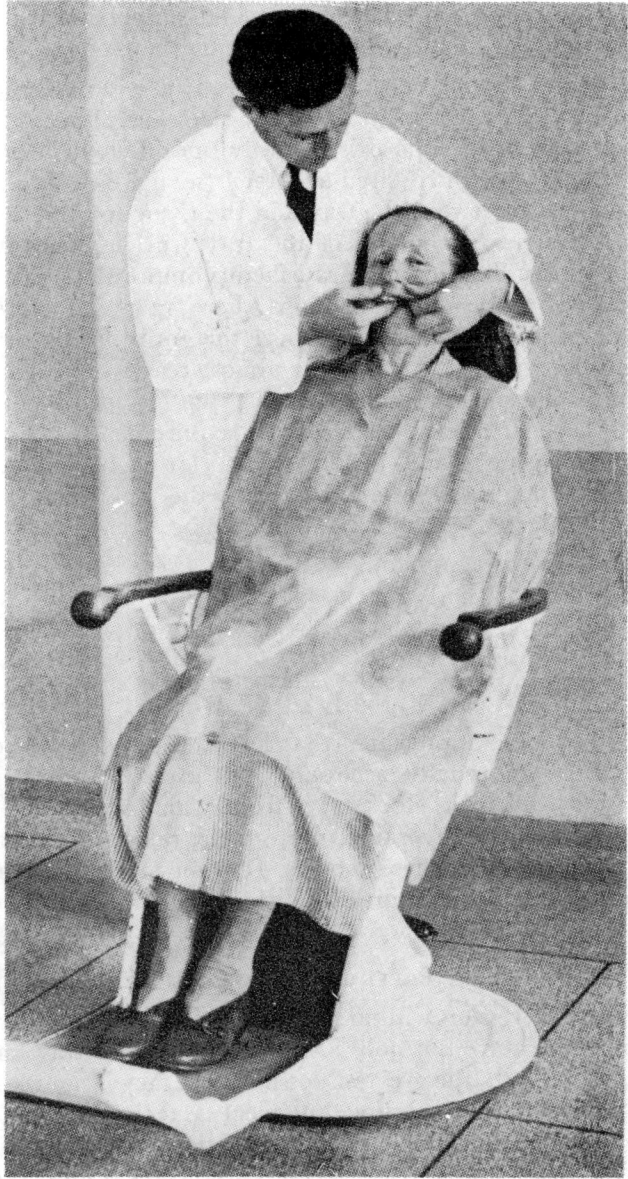

FIG. 82. – Illustrating the position of the operator when taking an upper impression.

position during setting or hardening and supporting it during removal from the mouth and when casting the model.

The dental supply houses manufacture a wide selection of impression trays but variations in the sizes and shapes of jaws are such that little hope exists of any one of them fitting an arch contour with the desired accuracy (*see* fig. 83). Too much space will exist between the tray and the tissue in some regions whilst in others the flanges of the tray will impinge on the ridge or sulcus. To produce a satisfactory impression and avoid variations in transmitted pressure there must be an equal thickness of impression material over the entire fitting surface, also the flanges of the tray must almost reach the functional position of the sulci and fraena and yet not displace them. It is unusual for a stock tray to fulfil these requirements and, therefore, special trays should be constructed for each patient. The special tray materials vary according to the type of impression technique selected, the more common being:

(1) Shellac or a similar proprietary material
(2) Acrylic resin either heat or cold cured   (*see* figs. 84–85).
(3) Tin lead alloy

It will thus be appreciated that for each patient two sets of impressions are usually necessary, the first, the preliminary impressions, taken in stock trays from which models are cast and the second, the working impressions, taken in the special trays constructed to these models. It is on models cast in the second, or working impressions that the dentures will be constructed.

The Preliminary Impression

Since this impression will not be used directly in the construction of the denture but only for making a special tray for one individual mouth, the greatest possible accuracy is not required and it is, therefore, possible to select a technique which is simple, quick and which gives the patient the minimum of discomfort. For these reasons composition has been chosen as the impression material, but it must be emphasized that this is

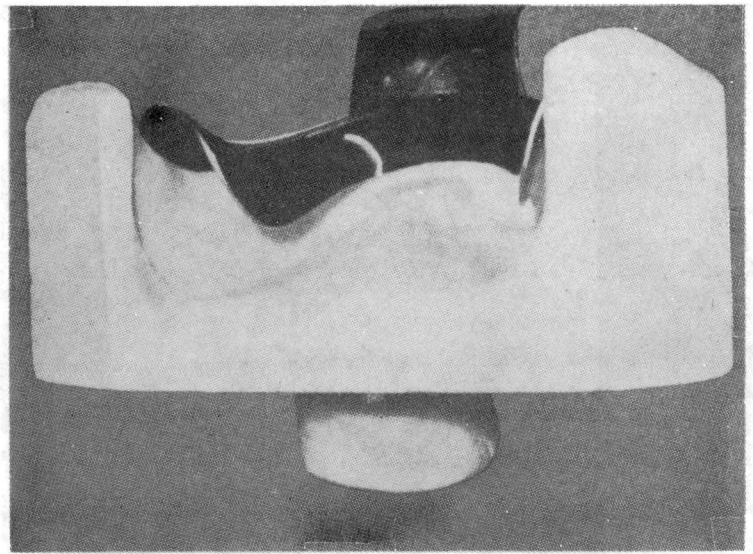

(a) Note shortness in lingual pouch and retromolar pad areas.

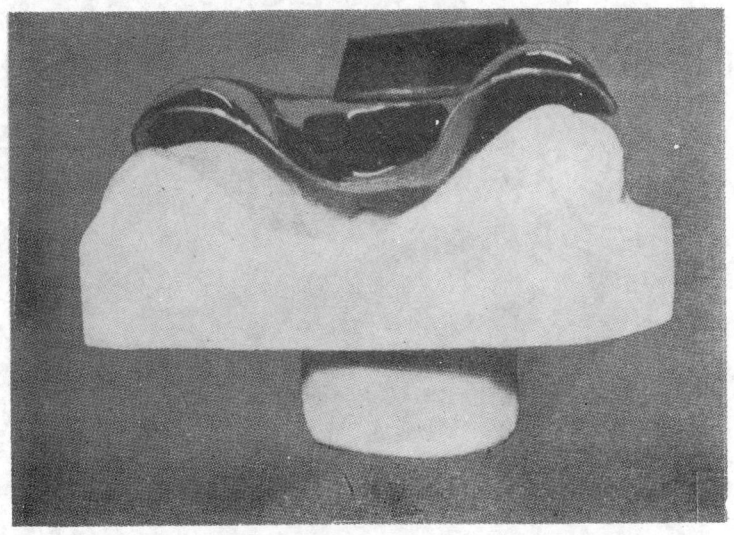

(b) Note poor fit in palate and poor adaptation to ridges.

FIG. 83. – The inaccurate fit of stock trays.

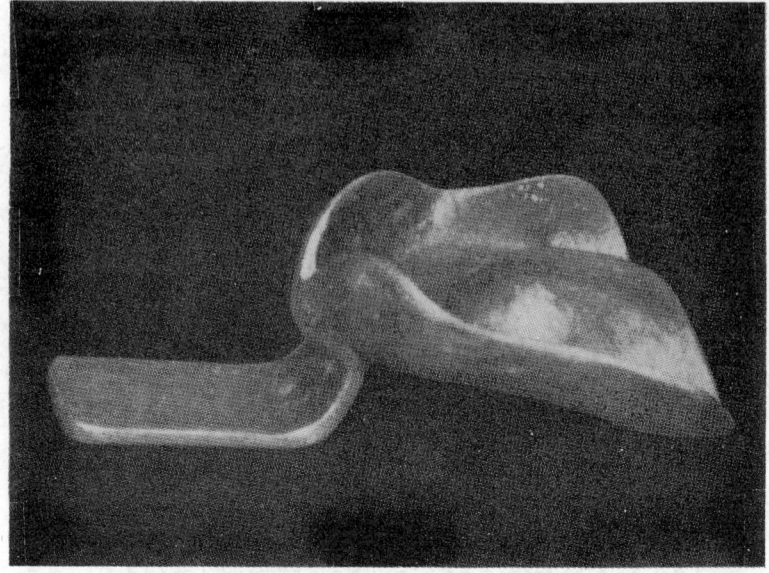

(*a*) Tin lead alloy.

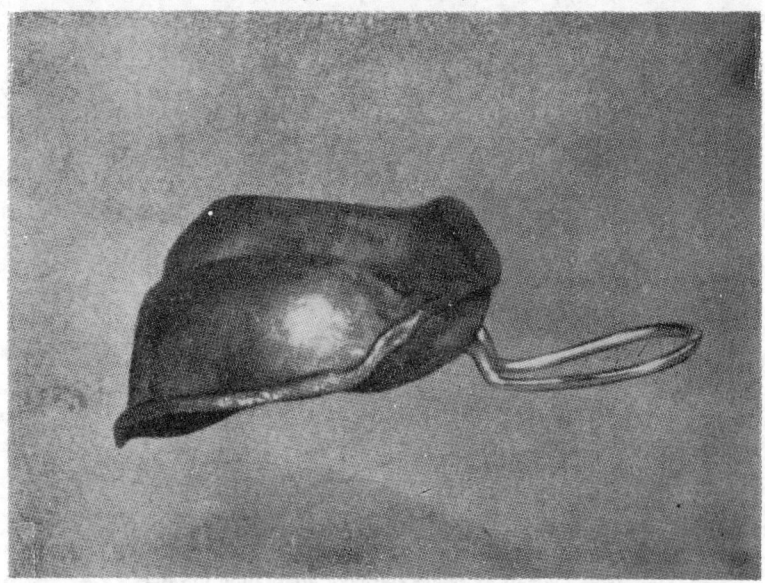

(*b*) Shellac.

FIG. 84. – Special trays – Note stepped handles.

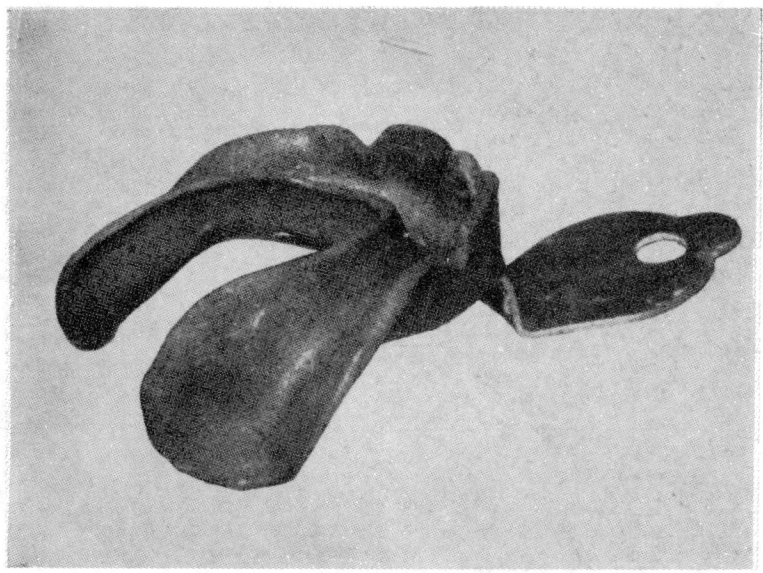

(c) Tray compound.
FIG. 84. – Special trays – Note stepped handles.

not a suitable technique for a working impression, though such an impression can be obtained with composition using a special technique as described later in this chapter.

Composition, sometimes called impression compound, is the name given to a class of thermoplastic materials containing various waxes, resins and fillers which soften in hot water and harden at or slightly above mouth temperature. Many proprietary brands are obtainable with optimum working temperatures varying from 110° F. to 140° F. at which temperatures they should flow easily. Whichever composition is selected for this primary impression the manufacturers' instructions regarding its working temperature should be strictly observed.

Selection of the Stock Tray

The alveolar ridges and palate are examined for shape and size, and from a selection of previously sterilized stock trays a suitable upper and lower are chosen and tested in the mouth for their approximation to the oral structures, as follows.

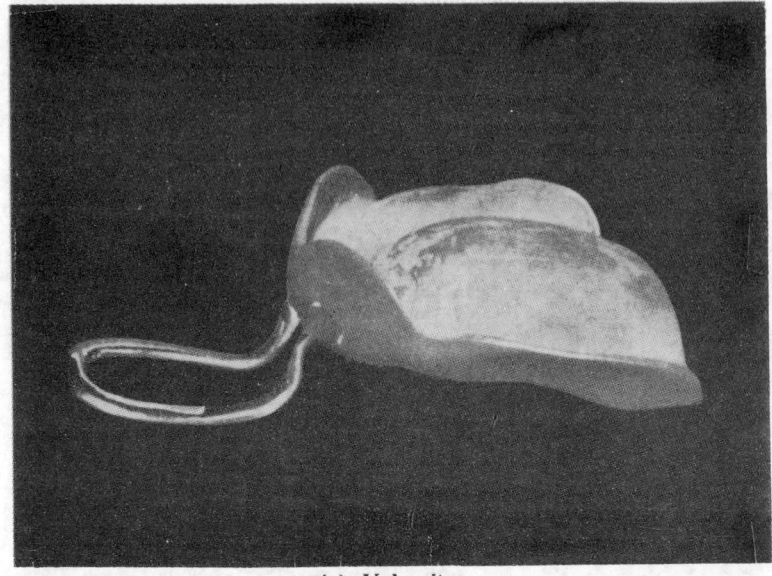

(a) Vulcanite.
FIG. 85. – Special Trays.

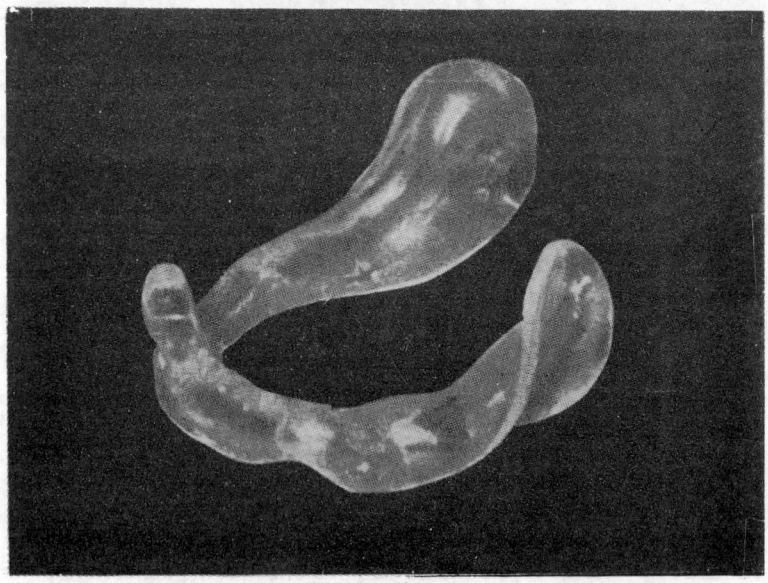

(b) Acrylic resin.
FIG. 85. – Special Trays.

The Upper Tray

The tray is inserted in the mouth, the posterior border, raised to make contact with the anterior part of the soft palate and it can then easily be seen if the tray will cover the maxillary tuberosities allowing enough room for the impression material. The tray is then slowly raised anteriorly and the lateral flanges watched for clearance of the alveolar ridges and, as the tray is brought right up at the front, the upper lip is lifted so that the labial flange can be checked for fit in this region (*see* fig. 86). The tray must not be pulled forward during examination for buccal and labial clearance. Sufficient space must exist between the tray and the tissues for the impression material and, in some cases, it may be necessary to bend the tray slightly with pliers to provide adequate space and in others to cut and trim the flange to accommodate fraena and

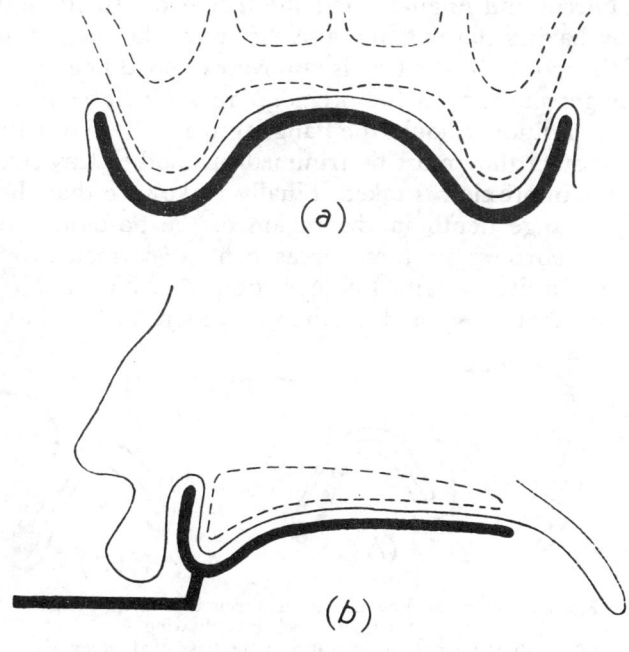

FIG. 86

(*a*) Coronal, and (*b*) Sagittal diagrams showing correct extension of an edentulous upper tray.

prevent pressure on bony structures such as the zygomatic process of the maxilla. Finally the tray should be checked to make sure that it does not rock from side to side through making contact with the hard palate since, when seated, it should make contact with the crest of the alveolar ridges.

The Lower Tray

Insert the selected tray in the mouth and pass it backwards until the distal ends cover the retromolar pads, whilst at the same time the patient protrudes the tongue slightly to facilitate placing the tray between it and the lingual surfaces of the ridge. Lift the tray anteriorly and slowly lower again observing its approximation to the ridge both lingually, buccally and in front. When satisfied that the selected tray covers the ridge and allows sufficient space for the impression material the flanges are checked for over-extension into the labial, buccal and lingual sulci; the first two visually and the latter by having the patient raise the tip of the tongue to the roof of the mouth. If the tray is not overextended lingually only slight finger pressure in the premolar region will be needed to keep it in position. Should the flanges grossly interfere with the fraena or sulci they must be trimmed or another tray selected before the impression is taken. Finally make sure that there is sufficient flange depth in the region of the posterior lingual pouches. Shortness in these areas can be corrected by the addition of a little warmed composition (of a higher softening point than that to be used for the impression), attached to the

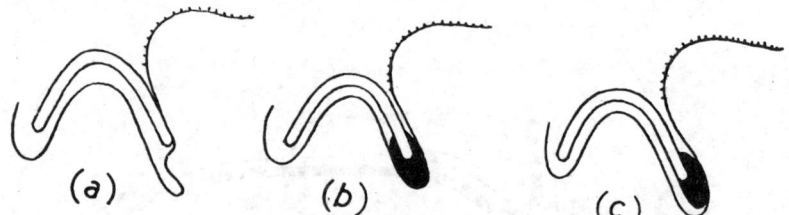

Fig. 87. – Coronal diagrams taken through the 2nd molar region of a lower stock tray showing –
(a) A short lingual flange trapping the base of the tongue.
(b) The flange extended with composition.
(c) The added composition displaced lingually to allow room for the impression material.

lingual flanges of the dried tray (*see* fig. 87). Reinsert the corrected tray in the mouth and ask the patient to protrude the tongue slightly, this will trim the added composition to the functional depth of the pouches by raising the floor of the mouth and drawing forward the palatoglossus muscles. On removing the tray from the mouth displace the composition lingually to provide space for the impression material and then chill thoroughly. A short tray can be extended distally in the same way, to cover the retromolar pads (*see* fig. 88). Unless sufficient tray extension exists distally and lingually to push the tongue aside, when the impression is seated there is considerable possibility that this highly muscular structure will be trapped beneath the lingual flanges resulting in an impression which is short in the pouch area.

The Order of Impression Taking

The trays having been selected and necessary adjustments carried out the next consideration is whether the upper or lower impression should be taken first. From the patient's point of view the upper impression usually causes the greater

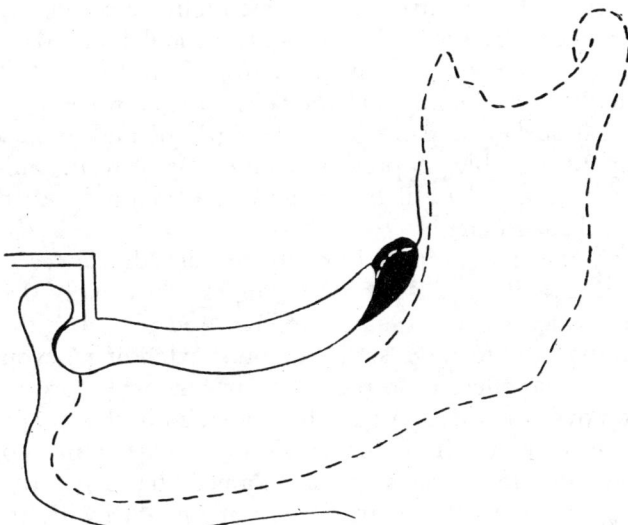

FIG. 88. – Composition added to the distal end of a lower tray to cover the retromolar pad.

discomfort and anxiety, either through stimulation of the retching reflex or from fear of being choked by the material, but these symptoms are usually absent when taking the lower impression. Some operators prefer to take the more troublesome impression first assuring the patient that although the upper may be a little unpleasant no such reactions will be experienced with the lower. However, there are some patients who, having felt sick once will do so again even with a lower impression, so it is advocated that in most cases the lower impression should be taken first. A further reason for this is that a foreign body placed in the mouth produces an increase in the rate of salivation and it is, therefore, preferable to have the lower impression seated in position before this takes place. If the upper precedes the lower the operator and the patient may be embarrassed by the accumulation of saliva in the floor of the mouth, the result being a poor impression particularly when using plaster of Paris.

The Lower Impression

The selected composition is placed in a water bath, preferably thermostatically controlled to maintain the temperature recommended by the makers of that particular brand. After a few minutes the composition is removed from the bath, folded repeatedly from the edges to the centre thus always presenting a smooth surface on one side (*see* fig. 89), and replaced as quickly as possible to prevent undue loss of heat. This procedure is repeated until the material has acquired a uniform softness throughout.

When the composition is ready for use the lower tray is warmed in a Bunsen flame, the composition rapidly dried on gauze, formed into a suitable-sized roll and placed in the tray. It is important to have sufficient bulk extending beyond the flanges so that there is no restriction in flow when pressed into position over the ridge. A trough is indented in the composition with the finger to simulate the ultimate ridge impression (*see* fig. 90), and the surface quickly flamed, tempered to avoid burning the patient, by immersing momentarily in the hot water bath and lightly smeared with vaseline. The tray is now placed in the mouth and when the operator is satisfied that it

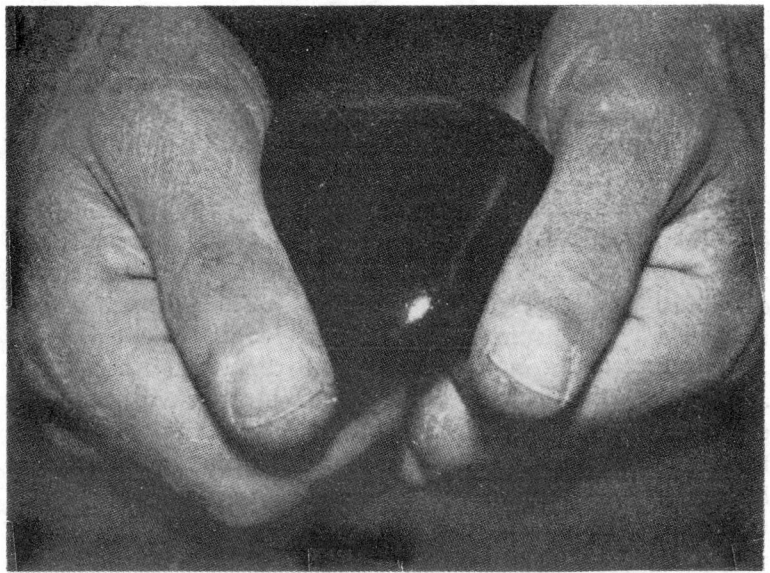

FIG. 89. – Preparing composition to present a smooth surface.
The thumbs move away from one another.

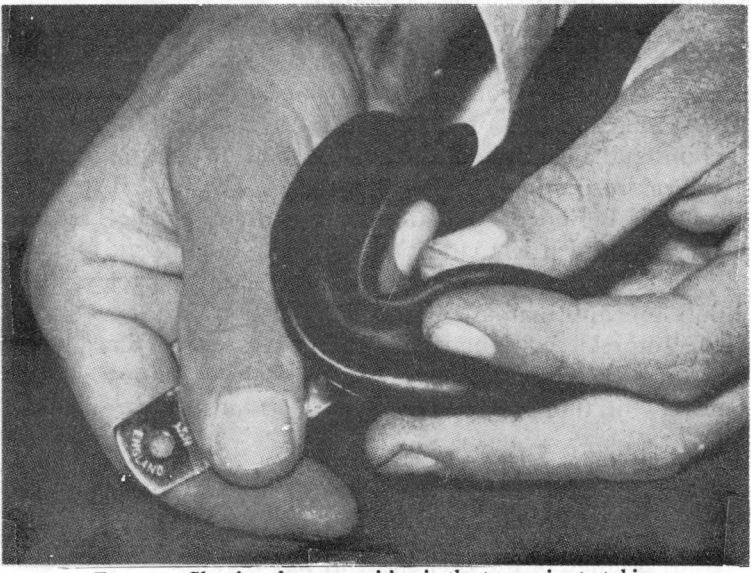

FIG. 90. – Shaping the composition in the tray prior to taking
preliminary impressions.

is in the correct position in relation to the ridge, the patient is instructed to raise and slightly protrude the tongue and as this movement begins the tray is pressed vertically downwards to seat the impression to the desired depth. Pressure in a backward direction, may also be required to counter the forward thrust from the tongue when protruded.

As soon as the impression is seated in position it must be held there quite firmly but without any increase in pressure, in other words the maximum pressure must be exerted when the composition is nearest to the optimum working temperature as the farther it drops below that, the less readily will it flow.

The impression obtained so far will reproduce, though not accurately, the denture-bearing surface, but will be over-extended round the periphery and a special tray constructed from it would require considerable time-consuming adjustment before it could be used for taking a working impression. This reduction of the special tray can be eliminated, or at least very considerably reduced, if the muscles around the periphery are brought into play to mould the impression into their functional positions, and this is done as follows:

The tray is held firmly in position whilst the patient protrudes the tongue and then moves it from side to side. This movement of the tongue draws forward the palatoglossal arches, raises the floor of the mouth and tenses the lingual fraenum and thus moulds the composition in the lingual sulcus to the raised position of these structures. The buccal sulci and fraena are moulded by manipulating alternate cheeks downwards and outwards, to free any trapped folds of tissue and then pulling gently upwards, inwards and slightly backwards to obtain the approximate functional position.

The impression taking is now completed and all that remains is to hold it lightly but firmly in place for a minute or two, remove, chill thoroughly in cold water and inspect (*see* fig. 91).

Common Faults in Lower Impressions

(1) Insufficient depth, in the posterior lingual pouch.

CAUSES:

(*a*) Flange of the tray short in this region.

(*b*) Lack of composition in the tray.

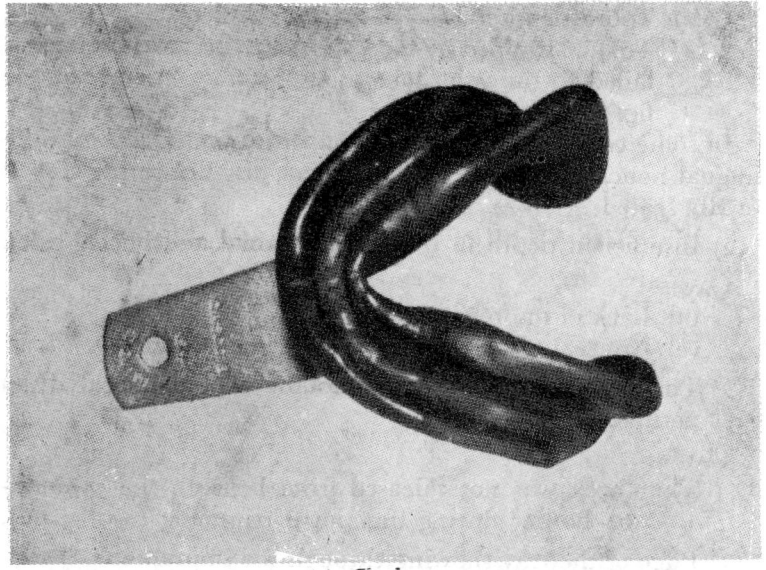

(a) The lower.

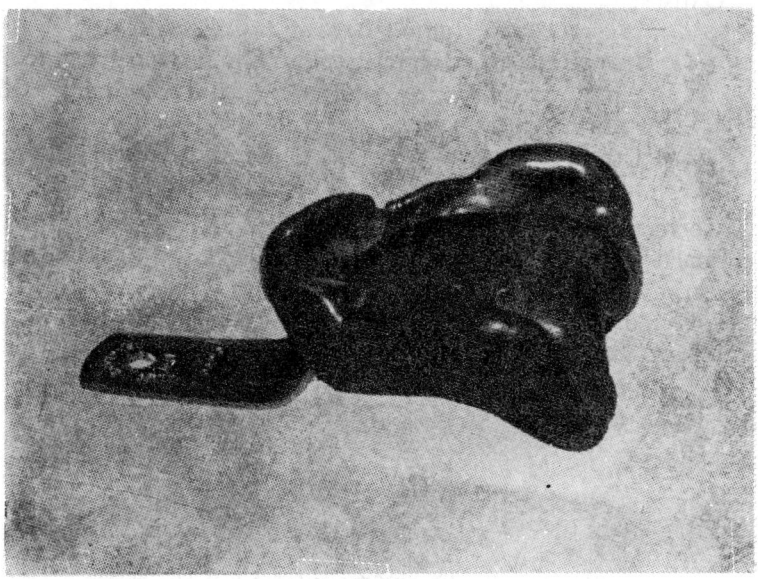

(b) The upper.

FIG. 91. - Completed preliminary composition impressions.

(c) Too little force used in seating the tray.

(d) Tongue trapped by the tray flanges because the patient failed to raise the tongue as the tray was seated (*see* fig. 92).

In some cases it is necessary to push the compound into the lingual pouch area with the fore-finger just before the tray is finally seated.

(2) Insufficient depth in the lingual, labial and buccal sulci.

CAUSES:

(a) Lack of impression material.

(b) Not seating the tray with sufficient pressure.

(3) The presence of a smooth hollow in the buccal distal periphery.

CAUSE:

The cheek was not released from beneath the composition border during functional trimming (*see* fig. 92).

(4) Edge of the tray showing through the impression.

CAUSES:

(a) Incorrect centring of the tray before seating.

(b) In the anterior lingual region. The forward thrust of the tongue not being countered by sufficient backward pressure on the tray.

(c) Use of too large a tray for the mouth or failure to trim the flanges adequately.

Corrections to faults 1 and 2 may be made by adding small softened pieces of composition to the imperfect areas and then reseating and re-moulding the impression. The error due to cheek folds, (3), should be corrected by re-heating the im-

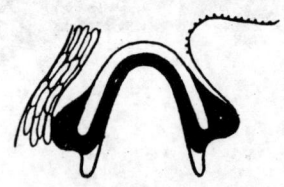

FIG. 92. – Showing how tongue and cheek may be trapped under impression material if correct trimming movements are omitted.

pression in that area and re-adapting, whilst fault number (4) usually requires an entirely new impression.

When adding composition to an impression the latter should first be thoroughly chilled and dried and the area requiring correction flamed sufficiently to make it sticky. A piece of the softened material is then taken, lightly flamed and attached to the main impression and moulded to the approximate shape required. Its surface is again flamed and then momentarily plunged into the hot water bath before being reseated in the mouth. Only the area to be re-adapted should be heated, the remainder being kept as cool as possible to avoid distortion on reinsertion.

The Upper Impression

The composition is softened and prepared in the way already described for the lower impression. When ready it is formed into a ball, dried on gauze and placed in the centre of the palate of the warmed tray. It is then moulded outwards to the periphery until the whole tray is filled, leaving a smooth, uncreased

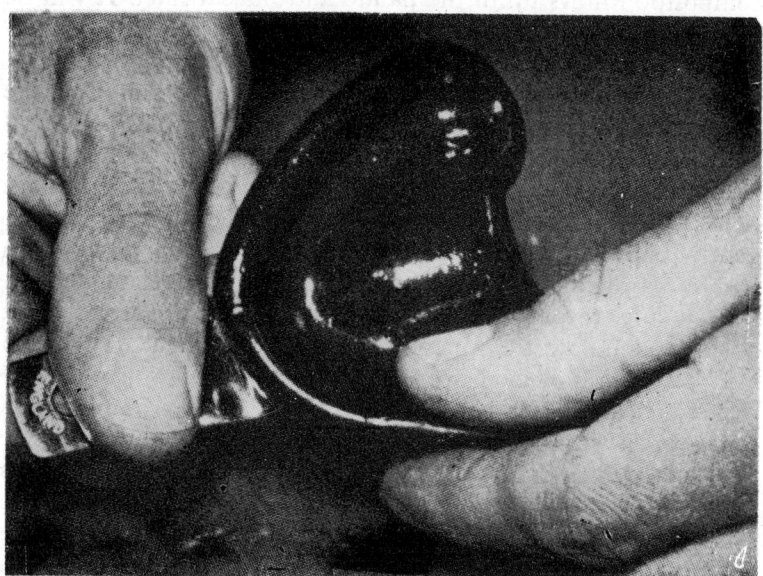

FIG. 93. – Shaping the composition in the tray prior to taking an upper preliminary impression.

surface indented to form a trough for the ridge and slightly raised in the middle for the palate (*see* fig. 93). Sufficient composition must be moulded along the periphery to enable the depth of the buccal and labial sulci to be reached without having to force the tray upwards too far. This is because excessive pressure together with an abundance of composition in the palatal region will cause it to flow backwards so far over the soft palate that retching and vomiting may result.

The diagram (*see* fig. 94) illustrates the manner in which the

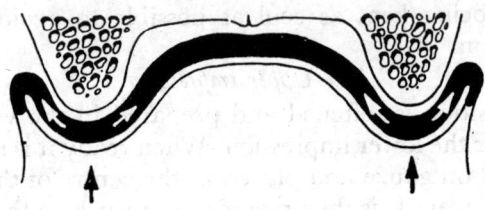

FIG. 94

composition flows to fill the palate and buccal sulci. It will be seen that the palatal area receives composition from two directions whilst the sulci are filled from only one.

Once the composition has been adapted to the tray the surface is lightly flamed, tempered in the water bath, smeared with vaseline, inserted in the mouth and centred under the ridge. Firm upward pressure now seats the impression in place ready for the peripheral moulding. Alternate cheeks are gently pulled upwards and outwards, and then downwards and inwards and slightly backwards. The first movements release any trapped air or folds of tissue, the latter three positions simulate the function of the cheek when drawn in to aid the placing of food over the occlusal surfaces of the teeth, and to clear the sulci of debris. The labial trimming can similarly be carried out by manipulations by the operator or the patient can be asked to purse up the lips as tightly as possible, then to retract them forcibly and finally to try to push the impression down with pressure of the upper lip. During these manoeuvres the tray is firmly held in position and for a further two minutes before being removed, chilled and inspected (*see* fig. (91*b*)).

Common Faults in Upper Impressions.

(1) A crevice in the mid-line of the palatal posterior third.

CAUSES:

    (*a*) Insufficient composition in the palatal area when filling the tray.

    (*b*) Insufficient pressure.

(2) Excess composition extending well beyond the posterior palatal border of the tray.

CAUSES:

    (*a*) Excessive pressure or too prolonged pressure when seating the tray.

    (*b*) Too much composition in the palatal area when filling the tray.

Composition which is unsupported by the tray will fall away from the palate by its own weight dragging some of the supported composition with it and producing an inaccurate impression. Upward pressure on the tray should cease when the impression material is approximately 1 cm. beyond the posterior border of the tray.

(3) An impression short in one or more regions of the sulci, especially the areas of the tuberosities or the labial sulcus.

CAUSES:

    (*a*) Insufficient material in the tray.

    (*b*) Failure to mould the peripheral composition in this region when filling the tray so that it will slip up between the cheek and the tuberosity or the lip and the alveolar ridge.

    (*c*) Failure to pull the upper lip outwards and upwards sufficient to allow the composition to flow into the labial sulcus.

    (*d*) Insufficient pressure.

(4) Tray flange showing through the composition.

CAUSES:

    (*a*) Poorly selected or adapted tray.

    (*b*) Incorrect centring of the tray.

Most deficiencies can be corrected by the addition of small amounts of composition, as described for the lower impression, but if the tray has been malpositioned or is too small it is better to retake the impression than to attempt adjustments. Palatal excess should be avoided and, therefore, is not considered.

A Warning

Be sure that composition does not burn the patient. Check the tray temperature against the back of the hand before inserting in the mouth and, whenever composition has been softened in a flame, it must be immersed for a moment in hot water before being put in the mouth otherwise a serious burn will result.

THE WORKING IMPRESSIONS

Four groups of impression materials are available to the prosthetist for obtaining the final working model. The impression techniques advocated for these materials are innumerable, though often differing only in minor details, so a selection will be described to cover sufficient general techniques suitable for any mouth conditions which are likely to be met with in a general dental practice.

The techniques to be described are:

1. The plaster impression.
2. The alginate impression.
3. The zinc oxide-eugenol paste impression.
4. The functionally trimmed lower impression.
5. The composition impression peripherally adapted.

PLASTER OF PARIS

There are two properties of plaster of Paris which would normally render it unsuitable for use as an impression material, these are:

(a) the length of time it takes to set, about fifteen minutes.
(b) the fact that it expands on setting.

Fortunately both these faults can be remedied easily. Commercial plaster as obtained from the manufacturers contains from 3 to 10 per cent of anhydrous calcium sulphate resulting from local overheating during manufacture and the presence of this will cause a variable setting time which is undesirable in any exact technique. If, however, the plaster as purchased is spread out in layers of approximately 2 cm. to 3 cm. thick and exposed to the air for a week the anhydrous sulphate will absorb water from the atmosphere and so become converted into plaster of Paris. All commercial plaster to be used for impression taking should be so conditioned.

Heat will materially shorten the setting time of plaster but will not lessen its setting expansion. The salts of most metals will also reduce the setting time of plaster and many of them also reduce the setting expansion. The addition of 4 per cent potassium sulphate to the water with which the plaster is mixed will make its setting expansion clinically negligible, but at the same time will reduce its setting time to about $1\frac{1}{2}$ minutes. If borax is also added to the water the setting time is increased and, by varying the quantity of borax in the solution, mixes of plaster can be obtained which set in anything from $1\frac{1}{2}$ minutes to many hours. Addition of 0·4 per cent of borax to the potassium sulphate solution will, with conditioned plaster, give a setting time of about four minutes which is a convenient time for most operators but which can be shortened or lengthened as desired by adding less or more borax.

Thus if the following solution, which is usually referred to as an anti-expansion solution, is used in the correct proportions with conditioned plaster of Paris a constant setting time will result and so a consistent technique can be developed.

Potassium sulphate	4	grammes	4%·
Borax	0·4	,,	0·4%
Colouring matter ..	0·04	,,	0·04%
Distilled water to .. . 100 c.c.			

50 grammes of plaster to 30 c.c. of solution

Setting time four minutes.

This setting time of four minutes is only constant when the stated proportion of conditioned plaster to solution is maintained and the use of unconditioned plaster, with water containing a pinch of sodium chloride, will never allow an exact technique to be developed.

Special Plasters

Special plasters are obtainable for impression taking, most ot
them having a finer texture than ordinary plaster of Paris;
some contain the potassium sulphate and borax in the solid
form and so have only to be mixed with water. A special
·class of impression plaster contains up to 20 per cent of starch
which makes a very smooth mix with the added advantage
that it is slightly sticky and so will adhere to the tray even
when in a thin wafer. Also such impressions can be readily
removed from the model by boiling water which causes the
starch granules to swell and so disintegrate the whole
impression.

Mixing Plaster for Impressions

The setting time of plaster of Paris is constant under constant
conditions but vigorous spatulation will delay the initial
setting though having little effect on the final setting time. This
is because spatulation prevents the quickly growing crystals of
gypsum which develop from numerous centres of crystallization
from joining up until crystal growth has reached such an
advanced stage that the final set is imminent.

Below the point A in the diagram the mixture is too liquid
for impression taking and above point B it is too thick so it will
be seen that with a setting time of four minutes the operating
time is only two minutes (see fig. 95). Although spatulation
retards the initial set the setting is again constant from the time
spatulation ceases.

The second diagram, though not scientifically accurate,
illustrates how spatulation for the first two minutes will reduce
the operating time to about one minute which is insufficient
for most operators (see fig. 96).

The correct technique for mixing plaster for impression
taking is as follows: Place 30 c.c. of anti-expansion solution in
a dry bowl and quickly sift into it 50 grammes of conditioned
plaster allowing it to stand for thirty seconds without disturbance other than to flick any mound of dry plaster on to
the solution. At the end of half a minute it will be found that
the plaster is moistened throughout and one or two gentle
stirs with a spatula will render the mass homogeneous.

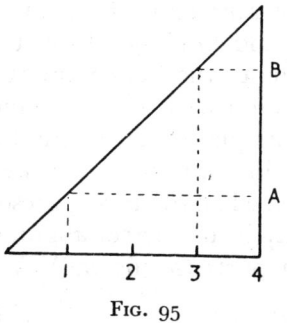

FIG. 95

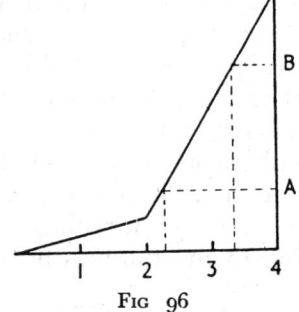

FIG 96

These quantities will result in more plaster than will be necessary for even the largest edentulous jaw and are suggested only for beginners; obviously any smaller quantities can be used with the same results provided that the plaster/solution ratio is kept the same.

Special Trays

These may be constructed of any one of the materials already mentioned although the commonest is shellac or a shellac based proprietary material. The handle must be staggered so as to clear the lip and avoid its distortion. The clearance between the tray and the model should be approximately 2 mm. which is attained by using a spacer between the model and the tray when constructing the latter (*see* fig. 97).

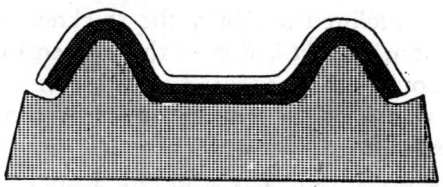

FIG. 97

Checking and Trimming the Trays

The Lower

The tray should be placed in the mouth and centred over the lower ridge. It should first be checked for correct extension posteriorly and in this region it must just cover the retromolar pads. If it extends farther it should be trimmed and, if short, be extended with a little composition.

Next, the front of the tray should be raised and the clearance between its posterior lingual flanges and the lingual aspect of the ridge checked; if this is inadequate, the flanges must be bent towards the tongue until adequate clearance is obtained, as this region is often undercut and the plaster frequently fractures here on withdrawing the impression; if the tray fits closely only a thin layer of plaster exists which, when fractured, presents some difficulty in replacing in the tray in its correct alignment owing to the thinness of the broken parts (*see* fig. 98). With

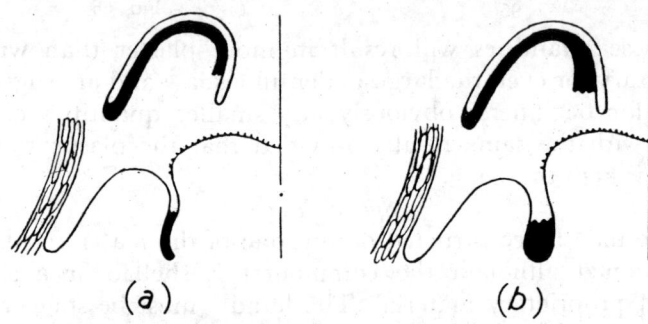

(a) (b)

Fig. 98. – Diagram through lower second molar region.
(*a*) Lingual flange of tray fitting too closely; very thin flake of plaster left under tongue.
(*b*) Lingual flange of tray correctly inclined lingually, a much bulkier piece of plaster left under tongue.

the tray flange inclined medially the thickness of plaster thus obtained aids the correct union of the broken impression.

The tray should now be seated on the ridge and while it is held in this position, the cheeks and lips should be gently pulled upwards and outwards so that the sulci simulate their functional positions. The edges of the seated tray should be almost in contact with the sulci and fraenae all round during these movements and thus will be 2 to 3 mm. short when the original spacing of the spacer is replaced by plaster when taking the impression. Any overextension present must be corrected by trimming and any gross shortness remedied by the addition of composition. Next the lingual periphery should be checked. This is done by requesting the patient to raise and slightly protrude the tongue and if excessive pressure is required to maintain the tray in place it indicates that the tray is over-extended, usually in the premolar or first molar regions, or in that of the palato-glossal arch, and should be corrected by trimming. If any doubt exists regarding its final accuracy some composition may be added to the edge of the lingual flange and the tray replaced in the mouth and the patient instructed to protrude the tongue slightly. If, on removal of the tray, the composition is found to have been swept up on to the lingual side of the flange so that the edge of the flange shows or almost shows, then it may be assumed that the depth of the tray is adequate and the composition may be removed. If, however, the composition has remained in place and merely shows signs of having been moulded by the tissues it should be gently bent lingually so as to provide space for the plaster, chilled and left in position.

The Upper

The tray should be placed in the mouth and the position of the back-edge checked. This should extend just on to the soft palate. The position of the junction of the hard and soft palate is usually delineated by the two foviae palatinae but this should be verified by gently palpating for the back-edge of the hard palate with a blunt instrument such as a burnisher, and the tray should be trimmed to this position.

Next the front of the tray should be lowered and it should be observed if there is sufficient clearance between the tray flanges and the buccal aspects of the ridge. If not, room must be made by bending the flanges outwards. Finally the cheeks and lips should be pulled gently downwards so that the sulci simulate their functional positions: this enables the periphery of the tray to be adjusted in the same way as was done for the lower. Special attention should be paid to ensure that adequate clearance is provided for the root of the zygoma.

The correct trimming and adaptation of special trays is a primary factor in obtaining a good working impression and it cannot be emphasized too forcibly that time spent on this is invariably saved by obtaining a good impression at the first attempt.

Plaster of Paris Impressions

There are a variety of techniques in common use for taking

plaster impressions. For instance some operators favour the placing of plaster in those areas of the mouth in which difficulty is experienced in obtaining an impression, before inserting the tray. Others disagree with this method and rely on manipulating the tray and the tissues so that the plaster flows into the difficult areas without the necessity of having to place it there beforehand.

Some operators favour raising the front of the upper tray first and others the back whilst some keep the tray horizontal and raise it evenly.

The treatment of the back edge of the upper tray also varies. Some operators favour post-damming with soft wax or composition to compress the tissues in this region and also to prevent the escape of plaster towards the throat. Post-damming is a means of increasing pressure over an area in order, either to control an impression material, or to improve peripheral seal (see fig. 99). Others fix cotton-wool with sticky wax to the tray to prevent this escape of plaster whilst some prefer to leave the back-edge as it is and trust to their judgment

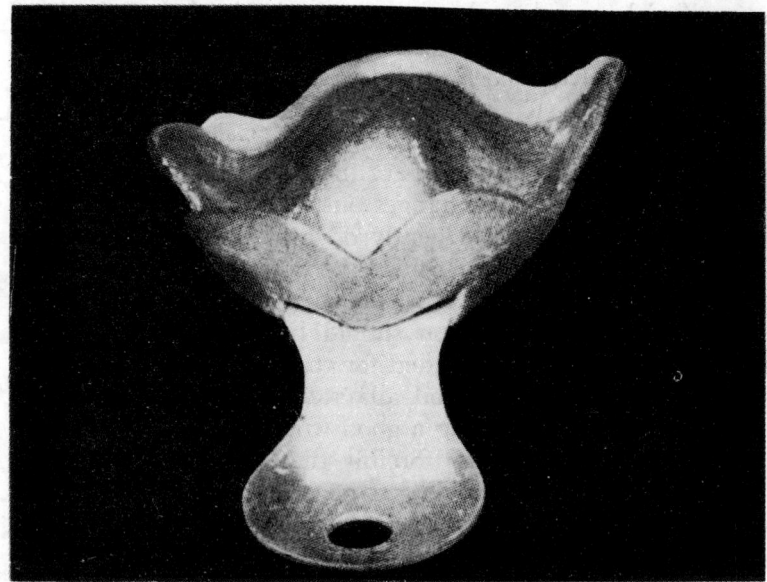

FIG. 99. – An upper tray post-dammed with a strip of wax.

of the volume of plaster required and manipulative skill to prevent an excess of plaster escaping posteriorly.

The technique described below has been developed over many years and is designed for teaching students to obtain satisfactory plaster impressions before they have gained the manipulative skill which comes with experience.

The Lower Working Impression

When the mixed plaster is beginning to thicken slightly the lower tray is filled by means of a spatula, spreading the plaster evenly over the tray surface so that it tends to form a trough for the ridge. If the tray is loaded too soon the plaster being liquid will merely run out.

By the time the tray has been filled the plaster in the mixing bowl will have thickened sufficiently to support its own weight. This may be tested by picking some plaster up on the spatula and turning it upside down so that the plaster hangs; it should

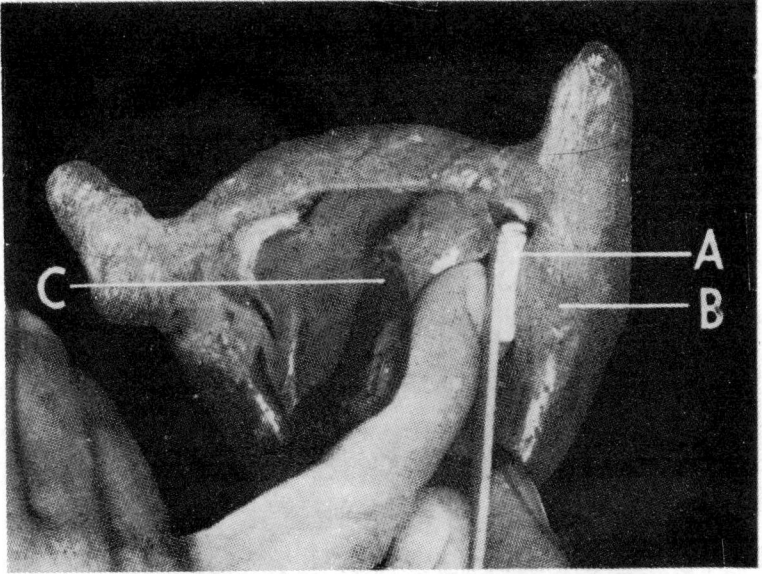

Fig. 100. – Method of placing plaster in the alveolingual sulcus. Photographed on a model.
A. – Plaster on the end of wooden spatula.
B. – Alveolar ridge.
C. – The tongue held away by the finger.

just fail to fall off the spatula. At this stage, and not before, is the time to start placing it in the mouth. If it is introduced into the mouth prematurely it will be too liquid to remain where it is placed.

A generous portion of plaster should be picked up on the spatula. The forefinger of the left hand should then be inserted into the left lingual sulcus as far back and as deeply as it will go and the tongue gently but forcefully pushed towards the centre of the mouth and held there while the plaster on the spatula is placed deep into the pouch under the mylohyoid ridge (*see* fig. 100). As the spatula is withdrawn the tongue should be allowed to resume its normal position thus covering the plaster and holding it in place. The opposite side is dealt with in a similar manner.

Next the lower lip should be pulled gently forward and some plaster placed between it and the ridge, and while the lip is held well forwards the previously filled tray should be rotated into the mouth (*see* fig. 101) and centred over the ridge and then with a very definite wriggling or puddling movement it should be pushed downwards and slightly backwards until fully

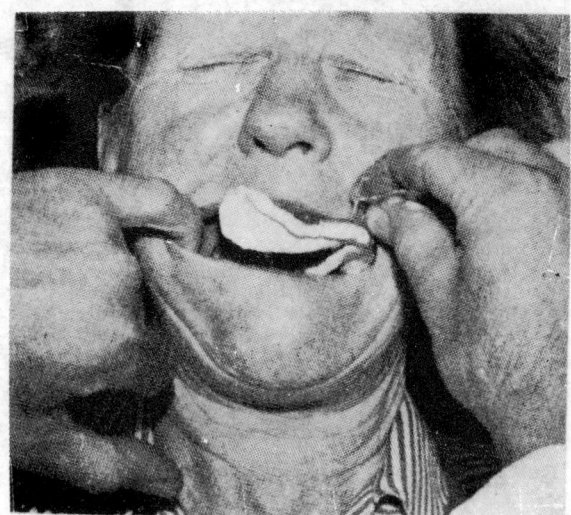

Fig. 101. – Method of rotating lower tray into or out of the mouth.

in place. As the tray is wriggled downwards the patient should be instructed to raise the tongue, this will prevent the edges of the tongue or folds in the floor of the mouth being caught under the lingual flanges of the tray.

When the tray is fully in place the periphery of the impression must be trimmed. For the lingual trimming the patient is instructed to protrude and raise the tongue slightly and move it gently from side to side. Protrusion and sideways movement of the tongue draws the palato-glossal arches forwards and raises the floor of the mouth. The elevation of the tongue tenses the lingual fraenum. The plaster lying in contact with these structures is, therefore, moulded by these movements so that the impression indicates them in the positions they assume when the tongue is functioning and thus prevents the lingual flange of the ultimate denture being overextended, and so impinging on these structures during tongue movement.

Buccal peripheral trimming is effected by, firstly, pulling the cheek outwards and downwards in order to release any air or folds of soft tissue trapped under the periphery. The second movement is upwards, inwards and slightly backwards thus raising the sulcus to the adjudged functional level and so moulding the plaster in contact with it. Finally the labial trimming is effected by drawing the lip upwards and backwards thus conforming the plaster to the functional position occupied by the labial sulcus and indicating the fraenum. It will be found impossible to perform correct labial trimming unless the tray has a stepped handle (*see* figs. 84 and 85).

Once the peripheral trimming is complete all that requires to be done is to instruct the patient to relax and for the operator to maintain the tray in position and support the jaw until the plaster has set.

The tray may be held in position by one of several ways.

(*a*) The tips of the forefingers of each hand may be placed on the top of the tray in the premolar region with the thumbs below the inferior border of the mandible, thus supporting the jaw (*see* fig. 102).

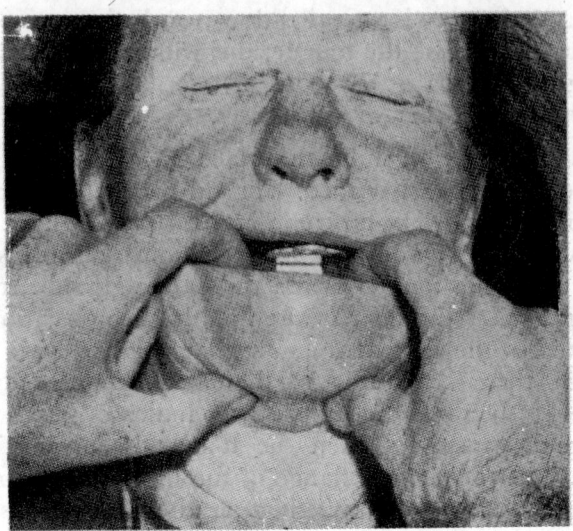

FIG. 102. – A method of holding a lower plaster impression in place.

(b) The first and second fingers of one hand may be placed on the top of the tray, one on either side in the premolar region, with the handle protruding between them and with the thumb under the chin supporting the mandible (*see* fig. 103).

(c) The mouth may be completely closed and the thumb and forefinger of one hand encircle the lower part of the face pressing the cheeks and lips on to the tray with sufficient pressure to hold it in place. The remaining fingers of the hand support the mandible from below (*see* fig. 104).

In no circumstances must the tray be held in place by mere downward pressure on an unsupported jaw as this is most tiring for the patient.

Removal of the Impression

During the time that the tray is held in the mouth the plaster in the mixing bowl is periodically tested for its degree of set, by breaking pieces between the fingers. When it frac-

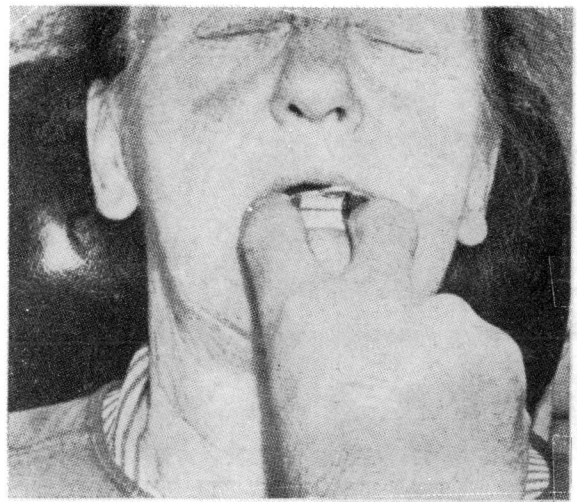

FIG. 103. – A method of holding a lower plaster impression in place. The thumb is under the chin.

tures with a clean break the impression is ready for removal from the mouth.

Before commencing removal the patient should be informed that it may break and that if it does, the broken pieces must be retrieved before rinsing can be allowed.

Removal of the impression is commenced by lifting the lips and cheeks away from the periphery to release the air seal which may have developed. A gentle upward movement applied to the handle of the tray will be sufficient to lift the impression from the ridge provided no gross undercuts exist. If undercuts are present, however, a sudden jerk may be required to fracture the plaster. When the tray is fully raised from the ridges it may be rotated out of the mouth (*see* fig. 101) when it should immediately be inspected to see if any pieces of plaster have fractured and remained in the mouth; if so, they should be carefully removed with tweezers.

The removal of pieces remaining in a posterior lingual pouch is facilitated if the patient places the tip of the tongue into the opposite cheek. This action raises the floor of the pouch and the piece of plaster with it.

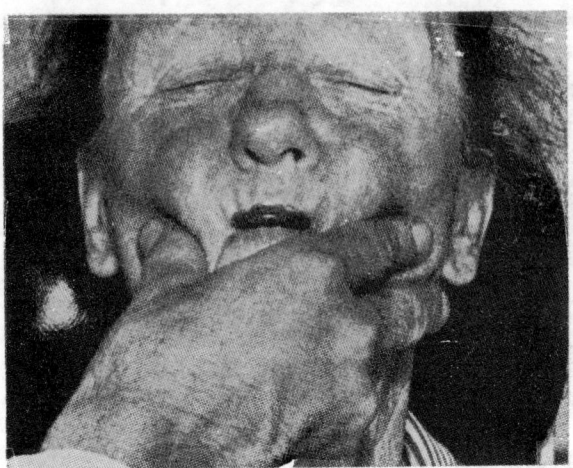

FIG. 104. – A method of holding a lower plaster impression in place. The third and fourth fingers are under the chin.

The impression, together with the pieces broken from it, should be placed on a napkin and left to harden and dry slightly. The broken surfaces are then lightly brushed with a camel hair brush and the small pieces fitted into the main impression, so that the fracture line is almost invisible, and secured with a little molten wax on the external surface. The pieces should be handled gently with tweezers as surface detail can easily be rubbed away.

If an impression fractures into many small pieces it is usually quicker and more accurate to take another rather than try to piece the first impression together.

The completed impression should embrace the entire surface which it is intended to cover with the denture. The periphery should be smooth and rounded and the impression surface smooth (see fig. 105). The only faults allowable are air bubbles small enough to be accurately filled with wax.

The Upper Working Impression

The ridge depression of the tray is filled with plaster, the palate being left free, or at the most covered with a very thin film; this is because plaster will be placed in the palate of the

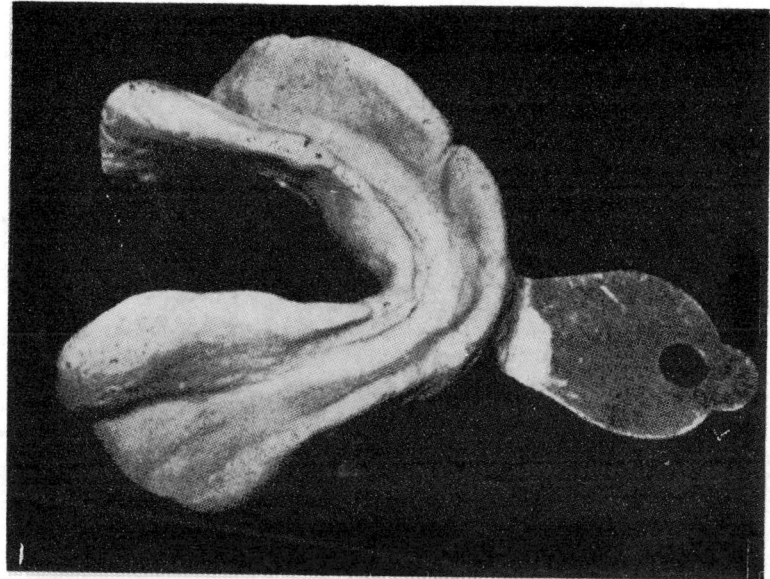

(a) The lower.

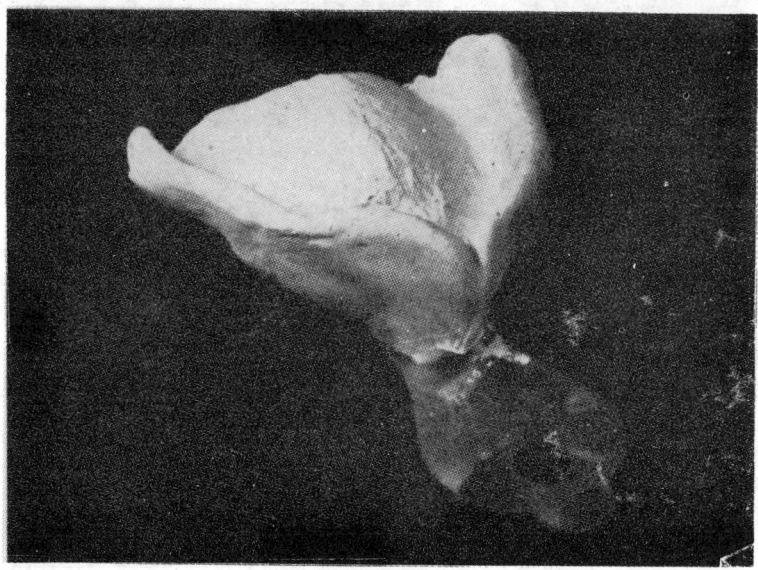

(b) The upper.

FIG. 105. – Completed plaster impressions.

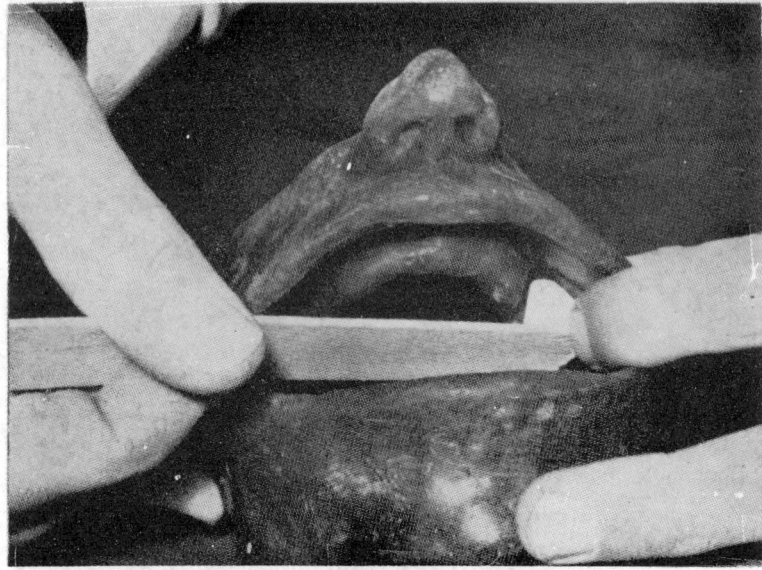

(*a*) In the region of the tuberosity.

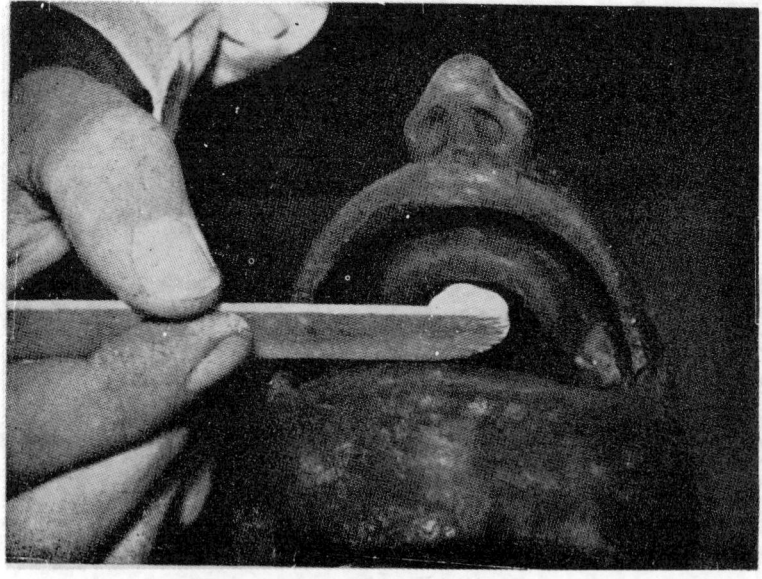

(*b*) In the centre of the palate.

FIG. 106. – Placing plaster in the mouth prior to the insertion
of the upper tray.

mouth to obviate air being trapped there. If much is also put on the palate of the tray an excess will be present which will flow towards the throat and cause retching.

When the plaster in the mixing bowl has reached the correct consistency for placing in the mouth, as described for the lower impression, some of it should be placed in the buccal and labial sulci and in the centre of the hard palate (*see* fig. 106). When placing plaster round the tuberosity the patient should be told not to open the mouth too widely, for the reason that the coronoid process is immediately lateral to the maxillary tuberosities when the mouth is fully open, and this will make it difficult to place the loose plaster in position in some patients.

The tray is then rotated into the mouth (*see* fig. 10⁷ (*a*)) and pushed backwards, the operator standing behind the patient and leaning forwards to do this and it is most important to observe that the tray is correctly centred; provided the handle of the tray has been attached squarely this may be used as a guide. The lip is lifted so that it may be clearly seen that the

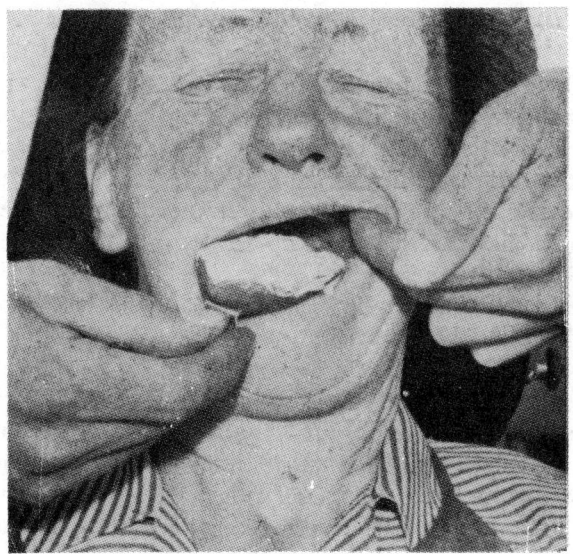

Fig. 107

(*a*) Method of rotating upper tray, filled with plaster, into the mouth.

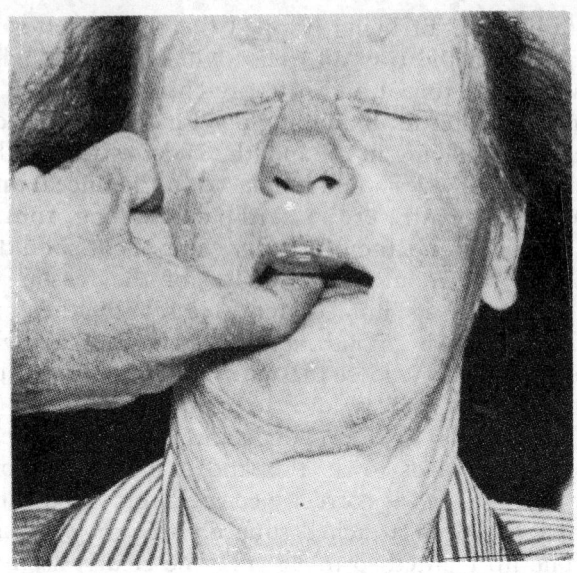

FIG. 107

(*b*)   Method of supporting upper tray when in position.

labial flange is in a position to pass up outside the ridge. The front of the tray is then raised with a wriggling motion until it is fully in position. The back of the tray is still low, resting just above the tongue and when the front is in position the back is puddled into place until the plaster just flows out behind the edge for a distance of approximately 3 mm. When this occurs the raising of the tray should cease.

When the tray is finally in place peripheral trimming should be performed. This may be carried out by first raising the cheeks and lips to release any trapped air or folds of tissue and then drawing the sulcus gently downwards, inwards and slightly backwards to obtain the functional position. When trimming, care should be taken not to draw the cheeks and lips away from the underlying ridges but to keep the plaster always in contact with them, thus obtaining a satisfactory peripheral seal.

The impression must be supported without pressure until the plaster has set (*see* fig. 107 (*b*)).

Removal of the Impression

The patient should be warned that the impression may break and the peripheral seal should be released as in the case of the lower impression. The removal should be effected by placing a finger of each hand on the periphery in the pre-molar region and the thumbs under the handle of the tray and then applying pressure downwards with the fingers and upwards with the thumbs. This action rotates the posterior border down first. An upper plaster impression is sometimes difficult to remove because undercut areas are frequent and also because the saliva may have been absorbed by the plaster which then tends to stick to the tissues. A little water ejected from a syringe around the periphery will wet the tissues again and simplify removal of the impression.

If the tray comes away leaving the impression in the mouth downward pressure with the fingers on the periphery will usually break the impression along the mid-line when it can be removed easily.

When an impression is difficult to remove it should be remembered that long continued pulling will only hurt the patient and not effect its removal. A sudden powerful jerk is what is required. This will hurt the patient once only and the impression will usually come away.

Puddling of Plaster

During the foregoing description of plaster impression technique the term puddling of plaster has been used. This action plays a most important part in the use of this material for impressions, in fact no satisfactory impression will ever be obtained without a clear understanding of what it implies. A comparison with wet sand will clarify what is meant. Firm pressure on a mound of wet sand will firstly express the water and then, if continued, cause the sand to break away still leaving the hand uncovered. If, however, instead of using firm direct pressure, the hand is wriggled and puddled into the mass with a gentle vibratory movement the wet sand will flow round and over it without any tendency to break away. Plaster impressions should always be treated as if they were composed of wet sand.

Failures

Failures with plaster impressions are due usually to one, or a combination of, the following:

(1) Placing insufficient plaster in the mouth.

(2) Insufficient plaster in the tray.

(3) Too much plaster in the tray.

(4) Slowness on the part of the operator allowing the plaster to set before the tray is adequately seated in place.

(5) Incorrect centring resulting in the flanges of the tray showing through the impression.

(6) Insufficient pressure when puddling the tray into position resulting in failure to seat the tray properly.

(7) Failure to observe the extrusion of sufficient plaster beyond the back edge of the upper tray.

(8) Direct pressure instead of puddling when seating the impression, and delayed peripheral trimming, result in cracks on the edges of the impression.

(9) Inclusion of some of the surrounding soft tissues such as the cheek or tongue.

(10) Trapped bubbles of air. These usually result from failure to place plaster in the sulci or palate.

(11) Trapped bubbles of mucous. In mouths which exhibit a lot of mucous bubbles in the sulci a far better impression will be secured if these bubbles are wiped away with a gauze napkin just prior to inserting the impression.

Plaster of Paris as an impression material gives exact reproduction of the denture-bearing surface at rest, with excellent surface detail. However, since it is semi-liquid when introduced into the mouth, very little compression of the soft tissue takes place and for this reason it is not the most suitable material for the case presenting grossly varying thicknesses of mucosa covering the denture bearing surface.

In spite of its disadvantages (*see* end of chapter), plaster will be found to be eminently suitable in most edentulous cases, especially as the technique is so simple, speedy, cheap and clean, points to be considered in a busy practice.

The Alginate Impression
Indications for Its Use in Edentulous Cases

A certain number of edentulous ridges exhibit severely undercut regions or irregularities resulting from recent extractions. The use of plaster in such cases frequently results in a badly fractured impression and the infliction of pain on the patient. These difficulties can be overcome by the use of a hydrocolloid material, which is sufficiently elastic when set, to spring over the bulbous areas of the ridge without becoming permanently deformed.

When there is an excessive amount of saliva in the floor of the mouth it tends to wash away plaster before it has set, leaving the impression with a rough crumbly surface. This disadvantage can be overcome by the use of an astringent mouth-wash and by allowing the plaster to thicken a little more than usual before putting it into the mouth. Some operators, however, prefer to use hydrocolloid for these cases and they undoubtedly produce excellent surface detai under these difficult conditions.

Sodium Alginate

Sodium alginate is capable of producing very accurate impressions if the several points in the technique requiring attention are meticulously observed.

The active ingredient is sodium alginate which, when mixed with water, produces a colloidal sol. If calcium ions are now added the sodium alginate is transformed into calcium alginate, which forms a gel, so setting occurs. If sodium alginate and calcium sulphate (a source of Ca ions) are mixed with water, gelation takes place so rapidly that no time is allowed for conforming the material to the impression tray and inserting it in the mouth. A controlling agent is, therefore, added in the form of trisodium phosphate. This substance has a greater affinity for Ca ions than has sodium alginate and by absorbing the Ca ions it is transformed into calcium phosphate, therefore, so long as any of it remains unchanged, it will delay the formation of calcium alginate. The set may thus be delayed for as long as required by the addition of the appropriate quantity of sodium phosphate which is done by the manufacturer.

The setting time is usually delayed one and a half minutes, which is ample time in which to mix it, conform it to the tray, and inset it in the mouth.

Method of Using

Several varieties of alginate impression material are available with slightly different methods of proportioning the water and powder. The manufacturer's instructions applying to the brand being used should be strictly adhered to because the reactions of alginate materials are sensitive to small variations in the powder/water ratio and the temperature of the water.

A straight-sided bowl and a straight metal spatula should be used for mixing so that the powder and liquid can be thoroughly incorporated by a firm rotary motion of the flat spatula against the side of the bowl. Thorough and speedy mixing is essential so that the tri-sodium phosphate is evenly dispersed throughout the mass and the mixing time should be that stated by the manufacturers.

Impression Trays

As with plaster, special trays are required, and these may be constructed of any of the materials already mentioned but they must of course be tried in the mouth and modified if necessary as described for plaster impressions. The alginates, unlike plaster, will not adhere to the tray of their own accord; fixation may be effected by one of the following methods:

(1) Sticky wax may be melted on to the surface of a metal tray immediately before the alginate is placed in it.

(2) Small holes may be bored in the tray through which some of the alginate will flow securing the impression firmly to the tray (see fig. 108(a)): holes made by a No. 10 rose-head bur or a $\frac{3}{32}''$ twist drill will be the minimum size suitable.

(3) Wisps of cotton-wool may be secured to the tray with sticky wax or sandarac varnish and will become incorporated in the alginate as it sets (see fig. 108(b)).

Attachment of the alginate to the tray is essential because if it pulls away a distorted impression will result which may easily pass unnoticed since the detail of the surface will remain unchanged (see fig. 109(b)).

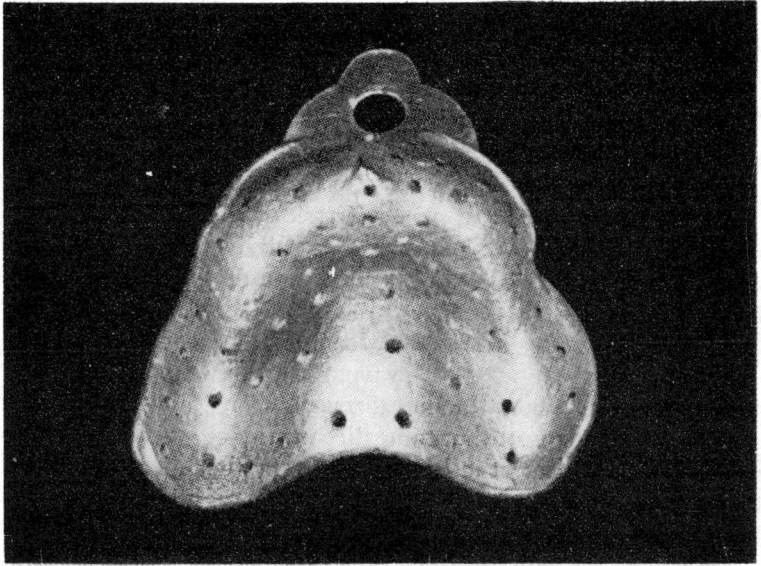

(*a*) Perforated tray with holes $^3/_{32}''$ diam.

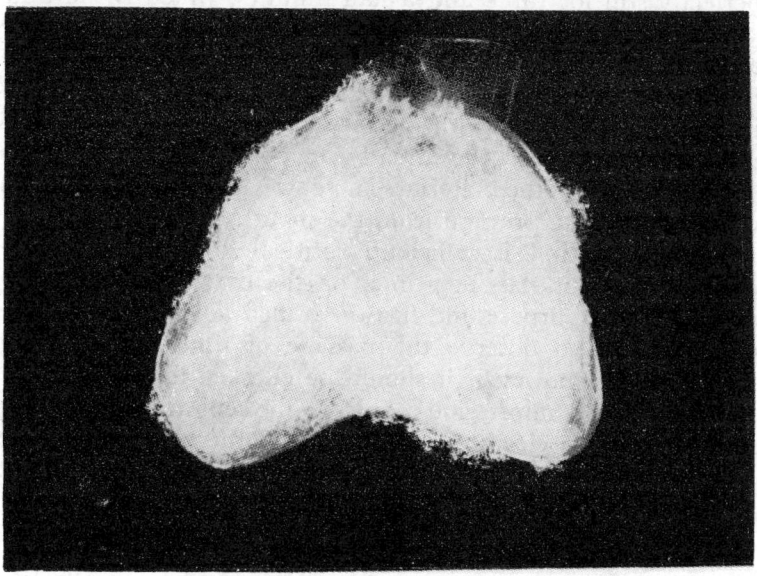

(*b*) Cotton-wool fixed to tray with sticky wax.

FIG. 108. – Methods of securing alginate to the tray.

Careful palpation may elicit an area similar to that illustrated and if such an area is found the impression must be discarded.

Taking Alginate Impressions

The technique of inserting and seating the impression material in the mouth is almost identical with that used for plaster.

With regard to the upper impression, however, one point requires stressing. It is most important to ensure that the minimum quantity of alginate flows past the back-edge of the tray. A mass of material in this region, unsupported by the tray, will pull away from the palate under the influence of its own weight, giving rise to warpage and strains which will affect the impression further forward. For this reason some operators favour post-damming the back-edge of the tray with soft wax and raising the back of the tray first so that the wax forms an effective seal with the palate and prevents the backward flow of the alginate (see fig. 99).

Once an alginate impression is in place it must be kept perfectly still for three and a half minutes, which is the time required for gelation. It is essential to keep the tray still because as heat accelerates the gelation of the alginate, that part of the impression in contact with the mucous membrane will set before that in contact with the tray and if the unset portion is moved in relation to the already set portion internal stresses will be induced in the material. These stresses will be released on removal of the impression from the mouth causing warpage.

The setting time is sufficiently critical to require accurate timing. An hour-glass egg-timer on the bracket table is very useful for this purpose and has the added advantage that the patient can also observe the passage of time. Before using such a device, however, it should be checked for accuracy.

As an alginate impression requires to be kept in the mouth for so long, a saliva ejector should be used otherwise the volume of saliva collecting in the floor of the mouth causes the patient considerable discomfort.

Removal of the Impression

An alginate impression, when set, develops a very effective peripheral seal so, before trying to remove it from the mouth,

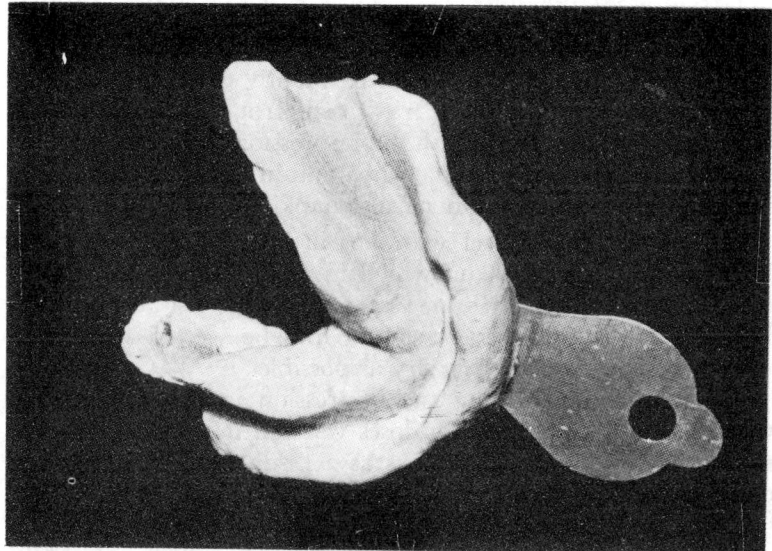

(a) A completed lower alginate impression.

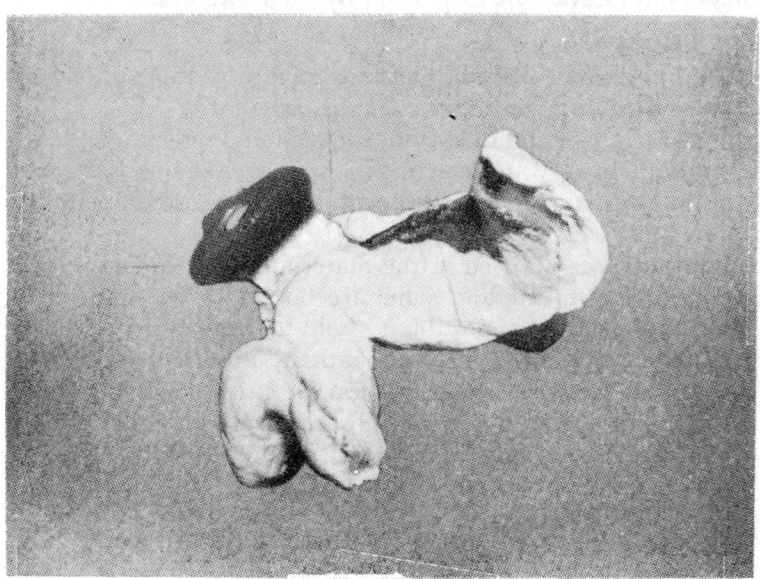

(b) A lower alginate impression pulled away from the tray
on the right side.

FIG. 109

this seal should be freed by running the finger round the periphery. Remove with a firm withdrawal movement. A gentle, long continued, pull will frequently cause the alginate to tear or pull away from the tray (*see* fig. 109 (*b*)). Immediately after removal from the mouth the impression should be washed under the cold tap, to remove saliva and immediately placed in the humidor or wrapped in a damp napkin.

A humidor is a vessel with an airtight lid, it contains a little water and a shelf on which impressions may be placed out of actual contact with the water but in a moist atmosphere. If a damp cloth is used it should first be wetted with cold water and then squeezed as dry as possible.

The reason for placing the impression in the humidor is that sodium alginate rapidly loses water if left exposed to the normal atmosphere and shrinks as a result. Another frequent cause of distortion of alginate impressions is that they are left standing on the bench, the whole weight of the impression and tray being taken by the back edge or heels of the impression. They should always be suspended by their handles.

Casting Alginate Impressions

The impressions should be cast as soon as possible after they have been taken. The reasons for this are that:

(1) Even in the humidor an impression tends to undergo alteration in water content and changes shape as a result (imbibition, i.e. water absorption, will cause alginates to swell).

(2) The stresses induced in the material, when the impression was being taken, and some are bound to be induced as it is physically impossible to hold an impression perfectly still in the mouth of the patient, are released slowly, and the sooner it is cast, the less the stresses will have been released and so the less it will have warped. Half an hour is the maximum time which should elapse between taking the impression and casting it.

The technique of casting is similar to that used for any other impression and no separating medium is needed. The one point to watch is that no force, sufficient to distort the alginate is allowed to develop. For example, if the mound of plaster built on the bench is allowed to become too stiff before inverting the impression into it, it will be necessary to use force to seat the impression, and the alginate will be distorted. It should also be ensured that the flanges of the impression are never forced into contact with the bench.

THE ZINC OXIDE-EUGENOL PASTE IMPRESSION

This paste is basically a mixture of zinc oxide, white powdered resin, eugenol or oil of cloves, and lanoline. It is smooth, flows readily, and is very sticky until it has set, which takes three and a half to four minutes in the mouth. Because of its stickiness this material is admirably suited for wash impressions. Such impressions, as their name implies, are very thin and are taken in a base-plate, denture, or preliminary composition impression. Special trays for this material require no clearance and are adapted directly on to the preliminary model.

The special tray must be very carefully adapted to the mouth, particular attention being paid to ensure that the paste is everywhere carried to the full functional depth of the sulci.

The proprietary brands of paste are mostly supplied in two tubes, one containing basically zinc oxide and the other basically eugenol. For the lower impression about 6 cm. and for the upper 9 cm. of each are squeezed on to the mixing block, thoroughly spatulated, and evenly distributed over the fitting surface of the carefully dried tray.

Before starting to mix the paste the patient's lips and neighbouring skin should be lightly covered with face-cream or vaseline to prevent the paste adhering to these dry surfaces should it touch them during the insertion of the tray. Many operators also treat their own fingers in the same way. Should some zinc-oxide paste inadvertently touch a patient's or operator's dry skin, it can readily be removed by a napkin moistened with chloroform.

The Technique of Impression Taking

Owing to its more sluggish flow, and smaller bulk, it cannot be puddled into place like plaster or sodium alginate but as soon as the tray has been centred in the mouth, it should be seated by a firm constant pressure which should be maintained for a short time before peripheral trimming is carried out in the usual manner.

Removal of the impression is sometimes a little difficult owing to the excellent peripheral seal obtained, but it can be facilitated by introducing a few drops of water from the syringe as previously described for plaster of Paris.

Some patients will complain of a burning sensation when the impression is in the mouth, this is due to the slight irritation caused by the oil of cloves or eugenol. Fortunately true allergy to oil of cloves is very rare though a hyperaemia lasting several days may occasionally be met; treatment by bland mouth-washes is all that is required.

THE FUNCTIONALLY TRIMMED LOWER IMPRESSION

This type of impression, first described by Fournet and Tuller, requires extremely careful attention to detail, probably more so than any other technique, and is therefore rather a time-consuming procedure. It is one, however, which is fully justified by the results obtained. It is chiefly used in those cases where the ridge, as such, is very poorly defined, and where the factors of retention and tongue control are adverse. The excellent results obtained with this technique are due to the more perfect functional adaptation and meticulous care in covering the maximum possible area.

It is an advantage if the primary impression is taken in plaster of Paris, with functional trimming, as there is then less likelihood of the special tray being grossly over-extended but a carefully adapted composition impression is quite suitable. Mark on the model taken from the primary impression the approximate functional position of the periphery and construct a fitting base-plate in acrylic to this outline. A small vertical handle should be fitted in the incisor region, designed so as not to interfere with the movement of the tongue and lips (*see* fig. 110).

The steps in taking the impression are as follows:

(1) Examine the mouth to discover the position occupied by the buccal sulcus in function by gentle manipulation of the cheek (*see* fig. 111).

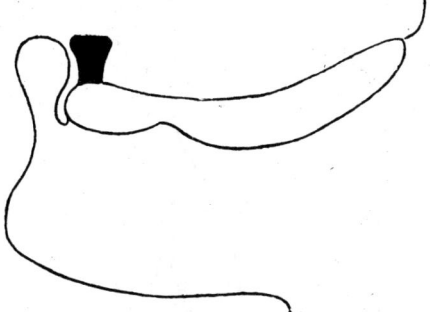

Fig. 110. – Tray for a functionally trimmed lower impression.
Note form of handle.

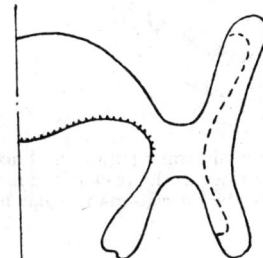

Fig. 111. – Position of Sulci.
Continuous line illustrates their relaxed position;
Dotted line their approximate functional position.

Towards the back of the mouth the contraction of
the buccinator and masseter muscles almost completely
obliterates the sulcus. This is because the former muscle
crosses the ridge to gain its attachment to the pterygo-
mandibular ligament (*see* fig. 112).

(2) With a revolving carborundum stone in the dental
engine trim the buccal periphery of the tray so that it is
about 2 mm. short of the position occupied by the buccal
sulcus in function (*see* fig. 113).

(3) Examine the position occupied by the labial sulcus in
function by gently pulling up the lip and trim the tray
just short of this position.

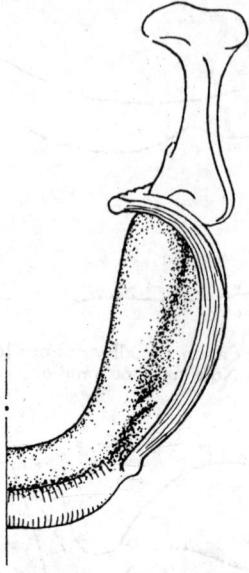

Fig. 112. – Diagram illustrating how the buccinator muscle crosses the alveolar ridge at the back of the mouth to gain its insertion into the pterygo-mandibular ligament.

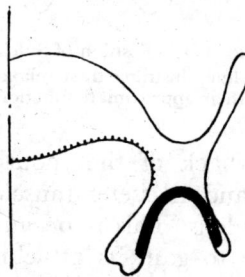

Fig. 113. – Correctly trimmed tray 2 mm. short of the functional positions of the sulci.

(4) Trim the distolingual aspect of the special tray so that it is just short of the position occupied by the palato-glossus muscle when the tongue is protruded to touch the lips (*see* fig. 114). This is most easily accomplished by placing the tray in position in the mouth, then placing the finger in the posterior lingual pouch over the tray; ask the

patient to protrude the tongue and it can be felt if the palatoglossus muscle comes into contact with the tray. Trim until the muscle just fails to reach the tray.

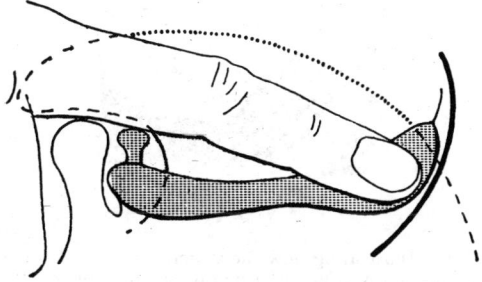

FIG. 114. – The thick curved line represents the position of the palato-glossal arch when the tongue (shown by dotted line) is protruded.
The tray as illustrated is correctly trimmed and the position of the palpating finger shown.

(5) To examine the functional position of the floor of the mouth ask the patient to place the tip of the tongue in the superior buccal sulcus opposite the side it is wished to examine. In the majority of cases the whole floor of the mouth will rise up and overlap the ridge and it will appear as if no lingual sulcus exists; this appearance, however, is usually false. The structures in the floor of the mouth immediately under the mucous membrane consist, for the most part, of the sublingual salivary gland, from about the 1st molar region forwards, and the deep part of the submandibular salivary gland further back. As these glands are pulled upwards by the action of the tongue they overlap the ridge and mask the sulcus (*see* fig. 115).

The most satisfactory way to trim the tray to the functional position of the lingual sulcus is to place the finger on top of the tray in the area under examination, and ask the patient to repeat the tongue movement. If the tray is too deep the lingual tissues will exert an upward pressure, the degree of which can be judged by the force required to keep the tray in contact with the

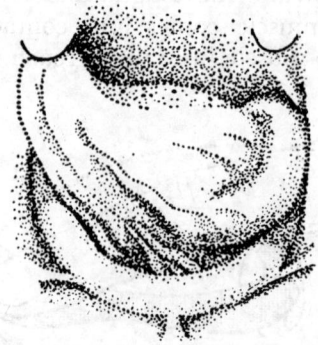

FIG. 115. – Illustrating how the structures of the floor of the mouth rise and overlap the ridge when the tongue is raised.

alveolar ridge. Trimming should be continued until only the slightest finger pressure is needed to hold the tray in position. A little practice is needed to gain this sense of touch trimming, but by running the finger along the top of the tray while the patient keeps the tongue elevated, it will soon be learnt where adjustment is required. Final test for stability should be made by holding the tray lightly with the index fingers in the premolar region on both sides and asking the patient to moisten the lips and then place the tip of the tongue in each upper molar region in turn.

(6) Trim the tray posteriorly so that it crosses the middle of the retromolar pads. This is very important because the excellent retention exhibited by the final denture cannot be obtained without a perfect peripheral seal being effected in the retromolar area, and this can only be attained on compressible tissue.

(7) Trim the tray so that it is clear of the fraenum of the tongue both when it is protruded and when the tip of the tongue is in contact with the junction of the hard and soft palates.

The correct trimming of the tray is essential to the success of this type of impression. When the tray has been satisfactorily trimmed the next procedure is accurately to adapt the entire periphery to the functional positions of the various sulci; this is done by tracing on to the periphery of the tray a low fusing composition and while this is soft placing the tray in the mouth. This softened composition is then moulded by the movement of the various sulci and adapts itself closely to their functional positions.

The Technique of Adapting the Periphery

Apparatus required.

Bunsen burner.

Pin-point flame.

Bowl of water temperature 120° F.

Bowl of cold water.

Tracing stick (this is a pencil-shaped stick, of special composition which softens at a temperature of 110°–120° F. It is usually coloured to differentiate it from ordinary impression composition).

(1) Soften the end of the tracing stick in the Bunsen flame. Commencing at the distal aspect of the left buccal periphery, 'paint' the trimmed tray with the softened tracing stick for a distance of about 3 cm. The softened composition will adhere to the periphery of the tray (*see* fig. 116).

The procedure of 'painting', or sticking the special composition to the periphery of the tray, is termed tracing.

(2) Brush the traced composition with the pin-point flame to re-soften it, as it will have commenced to harden while it was being traced, plunge it into the bowl of hot water and quickly place the tray in the mouth. It is most important to remember that whenever composition is heated with a flame it must always be immersed for a few seconds in hot water to equalize the temperature, otherwise the patient's mouth may be seriously burned.

Using one hand to hold the tray in place and support the jaw, mould the softened periphery to the correct level by carrying out functional movements of the cheek with the other hand, or by asking the patient to suck the cheeks gently inwards. This operation will adapt the composition into close intimacy with that part of the buccal sulcus adjacent to it.

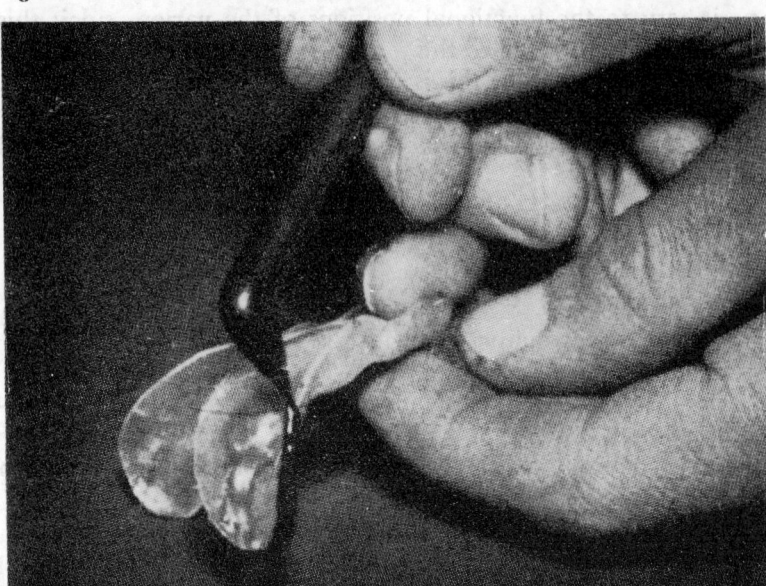

FIG. 116. – Tracing the periphery of an acrylic tray with low
fusing tracing compound.

(3) Remove the tray from the mouth, place it in the bowl of
cold water, and leave it there for a few moments to chill.
Remove the tray from the water to examine the composition which, if correctly adapted, should show a smooth,
matt rolled everted edge (*see* fig. 117 (*a*)).

If it does not appear everted, or looks rough or is shiny
instead of matt there was not sufficient composition present
to fill the sulcus in its functional position (*see* figs. 117 (*b*)
and 118).

To correct this error, dry the original composition with
gauze and add to it by tracing on another layer and
re-adapt to the sulcus. (If the tray has not been trimmed
sufficiently short of the functional position of the sulcus
the composition will be everted completely, and the edge
of the tray will show through (*see* fig. 119). In this case
the tray must be trimmed further.

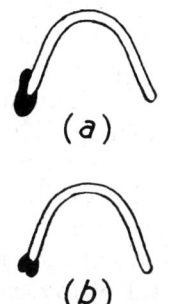

FIG. 117. – Section through lower tray showing traced
periphery.
(a) Composition smooth, rolled and everted.
(b) Composition rough and not everted.

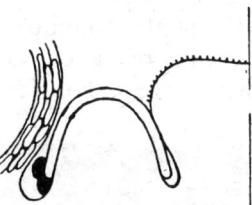

FIG. 118. – Illustrating how the error shown in 117 (b) occurs.

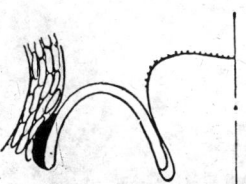

FIG. 119. – Tray overextended, composition completely
everted.

(4) Adapt the whole of the buccal and labial periphery,
working in sections of about 3 cm. at a time. Pay particular
attention to the adaptation around the fraenal attachments.

(5) When the buccal and labial tracing is complete, commence
the lingual tracing, starting with the distal border
adjacent to the left palatoglossal muscle. Trace on the
composition, flame, dip in hot water and place the tray
in the mouth taking care not to brush off the composition

against the side of the tongue, as the tray goes into place. Hold the tray in place with the fingers in each premolar region, at the same time asking the patient to place the tip of the tongue in the right superior buccal sulcus and then protrude the tongue. These actions pull forward the palatoglossal arch and conform the composition to its correct shape. The position of the tongue in the former of these movements is one commonly assumed during meals, as the tip of the tongue frequently traverses the superior buccal sulcus to clear it of accumulated food.

(6) Continue the lingual tracing, section by section, trimming with the tip of the tongue in the buccal sulcus because in addition to pulling the palatoglossal muscle forwards this action also raises the floor of the mouth on the side opposite to the tip of the tongue.

The lateral aspect of a correctly trimmed lingual periphery is shown in fig. 120. The notch discernible in

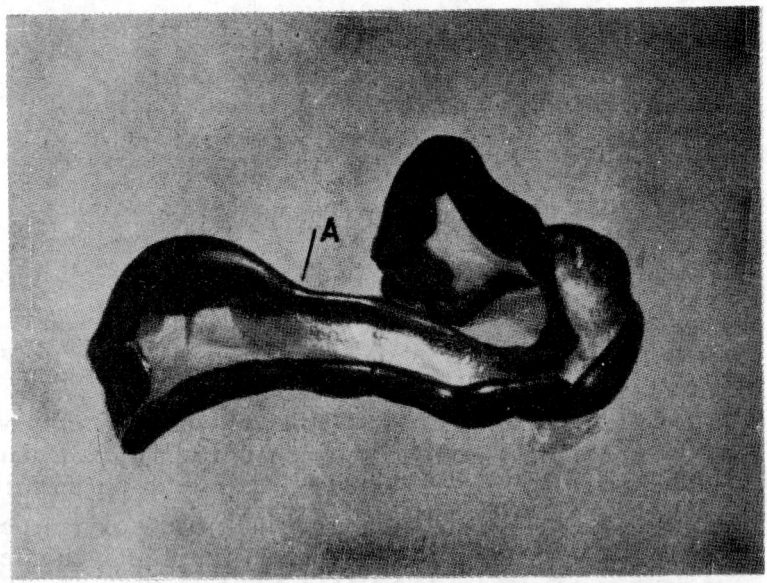

Fig. 120. – Illustrating the lateral aspect of a correctly trimmed periphery.
A indicates the depression made by the posterior fibres of the mylohyoid muscle.

the region of the second molar is made by the mylohyoid muscle which, in this region, is just a thin slip merging with the posterior aspect of the mylohyoid ridge.

The most satisfactory way to trim the lingual periphery is to work forward from the left palatoglossal muscle to the region of the left canine; then forward from the right palatoglossal muscle to the right canine, leaving the area of the lingual fraenum to be trimmed last.

(7) When adapting the antero-lingual periphery, instruct the patient first to protrude the tongue and then roll it back and touch the junction of the hard and soft palate with its tip.

(8) The final areas to be adapted are over the retromolar pads. Trace both these areas together by dropping composition into the ntting surface, and then place the tray in the mouth and hold it with a firm pressure for about 30 seconds. If the tracing of the entire periphery has been carried out correctly the tray should resist removal and come away with a definite sucking sound.

Retention Tests

Tests for retention and methods of correcting faults are as ollows:

(1) Protrude the tongue. The tray should remain in place but if it lifts soften the tracing in the palatoglossal areas and readapt.

(2) Place the tongue successively in each superior buccal sulcus. The tray should remain in place but if it lifts, the lingual extension is too deep. Soften the tracing on the side which lifts and readapt.

(3) Roll the tongue back to touch the junction of the hard and soft palates. The tray should remain in place but if it lifts the lingual extension anteriorly is too deep, and should be softened and readapted.

(4) Open the mouth to the fullest extent. If the tray lifts, soften and readapt the buccal and labial peripheries.

(5) Grasp the handle and exert a vertical upward pull.

Resistance should be felt but if the tray comes away easily tracing stick should be added to the lingual periphery in the premolar regions and readapted.

(6) Exert forward pressure on the distal aspect of the handle. The tray should resist and only come free with a sucking sound.

   If there is no resistance add composition over the retromolar areas and recompress.

Completing the Impression

Having carefully adapted the periphery, there still remains to be obtained the impression of the bearing surface of the ridge. This is most satisfactorily done by using an impression paste.

Spread a thin layer over the dry tray, place the tray in the mouth and seat firmly. Instruct the patient to repeat all the tongue movements made during the peripheral trimming, to trim the buccal and labial peripheries. Hold the tray in place for four minutes and then ask the patient to rinse his mouth with cold water several times. Remove the impression and place in a bowl of cold water, fitting surface upwards, supported by a submerged gauze square to prevent its edges being spoiled by contact with the bowl.

Examine the periphery of the completed impression (*see* fig. 121). It may be found that areas of the periphery show the composition tracing free of paste, while in other areas the paste has covered the composition and corrected the slight inaccuracies of adaptation. The surface of the paste impression should appear smooth and accurately duplicate the surface details. Faults in a paste impression are easily corrected by drying the inaccurate area, spreading over it a thin layer of freshly mixed paste, and re-seating. The completed impression may be placed in the mouth and tested, it should be practically impossible for the patient to dislodge it by any of the usual movements of the tongue, cheeks or lips.

Casting the Impression

In casting the impression the plaster is brought up the external surfaces of the flanges to a height of approximately 3 mm. in order that the peripheral contour, including its actual thickness,

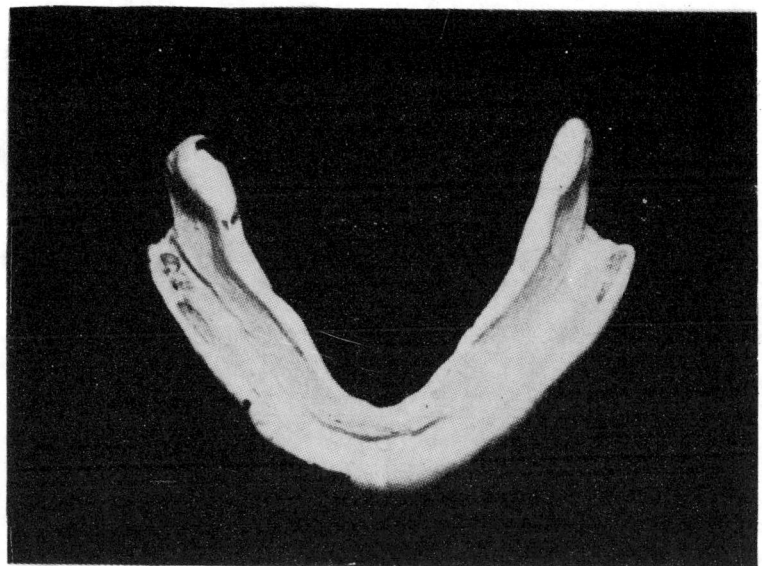

(a) seen from above,

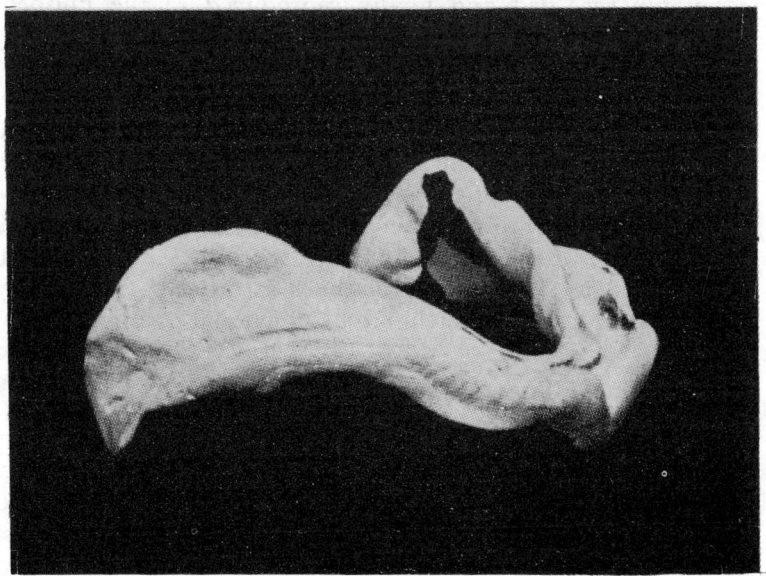

(b) seen from the side.
FIG. 121. – The completed lower impression.

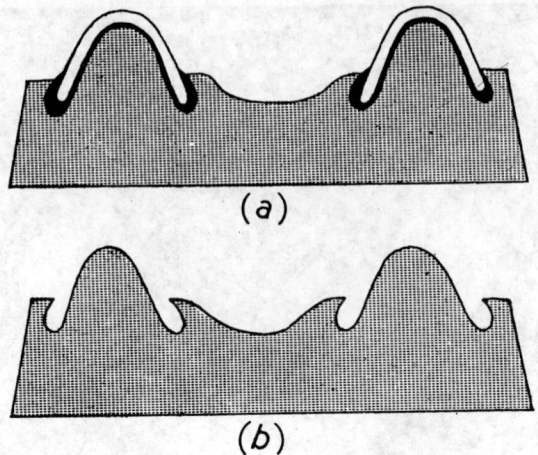

FIG. 122

(a) Plaster model cast with impression in place.
(b) Plaster model after impression has been removed. Note how the peripheries of the impression have been reproduced on the model.

is suitably recorded and finally reproduced in the finished denture (*see* fig. 122).

A similar technique can be used for taking an upper impression (*see* fig. 123), but this must be post-dammed along the palatal border. The technique for post-damming is to add a tracing of composition along the fitting surface of the posterior palatal border, joining the buccal tracings round the tuberosities. This composition is then softened in the usual way, and the impression inserted and held firmly in place. The patient is instructed to swallow several times in order to mould the tracing in the hamular notches to its functional position.

THE COMPOSITION IMPRESSION

Compression Impression

There are often considerable differences in density and thickness of the mucous membrane in different parts of the denture-bearing area, usually, though by no means always, more marked in the upper than in the lower. The following technique, which has been described by many writers, each

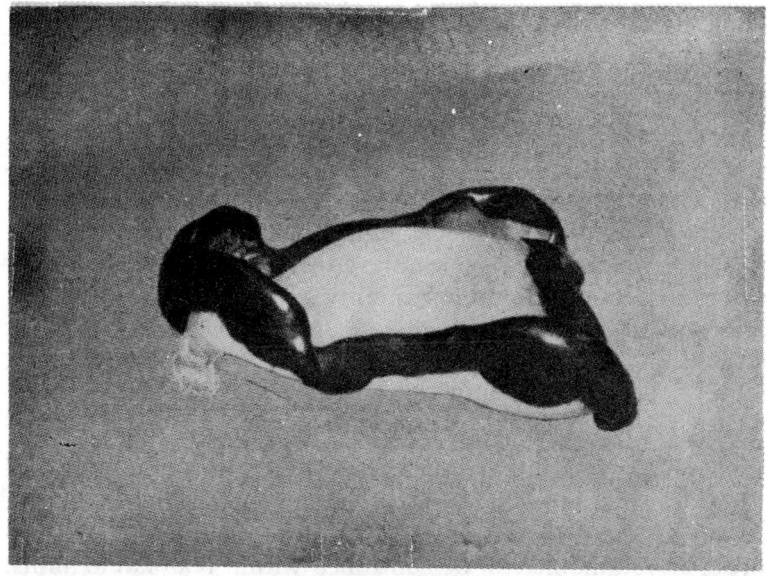

(*a*) The completed tracing.

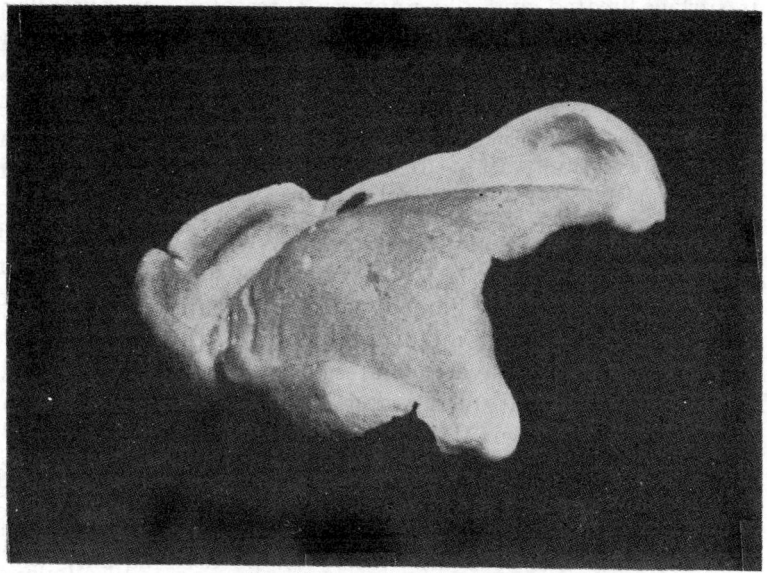

(*b*) The completed impression.
FIG. 123. – A peripherally adapted upper impression.

with slight variations, is designed to take an impression of these tissues under pressure so that, under the stresses of mastication, the pressure transmitted through the entire mucosa on to the underlying bone is approximately equal over its whole surface. Unfortunately this ideal can never be attained since pressure can only be evenly transmitted to the bone when all the mucous membrane is fully compressed and this state may not be achieved by the operator when taking the impression. Further, masticatory stress is very variable which will result in variable compressibility of the mucosa and uneven pressure on the supporting bone. Nevertheless this type of impression results in a denture which is extremely stable, requires no relieving and since the periphery is functionally adapted it possesses excellent retention.

Composition, with its high viscosity, is the only material which is suitable for this technique and by varying its degree of softness, and thereby its rate of flow, the amount of compression obtainable can be controlled within reasonable limits. A composition impression which has been thoroughly chilled, its surface heated and the impression reseated can exert far greater compression than one in which the composition is equally softened throughout its entire mass. A criticism levelled at this type of impression is that sometimes rapid absorption of the ridges with consequent flabbiness of the mucosa results from the extremely tight fit of a denture made to such an impression.

A composition should be selected which softens at a temperature between 120° F. and 140° F., flows readily when softened, can be flamed without burning or blistering and which sets hard at mouth temperature. It is a help, and a considerable time saver, to have an electrically heated and thermostatically controlled water bath set at the optimum temperature for the material being used. This is not essential if a thermometer is used constantly to check the temperature of the water which should not be allowed to vary more than 5° F. A bowl of iced water to chill the impression will save chairside time but cold tap water can be used equally well except that it takes longer.

The Special Tray

A special tray is always required for this technique and it should be made in the following way:

Cover the whole model with an even thickness of new composition; composition which has been used even once is quite useless for this purpose as many of the more volatile constituents have been lost, thus altering its working properties, raising its softening point, and decreasing its ability to flow. This layer must extend to the full depth of the sulcus all round as it is to be moulded by the soft tissues of the mouth. Next cover the composition with a swaged or cast metal base, so that the composition will be retained in shape when softened (*see* fig. 124).

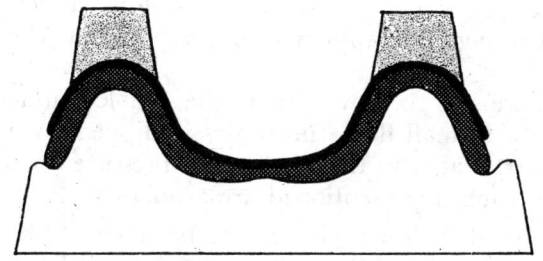

Fig.124. – Details of the construction of an upper special tray for taking a compression impression.

This stiffener must be left 4 mm. short of the periphery everywhere except at the posterior border; if extended to the periphery it will interfere with the moulding of this area and if it does not support the softened composition at the junction of hard and soft palates, gravity will tend to pull the composition away from the tissues and adequate post-damming cannot be obtained. A handle in the form of a rim, such as is used in bite registration, is convenient, it may be made of old composition and is only really needed anteriorly.

The Impression

Besides bowls of hot and cold water, a small pin-point flame, either of gas or a spirit blowpipe, will be required.

Only the upper impression will be described as the technique for the lower is similar.

Soften the composition lining of the special tray either by immersing in hot water or by pouring the hot water over it by means of a ladle or syringe; this latter is probably the better technique as there is then no risk of softening the composition rim used as a handle. As soon as the composition has become soft, it is seated in the mouth with only gentle pressure, and no precautions are taken against distorting the surrounding soft tissues by over-extension, this will be corrected at a later stage. The impression should be held in place until it has hardened, which usually takes about three minutes, it is then withdrawn and immediately placed in the bowl of cold water, being left there until it is thoroughly hard right through. Composition is a very poor thermal conductor and if cold tap water is being used, it should be chilled for at least as long as was spent in heating; this applies to every occasion when heat is applied.

The impression is now dried, the whole surface heated rapidly with a small flame until glossy, dipped for a moment in hot water, seated in the mouth and pressure applied. The reasons for each step mentioned are as follows:

(1) It is dried, as otherwise it will be unevenly heated and softened, i.e. 212° F., where wet and much higher elsewhere.

(2) Rapid heating of the surface will leave the remainder of the composition hard so that pressure can be applied without distorting it.

(3) Flamed composition, like hot sealing-wax, will stick and burn and, on removal, will bring the surface tissues with it so that every time a flame is used the impression must be dipped into hot water before being inserted in the mouth (this process is often referred to as 'tempering').

The pressure in the upper must be directed upwards and backwards towards the crown of the head, and a more evenly balanced pressure is obtained by most operators when pressing with one finger in the centre of the palate, than when using one finger of each hand on either side. This is because right-handed people unconsciously tend to press harder with the right hand, and this would make for instability of the denture.

If both hands are used, however, uneven pressure may be checked by reference to the patient, and if the pressure appeared to him to be less on one side than the other, then the whole of this step must be repeated with greater care.

Remove the impression when hard and place at once in cold water; this cooling immediately on removal from the mouth must be carried out throughout the whole technique, as the residual heat in the deeper layers will easily cause distortion, even during handling.

So far an impression has been obtained which, under an upward and backward load of unknown quantity, will bear equally on hard and soft areas, but which is somewhat over-extended and has no peripheral seal (*see* fig. 125 (*a*)).

The peripheral borders are now trimmed with a sharp knife until they are approximately 3 mm. short of the functional position of the sulci and fraena, and the thickness is also reduced to about 3 mm. by removing part of the rolled border in contact with the cheeks and lip (*see* fig. 125 (*b*)). Particular attention must be paid to this stage of the technique as any composition that impinges on the sulci or fraena will result in the finished denture being dislodged by muscular pull: if retention is good enough to prevent this the consequence will be pain and inflammation at that point.

Once this trimming of the impression is completed, the periphery is rebuilt and adapted section by section, using a low-fusing tracing composition in stick form. Begin at the distal end of one buccal border, dry, add tracing composition for 2 cm. to 3 cm., flame, temper, insert and mould for the functional position. Details of trimming for the functional position have already been given in previous techniques, but emphasis must be laid on the fact that some pressure must be maintained to keep the soft composition in contact with the mucous membrane of the ridge so that excess composition will be rolled to the correct position and not pulled away (*see* fig. 126).

Repeat the procedure until the whole periphery from tuberosity to tuberosity has been readapted and after each section has been trimmed, place the impression in cold water until it is thoroughly hard.

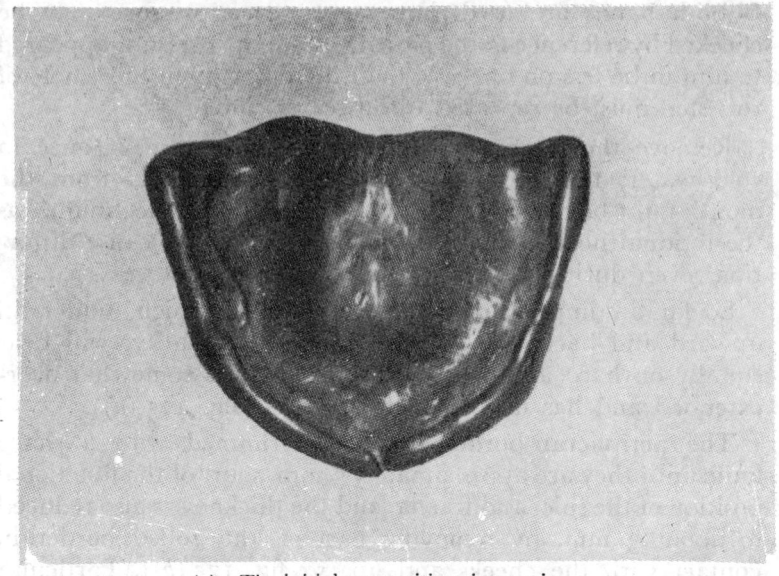

(*a*)   The initial composition impression.

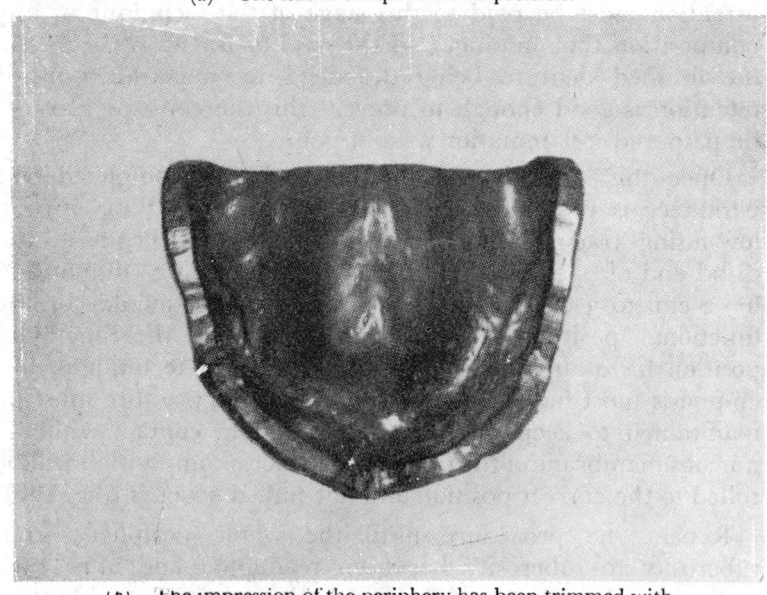

(*b*)   The impression of the periphery has been trimmed with
a knife prior to tracing.

FIG. 125. – An upper compression impression.

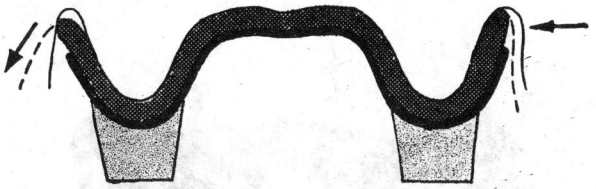

FIG. 126. – Right side of diagram illustrates the direction in which pressure must be applied to keep the composition in contact with the tissues when functional trimming is being carried out.

Left side illustrates what occurs if the cheek is merely pulled outwards and downwards.

The posterior palatal border still remains to be adapted and this is done as follows:

The vibrating line of the soft palate is first located, usually by asking the patient to open his mouth widely and say a prolonged 'ah' when the movement of the palate is easily seen. This line may be marked in the mouth with an indelible pencil and the impression cut or added to so that it terminates just anterior to this vibrating line, but posterior to the hard palate. Again dry the impression, add a tracing on the fitting surface just anterior to the palatal border, flame, temper, place in the mouth and hold with a firm pressure. Chill thoroughly after removal.

There remain two areas which so far have received no attention, the hamular notches, and it is here that the final seal is produced. Place a tracing in both these areas and, after the usual routine, seat the impression firmly in position and ask the patient to swallow several times which will trim the soft tissues in these regions.

The impression should now be complete (*see* fig. 127) and it should be impossible for the patient to dislodge it by any normal movement of the lips and cheeks.

Tests for Retention

(1) Upward and outward pressure in the incisor region. If the impression can be dislodged without great difficulty the posterior border requires further post-damming.

(2) Upward and outward pressure in the premolar regions. If the impression falls, then further peripheral seal is

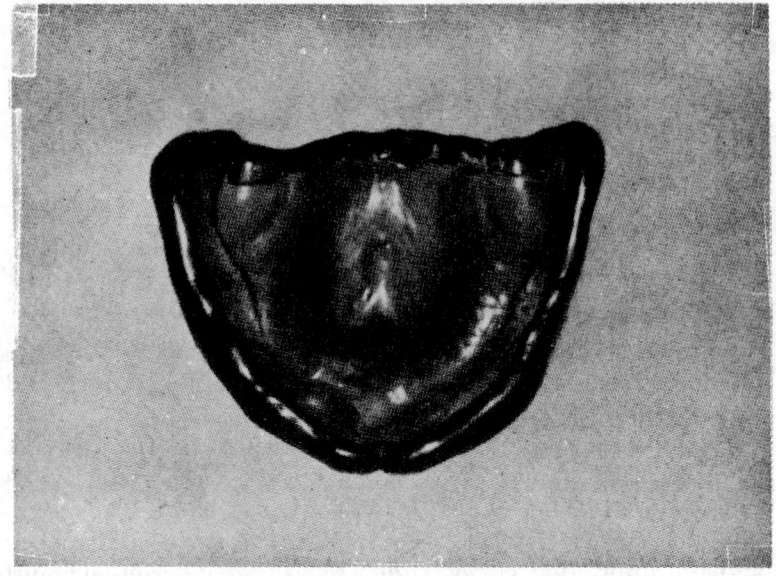

FIG. 127. – A completed upper compression impression.

required on the opposite side, usually around the tuberosity.

Sometimes a difficult air leak can be spotted by seeing a small collection of bubbles at one spot on the periphery and this must be corrected in the usual way.

(3) Pulling down the upper lip. Overextension in the labial sulcus is common and if this test dislodges the impression the labial periphery must be readapted.

At some point during the taking of the impression the air seal will become sufficiently good to make removal of the impression difficult, and this can be overcome by asking the patient to close the lips and blow out the cheeks, thus forcing air under the impression and allowing it to drop.

Difficulties

The commonest cause of failure with this technique is impatience on the part of the operator at the time spent in chilling the impression but, unless it is thoroughly hardened after each insertion in the mouth, warpage will occur and the only remedy for this warpage is to start the impression over again from the very first step, there are no short cuts.

GENERAL REMARKS ON IMPRESSION TAKING

Most of the difficulties encountered in impression taking can be traced to the operator's lack of attention to details of technique, and especially the acceptance of a poor stock tray impression with the comment that, 'it will be good enough for making a special tray'. It is of extreme importance that the primary impression should record the entire possible denture-bearing surface but, at the same time, does not encroach on the movable muscular tissues.

Special trays must be carefully checked for possible over-extension and, if plaster is the material of choice, it is necessary to ensure that sufficient space exists in all regions, between the fitting surface of the tray and the tissues to be recorded. A suitable thickness of material is necessary so that fractured areas may be accurately reunited.

Nausea

A disturbing factor experienced by some patients is the sensitivity of the soft palate and the dorsum of the tongue to foreign bodies; such conditions may produce retching and in rare instances actual vomiting. This is a normal reaction to gentle, intermittent stimulation of these parts and many patients are more affected during the selection of a standard tray than during the actual taking of the impression with its firmer contact over a more restricted area and its avoidance of the dorsum of the tongue. Unfortunately with the more difficult cases there is always a psychological factor present as well, probably connected with a fear of choking, but a successful operation can be assured by adopting one or more of the following methods:

(1) A firm, sympathetic manner of self-confidence on the operator's part.

(2) Assure the patient that no difficulty will be experienced if instructions are followed, and that the discomfort will be minimized as much as possible, being in any case only for a short time.

(3) The patient should blow the nose to clear any nasal obstruction and then be encouraged in deep, nasal breathing.

(4) Explain to the patient that, as soon as the impression is seated, the head may be brought well forward over the lap and that a bowl will be provided to hold under the chin to catch any saliva that may run out of the mouth. This will reduce the fear of being choked and will also help by keeping the patient's hands occupied, and any pieces of plaster which do drop from the back edge of the impression will fall on to the front, not the back, of the tongue, and so will be under control as explained in the chapter on applied anatomy.

(5) Carry out the impression technique using as little material as is commensurate with procuring a satisfactory impression. Avoid touching the dorsum of the tongue with the back of the tray and seat the impression as quickly as possible.

(6) Desensitize the surface of the mucous membrane with:

    (a) A phenol mouth-wash of one part phenol to eighty parts of water as cold as can be procured.

    (b) Sucking a tablet made for this purpose.

    (c) The application of a surface type of local anaesthetic either in the form of a cream or a spray.

As sensitive patients will experience the same difficulty at each succeeding visit and as the wearing of the finished denture will be difficult, it is advisable to construct a fitting base-plate in acrylic on the first impression and give it to the patient with instructions to practise wearing it for increasingly longer periods each day until it can be worn for at least an hour without discomfort.

Impression materials vary in their nauseating effects, partly owing to their viscosity and hence their controllability and partly owing to their consistency and flavour. Patients dislike plaster of Paris more than any other material, even when it is flavoured; the alginates are tolerated slightly better; composition is usually tolerated well, probably owing to its putty-like consistency and its heat; zinc oxide paste seems to be disliked least of any but this may be largely due to its only being used in a tray which already fits, though its flavour of cloves undoubtedly helps in some cases.

Impressions for Bedridden Patients

Occasionally the prosthetist is called upon to take impressions for a patient who is confined to bed. The first thing to do if possible is to turn the patient round in bed so that his head is at the foot, then the head board of the bed will not obstruct the operator. The use of plaster or hydrocolloid is contra-indicated as these easy-flowing materials are difficult to control, but composition or zinc oxide paste have a relatively high viscosity and can be more readily controlled. Lengthy techniques cause undue fatigue and should be avoided.

SUMMARY OF ADVANTAGES AND DISADVANTAGES OF VARIOUS IMPRESSION MATERIALS

In conclusion, it is felt that it may be useful to summarize the advantages and disadvantages of the various impression materials which have been discussed.

Plaster of Paris

Advantages

(a) It produces excellent surface detail.

(b) It is dimensionally accurate if used with an anti-expansion solution.

(c) It does not distort on removal from the mouth but fractures if deep undercuts exist and may be accurately assembled out of the mouth.

(d) The rate of set is under the control of the operator.

(e) It is compatible with all materials commonly used for making models and is the only material into which metal can be poured.

(f) It is hygienic, as fresh plaster must be used for each impression.

(g) It is cheap.

Disadvantages

(a) It cannot be used for compressing the tissues.

(b) In very wet mouths the surface of the plaster tends to be washed away spoiling the surface detail.

(c) It cannot be added to if faulty.

(d) Its taste and rough feel when in the mouth induce nausea in some patients.

(e) It is disliked by many patients.

Indications for Use

(a) In all normal mouths when the factors affecting retention are favourable.

(b) Whenever excessive flabby tissue covers the ridges.

Sodium Alginate

Advantages

(a) It produces excellent surface detail.

(b) It is dimensionally accurate if cast within a short time of removal from the mouth.

(c) It is elastic and will spring over bulbous areas returning to its correct position when removed from the mouth. This only applies if the undercuts are not too deep.

(d) It is hygienic, as fresh material must be used for each impression.

(e) It does not lose surface detan very wet mouths.

Disadvantages

(a) It cannot be used alone for compressing the tissues.

(b) It cannot be added to if faulty.

(c) Distortion may occur without it being obvious. It must be held stationary in relation to the tissues throughout its setting period, and it must remain adherent to the tray during removal.

Indications for Use

(a) Whenever there are undercuts which are too severe for plaster.

(b) In mouths with an excessive flow of saliva.

Zinc Oxide and Eugenol Paste

Advantages

(a) It produces excellent surface detail.

(b) It is dimensionally accurate as it is only used in a thin layer.

(c) It is hygienic, as fresh material must be used for each impression.

(d) It does not lose surface detail in wet mouths.

(e) It can be added to and readapted if faulty.

(f) It can be used for compressing soft tissues.

(g) It reduces nausea to a minimum.

(h) It adheres well to a dried surface so that when the minimum of material is used there is little degree of flaking on removal from the mouth.

Disadvantages

(a) It cannot be used when more than a slight undercut exists.

(b) Only sets rapidly when in a thin layer and therefore can only be used as a wash material.

(c) Will not produce a satisfactory impression of the periphery unless supported by a very accurately adapted tray.

(d) Some patients are allergic to eugenol and in these cases it may cause a chemical burn.

Indications for Use

(a) As a final wash material when using techniques which have produced a closely adapted periphery.

(b) In cases exhibiting pronounced nausea.

Composition

Advantages

(a) It can be used for compressing soft tissues.

(b) It can be added to and readapted.

(c) It can be used for any technique requiring a close peripheral seal.

(d) It can be used in combination with other materials.

Disadvantages

(a) It distorts easily and should not be used where excessive undercuts exist. It may also be distorted if any pressure is applied to it out of the mouth before it has been chilled.

(b) It does not reproduce fine surface detail.

(c) As it can be re-softened and used again it tends to be unhygienic because it cannot be sterilized easily without destroying its properties.

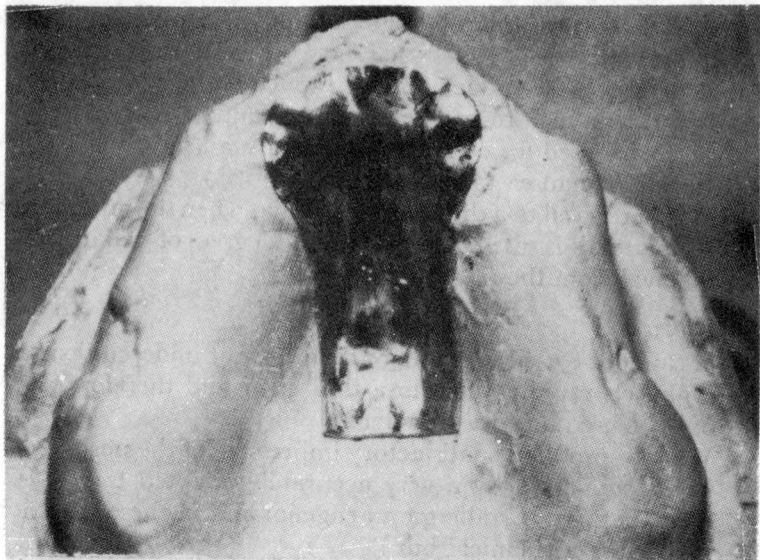

FIG. 128. - A tin foil relief for the hard tissue in the midline of the palate.

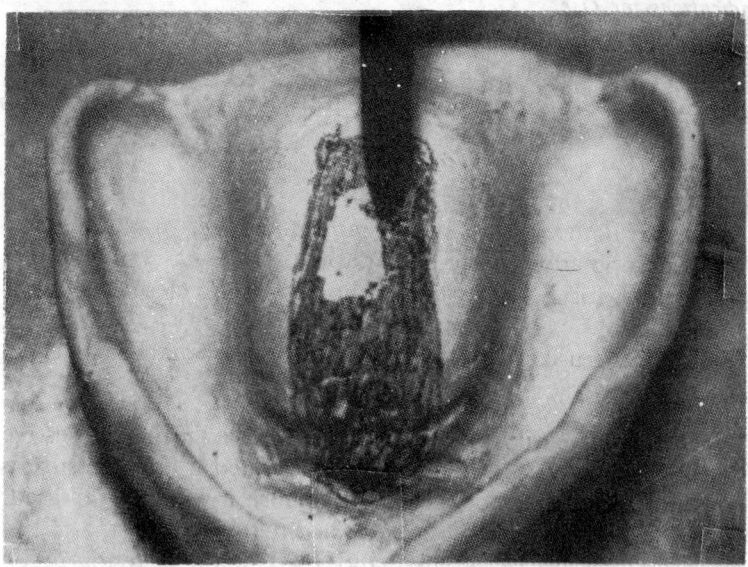

FIG. 129. - Providing relief for the hard tissues in the midline of the palate by scraping the plaster impression which has been covered with pencil lead to define the relief area.

(*d*) It can only give an accurate impression with a long and difficult technique.

Indications for Use
(*a*) For compression impressions.
(*b*) As a base in wash impression techniques.
(*c*) To obtain the maximum peripheral seal.
(*d*) As a first impression for the construction of special trays.

Relief Areas
Owing to the varying thickness of the mucous membrane on which the denture rests it is frequently necessary to relieve the denture over areas of thin mucosa in order to avoid pain and/or rocking of the denture and the commonest position requiring such relief is the mid-line raphé of the palate. Most technicians empirically relieve the centre of the palate but this leads to many unsatisfactory results as the areas needing relief are neither uniform in shape nor in position nor in the depth of relief required. The operator palpates the denture bearing area when first examining the mouth and probably decides which area will require relieving. Having taken the working impression all areas to be relieved should again be determined by careful palpation and their outline shown on the model used for constructing the special tray. The depth of the relief is dependent on the compressibility of the areas of thick mucous membrane and should be sufficient to prevent the denture from pressing on the areas of thin mucosal coverage when full masticatory loads are imposed. A simple means of conveying the information regarding depth, to the technician is to write on the model, within the outline of the relief area, the number of sheets of thin tin-foil to be used in constructing the relief (*see* fig. 128). If the working impression has been taken in plaster of Paris the outline and depth of relief can be drawn directly on the impression and the technician will blacken the whole area marked, with a soft graphite pencil and then scrape the blackened plaster away repeating the operation as many times as the figure instructs (*see* fig. 129).

Relief areas on dentures should always merge into the surrounding fitting surface and should never have a clearly defined outline such as is found in a suction chamber.

CHAPTER VI

RECORDING THE POSITION OF CENTRIC OCCLUSION

From time immemorial the procedure of recording the relationship of the mandible to the maxilla in the position of occlusion has been termed 'taking the bite'. This term is misleading for the relationship which one seeks to record is not that employed in biting or incising. A suitable term for this procedure is 'recording the position of occlusion' and therefore throughout this volume this term will be substituted for 'taking the bite' and when discussing those pieces of apparatus commonly termed 'bite blocks' the term 'record blocks' will be used which is short for blocks employed for recording the position of occlusion.

The first stage in the construction of full dentures has been described in the preceding chapter and has resulted in two models which are accurate reproductions of the denture-bearing area of the patient's mouth. Whilst the natural jaws bear a very definite relation to each other, both at rest and when functioning, the two models do not. It is the purpose of this chapter to explain how the models may be related to each other in the exact manner of their natural counterparts.

THE MAXILLO-MANDIBULAR RELATIONS

There are three relationships of the mandible to the maxilla:

(1) With the teeth in centric occlusion.
(2) With the mandible in its rest position when the teeth are always out of contact (relaxed relation).
(3) The dynamic relationship of the jaws during function.

Centric Occlusion

The maxilla is firmly united to the skull and only moves with this structure. The mandible on the other hand is attached to the skull by the two temporo-mandibular joints and is capable of opening, closing, protrusive, retrusive and lateral movements, and also combinations of any of these. The mandible is prevented from overclosing by the occlusion of the natural teeth, and it is also necessary to retrude the mandible at the conclusion of all functional movements, in order that the cusps may interdigitate. These two facts result in the mandible returning, at the conclusion of every masticatory stroke, to a position in which the cusps of the opposing teeth are in contact, and the heads of the condyles are placed as far back in the glenoid fossae as they can go without sacrificing their ability to make lateral movements. This maxillo-mandibular relation is termed centric occlusion (*see* fig. 130).

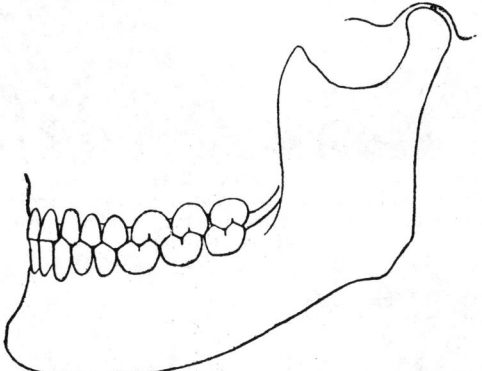

FIG. 130. – The centric occlusal position of the jaws.

The Relaxed Relation or Rest Position

When the mandible is not functioning, and provided the subject is not in a state of tension, and is breathing normally through the nose, the muscles and ligaments which are attached to the mandible support it in a relationship to the maxilla which is remarkably constant for any given individual. In this relation the heads of the condyles are fully retruded in the glenoid fossae to the extent that will allow freedom for lateral movements and the occlusal surfaces of the teeth are separated by 2–4 mm. (*see* fig. 131). The term relaxed relation is also commonly used for any relationship of the mandible to the maxilla from this physiological rest position up to but not including contact of the teeth.

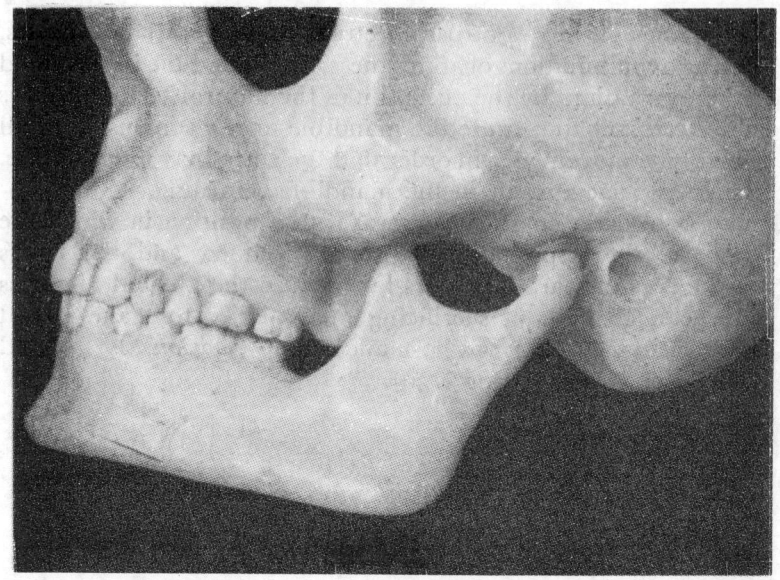

A, The relationship of the mandible to the maxilla both
vertically and horizontally dictated by the interdigitation
of the natural teeth. Note head of condyle retruded in
glenoid fossa.

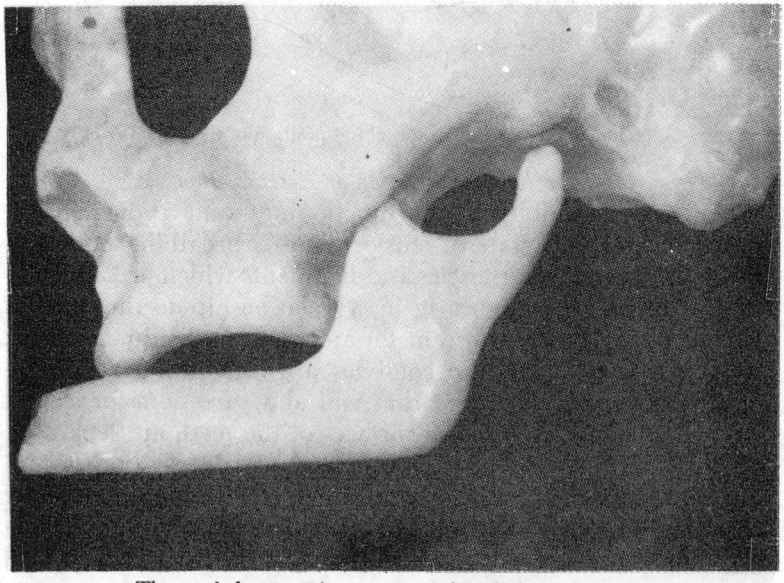

B, The teeth have all been extracted and the mandible has
no fixed relationship to the maxilla and can wander
widely both vertically and horizontally.

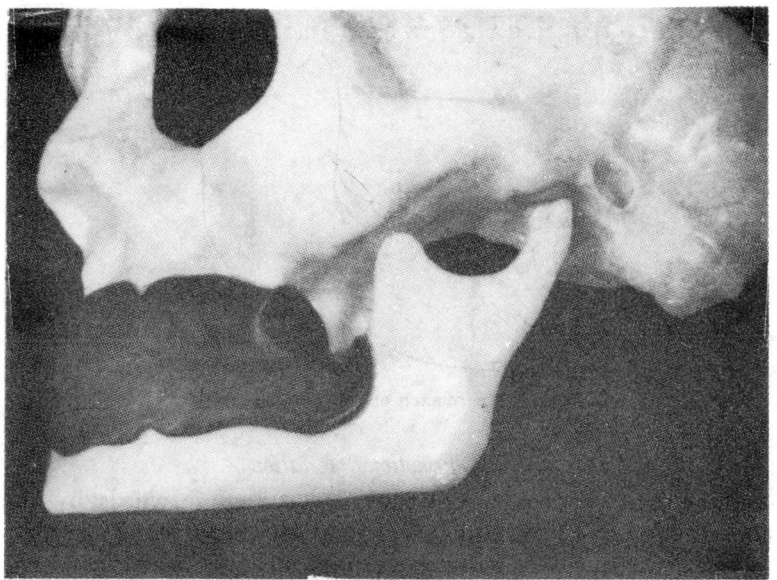

c, The record blocks have been trimmed and united to restore the relationship of the mandible to the maxilla both vertically and horizontally to that which pertained when the natural teeth were present (note the head of the condyle is retruded once again in the glenoid fossa).

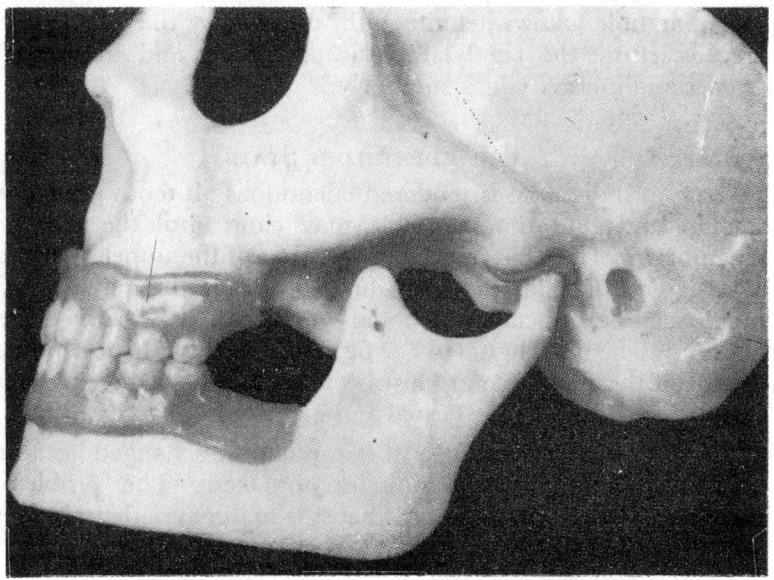

d, The finished dentures constructed to the jaw relationship given by the record blocks restore permanently the relationship of the mandible to the maxilla.

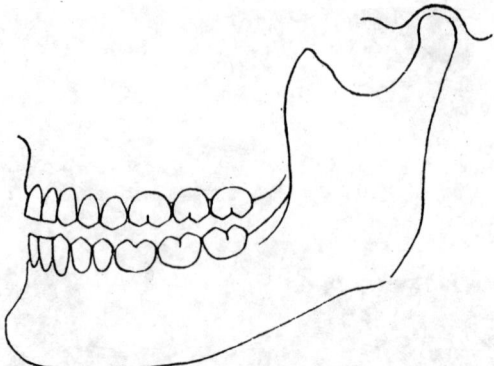

Fig. 131. – The relaxed or rest relation of the jaws.

The Functional Relation

When the mandibular condyles are drawn forwards by the contraction of the lateral pterygoid muscles, they are forced to move downwards because their superior articular surfaces, the eminentia articulares, are sloped downwards and forwards. When the occlusal surfaces of the teeth make eccentric contact during function, the cusps and incisive edges of the mandibular teeth slide up the cuspal inclines of the maxillary teeth. Thus the mandible follows definite paths dictated by the guidance it receives from the condylar paths posteriorly and the cuspal slopes and incisive edges anteriorly.

THE EDENTULOUS STATE

When an individual is rendered edentulous all tooth guidance is lost and thus the mandible may close until the mucous membrane of the lower ridge meets that of the upper. It is no longer necessary for the individual to retrude the mandible at the conclusion of each functional movement, because no cusps require to be interdigitated (see fig. 132). Finally, the functional paths of the mandible are lost because, although the condylar guidances still exist, the cuspal and incisal guides do not.

The relaxed relation is stated to remain unchanged because it is dependent on the muscles not teeth. The problem, therefore, which faces the prosthetist is to discover the relations which the mandible bore to the maxilla when the natural teeth were present and relate the models to each other in a like manner. The teeth may then be set up on the models with the knowledge that they will articulate correctly when placed in the mouth.

THE RELATIONS WHICH REQUIRE TO BE RECORDED

These depend on the type of articulator which is to be employed. Plane line articulators only require centric occlusion, while anatomical articulators require that the paths of the condyles and their relationship to the mandible be also recorded.

The difference between these two types of articulator is that the plane line permits only a hinge movement whilst the anatomical type copies functional movement (*see* figs. 133, 134).

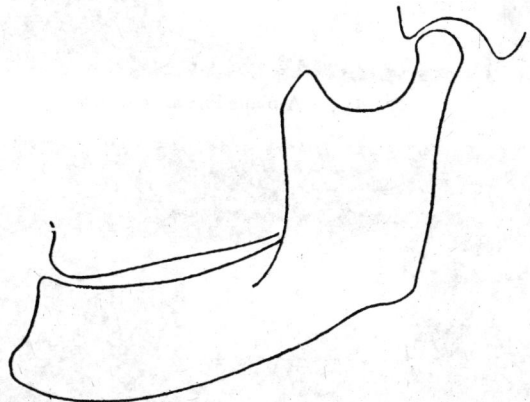

FIG. 132. – Complete loss of tooth guidance for the position of the mandible.

In addition, other facts required by the operator to enable him to construct the dentures are noted, and these will be described together with the technique employed to obtain the position of centric occlusion. Some form of simple, intra-oral apparatus is needed to register these various relationships of mandible and maxilla and before describing the technique for obtaining these positions, various types of record blocks used for this purpose will be discussed.

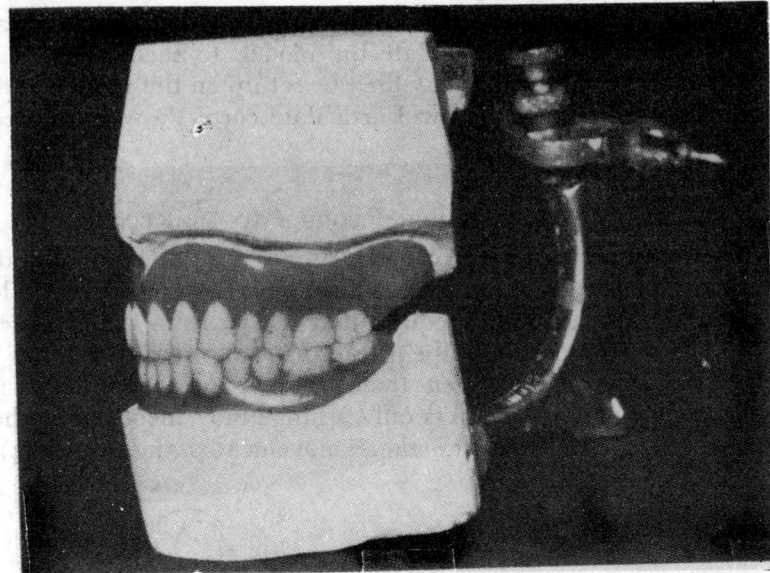

FIG. 133. – A plane line articulator.

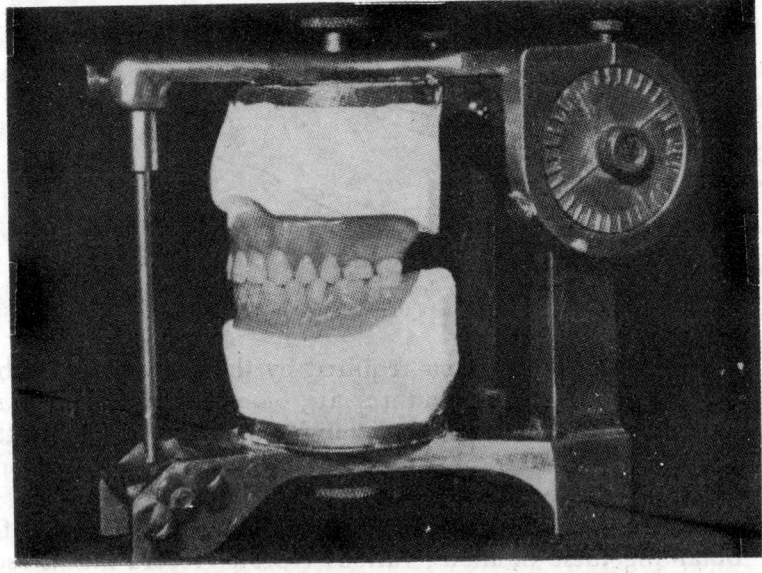

FIG. 134. – An anatomical articulator.

THE RECORD BLOCKS

These consist of two parts (*see* fig. 135):

   (1) The base-plate.
   (2) The rim.

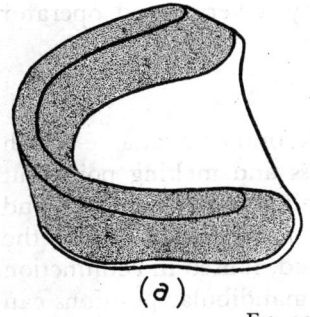
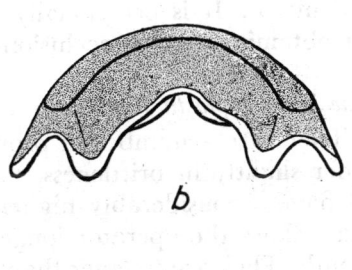

FIG. 135. – Record blocks.
(*a*) An upper.
(*b*) A lower.
In the diagram the base-plate is plain, the rim shaded.

The Base-plates

These may be divided into two classes.

   (1) Temporary.
   (2) Permanent.

Temporary base-plates are discarded and replaced by the denture base material, whilst those of the permanent group will ultimately form part of the finished denture.

Temporary base-plates may be made of:

   Wax.
   Thermo-plastic material.
   Swaged tin.
   Cold cure acrylic.

Permanent bases may be made of:

   Cast or swaged metal.
   Acrylic.

The Wax Base-plate

This type is used in conjunction with a wax rim, forming an

all wax record block, but it is a thoroughly unsuitable material for a base-plate. It softens readily at body temperature resulting in distortion during the record taking, thus preventing the accurate repositioning of the block on the model, leading to an incorrect occlusal relationship being established on the articulator. It is occasionally used by a very rapid operator for obtaining centric occlusion only.

The Thermo-plastic Base-plate

There are a number of proprietary brands available which differ slightly in brittleness, toughness and melting point but all have a considerably higher softening point than wax and thus allows the operator longer time for manipulation in the mouth. They are tougher than wax and, if used in conjunction with composition rims, recordings of mandibular positions can be obtained with a fair degree of accuracy. There are two criticisms which may be levelled against them. Firstly, being hard they tend to rub the model, and secondly they tend to warp slightly at ordinary room temperature, particularly if they were not thoroughly softened before being adapted to the model.

The Swaged Tin Base-plate

Three pieces of gauge 5 tin are swaged down, one on top of the other, on to a metal die made from the master model and trimmed similar in outline to a cast or swaged metal base. The layers of tin may be cemented together with a thin film of hard wax and the complete unit re-swaged for final adaptation to the model. The advantages of this type of base are:

(a) It does not soften at mouth temperature.

(b) It is a reasonably accurate fit.

(c) It gives a uniform thickness for the palate of the finished denture.

(d) It reproduces the rugae, to some extent.

Cold Cure Acrylic

This material may be purchased in bulk, specially for making base-plates and special trays.

The powder and liquid are mixed and allowed to form a

dough which is then pressed into a thin sheet between two pieces of polished metal or glass protected by cellophane. This sheet of acrylic is then conformed by hand or by a rubber swager to the plaster model which has previously had excessive undercuts waxed out and been painted with cold mould seal. The base-plate is roughly trimmed to shape with scissors while still soft and the final trimming is done with a revolving stone when the acrylic has polymerised.

Acrylic bases have the advantage of being a close fit and not softening or warping in the mouth.

Cast or Swaged Metal Bases

Such bases will form part of the finished denture and are, therefore, classified as permanent; any type of rim can be mounted on them according to the requirements of the case.

They are designed to cover the palate in the normal way and usually terminate at the crest of the alveolar ridges, though when there are no undercuts the ridges may be covered (see fig. 136). Buccal and labial flanges are rarely extended to the full depth of the sulci because of the difficulty of obtaining a good peripheral seal or of easing the finished denture.

They are resistant to the influences of mouth temperature and capable of withstanding the stresses and strains exerted during the trimming and recording of the occlusal relationship without distortion. The accurate fit of these bases enables the prosthetist to record mandibular movements under the best conditions possible, as displacement of the bases from the alveolar ridges is minimized, and possible error from that source avoided.

Acrylic Base (Heat Cured)

This base has the unique advantage that it enables the retention of the finished denture to be determined at this early stage, when steps can be taken to improve it if it is unsatisfactory. Its only disadvantage is that a second processing to attach the teeth causes warpage which can only be prevented by attaching the teeth to the base with cold cure acrylic.

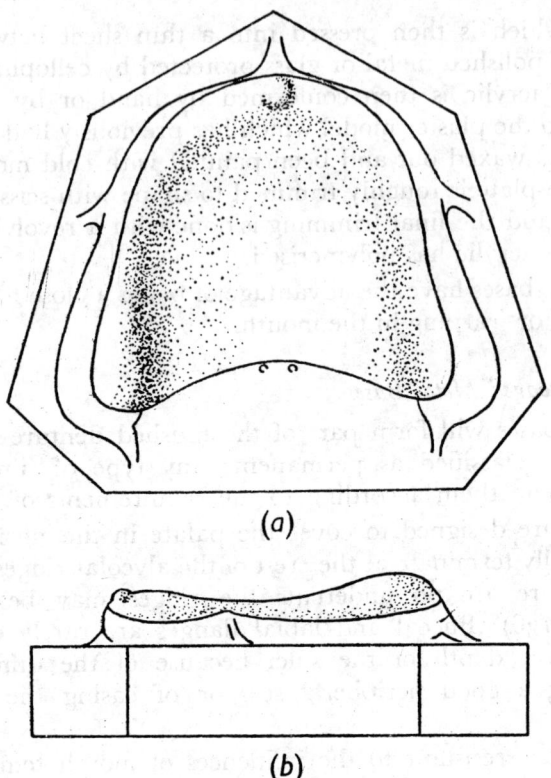

Fig. 136. – The area covered by a metal palate

(a) From above.

(b) From the side.

Record Rims

Three materials are in general use for the construction of the rims, they are:

(1) Wax.

(2) Composition.

(3) A mixture of plaster with an abrasive, such as pumice, sand, emery or carborundum.

Wax Rims

These are often used for recording the position of occlusion of those cases which will be set up on a simple, plane line type of articulator.

Advantages

(*a*) Quick.

(*b*) Simple.

Disadvantages

(*a*) They distort considerably if kept in the mouth for more than a few minutes without removal and chilling, and so can only be used satisfactorily by a rapid operator

(*b*) They are inaccurate for patients who bite hard on the blocks which readily distort under pressure and are slightly resilient.

(*c*) They soften too easily to be used with accuracy for recording lateral and protrusive positions of the mandible in addition to centric occlusion.

Composition Rims

Suitable for most cases and techniques.

Advantages

(*a*) They have a sufficiently high softening point for them to be used for any intra-oral records.

(*b*) They are not readily distorted under pressure.

Disadvantages. – Composition takes rather longer to cut and trim than does wax but the chairside time spent on trimming the rims can be very considerably reduced if a squash record is taken at the same time as the impressions. A squash record is taken by placing a roll of softened wax on the lower alveolar ridge and requesting the patient to relax and close the jaws slowly. When the operator considers that the jaws are separated by the correct distance, he tells the patient to stop closing. The wax is removed from the mouth and chilled. This does not give an accurate relationship of the jaws but enables the technician to mount the models on a plane-line articulator in approximately the correct position, and then to construct composition rims of almost the correct vertical height.

The simplest method of trimming a composition rim is to soften the occlusal surface with a pin-point flame, press it against a smooth, flat, wet surface, a glass or porcelain slab for example, and then cut away the excess which will have been squeezed out sideways before it has hardened.

Plaster and Abrasive Rims

Such rims are preformed when mandibular movements are to be recorded by the patient grinding the lower rim against the upper until an even gliding contact is produced, so shaping the surface of the rims to correspond with the path taken by the mandible in movement.

A description of this technique will be found in Chapter IX.

RECORDING CENTRIC OCCLUSION
Testing the Upper Record Block

It is essential that both the retention and the stability of the blocks are good if accurate results are to be obtained and both must be checked before starting to trim the rims. The terms retention and stability are frequently used in the following pages so in order to avoid ambiguity they will have the following meanings: Retention is the ability of a denture to remain in contact with its supporting mucosa. Stability is the ability of a denture to remain stationary in relation to its bony support. This is unobtainable with full dentures owing to the very slight compressibility of even normal mucosa when subjected to masticatory pressure but a denture is considered to be clinically stable if it remains stationary in relation to its bony support, within the bounds of compressibility of normal mucous membrane. Both these descriptions must remain true during all normal movements of mastication and speech.

Retention

The retention of an accurately adapted base is usually quite good, but it should invariably be checked for over-extension since the movement of the lips, cheeks and fraenal attachments will dislodge it if the flanges are too deep.

If the retention is not good and the base is of wax, or some other thermoplastic, distortion of the base is at once suspect, and the fit of the base on the model should be carefully inspected. When retention is poor, even with a well-fitting wax or shellac base, or any of the other materials, and there is no overextension of the flanges then the use of a little gum tragacanth to retain the record block is indicated, provided that the operator does not suspect an inaccurate impression as being the cause of the lack of retention.

Stability

This may be tested by alternate finger pressure on the rim of either side of the mouth and if the base tends to rock it may be due to the rim being mounted outside the centre of the ridge or to insufficient relief in the centre of the palate. Whichever is the cause it must be corrected before proceeding.

A word of explanation is required here since the above paragraph apparently contradicts the statements regarding the position to be occupied by the artificial teeth (p. 236 *et seq.*). Record blocks are constructed with flat occlusal surfaces and therefore any pressure on them will be almost vertical: in order to resist this pressure they must be placed over the centres of the supporting ridges though this may not be the position which the artificial teeth will occupy. Encroachment on the tongue space with resultant instability is of minor importance at this stage as no functional movements will be required.

Trimming the Upper Record Block

When trimming the rim there are four main considerations and they must be taken in the following order:

1. *Labial Fullness*

The lip is normally supported by the alveolar ridge and teeth, which at this stage are represented by the base and rim of the record block, therefore the labial surface must be cut down or added to until a natural and pleasing position of the upper lips is obtained. The lip line (that is, a straight line just in contact with the inferior border of the upper lip when relaxed) will be raised if the labial surface of the block is too bulky and will be lowered if the support is inadequate (*see* fig. 137).

2. *The Height of the Rim*

The technician will mount the incisor teeth with their incisive edges in the same position as the occlusal surface of the upper record rim which must, therefore, be trimmed vertically until it represents the amount of the anterior teeth which it is desired to show below the lip at rest. The average adult

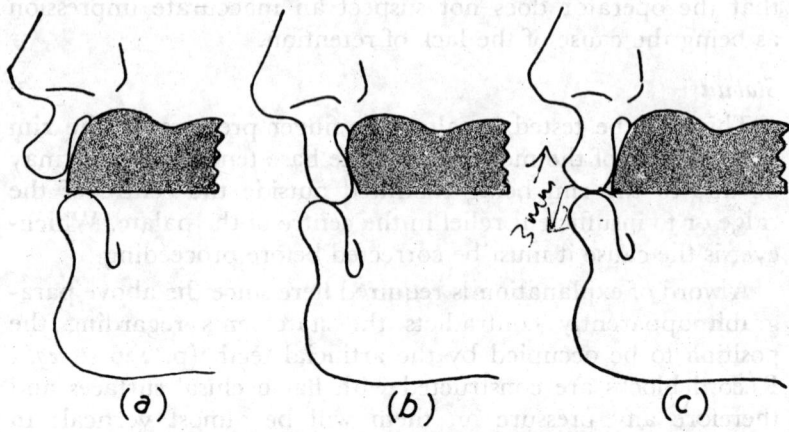

FIG. 137. – Diagram illustrating the effect of the labial bulk of the upper record block on the position of the upper lip and its inferior border.

(a) Too full.
(b) Not full enough.
(c) Correct.

shows approximately 3 mm. of the upper central incisors when the lips are just parted, but there are many variations from this amount which should be accepted as a guide rather than a rule (see fig. 138). A greater length of tooth than normal will be shown if the patient has:

(a) A short upper lip.
(b) Superior protrusion.

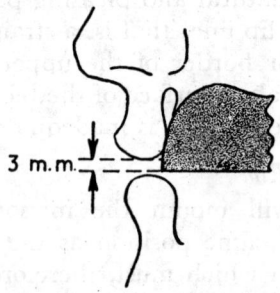

3 m.m.

FIG. 138. – Illustrating the amount of the upper record rim which should be visible below the upper lip in the average case.

And less will be shown:

(*a*) With a long upper lip.

(*b*) In most old people, owing to the attrition of the natural teeth and some loss of tone of the orbicularis oris muscle.

3. The Anterior Plane

Since the upper anterior teeth are set-up with their incisive edges in the same position as the occlusal surface of the record rim, it is important for the anterior plane of this rim to be trimmed level. If the anterior teeth are set to a plane which drops to one side of the mouth the appearance may be displeasing. Generally the plane to which the anterior teeth should be set, and to which the rim must be trimmed, is parallel to an imaginary line joining the pupils of the eyes or the supra-orbital ridge (*see* fig. 139). Sometimes the lip line or, very

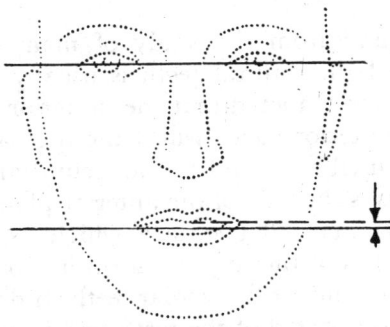

Fig. 139. – Illustrating the plane parallel to which the upper record rim should be trimmed. Space between arrows indicates the amount of rim showing below upper lip.

rarely the interpupillary line, will be found to have a distinct drop to one side of the face, in which case the operator will have to locate his anterior plane by his aesthetic judgment.

4. The Anteroposterior Plane

This plane indicates the position of the occlusal surfaces of the posterior teeth and is obtained in conjunction with the anterior plane. The rim is trimmed parallel to the naso-auricular line (*see* fig. 140) (an imaginary line running from the external auditory meatus to the lower border of the ala of the nose).

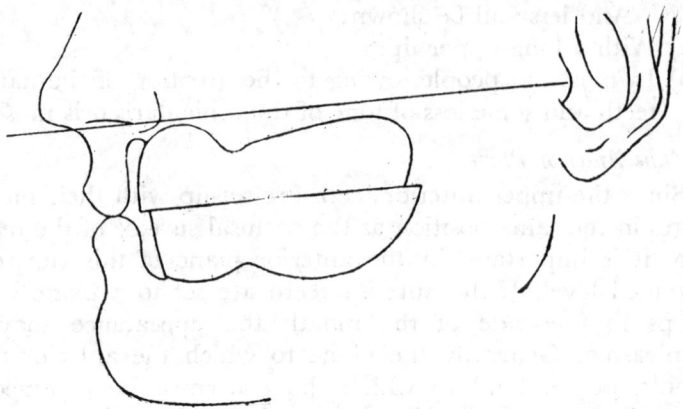

Fig. 140. – Illustrating the imaginary naso-auricular line and the manner in which the rims are trimmed parallel to this line.

It has been found from the study of many cases that the occlusal plane of the natural teeth is usually parallel to this line It must be remembered that the posterior teeth are set to a slight anteroposterior curve whilst the naso-auricular line is straight, and is used as an aid to the technician rather than a fixed position, as is the case of the anterior plane. The occlusal plane is an imaginary flat surface which extends from the mesio-incisal angles of the upper central incisors to the mesio-palatal cusps of the upper first molar teeth. It does not coincide with the occlusal surfaces of the teeth and its main use is as a fixed position to which to refer when describing the position of individual teeth or other structures.

Thus, when the rim has been trimmed to these planes it indicates the plane of orientation for setting-up the artificial teeth, and when this has been done to the satisfaction of the operator, attention is focused on the position occupied by the posterior palatal border of the base.

The Position of the Posterior Palatal Border

It will be remembered from the discussion on the retention of full dentures that an adequate seal must be obtained along this border if the upper denture is to be prevented from tipping when pressure is applied to the palatal surfaces, or incisive

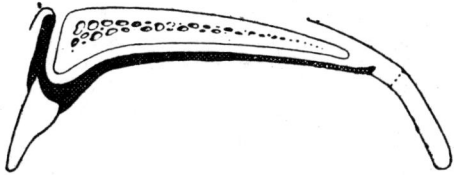

FIG. 141. – Correct placing of the posterior border of the upper denture just on to the non-movable part of the soft palate. The dotted line indicates the vibrating line, the point behind which movement of the soft palate occurs.

edges, of the front teeth. The seal must be situated in the region of compressible tissue just distal to the hard palate, but it must be anterior to the vibrating line (the line from which visible movement of the soft palate takes place), and this is of great importance (*see* fig. 141). If the back edge of the denture extends posteriorly beyond this vibrating line, the seal will be broken when the soft palate rises during deglutition and speech, and the denture will momentarily become loose and may drop; the patient is also likely to complain of nausea. If the posterior palatal border does not reach this compressible area, retention will be poor because the seal will be inefficient and again the patient may complain of nausea since the edge of the denture may irritate the posterior third of the tongue as it will not bed into the tissues.

The operator first discovers the position of this vibrating line by asking the patient to say a prolonged 'ah', with the mouth widely opened, and noting the line from which the soft palate moves. For future reference it is useful to mark this line on the palate with an indelible pencil. The tissue in front of this line is explored with a blunt instrument and the area of soft compressible tissue noted. In some cases this area may extend for several millimetres before merging with the thinner and denser tissue which commonly covers the hard palate, whilst in other cases only a small margin between the vibrating line and the less compressible tissue of the hard palate will exist (*see* fig. 142).

Another method of finding the post-dam area is to press the blunt surface of a ball-ended instrument, gently against the hard palate and gradually work backwards until a compressible area

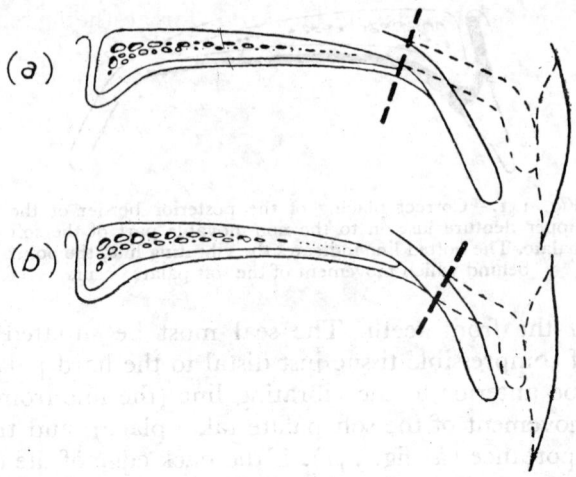

FIG. 142. – Sagittal diagram illustrating variations in the position of the vibrating line of the soft palate (marked by broken line).

(a) Movement occurs at the soft-hard palate junction.

(b) Movement occurs some distance behind the soft-hard palate junction.

is discovered, then note its relation to the previously marked vibrating line.

The posterior border can be located with great accuracy if it is possible to see the two small pits (foveae palatinae) one on either side of the mid-line on the anterior part of the soft palate. The foveae are usually, though not invariably, present, and are situated just anterior to the vibrating line, thus marking the posterior limit of the denture.

The posterior border of the record block is adjusted by trimming or by adding wax, to coincide with the position which has been selected for post-damming.

The adjustments to the upper block are complete with the recording of certain guide lines of which the first to be mentioned is essential, and the other two optional.

Guide Lines

(1) *The Centre Line*

In the normal natural dentition the upper central incisors have their mesial surfaces in contact with an imaginary vertical line which bisects the face and, for aesthetic reasons, it is desirable that the artificial substitutes should occupy the same position. If this centre line is not clearly marked on the labial surface of the upper record rim, the technician has tc depend on the position of the incisive papilla or the labial fraenum as denoted on his model, and whilst these landmarks are usually found in the mid-line this is not invariable. If, at the try-in stage, the mid-line is found to be incorrect, then both the upper and lower dentures will have to be entirely re-set to correct it, a considerable waste of time for patient, operator and technician.

No human face is symmetrical, therefore there can be no hard and fast rule for determining the centre line, which thus depends upon the artistic judgment of the individual operator. The following aids have been suggested as being likely to help the prosthetist in coming to a decision.

A vertical line is scored on the labial surface of the upper rim:

(a) Where it is crossed by an imaginary line from the centre of the brows to the centre of the chin.

(b) Immediately below the centre of the philtrum.

(c) Immediately below the centre of the labial tubercle.

(d) At the bisection of the line from corner to corner of the mouth when the lips are relaxed.

(e) Where it is crossed by a line at right angles to the inter-pupillary line from a point mid-way between the pupils when the patient is looking directly forwards (*see* fig. 143).

The accuracy of the centre line marking is best judged from a position directly in front of the patient and a little distance away.

(2) *The High Lip Line*

This is a line just in contact with the lower border of the upper lip when it is raised as high as possible unaided, as in smiling or laughing. It is marked on the labial surface of the rim and indicates the amount of the denture which may be seen under normal conditions, and thus assists in determining

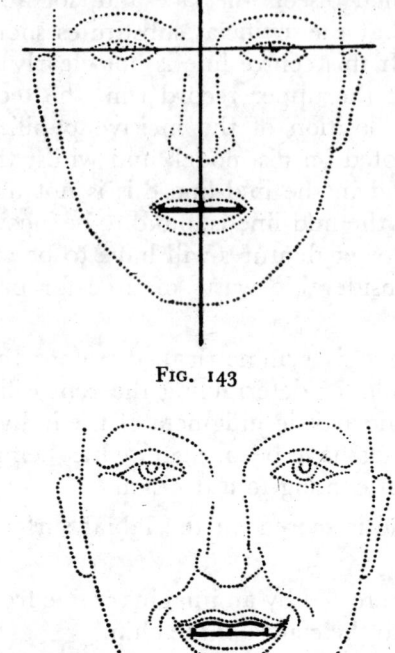

FIG. 143

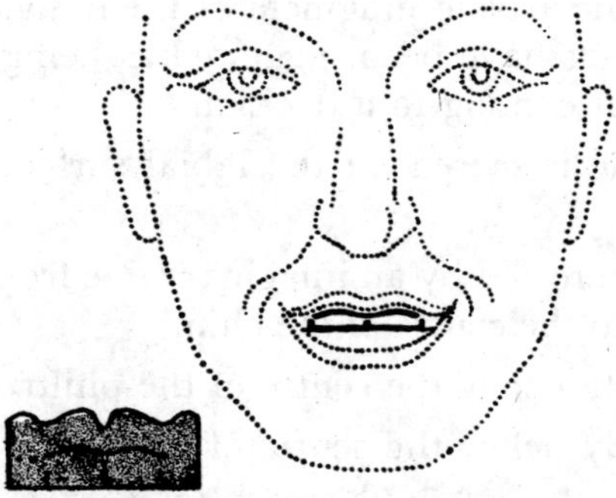

FIG. 144. – Illustrating the high lip line, centre line, and two corner lines, marked on the record rim, both in and out of the mouth.

the length of tooth needed (*see* fig. 144). This line was of considerable importance when pink vulcanite was the only facing material available and its unnatural appearance made longer teeth preferable. Methyl-methacrylate does not suffer from this disadvantage.

(3) *The Corner Lines*

These mark the corners of the mouth when the lips are relaxed and are supposed to coincide with the tips of the upper canine teeth but are only accurate to within 3 or 4 mm. These lines give some indication of the width to be taken up by the six anterior teeth from tip to tip of the canines (*see* fig. 144).

Having trimmed and marked the upper block, all that now requires to be done is to trim the lower so that when it occludes evenly with the upper, the lower jaw will be separated from the upper by the same distance that it was when the natural teeth were in occlusion; or as near to this distance as it is possible to obtain. If, now, the mandible is made to assume its retruded position with the rims of the blocks in contact, and these are sealed together in this position, then the position of centric occlusion will have been recorded.

It will be appreciated, therefore, that two dimensions are involved in the recording of centric occlusion, these are:

(1) The vertical dimension. This is the distance by which the jaws are separated.

(2) The horizontal relationship. This is the relationship of the mandible to the maxilla (in the horizontal plane) when the condyles of the mandible are as fully retruded in the glenoid fossae as is possible without sacrificing their ability to make lateral movements.

There are thus two more stages to be completed in recording centric occlusion. The first is to trim the lower block so that it occludes evenly with the upper at the correct vertical height, and the second is to unite the blocks with the mandible retruded.

Trimming the Lower Record Block

The block should first be tested for retention and stability as was done for the upper, and if these are unsatisfactory they must be remedied before proceeding.

Next, the occlusal surface of the rim is adjusted so that when it is in even contact all round with the upper rim the jaws are separated by the required distance. In most instances the rim of the lower block will be too high and require to be reduced, but occasionally it may be too low and require building up by the addition of wax or composition.

The Vertical Dimension

As mentioned at the beginning of this chapter, there is normally a gap of 2 to 3 mm. between the occlusal surfaces of the teeth when the mandible is in the rest position, and this gap is called

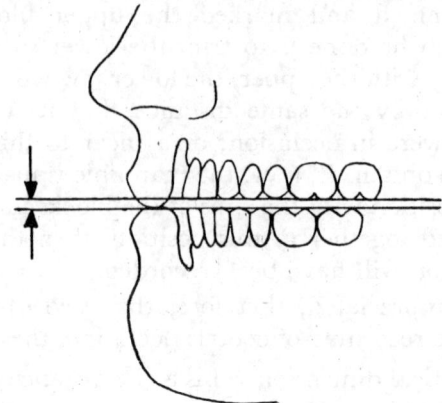

FIG. 145(*a*). – The freeway space.

the freeway space (*see* figs. 145 (*a*) and (*b*)). Probably the best technique is to record the rest position with the rims in contact and then remove the thickness of the desired freeway space from the occlusal surface of the lower block (*see* fig. 146).

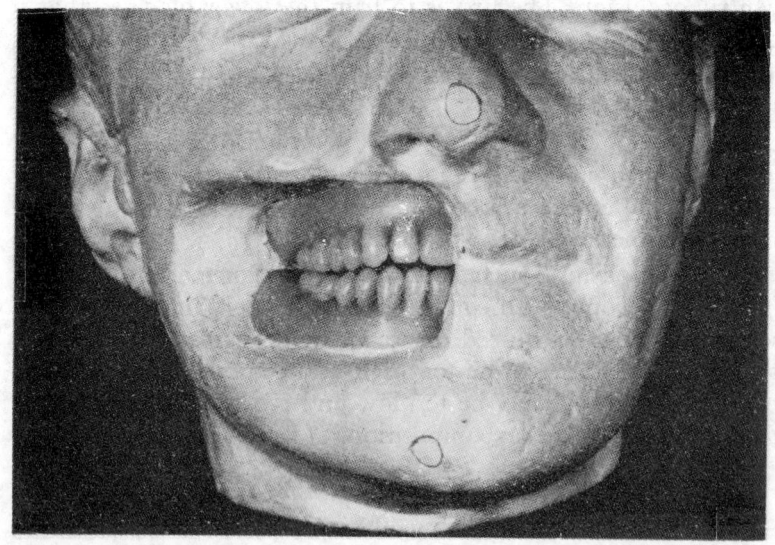

FIG. 145(*b*). – Dentures in mouth : mandible in relaxed position.
Note freeway space.

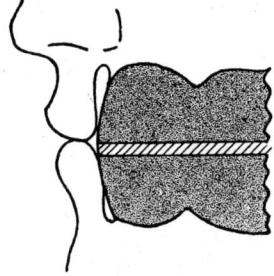

FIG. 146. – Illustrating the rest position of the mandible with the rims in contact. If the ruled section is removed from the lower rim that amount of freeway space will be provided.

Whilst many operators of experience rely solely on their judgment of the patient's appearance for obtaining this vertical dimension, many aids are available to help the less skilful or less artistic operator, but these are 'aids' and not accurate measurements.

(1) *Freeway Space Measurement*

Of the several aids about to be described, this is probably the most useful, but it must be remembered that this is merely a help and must not be relied on as being accurate. The technique is split up into stages for ease of description.

(*a*) Make a thin horizontal line or pin-head-sized mark on the tip of the patient's nose and another on the point of his chin selecting, in the latter position, an area where there is the least movement of the soft tissues (*see* fig. 147). These marks should not be made with an indelible pencil as they are too difficult to remove, but grease paint or charcoal will be found to be quite suitable. Alternatively, a piece of adhesive plaster may be placed on the nose and chin and the marks made on these.

(*b*) The patient must be comfortably seated in the chair and asked to relax his whole body as completely as possible and allow his jaw to rest in a comfortable position with the lips closed. When this position is achieved, measure the distance between the marks either with a pair of dividers or a millimetre rule (*see* fig. 147).

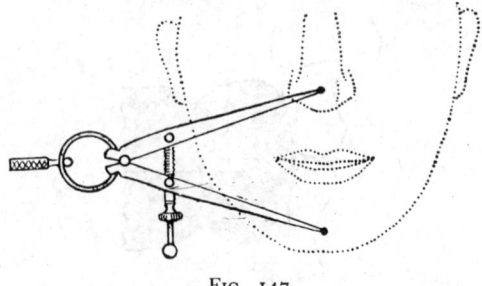

FIG. 147

(*c*) Ask the patient to moisten his lips with his tongue and then close them to a comfortable position. Check the measurement previously obtained.

(*d*) Ask the patient to swallow and relax without separating the lips. Again check the measurements.

(*e*) Ask the patient to repeat the letter 'M' several times, finishing in the middle of the last 'M': that is, not completing the sound by separating the lips. Again check. Any, or all, of these methods of obtaining a relaxed position must be repeated, until at least three constant readings are obtained.

(*f*) Insert the record blocks and trim the occlusal surface of the lower until it occludes evenly with that of the upper, when the distance between the marks is that of the constant reading. Such trimming may be facilitated if the surface of the lower block is softened by flaming and the patient asked to close it against the upper (*see* fig. 148).

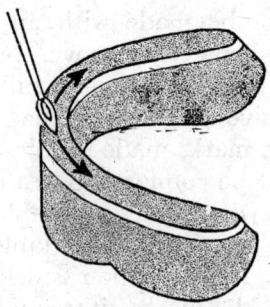

FIG 148. - Heating the surface of the record rim.

(g) Produce a freeway space by removing a further 2 or 3 mm. from the lower record rim.

(h) Check the existence of this freeway space by asking the patient to relax with the record blocks in his mouth and with his lips closed. Then ask the patient to close the blocks together, when a slight but definite movement of the chin will take place, if there is an adequate freeway space (*see* fig. 149). An intelligent patient may be questioned as to whether the blocks are in contact or not, when he is relaxed.

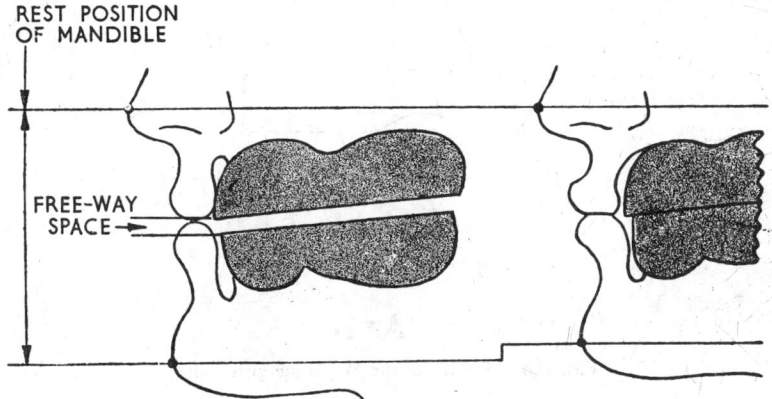

REST POSITION OF MANDIBLE

FREE-WAY SPACE →

FIG. 149. – The freeway space.

The first diagram illustrates the rest position of the mandible showing the rims parted.
The second diagram illustrates the small upward movement of the chin which occurs when the rims occlude.

Errors in this technique are due to the marks having to be made on soft tissue which is always movable to some extent.

(2) *Willis' Measurement*

This is a proportional measurement which is taught in art schools, and whilst it is true that a drawing made to these dimensions will be pleasing in its proportions there are many individuals whose faces, though not appearing in any way distorted, do not conform to these somewhat ideal limits. It is easy to take these measurements with accuracy on a two-dimensional drawing, but two different operators will rarely agree on a patient's measurements to within a few millimetres.

The theory of this measurement is that the distance from the lower border of the septum of the nose to the lower border of the chin is equal to the distance from the outer canthus of the eye to the corner of the relaxed lips in each case with the mandible in its position of rest with the teeth out of occlusion (*see* fig. 150).

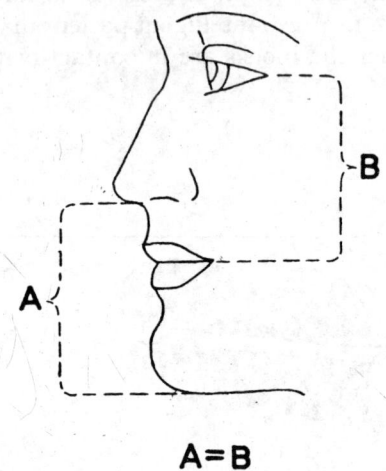

A=B

FIG. 150. – Details of the Willis measurement.

(3) *Ridge Relationship*

Sears suggests that an indication of the correct vertical height can be obtained from the parallelism of the upper and lower posterior ridges. Excessive divergence from the parallel, seen when the models have been set on an articulator, indicates that the vertical height is probably wrong and should again be checked.

INCORRECT VERTICAL DIMENSION

Up to this point the emphasis has been on the patient's facial appearance, because it is largely by this means that the correct vertical height is judged, but the effects of an incorrect height are greater than merely an unsatisfactory appearance. The degree of error, either of over-opening or of over-closing, necessary to produce any of the following results, cannot be given because a very small deviation from the normal occlusal position will produce symptoms in one patient, whilst a greater deviation will be tolerated with comfort by another.

EFFECTS OF EXCESSIVELY INCREASING THE VERTICAL DIMENSION

1. *Discomfort*

The patient has acquired, over a period of many years, a cortical pattern which controls, automatically and unconsciously, certain muscular movements, amongst them being those of the tongue and mandible when eating and talking. An example, which can be readily appreciated, of this unconscious control will be found in the act of running up a flight of stairs. The steps being all the same distance apart, one's weight is taken evenly and smoothly on each successive stair without any conscious thought, but if, without one's previous knowledge, one tread is at a different height from the others, a very nasty jar will result. In an exactly similar way, the pressure is smoothly and gradually applied to the food between the teeth when eating, but if the height of a tooth is altered, for example by a lead shot resting on the occlusal surface, a very unpleasant jar will draw attention to what is normally a purely automatic movement. By altering the vertical height the environment in which these unconscious movements take place has been altered and, until a new cortical pattern has been established, considerable discomfort will be caused.

2. *Trauma*

The jarring effect of the teeth coming into contact sooner than expected may cause only discomfort, but in most cases it will also cause pain owing to the bruising of the mucous membrane by these sudden and frequent blows. Particularly is this so under the lower denture whose area to resist pressure is so much less than the upper. Easing the fitting surface over sore areas does not cure this trouble, it only destroys the fit in one part and increases the pressure in another.

3. *Loss of Freeway Space*

Loss of the normal space between the occlusal surfaces of

the teeth, when the mandible is in the rest position, may have several effects, one of which is nearly always annoyance from the inability to find a comfortable resting position. Other effects may be trauma caused by the constant pressure on the mucous membrane, and muscular fatigue of any one, or any group, of the muscles of mastication.

4. Clicking Teeth

The tongue has become accustomed to the presence of teeth in certain fixed positions, and during speech helps to produce sounds without the teeth coming into contact. When, however, these teeth are raised, due to too great a vertical height, opposing cusps frequently meet each other, producing an embarrassing clicking or clattering sound. This same effect is also often produced during eating, but is not so obvious as it is muffled by the food.

5. Appearance

The result of over-opening must be an elongation of the face, but if it is only slight it will usually pass unnoticed. What will, however, generally be obvious, is that at rest the lips are parted, and that closing them together will produce an expression of strain (see fig. 151).

EFFECTS OF EXCESSIVELY REDUCING THE VERTICAL DIMENSION

1. Inefficiency

This is due to the fact that the pressure which it is possible to exert with the teeth in contact decreases considerably with over-closure because the muscles of mastication are acting from attachments which have been brought closer together.

2. Cheek Biting

In some cases where there is a loss of muscular tone, as well as a reduced vertical height, the flabby cheeks tend to become trapped between the teeth and bitten during mastication. When the over-closure has been deliberate, it is possible to avoid this cheek biting by setting the upper posterior teeth more buccally than normal, thus producing a greater overjet. Also by plumping the buccal flange of the denture the cheek may be given added support (see fig. 152).

(a)

(b)

(c)

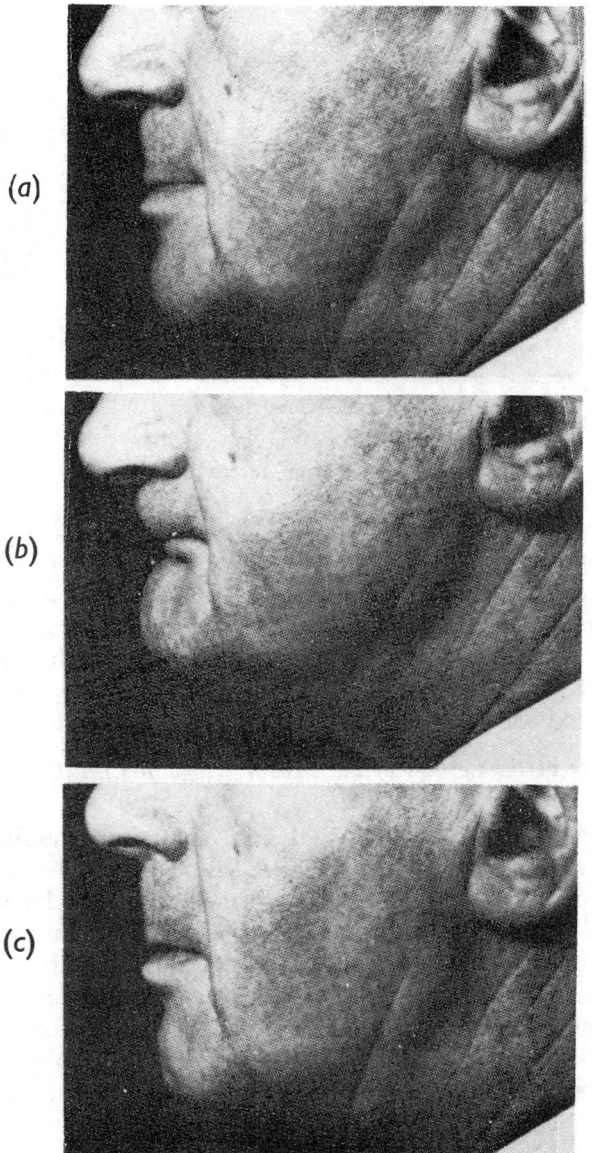

FIG. 151. – Profile view illustrating effect of alteration of
vertical dimension on appearance:
(a) Correct dimension.
(b) Closed.
(c) Open (note parting of lips).

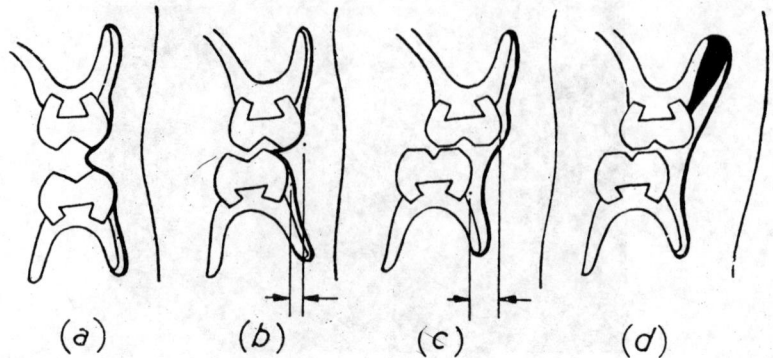

FIG. 152. – Cheek biting.
(a) How it occurs.
(b) Illustrating small buccal overjet.
(c) Increased buccal overjet to prevent biting.
(d) Plumping buccal flange.
          (Plumped part is shown in black.)

3. *Appearance*

The general effect of over-closure on facial appearance is of increased age: there is closer approximation of nose to chin, the soft tissues sag and fall in, and the lines on the face are deepened. The greater the degree of over-closure, the more exaggerated are these effects.

4. *Soreness at the Corners of the Mouth (Angular Cheilitis) (see* fig. 153)

Over closure of the vertical height sometimes results in a falling in of the corners of the mouth beyond the vermilion border and the deep fold thus formed becomes bathed in saliva: this area may become infected and sore and is then difficult to cure whilst it remains moist. Opening the vertical height restores the corners of the mouth to their normal position, sometimes producing a marked improvement or cure. A deep natural fold cannot be eliminated by this means and in no case must the increased vertical height excede the free way space.

5. *Pain in the Temporo-mandibular Joint*

In cases of gross over-closure of the jaws, pain in the temporo-mandibular joint may occur, probably due to strain of the

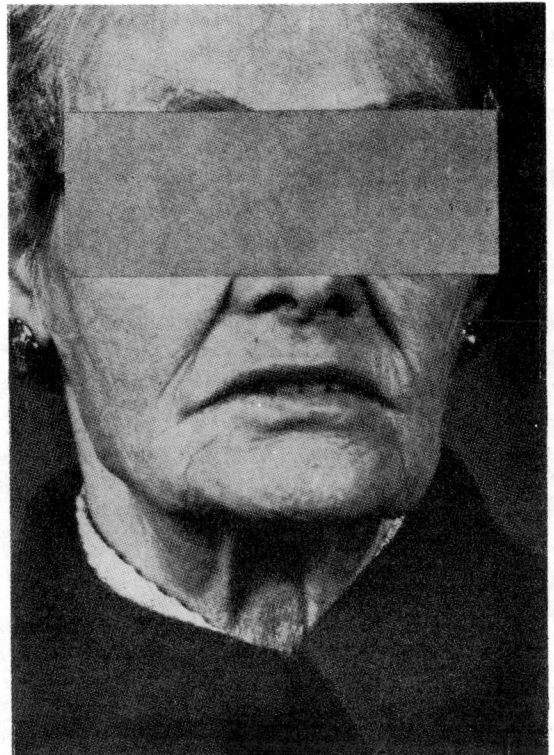

Fig. 153(*a*). – Soreness at the corners of the mouth. Note how the corners of the lips have fallen in.

joint and associated ligaments, which may be relieved by restoration of the correct vertical dimension

6. *Costen's Syndrome*

Costen's syndrome is stated to be the result of prolonged over-closure, though his explanation of how these symptoms are produced is now doubted. It consists of:

(*a*) Mild catarrhal deafness and dizzy spells which are relieved by inflation of the eustachian tubes.

(*b*) Tinnitus, or at times a snapping noise in the joint which is experienced while chewing. Painful, limited or excessive movements of the affected joint.

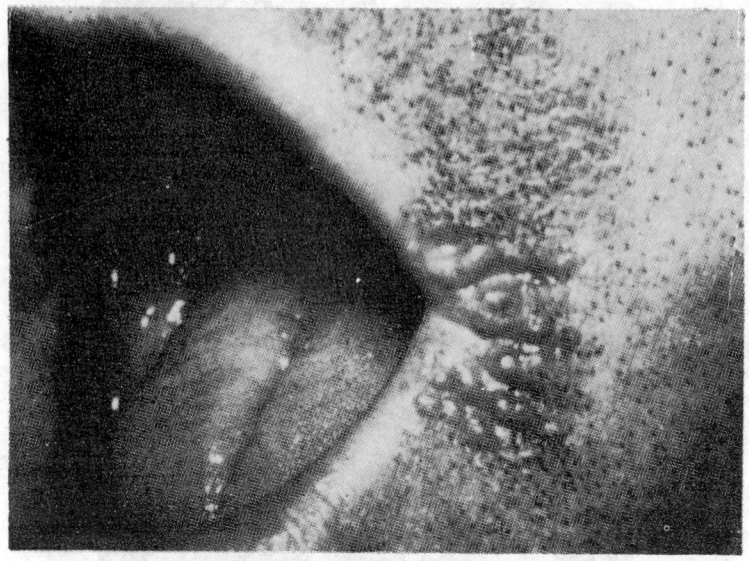

FIG. 153(*b*). – Close up of a chronic angular cheilitis.

(*c*) Tenderness to palpation over the temporo-mandibular joint or dull pains.

(*d*) Various neuralgic symptoms such as burning or prickling sensation of the tongue, throat and side of the nose. Various forms of atypical head pain, particularly that referred to the temporal region or the base of the skull.

(*e*) Dryness of the mouth due to disturbed salivary gland function.

PRE-EXTRACTION RECORDS

In practice the dental surgeon will usually either extract the teeth and construct dentures, or replace existing dentures; it is not often that patients present themselves for treatment without either natural or artificial teeth. When the dental surgeon is rendering a patient edentulous he has the opportunity for recording the vertical dimension and the position and shape of the teeth before they are extracted. The following methods may be used to obtain this information:

1. *The Dakometer*

This instrument records both the vertical dimension with the natural teeth in occlusion and the position of the upper central incisors; in most cases recordings can be obtained with an error range of $\pm$ 1 mm. The instrument is used as follows (*see* fig. 154):

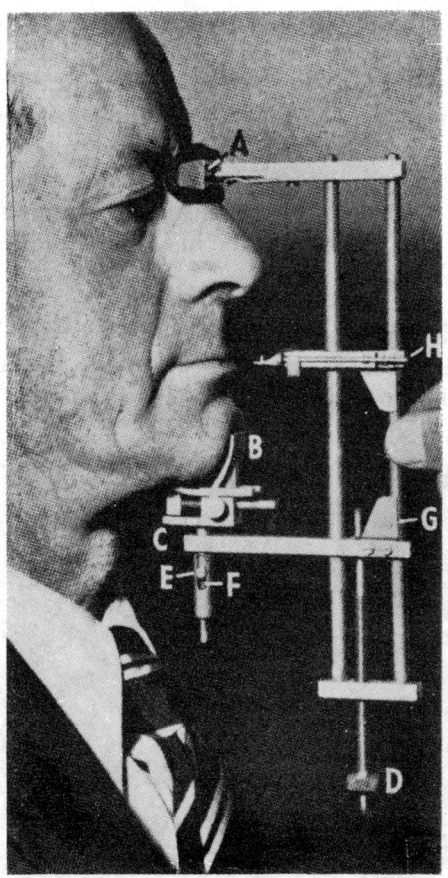

Fig. 154. – The Dakometer in position.

Press a piece of softened composition into the carrier (A) and, with the instrument in position, mould it into the depression at the bridge of the nose; the member (B) of the chin piece (C) is adjusted to rest on the skin covering the front of the chin. Remove the dakometer and chill the composition. Replace the instrument holding the composition carrier firmly in position, and, whilst the patient maintains centric occlusion, the chin-piece is screwed up by the screw (D) until the indicator on the spring pressure gauge (E) corresponds with the line on the sleeve (F). Take the readings on the vertical scale (G) and on the chin support (C). Finally, adjust and record the vertical and horizontal positions of the incisor attachment (H) by moving it until the 'L'-shaped terminal engages the incisal edges of the upper centrals. The readings are noted on the patient's chart and the composition nose-piece preserved for that patient, so that the whole instrument can be reassembled when taking the records after he has been rendered edentulous.

2. *The Willis' Gauge*

When this is used for recording the vertical height before extraction, the arm (A) (*see* fig. 155) is placed in contact with the base of the nose and the arm (B) is moved along the slide

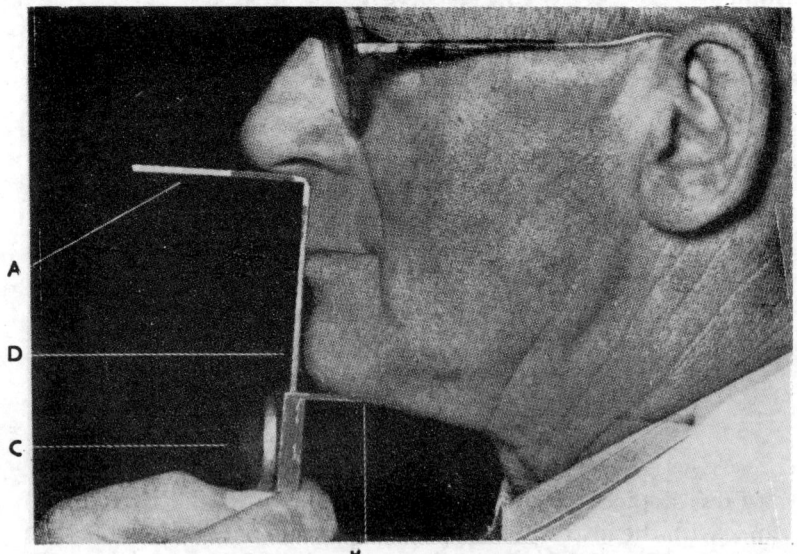

Fig. 155. – The Willis' gauge in place on the face.

(D) until it is lightly but firmly touching the lower border of the chin, when it is locked in position by the screw (C). The distance on the scale (D) is recorded on the patient's chart.

This is not a very accurate measurement; it depends on the operator always applying exactly the same degree of pressure when the instrument is making contact with the base of the nose and with the undersurface of the chin.

3. *Profile Tracing*

A piece of soft lead wire is moulded to the contour of the face starting on the brow, following down the nose and lips and ending just below the chin (*see* fig. 156). It is then carefully laid on a piece of stout card or thin wood, the outline pencilled in and the profile cut out. This template is then placed on the face to check its accuracy and to mark the position of the upper central incisors.

With the template held in contact with the face, a mark is made which corresponds with the incisive edge of the centrals. A line is drawn from this mark at right angles to the straight edge of the card, and on this line a second mark is made. The distance from the second mark to the labial surface of the central incisor is noted (*see* fig. 157).

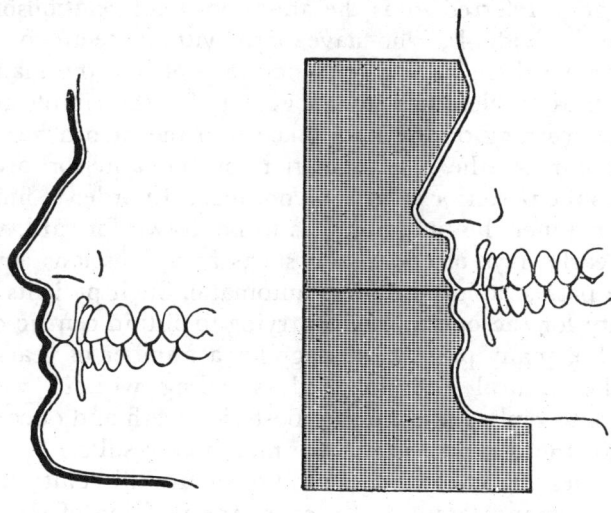

FIG. 156   FIG. 157

Any further information, such as name, address, date, colour and shape of the teeth, etc., can be entered on the template and filed away for future reference: being flat they take up little storage space.

With a little practice very useful measurements can be taken by this method which is probably one of the easiest and quickest ways for obtaining pre-extraction records.

4. Articulated Models

These will indicate the amount of overbite as well as assisting in the selection of size, shape and position of the teeth to be used for the dentures. An even more satisfactory method is to take composition impressions immediately prior to the extraction of the teeth, which are then extracted, sterilized, and inserted into the impression. The models thus obtained contain the natural teeth in their original position, but cannot be used as a record of their shade because this is changed due to loss of vitality.

THE HORIZONTAL RELATIONSHIP

Having discussed the vertical dimension there still remains the horizontal relation of the mandible to the maxilla to be found, often referred to as the anteroposterior relationship.

Many individuals, who have been without teeth for some considerable time, have a tendency to protrude the mandible when asked to close the jaws together, for the simple reason that the crushing of any food taken into the mouth has to be carried out by the approximation of the anterior alveolar ridges as the posterior ridges will not meet. In order to function in this manner the mandible has to be drawn forward, which in the early days of edentation starts as a conscious act, but as time passes rapidly becomes automatic. Such patients cause difficulty for the operator when trying to obtain centric occlusion. Also, many patients manage for a number of years with only the natural anterior teeth standing without wearing dentures to replace the missing posterior teeth and once again an unconscious protrusion of the mandible results.

Both these habit-forming conditions cause difficulty for the operator when attempting to secure the position of retrusion.

Sometimes it is desirable to record the acquired position instead of the true position, and this is discussed in Chapter III, but it is only the true retruded position which is being considered here.

Stress has purposely been laid on the difficulty to be expected in many cases in obtaining a correct retrusive record, because great patience will often be needed as satisfactory dentures cannot be constructed unless the record is correct.

There are many aids to help the prosthetist to obtain the retruded position and where one fails another may well succeed, such aids are·

1. *Instructions to the Patient*

Always ask the patient to 'close', never ask him to 'bite'. 'Bite' conveys the impression of incising, and to incise requires some protrusion of the jaw, which is just the reverse of what is required.

2. *Tongue Retrusion*

Ask the patient to place the tip of the tongue as far back on the palate as possible, to keep it there and close the blocks together until they meet (*see* fig. 158). Some patients have a tendency to let the tongue move forward and it is often helpful

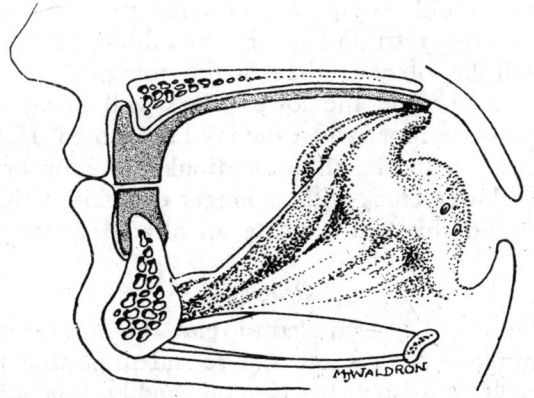

FIG. 158. – Illustrating the position which the tongue should assume when closing the blocks to obtain the retrusive record.

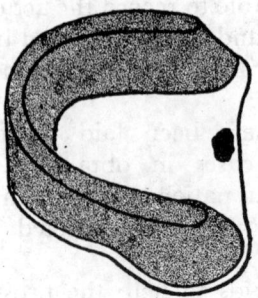

FIG. 159

to put a small knob of composition near the posterior border of the upper record block (*see* fig. 159). The position of the composition should be shown to the patient before the record block is inserted in the mouth and when the block is in place the patient is requested to place the tip of the tongue in contact with the composition and keep it there whilst he closes. The reason behind this suggestion is that the tongue, when in this position, will exert a muscular pull on the mandible, in a backward direction.

As soon as it is considered that the rims are in retrusive occlusion, two approximately vertical lines should be scored on their buccal aspects one on either side in the premolar region. These lines should extend across both rims and are used for checking the retrusion of the mandible by using other aids. It will be obvious that if the mandible is correctly retruded, the lines on the lower block will always coincide with those on the upper when the jaws are closed. If, however, any alteration in the maxillo-mandibular relation occurs, the lines on the lower block will no longer coincide with those on the upper, and this will indicate an altered relationship (*see* fig. 160).

3. *Relaxation*

If the patient can be persuaded to relax the muscles of the jaw it will automatically assume the retruded position and this will be greatly assisted by general bodily relaxation. The patient must be very comfortably seated in the chair and asked to relax as completely as possible with his arms hanging

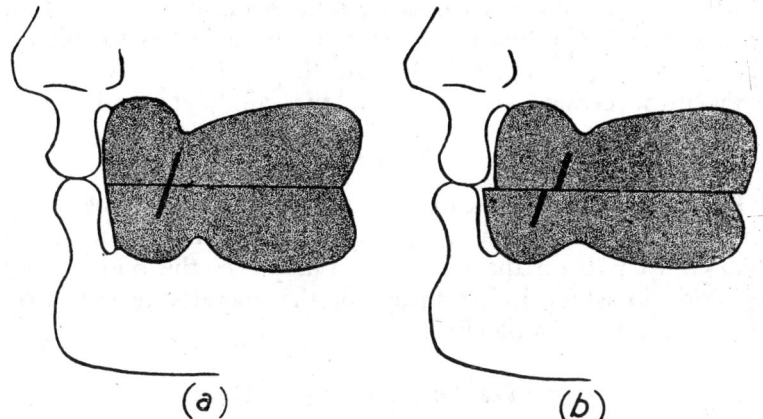

FIG. 160. – The use of guide lines to check the retrusive
position of the mandible.
(a) Line on upper and lower block coincide.
(b) Lines no longer coincide indicating that the mandible
is protruded.

outside the chair; relaxation is then tested by lifting the
patient's arm a few inches and if it does not drop when released,
relaxation is not complete and further persuasion will be
needed. The success of this 'aid' depends very largely on the
operator, some with a quiet, almost hypnotic manner, find it
almost invariably successful whilst others, because of too brisk
a manner, find it useless. When general relaxation is obtained
the patient is asked to close the blocks *slowly* together and the
continuity of the vertical lines made during the previous
technique are checked. If the mandible is now found to be
more retruded, fresh lines are made for further checking: if the
lines coincide it may be assumed that the position is correct,
or further checks as described below may be carried out as
desired.

4. *Swallowing*

Ask the patient to swallow and conclude the act with the
blocks in contact, this aid is based on the fact that with a
natural dentition the teeth are brought into centric occlusion
during swallowing.

5. *Fatigue*

Ask the patient to protrude and retrude the mandible continuously for as long as possible and to finish in a retrusive position with the blocks in contact. The object is to tire the lateral pterygoid muscles, so that they will relax when the movement ceases, and so allow the condylar heads to be retruded.

6. *Head Position*

Having lowered the head rest, ask the patient to bend the head backwards as far as possible. This will produce some backward pull on the mandible, but places the patient in a position in which it is difficult for the operator to check the relationship of the blocks.

7. *The Temporalis Muscle Check*

The anterior ·fibres of the temporalis muscle only contract on closure of the mandible if it is retruded. Thus if the fingers are placed on the temples and the patient closes the rims firmly the contraction or not of the anterior fibres of the temporalis may be used as an assessment of mandibular retrusion.

8. *The Gothic Arch Tracing*

This may be obtained either by intra-oral or extra-oral methods; both make use of the same principle and result in the most reliable assessment of centric occlusion. The technique shows the horizontal movement of the mandible in the form of a tracing, made by a pointed attachment fitted to one block on a recording plate fitted to the other (*see* figs. 161 and 162).

Consider for a moment the lateral movements of the mandible. Starting from the retruded position and moving to the right, the left condyle is drawn forwards down the eminentia whilst the right condyle acts as a pivoting point, and vice versa for the left lateral movement. If a tracing be taken from a given point in the mid-line of the mouth, two lines would result which would converge to a sharply pointed apex; if the mandible were then protruded, the tracing would also start and finish at this point, since it indicates the retruded position (*see* fig. 163). If this principle is applied, the point at which the tracings intersect and form a sharp, pointed arrow head will be the retruded mandibular position for a given individual.

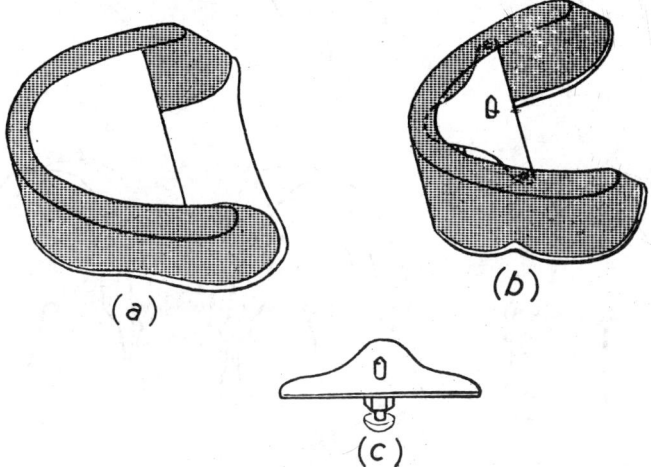

Fig. 161. – Details of intra-oral gothic arch tracing apparatus.
(a) Upper block with tracing plate inserted.
(b) Lower block with tracing point and holder inserted.
(c) Tracing point and holder.

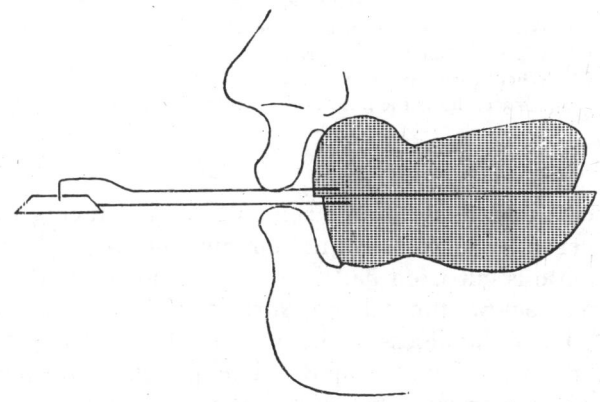

Fig. 162. – Details of extra-oral tracing apparatus, showing tracing stylus attached to the upper block and tracing plate attached to the lower block.

Tracing Devices and Technique

The intra-oral device consists of a carrier through the centre of which is threaded a pointed stylo controlled by a locking nut. After the correct vertical height has been obtained,

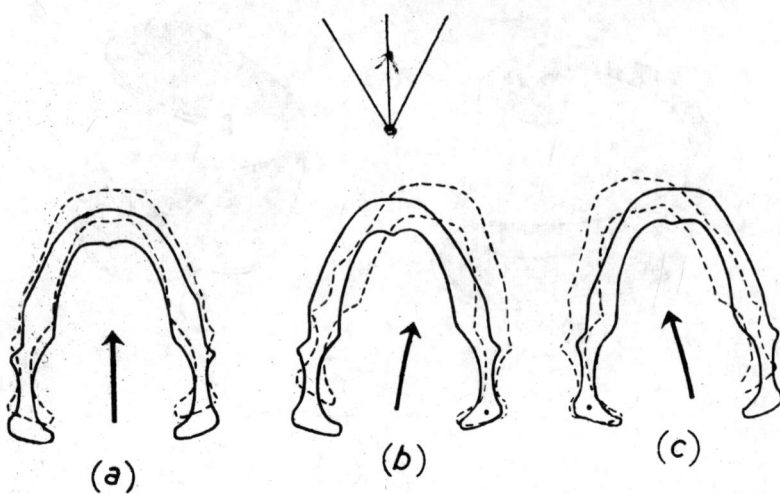

FIG. 163. – Illustrating how a gothic arch tracing is made.
The arrow indicates the direction of travel of a stylus attached
to a lower block, tracing on a plate fixed to the upper
block.

(*a*)   When the mandible is protruded.
(*b*)   When it is moved to the right.
(*c*)   When it is moved to the left.
        Insert shows the form of the completed tracing.

the unit is fitted to the lower rim so that the tracing point is
placed centrally across a line joining the premolars. The
tracing plate is cut from flat sheet metal and inserted parallel
to and just below, the occlusal surface of the upper rim (*see*
fig. 161). Place the blocks in the mouth with the stylo adjusted
to hold the rims slightly apart. The patient now performs
lateral jaw movements, keeping the tracing point in contact
with the plate the whole time. When the operator is satisfied
that the patient can perform these movements correctly, the
upper block is removed and after the tracing plate has been
filmed with black carding wax the block is replaced in the
mouth. Lateral and protrusive movements are made, the
tracings examined, and if a clearly defined arrow head has
been recorded the retruded position has been obtained. Drill a

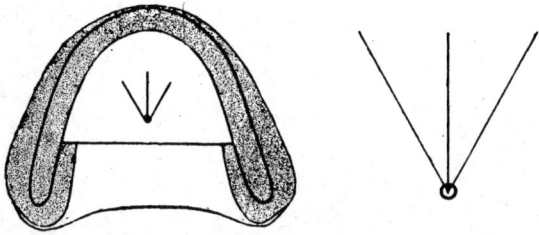

Fig. 164. – Upper block with completed gothic arch tracing and hole bored at apex. Insert shows enlarged view of
tracing and hole.

small hole through the apex (*see* fig. 164) to accommodate the
point of the stylo and ask the patient to move the mandible until
the point slips into the hole; the blocks should now be in
even contact and no longer held apart by the screw. The
blocks are united in the mouth with hot wire staples which are
inserted as shown in fig. 165, and care must be taken not to
burn the patient's lips.

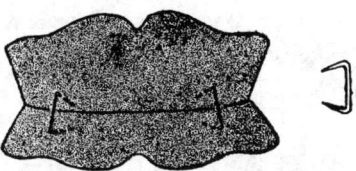

Fig. 165. – Illustrating the method of sealing the bite blocks
with hot wire staples.

The above description relates to a method of obtaining a
gothic arch tracing on conventional record blocks.

Such a tracing can be obtained perhaps more simply by
fixing the tracing plate and stylo directly to base plates made
of cold cure acrylic (*see* fig. 166).

The technique of using this apparatus is to obtain the
vertical jaw separation by screwing the stylo bolt up and down
and locking it at the correct height and then performing the
tracing as described above. The base plates are united in the
mouth in the retruded relationship by placing plaster of Paris
between them which, when set, firmly unites them in the
correct relationship (*see* fig. 167).

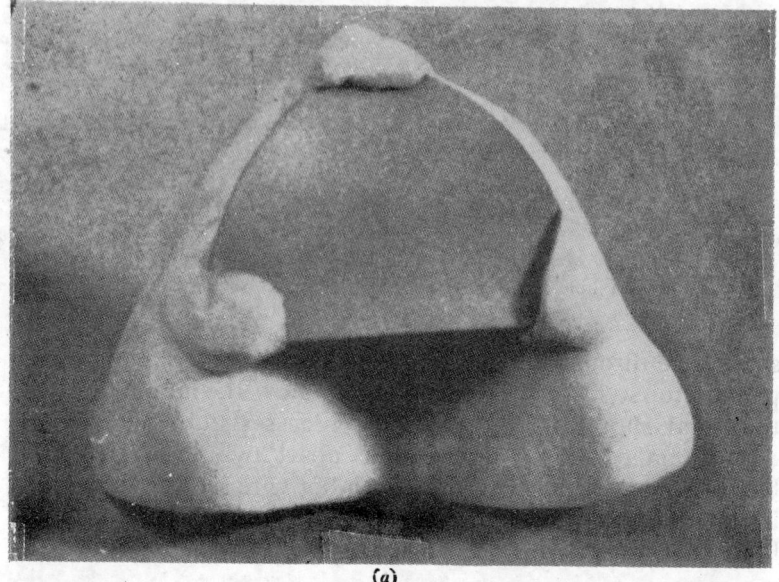

(a)

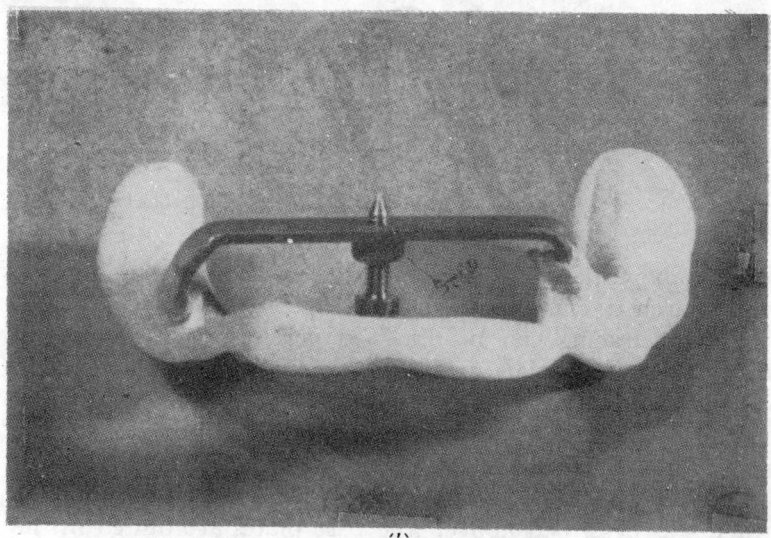

(b)

Fig. 166.– Gothic arch apparatus without conventional
rims. Base plates made of 'cold cure' acrylic.
(a) Upper.
(b) Lower.
(c) Upper covered with wax and tracing made.

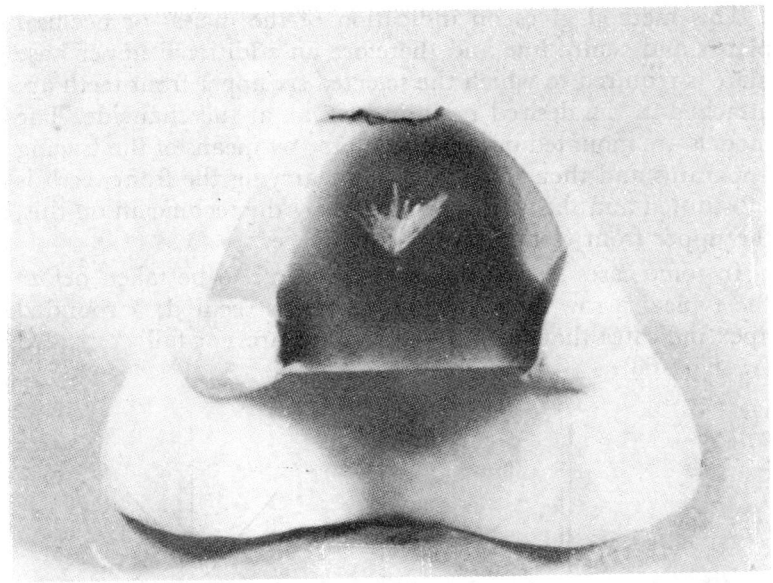

(c)

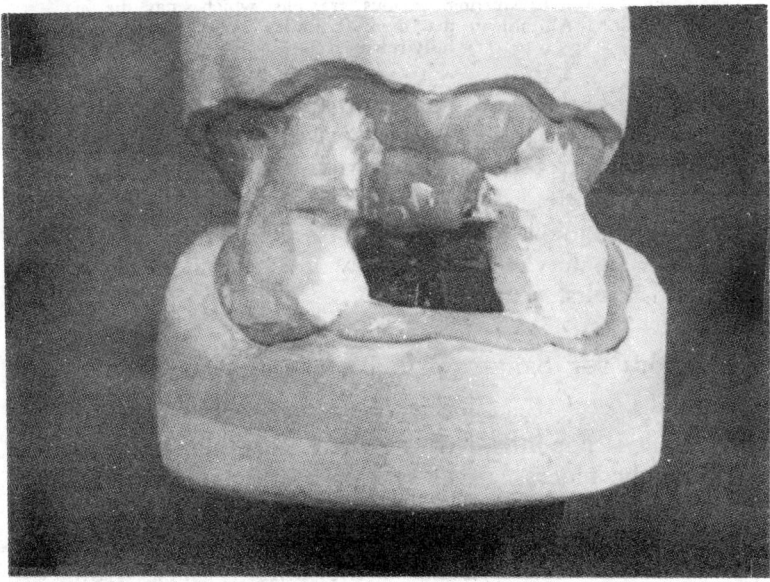

Fig. 167. – Gothic arch apparatus has been united in mouth
with plaster of Paris and models articulated.

This method gives no indication of the incisal or occlusal planes and centre line and therefore an additional upper base plate is required to which the selected six upper front teeth are attached in the desired position by wax at the chairside. The models are mounted on the articulator by means of the tracing apparatus and then the upper base carrying the front teeth is substituted and the set-up continued by the technician on this, the upper front teeth remaining in place.

In some cases several tracings will have to be taken before the typical arrow head or gothic arch is secured; a rounded apex indicates that the condylar heads are not fully retruded (*see* fig. 168).

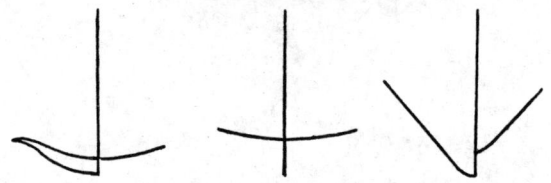

Fig. 168. – Illustrating various tracings which may be obtained. All indicate that the mandibular condyles are not fully retruded.

The extra-oral apparatus is similar to the intra-oral except that the stylo and tracing plate are outside the mouth, being attached to the record blocks by rods which pass between the lips (*see* fig. 162).

This technique is dependent on well-fitting, stable bases, and those of acrylic undoubtedly give the most uniformly successful results.

METHODS FOR SEALING THE RECORD BLOCKS TOGETHER

1. *Heat*

When it is not intended to record more than the retruded position, the blocks can be sealed together in the mouth by means of a hot wax-knife, care being taken that the knife is not hot enough to cause the wax to run. With this method it is sometimes difficult to remove the united blocks from the mouth, but if the patient is asked to open his mouth widely and to push the blocks out with his tongue, no difficulty will be encountered.

2. *Wax Template*

A few 'V'-shaped notches or circular pits are cut in the occlusal surfaces of the rims (*see* fig. 169) care being taken not to

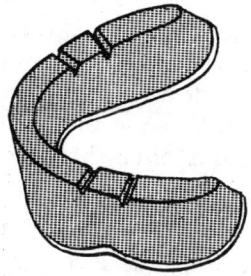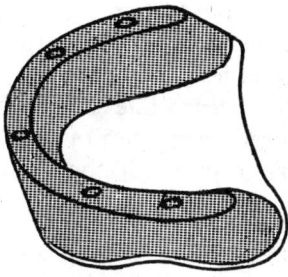

FIG. 169(*a*). – Illustrating the form of the notches and pits cut in the rims when recording centric occlusion with a wax template.

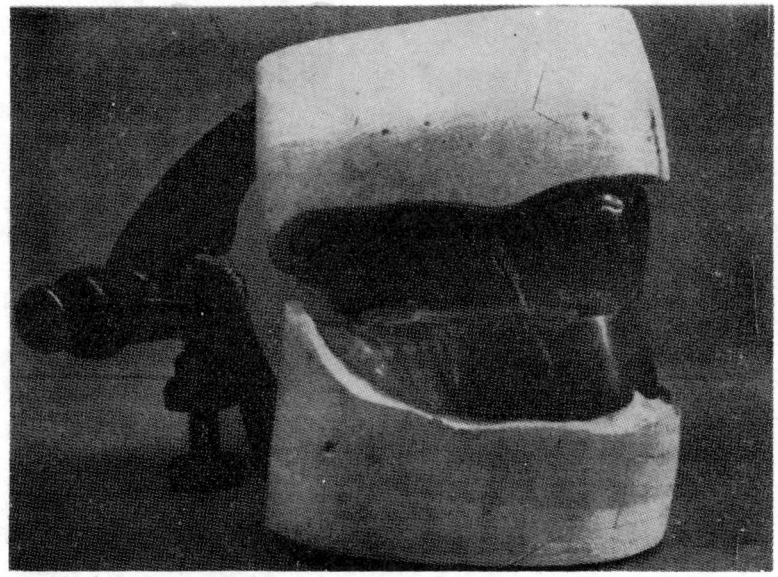

FIG. 169(*b*). – Conventional record rims united with wax.

obliterate the centre line marking. The blocks are placed in the mouth, the lower with a layer of softened pink wax covering its occlusal surface; this layer is usually made up of two thicknesses of pink sheet wax which must be thoroughly softened. The patient is asked to close the blocks together, using whatever 'aid' has been found most useful, and as soon as the operator has checked that the retrusive position is correct the patient is asked to close more firmly. Plaster of Paris may be substituted for wax (*see* fig. 170) and is helpful in those cases where the patient tends to slide the jaw forward as they close. The softness and lack of resistance of the plaster, thus reducing the pressure required to close, often inhibits the desire to protrude the jaw.

3. *Pinning*

Some patients tend to protrude the mandible when they have brought the record blocks into occlusion, and if a wax wafer is

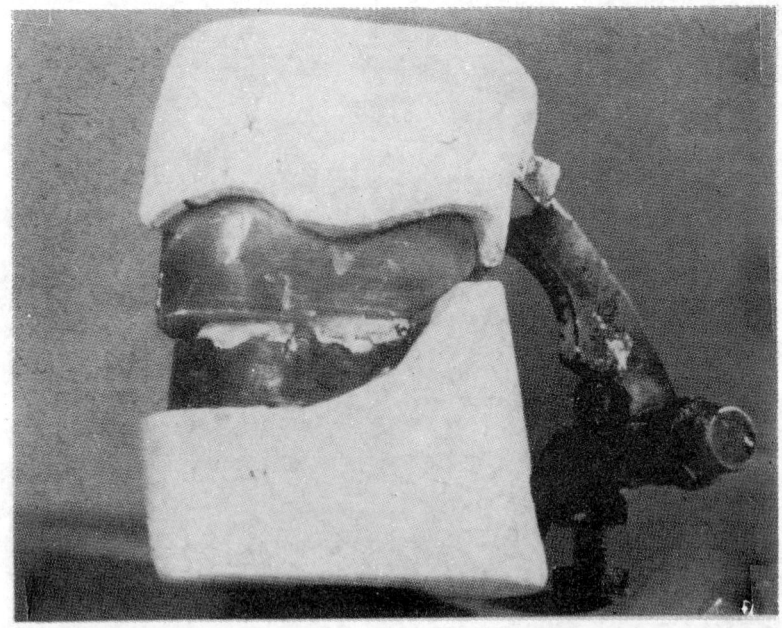

FIG. 170. – Record blocks united with Plaster of Paris.

used in these cases it acts as a lubricant between the rims and permits this sliding movement. In such cases the blocks may be fixed by means of pins instead of a wax wafer. Old gramophone needles are very useful for this purpose, two being warmed and inserted in each lower premolar area with their points protruding not more than 2 mm. above the occlusal surface (*see* fig. 171). The lower block is thoroughly chilled to

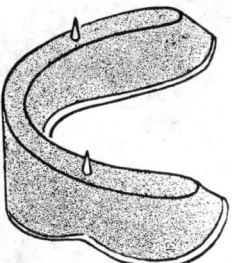

Fig. 171. – Illustrating the position and degree of protrusion of the pins when these are used for recording the position of centric occlusion.

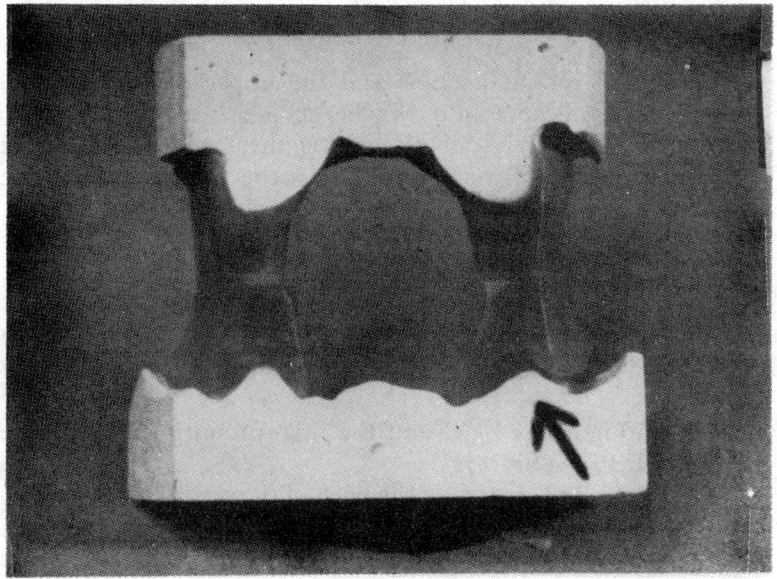

Fig. 172. – Coronal section illustrating how rims tilt off the ridge. Premature contact on right leads to tilt on left (arrowed).

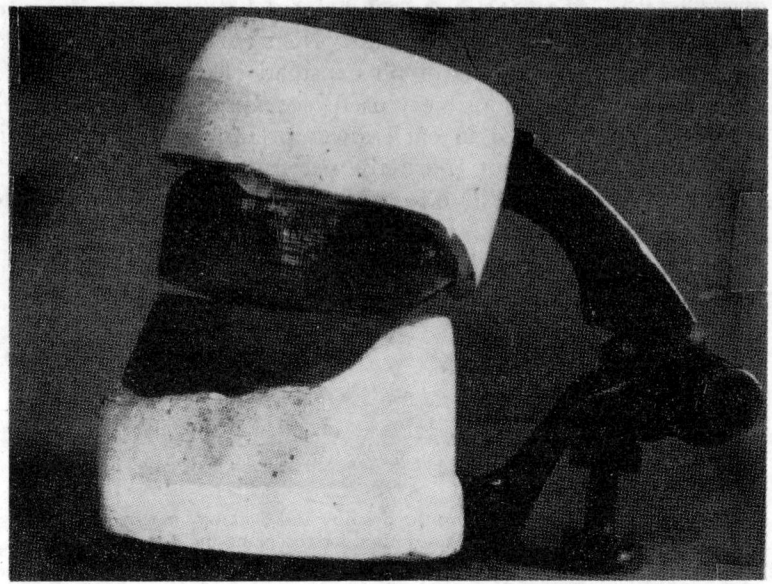

Fig. 173. – Premature contact of record blocks at heels.

support and retain the pins and the upper rim very slightly softened in the area into which the pins will be forced; the blocks are inserted and closed together, and the pins will prevent the sliding movement unless the upper rim has been over-softened.

Common Errors in Record Taking

Errors in occlusion of the finished dentures frequently arise as a result of errors at the record stage other than an incorrect vertical or antero-posterior dimension. The commonest of these are:

(a) Tilting of the blocks off the ridges resulting from uneven contact (see fig. 172).

(b) Premature contact of the heels of the record blocks leading to displacement or tilting of the blocks (see fig 173).

(c) Heavy contact of the heels of the plaster models which prevents them being accurately seated in the blocks (see fig. 174).

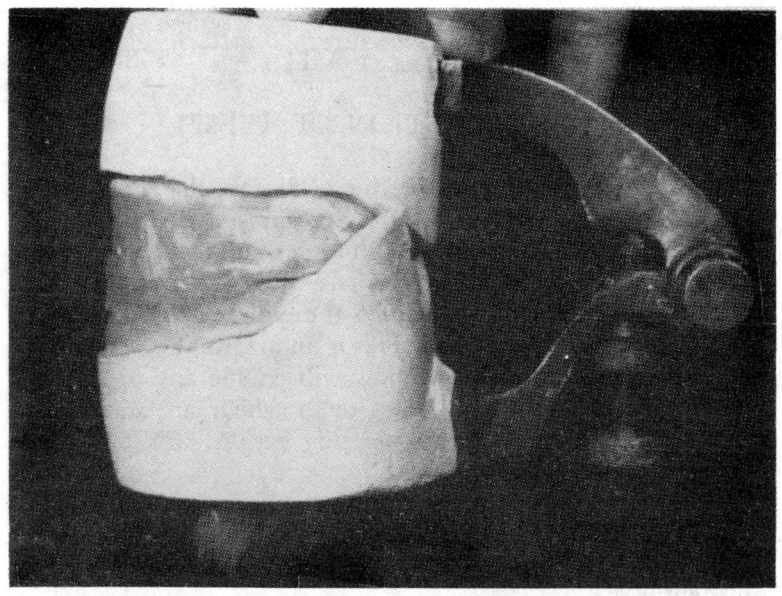

FIG. 174. – Note contact of the heels of the plaster models at the back preventing the record blocks from seating fully.

Chapter VII

THE SELECTION OF TEETH

At the conclusion of registering the occlusion, the choice of the teeth to be used on the dentures requires to be made. The selection of artificial teeth which are suitable in shape, size and colour is by no means an easy task for the tyro, and presents many difficulties even to the experienced operator if he lacks artistic appreciation. This is an art, not a science, and, whilst the principles which follow will enable any operator of average artistic ability to select teeth which are suitable for the average case, the most pleasing results will always be obtained by the artist.

Classification of Patients

There are three classes of patients who present themselves for full dentures:

(1) Those who still retain most of their upper anterior teeth and whom the prosthetist is going to render edentulous. This group are considered under 'Immediate Dentures'.

(2) Those who are already wearing full dentures. If the dentures have been worn for any length of time it is probable that the patient, and his immediate circle of relations and friends, are satisfied with the appearance of the dentures, which should thus be copied. It is rarely advisable to make very marked alterations in an individual's appearance, and improvements are best restricted to the selection of slightly larger teeth of a slightly darker shade.

(3) Those who have been rendered edentulous by another operator and who have not yet been supplied with dentures, or who have lost them. The selection of suitable teeth for this group will be considered under the headings:

    Shape.
    Size.
    Colour.

SHAPE

Soon after the introduction of porcelain teeth, to be used in conjunction with vulcanite for full dentures, it was realized that there was some relationship between the shape of the edentulous upper arch and the upper incisor teeth. For example, a V-shaped arch is associated with incisors which are much narrower at the neck than at the incisive edge; a squarish arch with almost parallel-sided incisors; and a round arch with ovoid teeth (*see* fig. 175).

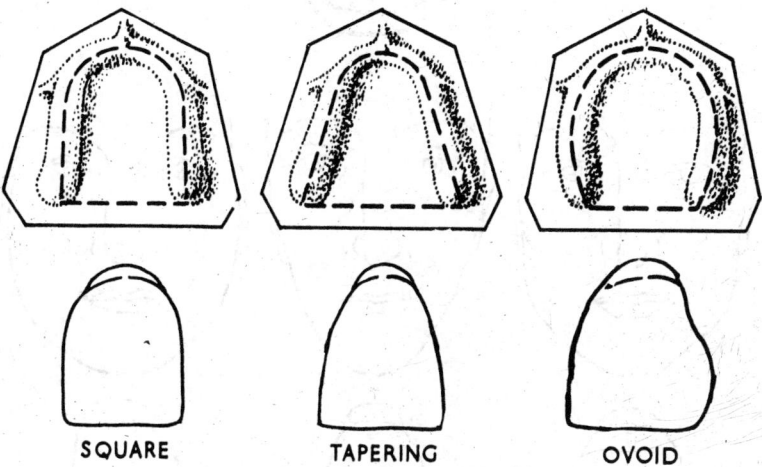

SQUARE   TAPERING   OVOID

FIG. 175. – Tooth form in relation to arch form.

Leon Williams' Classification

The classification of Leon Williams, though not scientifically correct, is undoubtedly the simplest and most useful guide yet suggested, with the added advantage that most manufacturers of artificial teeth have adopted it for their products.

Leon Williams claimed that the shape of the upper central incisors bears a definite relationship to the shape of the face. Thus if one of these teeth is enlarged, and the incisive edge placed above the brows with the neck of the tooth on the chin, then the outline of the tooth will nearly coincide with that of the face (*see* fig. 176). He classified the form of the human face, for simplicity, into three types: Square, tapering, and ovoid,

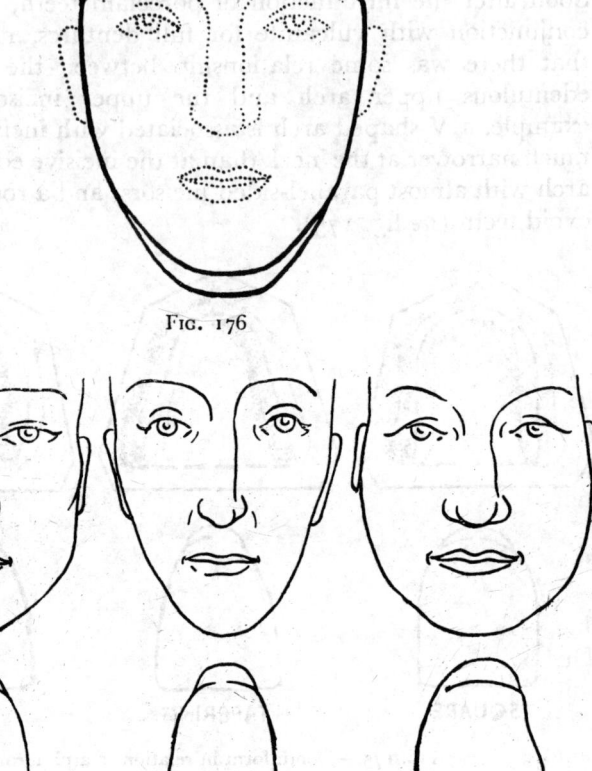

FIG. 176

FIG. 177. – Leon Williams' classification of facial and tooth
form.
(a) Square.
(b) Tapering.
(c) Ovoid.

each type merging into the others without any clear line of
demarcation. In order to determine to what type an individual
belongs the operator imagines two lines, one on either side of
the face, running about 2·5 cm. in front of the tragus of the

ear and through the angle of the jaw. If these lines are almost parallel the type is square, if they converge towards the chin the type is tapering, and if they diverge at the chin, ovoid (*see* fig. 177). Having determined the general type to which the patient belongs it only remains to select teeth which are suitable in length, width and colour, for that individual.

SIZE

Length and width are the only two dimensions which need to be considered at this stage, the thickness within reason being a variable of no aesthetic importance. This statement must not be taken to mean that the thickness of the anterior teeth is unimportant – it has a considerable bearing on phonetics – but it can be easily varied by the technician without alteration to the form, length or width.

Length

The length of the upper six anterior teeth is normally such that the necks of the teeth will overlap the anterior ridge by 2–3 mm. cervically, and the incisive edges of the centrals will show below the relaxed lip. The amount of the central incisors visible below the lip is about 3 mm. in a young person and less than half that amount in an elderly patient (*see* fig. 178). This is not a hard and fast rule, however, and wide variations will frequently be found necessary because the amount of tooth which an individual shows depends on the following factors:

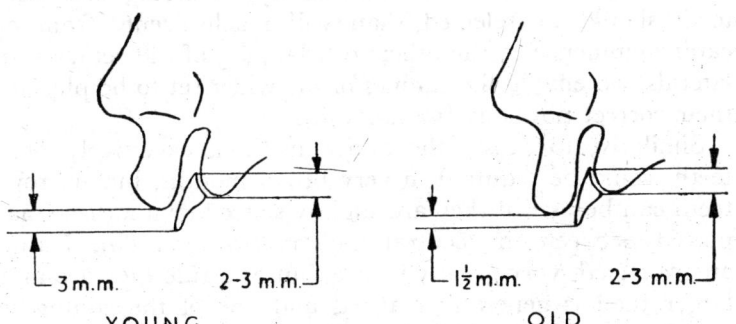

YOUNG   OLD

FIG. 178. – Amount of tooth visible below the upper lip in:
(*a*) a young patient.   (*b*) an elderly patient.

Length of the Upper Lip

Some people have long lips which almost completely cover their natural teeth whilst others have short, curved lips which, even in the relaxed position, expose sometimes more than half the length of the teeth.

Mobility of the Upper Lip

This also is a variable factor. Some individuals expose all the upper anterior teeth and a considerable amount of gum when they smile, others show very little tooth and merely stretch the lips laterally.

Vertical Height of Occlusion

Reduction in the vertical height will cause the lips to bunch up and cover the teeth, whilst an increase will cause an excessive amount of the teeth to show.

Overbite

A deep overbite results in the exposure of a much greater length of tooth than an edge-to-edge bite.

Width

Probably the most satisfactory way of selecting teeth of a suitable width for a given case is to choose a set which are wide enough to allow the canines to be mounted on the canine eminence when set up. When using this method, it must be remembered that in very narrow V-shaped mouths, the natural teeth were, in all probability, crowded, and wider teeth should be selected than will reach evenly from one canine eminence to the other: overlapping of the centrals and laterals will enable the canines of the wider set to be placed in their correct positions (*see* fig. 179).

Similarly, to satisfy the above method, excessively broad teeth would be required in very broad mouths, but narrower teeth can be used if they are slightly spaced or if a diastema is placed between the central incisors (*see* fig. 180). Natural anterior teeth vary greatly in size, but as a rule they are much larger than is generally realized and one of the commonest prosthetic errors is to use teeth which are too small, thus making them appear obviously false.

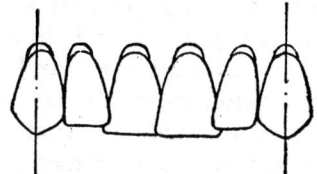

FIG. 179

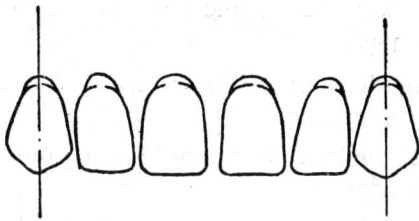

FIG. 180

Harmony

Having considered the length and breadth as individual factors, the final selection with regard to size should be made according to the general characteristics of the individual's features, bearing in mind that nature nearly always produces harmony in its work. The relationship between the length and breadth of the face and that of the selected teeth should be studied, and for this purpose the face-length is taken from the supra-orbital ridge line to the inferior border of the chin, and the breadth as the distance between the zygomatic processes, If the length and breadth of the face appear about equal, then the dimensions of the teeth should follow a similar pattern; the face which appears long in relation to its breadth would indicate teeth of those proportions, irrespective of their shape.

COLOUR

The natural teeth vary as much in colour as they do in size and shape, and the selection of a suitable shade for any edentulous person is a matter of individual judgment. There are, however, a few generalizations which help the novice whilst he is gaining experience. Fortunately colour is not critical for the edentulous patient provided that it is not inharmonious with the general colouring of the skin, hair and eyes, and harmony can be obtained over quite a wide range of colour. This statement will be obvious if it is remembered that the natural teeth remain almost constant in colour, merely darkening very slightly with age, but remain in harmony with hair which may first be black, then grey, then white. The colour of the skin may change from a ruddy complexion in health to a greenish-grey pallor in sickness, the same teeth remaining in harmony with both conditions.

The following facts are true of nearly all natural teeth, exceptions being very rare:

(a) The neck of the tooth has a more pronounced colour than the incisive edge.

(b) The incisive edge, if unworn, is more translucent than the body of the tooth and is usually of a bluish shade: this is due to the fact that it is composed entirely of enamel.

(c) $1|1$ are the lightest teeth in the mouth.

$$\frac{2\mid 2}{2\text{I}\mid 12}$$ are slightly darker.

$$\frac{3\mid 3}{3\mid 3}$$ are darker still.

Posterior teeth are usually uniform in colour and very slightly lighter than the canines. This variation in shade is appreciated by the manufacturers of artificial teeth, most of whom make the desired grading in each set of six anteriors, and the prosthetist selects only the shade of the centrals. More natural and pleasing effects can often be obtained by using canine teeth of an even darker shade than is supplied in a set of six anteriors.

(d) Teeth darken slightly with age. This change has never been satisfactorily explained

There are three dominant tooth colours – yellow, grey, and opal – and each is found in a wide variety of shades and intensity. Many classifications have been made in attempts to correlate tooth colour with that of the skin, hair and eyes, but only vague generalities have remained, for example:

(a) Yellow is dominant with fair hair, blue eyes and a fresh complexion.

(b) Grey sometimes tinged with blue is dominant with dark hair, brown eyes and dark complexion.

(c) Opal is dominant with a clear, pale complexion, irrespective of the colour of the hair and eyes.

(d) A person of powerful build and with large teeth usually has teeth of a darkish shade and a rather pronounced colour.

(e) Small, pearly-white teeth are so exceedingly rare that they always look false.

The following suggestions may be of some help:

(a) Always moisten the shade guide. When in the mouth the teeth are always moist, and this moistness has an effect on the reflection and refraction of light and hence the colour.

(b) Always place the tooth which is under consideration in the shade of the upper lip, in the position it is to occupy: it will appear lighter in this position than in the hand.

(c) When in doubt, select a tooth which is obviously too dark and view it in position, then try one which is obviously too light, gradually merging these two extremes till a pleasing shade is found.

(d) Always obtain the assistance of the patient and any friend or relation who may be available, but only let them see the tooth in the shadow of the upper lip, otherwise too light a colour will invariably be chosen.

(e) Attempt to look at the face as a whole rather than focus entirely on the teeth.

(f) Remember that the lighter the shade the more artificial does the tooth look. Many women patients will insist on lighter teeth than the operator thinks desirable but, unless they are glaringly bad, the prosthetist should give way to the patient – after all. it is she who will have to wear them.

POSTERIOR TOOTH FORM

Early artificial dentures were carved from solid blocks of ivory (*see* fig. 181(*a*)) and their fit, occlusion and articulation must all have been extremely poor, but with the discovery of vulcanite in 1839, followed soon after by the use of porcelain teeth, the modern conception of artificial teeth began. Operators found, before the end of the nineteenth century, that natural tooth forms with their interlocking cusps caused instability of the dentures, and investigations were begun on how this difficulty could be overcome. Research into this problem followed two quite distinct lines:

(1) To alter the shape of the posterior teeth so that cusps could be eliminated without sacrificing efficiency.

(2) To retain natural tooth forms and to prevent their causing instability. This was attempted by designing articulators which copied the mandibular movements of the individual and is discussed in Chapter IX.

A large number of tooth forms have made their appearance in the past, but as most of them have lapsed for various reasons they will not be discussed. For practical purposes the selection of posterior teeth at present available may be made as follows:

For Plane Line Articulation
Inverted Cusped Teeth (*see* fig. 181 (*b*))

The lack of projecting cusps reduces the lateral drag on the dentures when functioning. When setting teeth to ground-in plaster record rims or preformed templates, inverted cusped teeth should be used, otherwise the occlusal plane will not conform sufficiently closely to the curves of the block or template. Inverted cusped teeth may also be used whenever poor resistance to lateral movement of the dentures is anticipated.

Shallow Cusped Teeth

These teeth are still much used when setting up dentures on plane-line articulators, and provided the cusps are not too high they produce tolerable results. Patients will adapt themselves to the limitation of lateral mandibular movement imposed by any cuspal interference, and there is no doubt that

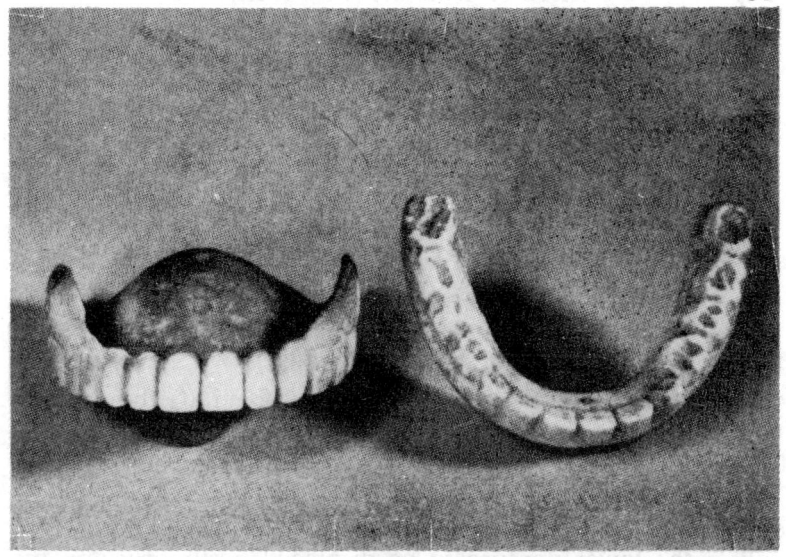

(i)

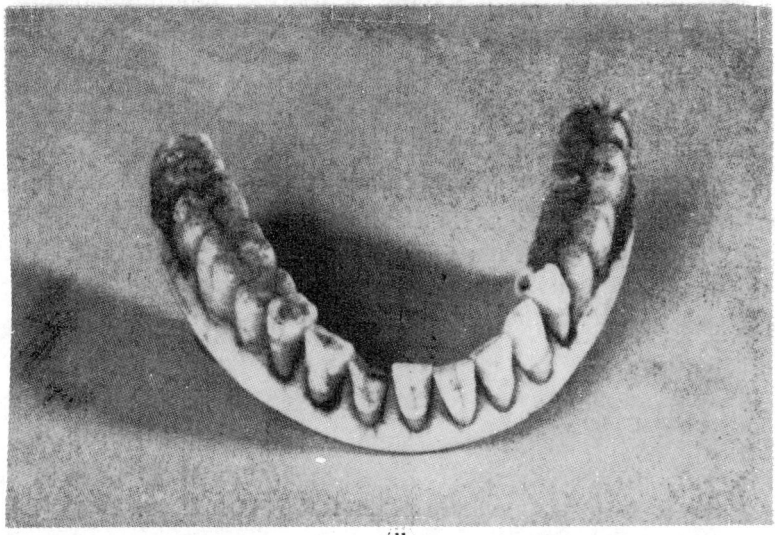

(ii)

FIG. 181(a). – Dentures carved from ivory circa 1800;
(i) Matching upper and lower carved from solid block.
(ii) Cheek teeth and base from ivory, front teeth are natural
ones riveted in place (probably not from the owner of the
denture). (Photographs by kind permission of Mr.
Adrian Halder.)

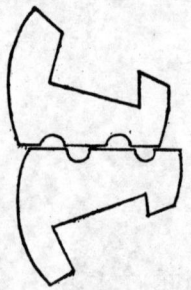

Fig. 181(*b*). – Inverted cusp teeth, illustrated in section.

the presence of normal raised cusps does facilitate the piercing of fibrous food.

One disadvantage of cusped teeth is that when alveolar absorption has progressed sufficiently to allow closure of the vertical occlusal dimension, the interlocking of the cusps causes the lower denture to be displaced posteriorly and the upper anteriorly, causing damage to the underlying tissues. The use of flat inverted cusped teeth obviates or reduces this.

For Anatomical Articulator

Ideally the cuspal angle and height of the cusps of all the posterior teeth should be accurately related to the paths of the mandible when functioning. Practically this is not possible, but certain teeth are available for which the manufacturers publish the cuspal angle, e.g. 20° posteriors and teeth of this type can be satisfactorily employed with most anatomical or lateral movement articulators. This is discussed further in Chapter IX.

CHAPTER VIII

SETTING-UP THE TEETH ON A PLANE-LINE ARTICULATOR

It is not intended that this chapter should in any way be an authoritative description of laboratory techniques, but in order to understand the necessity and value of oral records the clinician must know how they are used by the technician. Further, it is impossible for the operator to criticize intelligently and fairly his technician's work, or alter such work, without some knowledge of the technique of setting-up.

The Parts of a Denture

A denture (*see* fig. 182) consists essentially of two parts which, though united, serve different functions. These parts are:
The Base which may best be described by enumerating its functions which are:

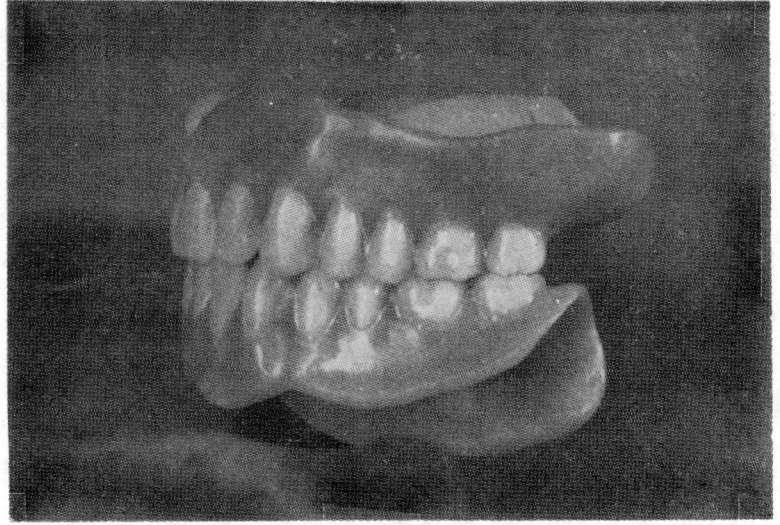

Fig. 182. – The denture bases and the teeth.

235

(*a*) To provide the retention and stability of the denture.
(*b*) To carry and support the teeth.
(*c*) To represent the gums.
(*d*) To assist the teeth in supporting the cheeks and lips.

The Teeth whose functions are:
(*a*) To assist in preparing food for deglutition.
(*b*) To impart a pleasing and natural appearance.
(*c*) To assist in speech.

In every case the artificial teeth arc first mounted in wax on a base-plate which may be either temporary or permanent (*see* Chapter VI). The process of arranging the teeth is termed 'setting-up'; that of moulding the wax supporting them 'waxing-up'.

THE POSITION OF THE TEETH

Before the artificial teeth can be arranged to form dentures the placing of each tooth, and the reasons why it is so placed, must be understood, because if each tooth is not positioned and angulated correctly, the dentures will be functionally inefficient and aesthetically poor.

The models, in their correct centric relationship, are mounted on a hinged piece of apparatus called an articulator (*see* figs. 133, 134). This is done to enable the technician to set up the teeth in correct relationship to each other. An articulator may be of the plane hinge type, producing 'plane-line' articulation, or it may imitate to some extent the mandibular movements and so produce 'anatomical' articulation.

It is only intended here to describe the position of each tooth when in centric occlusion.

The artificial teeth must be set-up in very definite positions which are only variable within rather small limits, and these will be described in relation to

The models.
The occlusal or horizontal plane
The vertical axis.
The other teeth.

The following description of the arrangement of the teeth is the normal, perfect occlusion unless otherwise stated. but this must frequently be modified for individual cases. This is particularly true of the upper anterior teeth where irregularities are frequently introduced for aesthetic reasons, and these alterations must be made at the chairside by the dental surgeon, or detailed instructions of what he wants given by him to his technician.

The Relationship of the Teeth to the Plaster Models

When the natural teeth are present in the mouth their crowns are situated over the centres of the alveolar ridges. In the

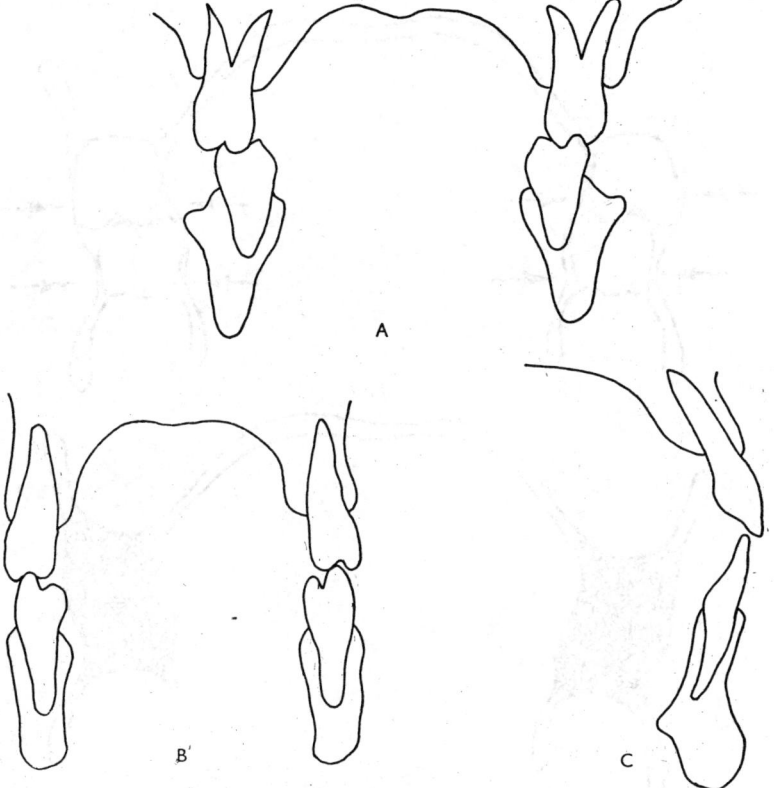

Fig. 183. – Illustrating the relationship of the natural teeth to their supporting bone in:
(a) The molar region.
(b) The premolar region.
(c) The incisor region.

mandible the alveolar ridge supporting the molar teeth forms a buttress of bone on the lingual aspect of the so-called basal bone or body of the mandible. The ridge supporting the pre-molars is immediately above the body of the mandible and the ridge supporting the lower incisors and the canines is slightly labial to the main body of the mandible. The maxillary alveolar process is situated on the external, inferior surface of the basal maxilla (*see* fig. 183).

The position, in the horizontal plane, of the teeth and the alveolar ridges which support them is determined by the inter-

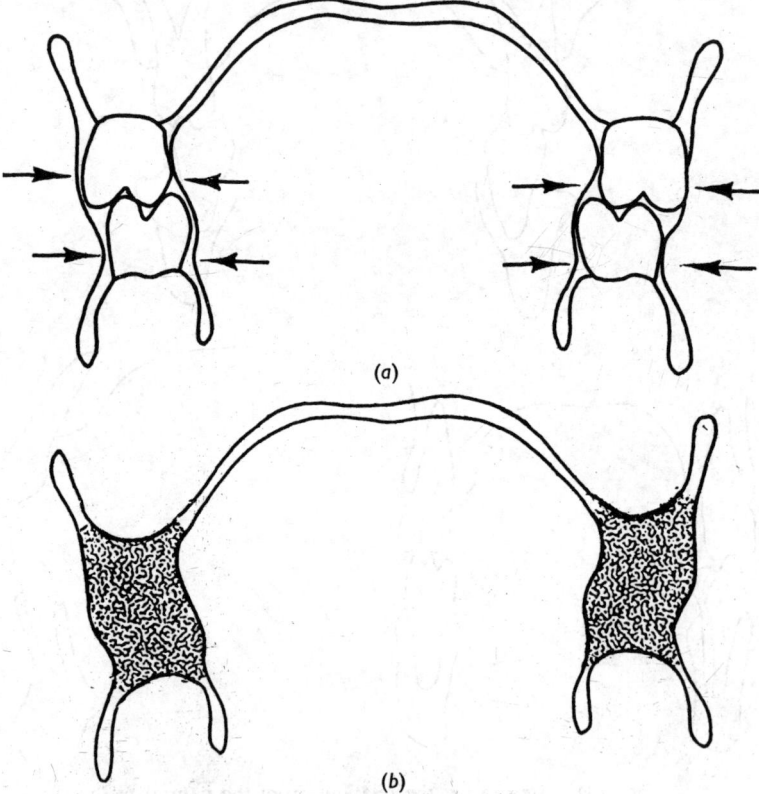

(a)

(b)

FIG. 184

(a) Arrows show how the pressure of the cheeks and tongue cause the teeth to lie in a zone of neutral pressure.

(b) Neutral zone after teeth are extracted (shaded).

action of the forces of the muscles surrounding them. Lingually this force is provided by the tongue and buccally and labially by the lips and cheeks; thus the teeth may be regarded as lying in a zone of neutral muscular force (*see* fig. 184), and if the development and function of the tongue, cheeks and lips are normal the teeth form two parabolic-shaped arches which when occluded interdigitate perfectly with one another. When the natural teeth are lost, the alveolar ridges, being no

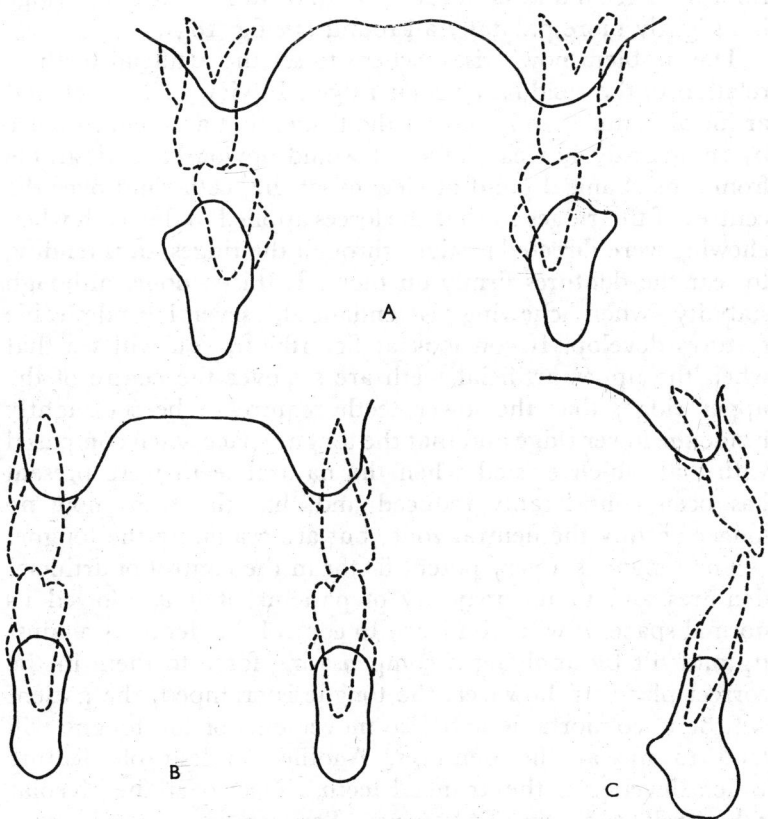

FIG. 185. – Illustrating the form of the residual alveolar ridge after the natural teeth have been extracted.
Dotted line illustrates tissue which is lost.
(*a*) Molar region.
(*b*) Premolar region.
(*c*) Incisor region.

longer required to support them, are absorbed. In the molar regions of the mandible this bone loss occurs from the lingual side; in the premolar region immediately downwards, while in the incisor region it occurs from the labial side, thus the residual alveolar ridge, by which the artificial dentures will be supported is situated slightly more buccally than was the original alveolar ridge in the molar regions and slightly more lingually in the incisor region. In the maxilla the loss is entirely from the buccal and labial surfaces and thus the residual ridge lies slightly more palatally all round (*see* fig. 185).

The problem now arises: where to set the artificial teeth in relation to the residual alveolar ridges. In view of the fact that artificial dentures only rest on the tissues and are held in place by comparatively weak forces, it would obviously be desirable from a mechanical point of view to set the teeth right over the centres of the ridges so that the forces applied to the teeth when chewing were directed straight through the ridges, thus tending to seat the dentures firmly on them. If this is done, although stability when chewing is enhanced, several undesirable features develop. If you look at fig. 186(*a*), you will see that when the upper artificial teeth are set over the centre of the upper ridge, that the lower teeth require to be set slightly inside the lower ridge and that the tongue space when compared with that which existed when the natural teeth were present has been considerably reduced and that the teeth now no longer occupy the neutral zone, but are cramping the tongue.

The tongue is a very potent factor in the control of artificial dentures and in the majority of patients, if it is allowed its normal space, it will soon learn to control the dentures against tip and tilt by applying a compensating force to them in the correct place. If, however, the tongue is cramped, the patient will be uncomfortable and also movements of the tongue will tend to unseat the dentures. Another undesirable feature which develops if the artificial teeth are set over the alveolar ridges relates to the appearance. Because the natural upper and lower front teeth are positioned outside the basal maxilla and mandible they support the lips and cheeks and give them a natural fullness. When the natural teeth are lost and the ridges absorbed, the cheeks and lips fall in and produce

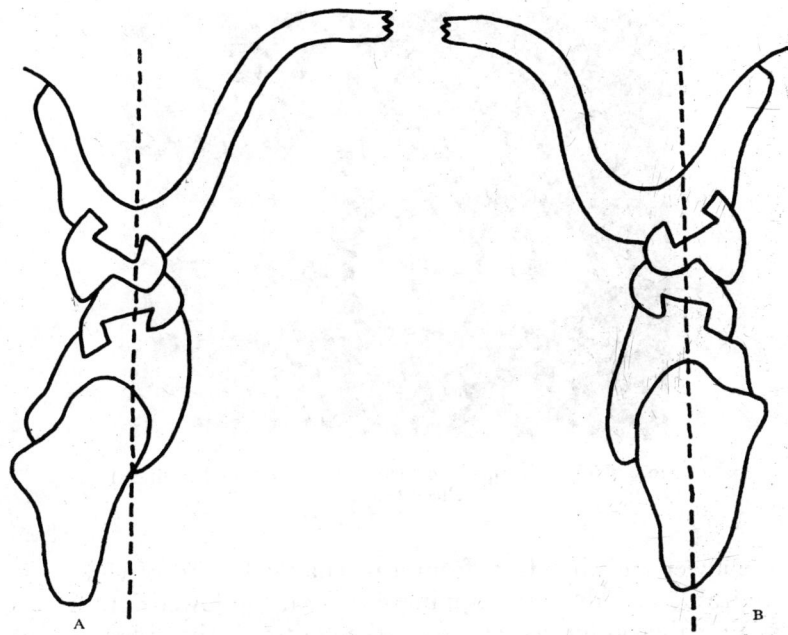

FIG. 186(*a*). – Showing the incorrect (A) and correct (B) relationships of the artificial cheek teeth to the ridges.

an aged and unpleasant appearance. If, however, the artificial teeth are placed as nearly as possible in the positions occupied by the natural teeth, support is once again provided for the lips and cheeks and the patient's appearance restored. It can be seen therefore that the correct position to set artificial teeth bears less relationship to the ridges than to the neutral space or the positions occupied by the natural teeth. This is not quite true, however, and when setting artificial teeth one endeavours to achieve a compromise of setting the teeth as near the ridges as possible without cramping the tongue or spoiling the appearance.

Artificial teeth are considerably narrower than natural teeth (*see* fig. 186(*b*)) and this allows some latitude in positioning them in the horizontal plane. It is also a fact that the forces retaining the lower denture in place are very much less than those retaining the upper, due to the smaller surface area of

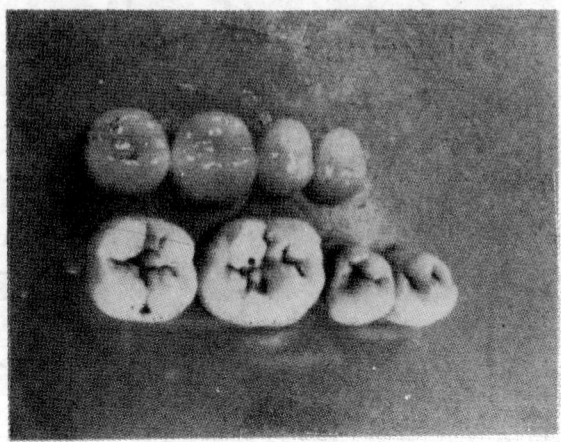

FIG. 186(*b*). – Comparison between natural and artificial cheek teeth.

the lower and therefore, from a mechanical point of view, it is desirable to reduce the tipping forces on the lower denture by setting the posterior teeth over the centre of the ridge and in view of the fact that absorption of the ridge in this region is mainly from the lingual side and that the artificial teeth are narrower than the natural teeth, they can usually be set right over the lower ridge without encroaching on the space occupied by the cheeks. This is the only rule which applies to setting up so far as the relationship of the teeth to the ridge is concerned. If the lower teeth are set in this position when the upper posterior teeth are set to occlude with them they will take up a position lateral to the upper ridge (*see* fig. 186(*a*)) the amount depending on the degree of absorption which has occurred and this varies with individual patients.

The anterior teeth, both upper and lower, are always set in front of the ridge, the amount depending on the degree of absorption which has occurred (*see* fig. 186(*c*)). The position of the labial surfaces of the anterior teeth is determined in the patient's mouth when the occlusion is being recorded. This information is available from the record blocks when setting up the teeth.

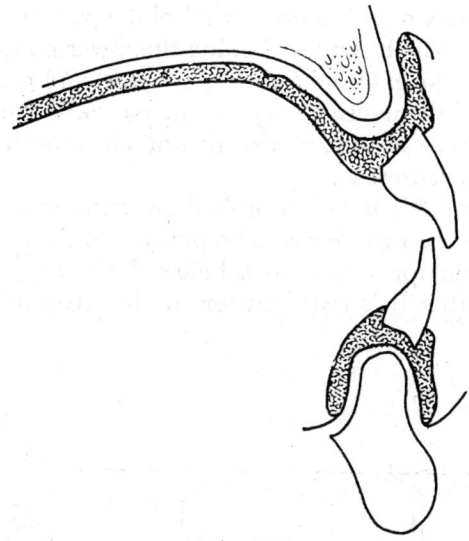

FIG. 186(c).

The Orientation of the Teeth in Relation to the Occlusal Plane and the Vertical Axis

When setting up, the teeth are placed one by one, not only in their correct positions in space, but with the correct angulation of their long axes and unless each tooth is correctly positioned and orientated the final set-up will be functionally useless and displeasing aesthetically.

The supremely important thing therefore, when beginning to set up, is to learn perfectly the position and angulation of each individual tooth, because if you know exactly where and with what slope you are going to place each tooth you will find that with patience you will soon be able to accomplish this.

Individuals who find setting-up difficult and who habitually produce ragged, functionless set-ups have never grasped the subtle but definite variations in the position and slope of individual teeth.

In order to describe the position and orientation of individual teeth, two imaginary references are employed: these are, The Occlusal or Horizontal Plane and The Vertical Axis. When recording the occlusion in the patient's mouth, the occlusal surfaces of the record blocks are trimmed parallel to the occlusal plane, which is a horizontal plane parallel to the naso-auricular line which is a line joining the lower border of the ala of the nose to the external auditory meatus, and positioned at a height so that the incisive edges of the patient's future artificial central incisors and the anterior palatal cusps of the upper first molars will just touch it.

In practice, this is accomplished by trimming the occlusal surfaces of the record blocks to be parallel to the naso-auricular line so that the upper rim shows below the relaxed upper lip by the amount that it is required for the future artificial incisors (*see* fig. 187).

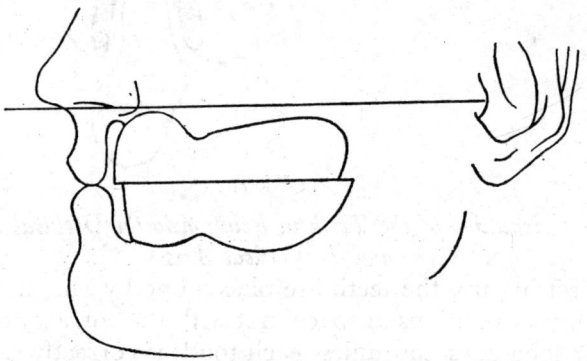

FIG. 187(*a*). – Occlusal rims of record blocks parallel to naso-auricular line.

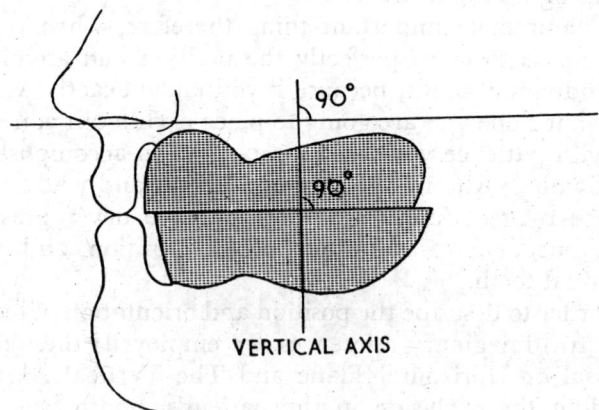

FIG. 187(*b*). – The vertical axis.

When the plaster models are articulated by means of the record blocks, the occlusal plane of the blocks is lined up parallel with the bench and thus the occlusal plane to which the occlusal or incisive edges of each tooth is referred as it is set can be imagined as a sheet of glass or perspex parallel with the bench and at a height just touching the incisive edges of the upper incisor teeth when they have been set. The set-up is commenced by placing the two upper incisor teeth with their incisive edges in the position indicated by the anterior occlusal plane of the upper record rim, so fixing the height of the occlusal plane of the set up (*see* fig. 188).

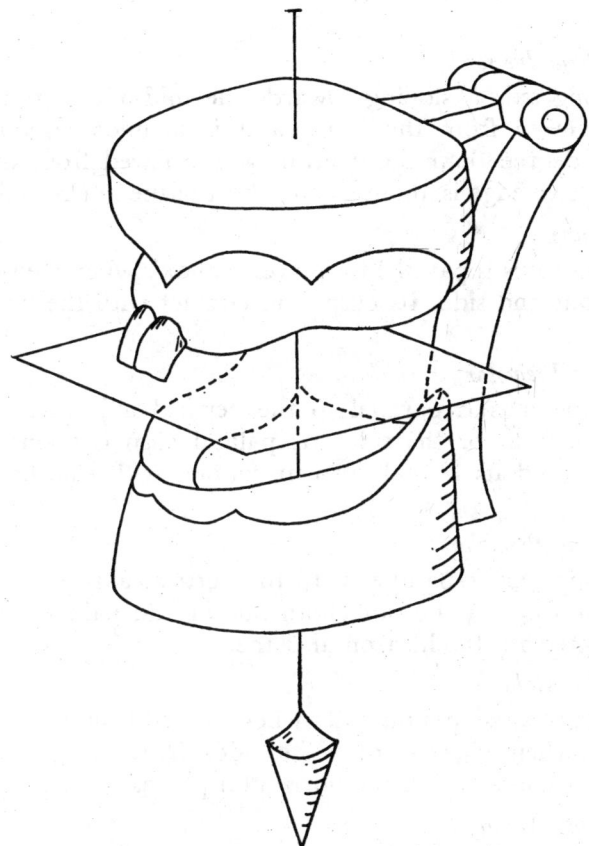

Fig. 188. – The imaginary vertical axis and occlusal plane.

The vertical axis can be imagined as a plumb-line, hanging and passing straight through the models when they are standing on the bench. Three points of reference now exist to which each tooth can be referred as it is set: the alveolar ridge, the occlusal plane and the vertical axis.

The Position of the Upper Teeth (see figs. 189, 190 and 191)

The Central Incisor

Its long axis is parallel to the vertical axis when viewed from the front, and sloping slightly labially when viewed from the side. The incisive edge is in contact with the horizontal plane.

The Lateral Incisor

Its long axis is sloping towards the mid-line of the mouth when viewed from the front, and is inclined labially to a greater degree than the central when viewed from the side. The incisive edge is about 2 mm. short of the horizontal plane.

The Canine

Its long axis is parallel to the vertical axis when viewed from both front and side. Its cusp is in contact with the horizontal plane.

The First Premolar

Its long axis is parallel to the vertical axis when viewed from the front or the side. Its palatal cusp is about 2 mm. short of, and its buccal cusp in contact with, the horizontal plane.

The Second Premolar

Its long axis is parallel with the vertical axis when viewed from the front or the side. Both buccal and palatal cusps are in contact with the horizontal plane.

The First Molar

Its long axis slopes buccally when viewed from in front, and distally when viewed from the side. Only its mesiopalatal cusp is in contact with the horizontal plane.

The Second Molar

Its long axis slopes buccally more steeply than the first

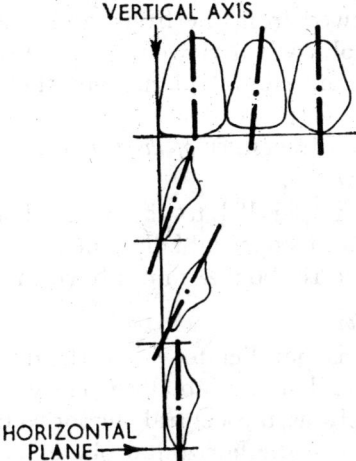

VERTICAL AXIS

HORIZONTAL PLANE

Fig. 189. – The relation of the upper front teeth to the horizontal plane and the vertical axis.

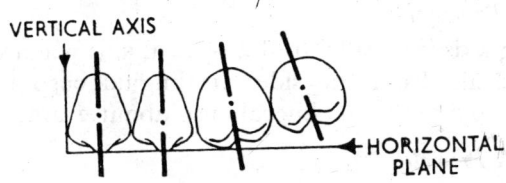

VERTICAL AXIS

HORIZONTAL PLANE

Fig. 190. – The relation of the upper posterior teeth to the horizontal plane and the vertical axis. Lateral view.

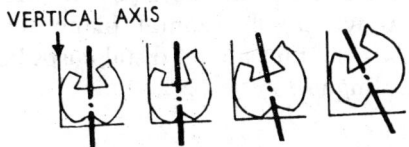

VERTICAL AXIS

Fig. 191. – The relation of the upper posterior teeth to the horizontal plane and the vertical axis, anterior view.

molar when viewed from the front, and distally more steeply than the first molar when viewed from the side. All four cusps are short of the horizontal plane, but the mesiopalatal cusp is nearest to it.

The Position of the Lower Teeth

The Central Incisor

Its long axis is parallel to the vertical axis when viewed from the front, and slopes labially when viewed from the side. The incisive edge is about 2 mm. above the horizontal plane.

The Lateral Incisor

Its long axis is parallel to the vertical axis when viewed from the front, and slopes labially when viewed from the side but not so steeply as the central incisor. The incisive edge is about 2 mm. above the horizontal plane.

The Canine

Its long axis leans very slightly towards the mid-line when viewed from the front, and very slightly lingually when viewed from the side. Its cusp is slightly more than 2 mm. above the horizontal plane.

The First Premolar

Its long axis is parallel to the vertical axis when viewed from the front and from the side. Its lingual cusp is below the horizontal plane and its buccal cusp about 2 mm. above it.

The Second Premolar

Its long axis is parallel to the vertical axis when viewed from the front and from the side. Both cusps are about 2 mm. above the horizontal plane.

The First Molar

Its long axis leans lingually when viewed from the front, and mesially when viewed from the side. All the cusps are at a higher level above the horizontal plane than those of the second premolar, the buccal and distal cusps being higher than the mesial and lingual.

The Second Molar

The lingual and mesial inclination of the long axis of this tooth is more pronounced than in the case of the first molar.

All the cusps are at a higher level above the horizontal plane than those of the first molar, the distal and buccal cusps more so than the mesial and lingual.

THE COMPENSATING CURVES

From the foregoing descriptions of the orientation of the teeth it will be seen that they are arranged so that the posterior teeth, when considered as a whole unit, form two curves, an anteroposterior and a lateral curve.

The Anteroposterior Curve

Compensating curves are the artificial curves introduced into dentures in order to facilitate the production of balanced articulation: they are the artificial counterparts of the curves of Spee and Monson which are found in the natural dentition. This curve follows an imaginary line touching the buccal cusps of all the lower teeth from the lower canine backwards, and approximates to the arc of a circle. A continuation of this curve backwards in the natural dentition (curve of Spee), will nearly always pass through the head of the condyle (*see* fig. 192).

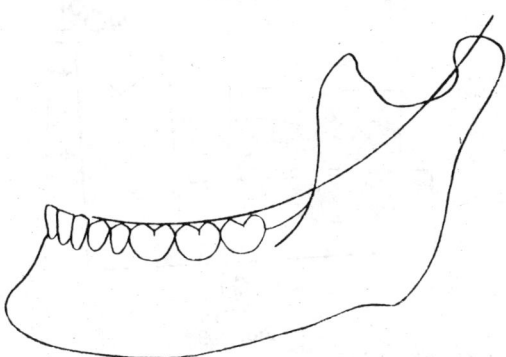

FIG. 192. – The curve of Spee.

This curved arrangement of the posterior teeth in this antero-posterior curved manner may best be appreciated by reference to the following diagrams (*see* fig. 193). If the path followed by the condyles is horizontal, then the teeth can be set to conform

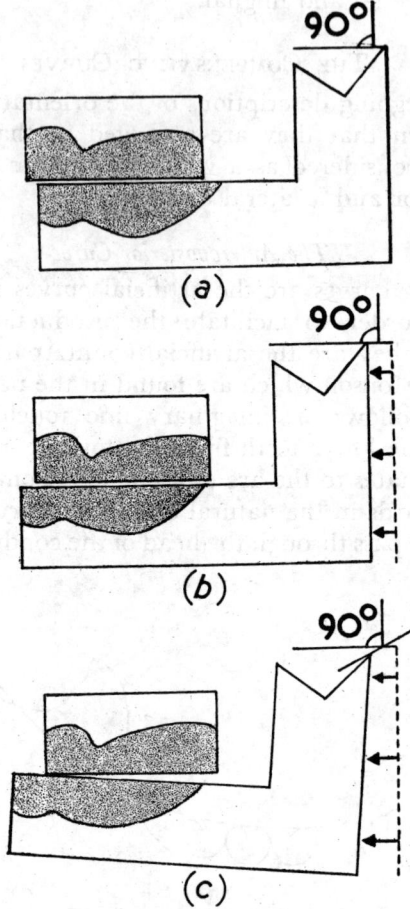

FIG. 193

(a) Centric occlusion.

(b) Protrusion with a condylar path parallel to the occlusal plane – contact maintained.

(c) Protrusion with a condylar path sloped at an angle to the occlusal plane - contact lost posteriorly.

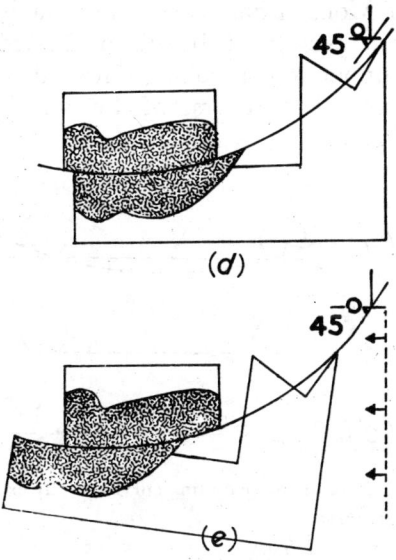

FIG. 193
(d) Centric occlusion with an occlusal surface which is an
    arc of the circle of which the condylar path is also an arc.
(e) Protrusion of (d), contact maintained.

to a horizontal plane. When the mandible moves forwards the
teeth will remain in contact.

If the path travelled by the condyles is sloped away from the
horizontal plane (as it always is to some degree), then as soon
as the mandible moves forwards the condyles commence to
descend, and the posterior teeth will lose contact if they have
been set to conform to a horizontal plane.

If the posterior teeth, instead of being set in a horizontal
plane, are set to an anteroposterior curve, then as the mandible
moves forwards and the condyles travel downwards all the
teeth can remain in contact.

The Lateral Curves

In the natural dentition there are two lateral curves, one
involving the molar teeth (the curve of Monson), and the
other involving the teeth anterior to the second premolars; the
second premolars being set on a horizontal plane surface.

The curve of Monson has its concavity facing upwards and increases in steepness from before backwards, the occlusal surfaces of the upper molars facing outwards and downwards. The anterior curve is a reverse of the curve of Monson just described (*see* fig. 194).

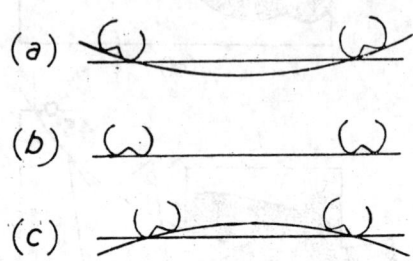

FIG. 194. – Lateral compensating curves greatly exaggerated.
(*a*) Molar curve.
(*b*) 2nd premolar 'curve'.
(*c*) 1st premolar curve.

When the mandible is moved laterally the condyle on the working side (i.e. the side towards which the mandible is moved) remains in the glenoid fossa and moves very slightly outwards and backwards (Bennett movement). The condyle on the other side (balancing side) travels downwards and forwards.

If the teeth are set on a horizontal plane, those on the balancing side will lose contact, due to the downward movement of the condyle on that side. If, however, the teeth are set to conform to a curve, the steepness of which relates to the steepness of the condylar path, then the teeth will remain in contact during the lateral and downward movements (*see* fig. 195).

THE POSITION OF THE TEETH RELATIVE TO ONE ANOTHER

The teeth of one jaw occlude with those of the other. Occlusion means 'the act of closing or the state of being closed' and relates to the position of the teeth when in contact.

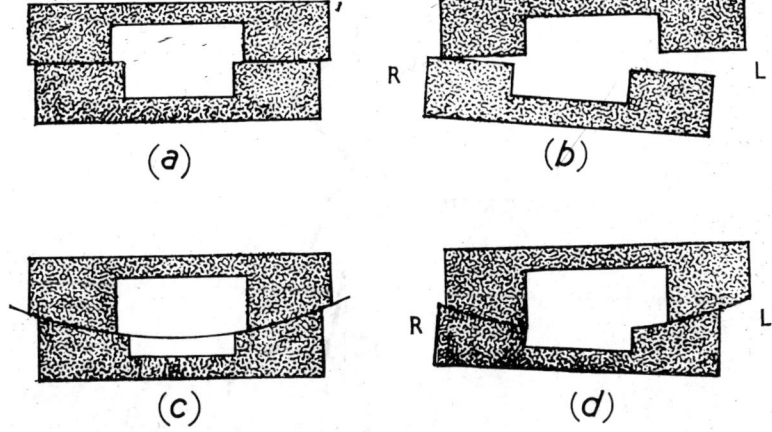

Fig. 195. – A diagrammatic representation of form of the occlusal surface in the molar region and its relation to lateral mandibular movement.

(a) Centric occlusion with a horizontal occlusal plane (seen from in front).

(b) Lateral movement of the mandible to the right, the left side loses contact.

(c) Centric occlusion with an occlusal surface forming an arc of a circle concentric to that followed by the mandible.

(d) Lateral movement of the mandible to the right, contact maintained on both sides.

Three types of occlusal relationship exist:

(1) Centric.

(2) Protrusive.

(3) Lateral.

These are dependent on the position of the mandible relative to the maxilla. When setting up teeth on a plane-line articulator the operator is only interested in the position of the teeth in centric occlusion, which is as follows:

(a) The six upper front teeth overlap the six lower front teeth by about 2 mm. This overlap is in both a horizontal and a vertical plane. In the vertical plane it is known as the OVERBITE and in the horizontal plane as the OVERJET (see fig. 196).

(b) The buccal cusps of the upper premolars and molars overlap those of the lower. The palatal cusps of the upper

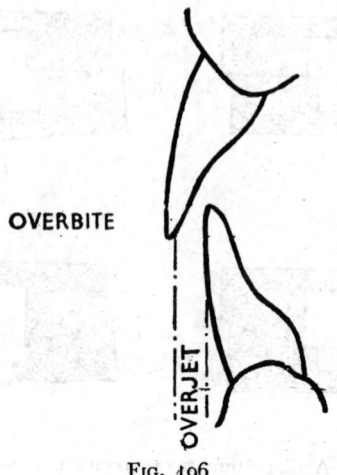

OVERBITE

OVERJET

Fig. 196

posterior teeth and the buccal cusps of the lower posteriors interdigitate with the opposing teeth (*see* fig. 197).

(*c*) Every tooth except the two lower central incisors and the two upper last molars occludes with two teeth in the opposing jaw. This may best be appreciated by reference to fig. 197.

(*d*) The labial surfaces of the six anterior teeth present a curve when viewed from the occlusal surface, the shape of this curve depending on the shape of the underlying alveolus.

The posterior teeth should be set-up in such a way that their buccal surfaces will make contact with a straight line drawn

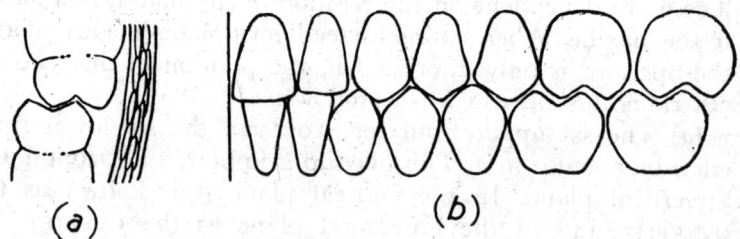

(*a*)   (*b*)

Fig. 197. – The occlusal relationship of the teeth.

(*a*) Anterior view.

(*b*) Lateral view.

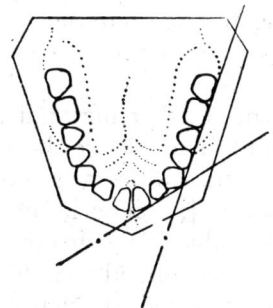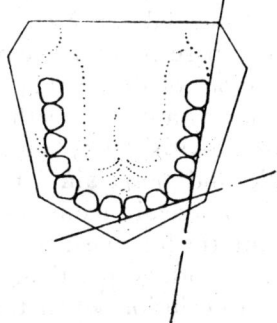

FIG. 198

from the labial surface of the canine, backwards (*see* fig. 198).

Articulation is a term which is constantly being used in relation to both natural and artificial teeth and is apt to be confused with the term occlusion. Occlusion is a static state used when opposing teeth are in contact without movement. Articulation is a dynamic state used when opposing teeth are in contact during movements of the mandible.

Materials from which Teeth are Made

Both anterior and posterior teeth may be made from either porcelain or acrylic resin. Each of these materials has advantages and disadvantages viz:

Porcelain is hard and resists abrasion and wear: the appearance of teeth made from it is reasonably natural but somewhat opaque and false, unless the very best quality teeth, which are expensive, are used.

Porcelain teeth cannot have stains and characterisation lines and fillings put in them easily. The bonding of porcelain teeth to the denture base is purely mechanical, the posterior teeth are held by the acrylic flowing into the diatoric holes in the teeth and the anterior teeth are held by their pins. The different coefficients of expansion of acrylic and porcelain results in the acrylic base being stressed in the regions of the teeth, but in practice this is of little significance.

Acrylic is soft and wears rapidly but the appearance of the teeth made from it is very natural even in the cheaper grades.

Acrylic teeth can be stained and have fillings inserted with ease in the laboratory. The bonding of this material to the denture base is by a chemical union and no stresses occur in the regions of the teeth.

So far as anterior teeth are concerned, either material may be used with safety and satisfaction. The choice between acrylic and porcelain for posterior teeth, however, is not so simple. Porcelain teeth being hard tend to jar on occlusion and transmit the full masticatory load to the ridge. They do not wear into a smooth even articulation easily to accommodate a slightly uneven occlusion when the dentures are fitted, or changes of articulation, due to bone resorption, throughout the life of the dentures, although polished facets do develop on them slowly. Porcelain teeth do, however, maintain the vertical occlusal dimension and are hard and sharp enough to produce efficient mastication.

Acrylic teeth produce a cushioning effect when chewing somewhat akin to that provided by the periodontal membrane in natural teeth. They wear to accommodate changes in occlusion, but unfortunately they usually wear so rapidly that they allow the vertical dimension to close (see fig. 199(a)), and they do not produce efficient mastication.

In the opinion of the authors the rapid wear of acrylic posterior teeth resulting in loss of vertical dimension and eventually uneven occlusion is a serious fault, and for this reason alone such teeth should not as a general rule be used. In cases presenting narrow painful ridges or in the aged, when the biting power is small, or where the ridge needs cushioning, a case may be made for them.

The claim that the wear of acrylic teeth is supposed to allow the occlusion to adjust itself to the gradual closure of the vertical dimension which occurs slowly throughout the life of the denture, due to the ridge absorption, is not in practice usually substantiated. Anyway dentures should never be worn for so long that gross closure of the vertical dimension due to ridge absorption is allowed to occur, for in these cases the denture bases will be so poor a fit on the ridges that they will cause damage. As a general rule most dentures require replacing within three to five years.

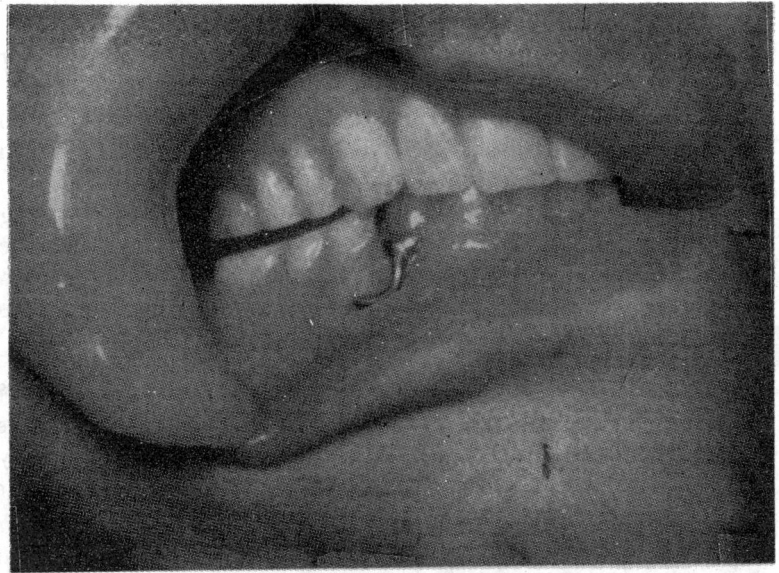

FIG. 199(a). – The wear of acrylic posterior teeth: note how the occlusion has been deranged and is now heavy on the lower natural anterior teeth.

WAXING-UP

When the teeth have been mounted in their correct positions and in proper occlusion, more wax is added to the base and the whole made to conform to certain definite requirements. The periphery of the upper denture must be thick and rounded, with the exception of the posterior palatal border which must be thinned down almost to a knife edge. The buccal and labial surfaces must be concave to allow for comfortable and free movement of the buccinator and orbicularis oris muscles.

The lower denture must be similarly finished on the buccal and labial surfaces and periphery, but the lingual surface must be inclined inwards, from above downwards, affording no undercut areas in which the tongue might lodge and unseat the denture. Further, the posterior lingual border must be finished to a thin edge so that the tongue can move over the mylohyoid ridge and up over the denture without encountering any distinct projection (*see* Chapter II).

GUM-FITTED ANTERIOR TEETH

In some patients the maxilla is overdeveloped in the incisor region, and if a wax flange is placed over this region it pushes the upper lip out, making the patient appear to have a swollen lip. In these cases the six upper front teeth are fitted directly on to the alveolar ridge without any labial flange (*see* fig. 199(*b*)).

Retention of this type of denture is usually impaired owing to the peripheral seal being more readily broken, and the loss of the stabilizing effect of the labial flange. Sometimes two extensions, known as 'wings', are added in an attempt to overcome these deficiencies (*see* fig. 199(*b*)).

SETTING UP THE TEETH FOR ABNORMAL JAW RELATIONSHIPS

When the models have been articulated, after taking the records it will be found in a considerable number of cases that they present deviations from the normal relationship and thus present problems in setting up and articulating the teeth.

Superior Protrusion

The lower ridge is narrower than the upper and associated with a receding chin.

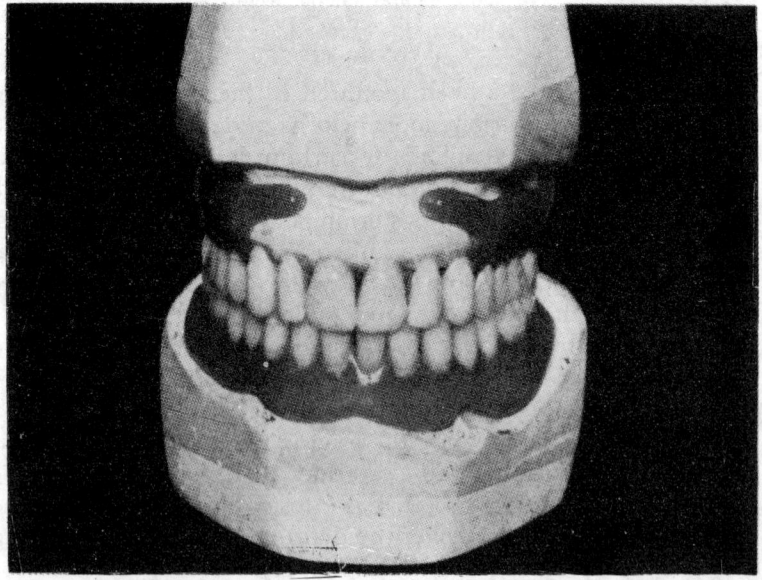

FIG. 199(*b*). – The upper six front teeth are fitted to the gum.

Setting the Posterior Teeth

The upper posterior teeth will need to be set inside the ridge, in order that they may occlude with the lower teeth. The lower teeth should never be set outside the ridge (*see* fig. 200).

Setting the upper teeth inside the ridge does not produce

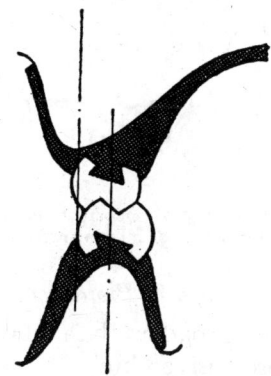

Fig. 200. – Upper posterior teeth set slightly inside the ridge.

marked instability, although it reduces the tongue space, but as the tongue is used to being cramped by the narrowness of the lower ridge this will not be serious. Setting the lower teeth outside the ridge, however, will lead to instability.

Setting the Anterior Teeth

Cases of superior protrusion always present a large overjet and no attempt should be made to reduce this by leaning the upper incisors backwards or the lowers forwards. Such angulation of the teeth will in the case of the upper give the patient a rabbity appearance and in the case of the lower tend to unstabilize the denture by placing the lower teeth in the way of the lower lip (*see* fig. 201).

A large overjet always exists in the natural dentition of individuals with a superior protrusion and they are rarely capable of approximating their upper and lower incisors, therefore it is neither necessary nor desirable to attempt to make that possible with the artificial teeth.

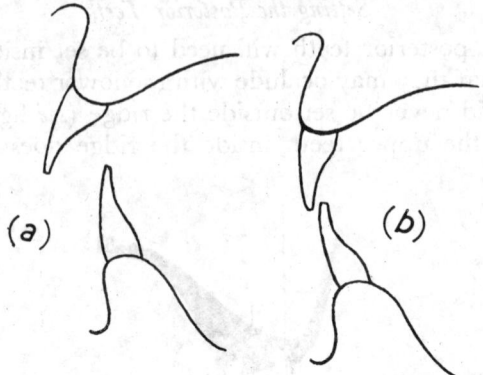

FIG. 201. – (a) Correct, (b) incorrect set up of the anterior
teeth for a case of inferior retrusion.

Inferior Protrusion

The lower ridge is broader than the upper and usually
associated with a protrusive chin.

Setting the Posterior Teeth

In these cases it will be necessary to cross the bite (*see* fig. 202).
This means that instead of the buccal cusps of the lower
molars fitting into the fossae of the upper molars, the reverse
occurs. Sometimes the crossing of the articulation has to be
applied to all the posterior teeth; but more commonly it is only

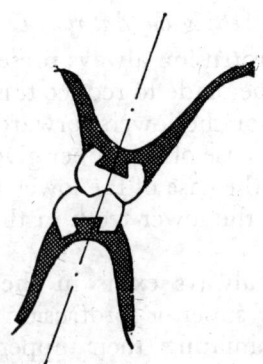

FIG. 202. – A crossed articulation shown in section. Note buccal
overjet of lower molar.

the molars which are affected. Occasionally the width of the lower ridge is so great in relation to the upper that the second molars cannot be made to occlude at all without moving the upper tooth outside the ridge. In such cases it is best left off the denture and as mastication is mainly performed in the premolar and first molar region its loss is not serious.

In cases presenting marked inferior protrusion it is frequently necessary to set the upper teeth outside the ridge. If the retention of the denture is satisfactory the only trouble likely to result from this is a mid-line fracture of the denture due to its continual flexion and if the jaw relationship requires the teeth to be set far outside the ridge a metal palate should be incorporated in the denture.

Setting the Anterior Teeth

To provide an overbite in a large number of cases of inferior protrusion will mean setting the upper incisor teeth so that their long axes are at a considerable angle to the vertical, giving the patient a hog-like appearance.

The anterior teeth in such cases are best set either edge to edge or with a negative overjet (*see* fig. 203).

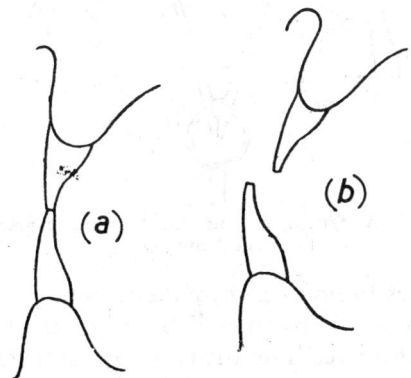

FIG. 203

(*a*) The method of setting the anterior teeth so that they occlude edge to edge in a moderate case of inferior protrusion.

(*b*) The method of setting the anterior teeth in a gross case of inferior protrusion.

Setting Up the Teeth for Patients who Already Possess Old Dentures which have Given Satisfactory Service

The most important fact to remember when setting up for patients who already possess satisfactory dentures is not to reduce the tongue space. If the tongue is cramped with new dentures they will never be successful. If the tongue has more space than in the old denture it is all right. A satisfactory method to ensure that the new dentures do not cramp the tongue is to measure the space provided by the old ones and copy it (*see* fig. 204). An even more satisfactory method is to take an impression in alginate of the existing dentures and the technician will then have a model of the dentures to guide him not only in relation to the position of the teeth but, of equal importance, enable him to reproduce the contour of the polished surfaces of the denture.

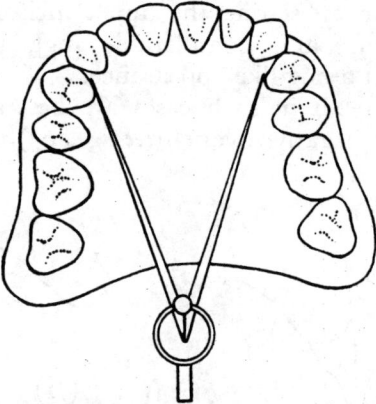

Fig. 204. – A method of measuring the tongue space on the old dentures.

In some cases in order to provide a similar tongue space to that which already exists it will be necessary to set the teeth off the ridge. If the teeth on the existing dentures have been set off the ridge it is usually safe to copy them, because the patient will have become used to manipulating dentures with teeth set in this position.

The Posterior Border of the Upper Denture

In many cases it will be found that the posterior border of an existing upper denture finishes far forward on to the hard palate and one must decide, when making a new denture, whether to place it in its correct location on the soft palate, or copy its old position. Although it is obviously desirable to place the posterior border correctly and so increase the retention of the denture, many patients who have been used to the back edge of their denture finishing on the hard palate will bitterly resent it being placed further back. It must be remembered in this connexion that people who have been wearing dentures for years have become very clever at holding them in position, subconsciously, with their tongue. The best way to discover a patient's reaction to the position of the posterior border is to carry the base-plate of the record block on to the soft palate and see what the patient has to say. If there is any protest or retching, finish the new denture to the same line as the old.

CHAPTER IX

ANATOMICAL ARTICULATION

The term 'anatomical articulation' is used to denote an arrangement of the artificial teeth whereby the wearer can make normal masticatory movements with comfort and efficiency. This result is obtained by setting-up the teeth in balanced occlusion, i.e. with as many teeth as possible in occlusion in any lateral or protrusive jaw position, (*see* figs. 205, 206, 207). The teeth must also be set-up to give balanced articulation, i.e. with the teeth arranged so that they maintain an even sliding contact during the final masticatory movements without causing any cuspal interference.

SHORTCOMINGS OF PLANE-LINE ARTICULATION

Provided the records have been taken correctly, dentures can be constructed on a plane-line articulator which will occlude perfectly in the centric position, but plane-line articulation is unsatisfactory for the following reasons:

1. *Tilting of the Dentures*

Pressure applied to only one or two teeth may cause tilting of the dentures (*see* fig. 208).

2. *Cuspal Interference*

Any attempt at lateral or protrusive movement, with the teeth in occlusion, will either prove impossible, or the dentures will be dragged bodily in the direction of mandibular movement. with consequent soreness of the tissues.

3. *Reduced Efficiency*

As a result of the above, patients wearing dentures with plane-line articulation learn to avoid making lateral and protrusive movements and to chew with a simple hinge-like action, ensuring that their teeth always occlude in the centric relationship. This hinge movement will only produce a

264

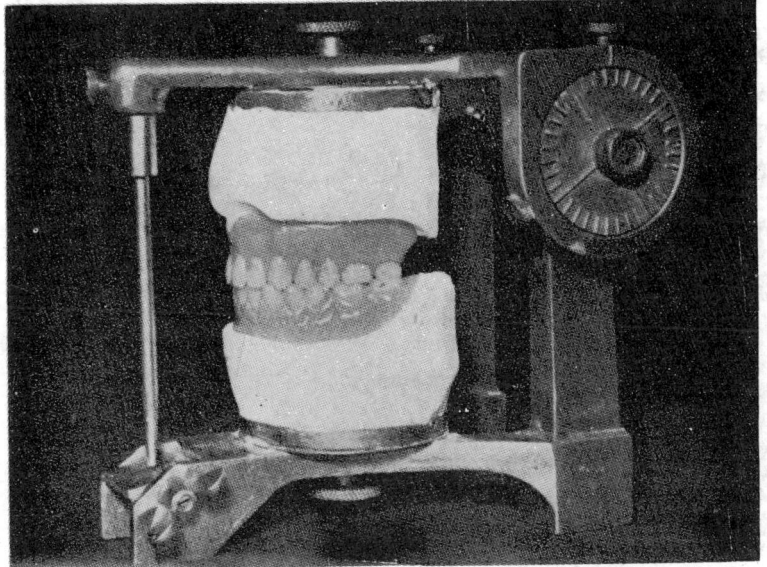

(a) Illustrating the occlusion of the teeth with the mandible in the position of centric occlusion.

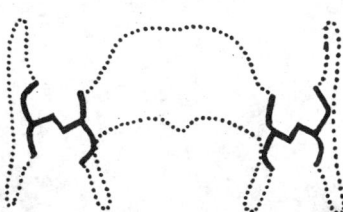

(b) Cross-sectional diagram of (a).

FIG. 205. – Anatomical articulation.

crushing of the food because cutting and grinding requires some lateral movement. A good example of grinding is that of the pestle and mortar where one surface is moved over another, whilst in cutting less pressure will be required if the knife-edge is drawn across the material which is being cut, than would be the case with direct pressure alone. From this explanation it can be readily understood why the efficiency of plane-line articulation is relatively poor.

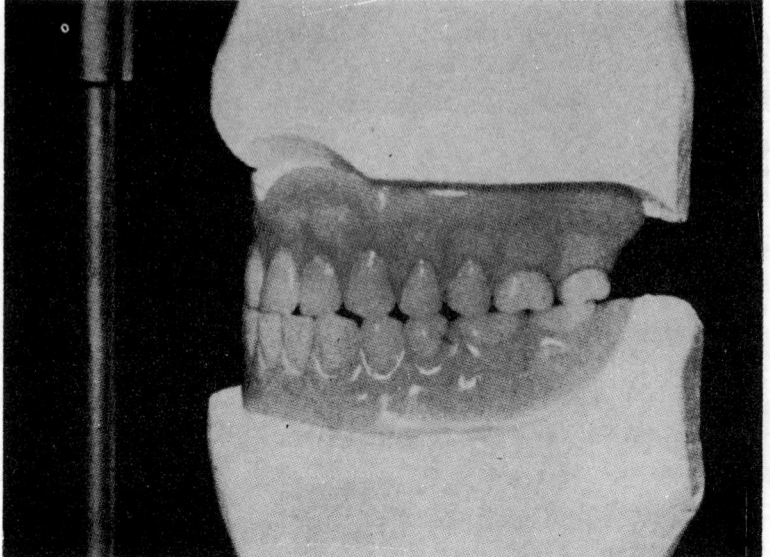

FIG. 206. – Anatomical articulation. Illustrating the occlusion
of the teeth with the mandible protruded.

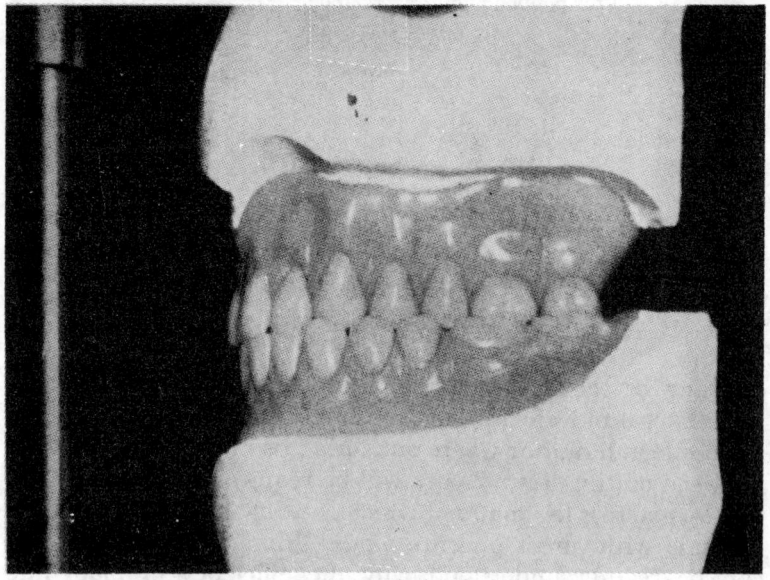

FIG. 207. – Anatomical articulation.
(a) Illustrating the occlusion of the teeth on the working
side with the mandible in a lateral position.

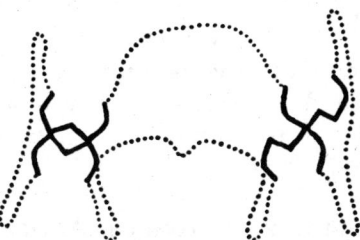

FIG. 207. – Anatomical articulation.
(b) Cross-sectional diagram illustrating how balance maintained in lateral occlusion.

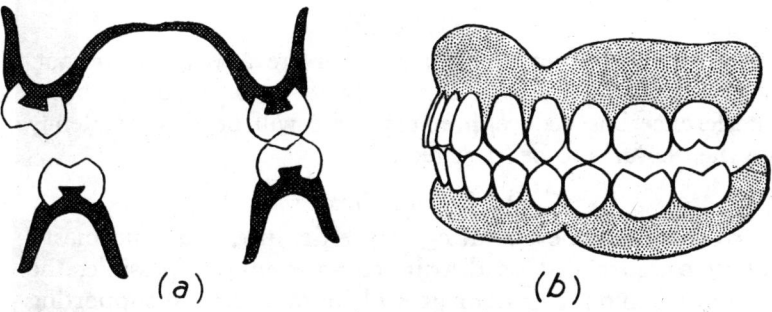

(a)   (b)

FIG. 208. – The unilateral and haphazard occlusion which occurs with plane line dentures in

(a) Lateral occlusion.

(b) Protrusive occlusion.

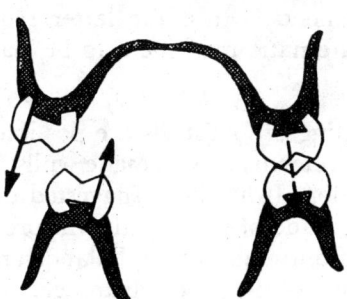

FIG. 209. – Tilting forces acting on dentures resulting from unbalanced occlusion.

4. *Pain*

In either lateral or protrusive positions only one or two teeth are in occlusion, and since these teeth will sustain the entire biting force, the tissues under them sometimes become painful (*see* fig. 209).

ADVANTAGES OF ANATOMICAL ARTICULATION

1. *Balanced Occlusion*

In any position of occlusion the maximum number of teeth are in contact and therefore the masticatory pressure is distributed over the supporting tissues.

2. *Stability*

Since the maximum number of teeth are always in contact, tilting of the dentures is less likely to occur, and as cuspal interference has been eliminated there will be little tendency for the dentures to be 'dragged'.

3. *Reduced Trauma*

Since there will be no tilting of the dentures, and the masticatory pressure will be distributed as evenly as possible, the minimum amount of damage will be done to the supporting tissues.

4. *Functional Movements*

Most patients will become accustomed to dentures which have been anatomically set-up far more readily than to plane-line dentures, because the former allow a continuation of normal masticatory movements, whilst the latter require an entirely new pattern of automatic movement to be learnt.

5. *Efficiency*

Grinding and cutting of foodstuffs are possible because lateral and protrusive movements can be made whilst still maintaining balanced articulation. It has been suggested that the introduction of food on one side of the mouth will prevent the teeth of the opposite side from maintaining balance and that therefore anatomical articulation is of no advantage. Whilst this statement is true for a large, hard morsel of food, it is not correct for the majority of foodstuffs which require much less pressure before the opposing cusps have penetrated it and have come into contact with each other. Maximum pressure is only exerted when the mandible encounters maximum resistance at the beginning of the return from a lateral position to that of centric occlusion, and at this stage the cusps have penetrated the food to some extent and are nearly in contact. From this it follows that very little tilting would be required before the teeth on the opposite side made contact and restored balance. This slight tilting is even further reduced by the fact that the soft tissues on the working side are under pressure and therefore are slightly compressed. Even if the statement, 'Enter food, exit balance, were correct, anatomical articulation would still be worth while, because any position of occlusion will re-seat such a denture but only in centric occlusion will this be possible with a plane-line set-up.

6. *Time Saving*

Balanced articulation having been obtained by the technician in the laboratory there remains only minor spot-grinding to be done and thus a considerable amount of time is saved.

BALANCED ARTICULATION

By balanced articulation is meant an arrangement of the teeth so that in any occlusal relationship as many teeth as possible are in occlusion, and when changing from one relationship to another they move with a smooth, sliding motion, free from cuspal interference and maintaining even contact.

In order that the teeth can be arranged so that they fulfil the requirements in the foregoing definition, four things are needed:

(1) An articulator which can be adjusted to copy the movements and reproduce the relationships of the jaws of the patient for whom the dentures are being made.

(2) A means whereby these movements and relationships can be measured and transferred to the articulator.

(3) An understanding of the factors which influence the arrangement of the teeth to produce balance.

(4) Posterior teeth with cusp angles which will permit of their being set-up to give balanced articulation.

These four points will now be described in greater detail.

1. *Anatomical Articulators*

There are many articulators which are designed to reproduce mandibular movements, but the majority of them are, for the sake of simplicity, arranged to give only the average of such movements. The more the patient differs from this average the less valuable do these fixed types become, and therefore only the type of articulator which is fully adjustable to individual movements will be considered. The influence of the Bennett movement on occlusal balance is small and, from a clinical point of view, can usually be ignored.

2. *Recording Jaw Relationships*

The anatomical relationships and the controlling factors in mandibular movement, which are peculiar to the individual patient, and which must be accurately transferred to the articulator before it can be used to set teeth in balanced occlusion, can best be appreciated from a study of fig. 210. This represents a schematic sagittal section of a patient with record blocks in place in centric occlusion, and a transverse section showing the maxillae and condyles. From it the following list of relationships, which are fixed for individual patients, but vary from patient to patient, can be drawn up:

(*a*) The relationship of the maxilla, A, to the head of condyle, B, in centric occlusion, is a fixed and unalterable factor peculiar to each patient.

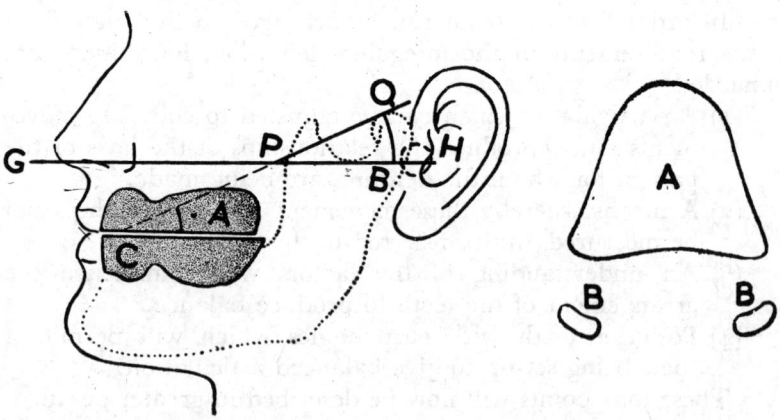

Fig. 210

(*b*) Once the vertical jaw relation has been determined, the relationship of the mandible, C, to the maxilla and to the head of the condyles in centric occlusion, is a fixed, unalterable factor and peculiar to each patient.

(*c*) The slope of the condylar path, PQ, is a fixed factor peculiar to each patient, and therefore the angle, QPH, which it makes with the horizontal plane will be constant.

In addition, the surfaces of the record blocks are parallel to the naso-auricular line, GH, and if all these factors are known and can be transferred to an articulator, it will be possible to reproduce the patient's masticatory mechanism.

Methods of Measuring the Patient's Fixed Factors

All the measurements are obtained through the agency of record blocks which have been trimmed parallel to the naso-auricular line and to the correct vertical height, as described in Chapter VI. The blocks must be notched ready to receive wax templates.

Relating the Mandible in Centric Occlusion to the Maxilla

This merely entails securing the normal centric relationship, as for plane-line articulation, by means of a wax template.

ecording the Condylar Angle

By condylar path is meant the path taken by the head of the condyle when moving up and down the articular eminence, (*see* fig. 211), and for practical purposes this is considered to be a straight line. The angle which this makes with the occlusal plane is known as the condylar angle.

(*a*) Place the upper record block in the mouth. Prepare a softened wax template as for normal record taking and place it on the lower block.

(*b*) Place the lower record block in the mouth and request the patient to move his jaw to the right lateral position and close the blocks together. Remove the united blocks from the mouth, chill under the cold tap, and separate the wax template from the blocks. (This separation is facilitated if the rims are smeared with a thin film of vaseline before recordings are taken.)

(a)

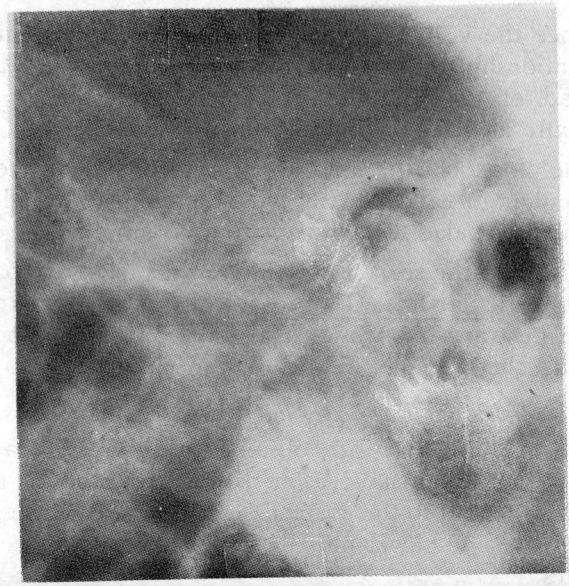

(b)

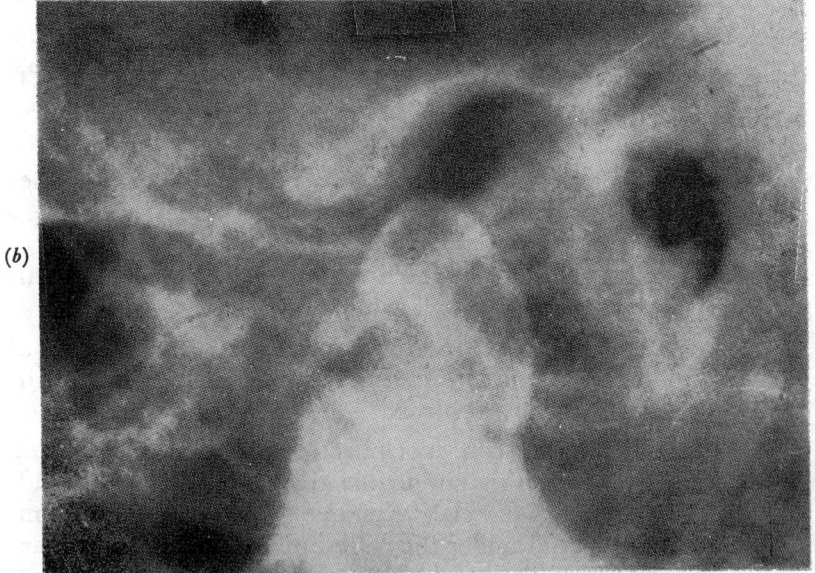

FIG. 211. — X-ray photographs showing head of condyle:
(a) In closed position.
(b) With mouth wide open.
Note the angulation of the path which it has travelled.

Using another template, record the position of the mandible in left lateral occlusion.

Instead of securing right and left lateral records it is possible to take one protrusive record which will give the forward positions of both condyles at the same time. This method does not usually give quite such accurate results but is useful in cases where it is difficult to persuade the patient to make true lateral movements. All movements must be of a considerable degree in order to be able to adjust the articulator satisfactorily.

Recording the Relation of the Maxilla to the Glenoid Fossae

For this a piece of apparatus called a face-bow is used, and this is illustrated in fig. 212.

It consists of a metal bow, A, carrying in channels at its extremities two graduated rods, B, which slide inwards and outwards for adjustment, and may be fixed by tightening the

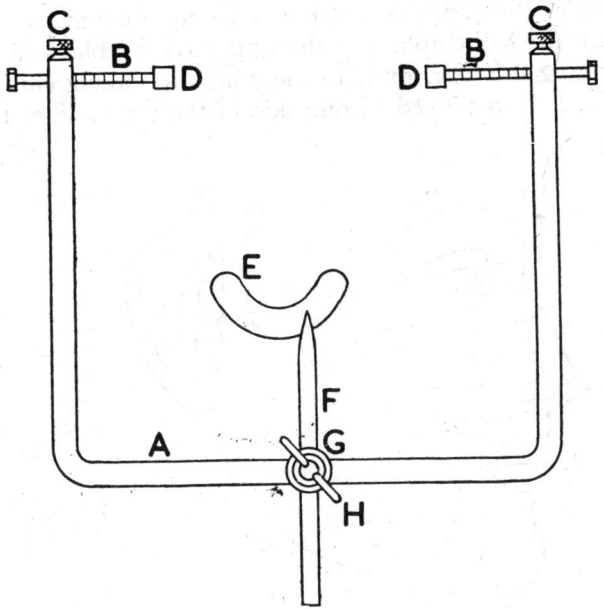

FIG. 212. – The face-bow.

finger screws, C. The rods bear at their inner ends two cups, D. A flat metal fork, E, is attached eccentrically to a rod, F, which is united to the centre region of the bow through the agency of a universal joint, G. This joint, G, can slide along, and rotate around the bow and may be fixed when required by tightening the finger screw, H. The construction of the face-bow endows it with considerable flexibility for adjustment. It is used as follows:

(*a*) The position of the glenoid fossae are marked on the patient's face. These positions may be arrived at by placing a straight edge from the outer canthus of the eye to the apex of the tragus of the ear, and marking a point on this edge 1 cm. in front of the tragus (*see* fig. 213). It is easier to measure the distance between two fixed points than between two moving ones, so the measurements are taken from the maxilla to the glenoid fossae rather than from the mandible to the heads of the condyles. Whilst taking these measurements the actual positions of the heads of the condyles must be entirely ignored.

(*b*) Adapt a wax template to the upper record block and by warming the fork, fix it to the template; taking care that the rod, F, is placed to one side of the centre line. Place

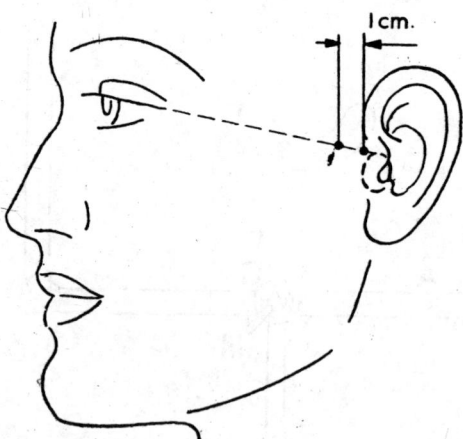

FIG. 213.– Determining the position of the glenoid fossae.

the upper record block, carrying the fork, into the patient's mouth and then insert the lower block and ask him to close. The position of the lower jaw in relation to the upper is of no importance, it is merely being used to hold the upper block in place.

(c) Loosen all the finger screws on the face-bow and slip the universal joint on to the rod, F, which is projecting from the mouth. Adjust the cups, D, so that they are in contact with the marks on the skin locating the glenoid fossae. Ensure that the face-bow is central in relation to the head by making certain that an equal number of graduations appear on both the rods, B. When the face-bow is correctly adjusted, tighten all the finger screws and it will then appear as in figs. 214 and 215.

(d) Loosen the finger screws, C, and remove the face-bow with the fork and the upper record block attached. Remove the record block, leaving the wax template

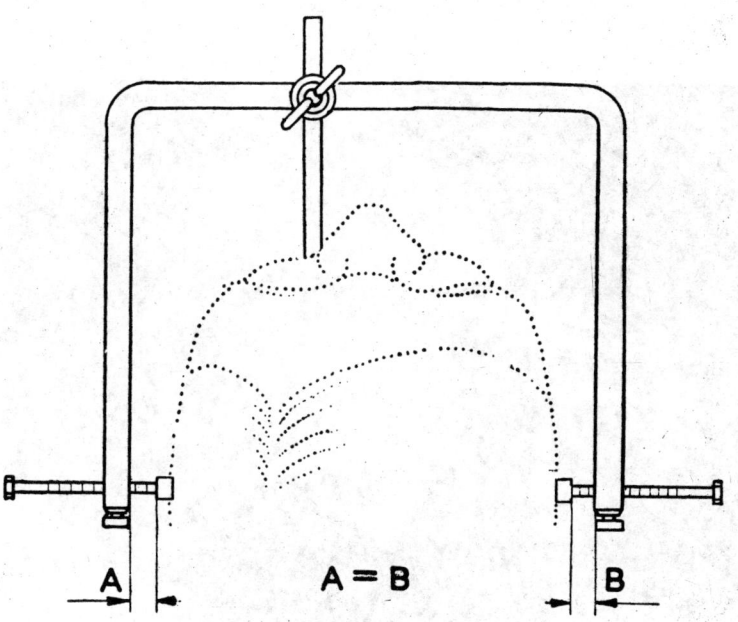

FIG. 214. – The face-bow in position. Seen from above.

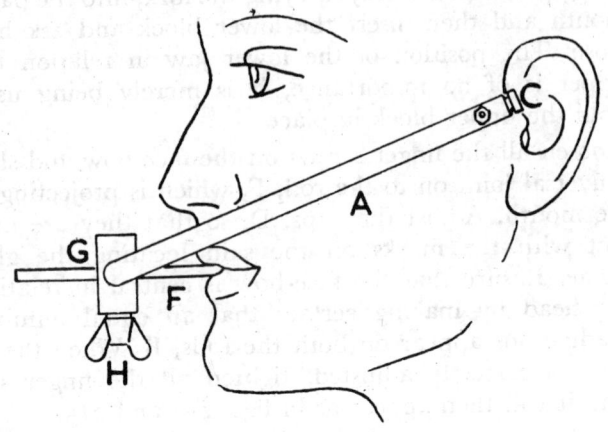

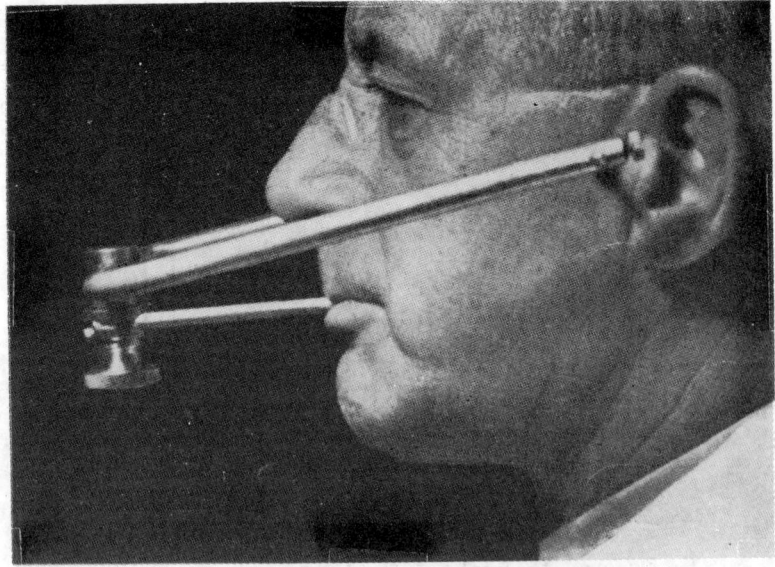

FIG. 215. – The face-bow in position. Seen from the side.

attached to the fork. The duplication in the template of the V-shaped grooves in the bite rims will enable it to be replaced in its correct position when required.

Mounting the Models on the Articulator

(*a*) Attach the face-bow to the articulator, making certain that it is correctly centred (*see* fig. 216).

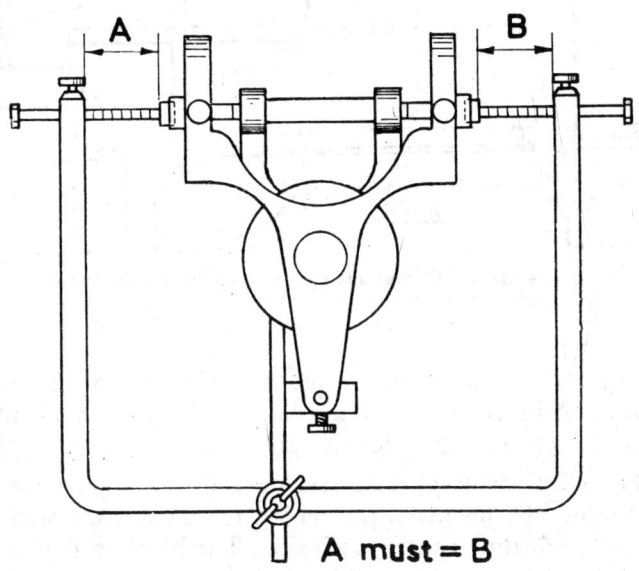

FIG. 216. – Attaching the face-bow to the articulator. Seen from above.

(*b*) Place the upper record block, together with the upper model, in place on the wax template of the face-bow fork and secure it firmly with molten wax. Raise or lower the front of the face-bow until the occlusal surface of the record block is parallel with the base of the articulator (*see* fig. 217). Support the face-bow in this position and, by means of plaster, attach the upper model to the upper member of the articulator which must also be parallel to the base.

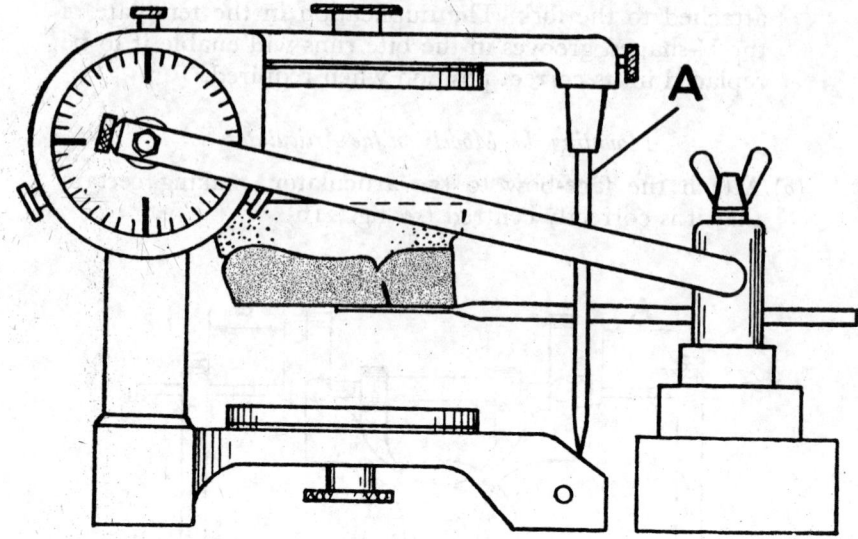

FIG. 217. – Method of positioning the upper model and record
block on the articulator by means of the face-bow.

(c) Adjust the hinge stop or incisal guide pin of the articulator, A in fig. 217, to maintain the upper arm parallel to the lower, and then remove the face-bow.

(d) The relationship of the lower model to the upper model is obtained by means of the record blocks and the wax template recording centric occlusion. The blocks are placed on the models, sealed to the template and the lower model then attached to the base of the articulator with plaster.

The upper model has now been fixed to the articulator in the same relationship to the hinge of the articulator as the patient's maxilla bears to his glenoid fossae (see fig. 218). Further, the lower model is now fixed to the articulator in the same relationship to the upper model as the patient's mandible bears to his maxilla in centric occlusion, and thus both models are related to one another and to the hinge of the articulator in a similar manner to the way the patient's maxilla and mandible are related to one another and to his condyles.

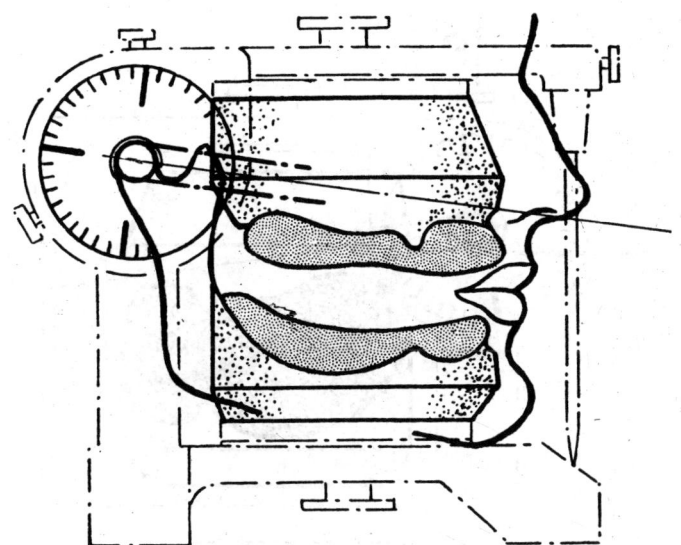

Fig. 218. – A face superimposed on an articulator to illustrate
how the maxillo-condylar relationship is copied on the
articulator by means of the face-bow.

Adjusting the Condylar Angle

(a) Loosen the articulator adjustments, B, and replace the
retrusive template, which is between the record blocks,
with one of the lateral templates (*see* fig. 219).

(b) Move the upper arm of the articulator and the adjustable
condylar path, C, until this template is accurately seated
between the record blocks. Lock the adjustment on the
opposite side to that to which the mandible has moved, i.e.
if the mandible has moved to the right, lock the left
condylar adjustment.

(c) Repeat the operation using the other lateral template.

When employing the single protrusive record to adjust the
articulator, the same procedure as for lateral recordings is
followed, except that both condylar paths are adjusted and
fixed by using the one template.

3. *Factors Influencing Balance*

For clarity of description, in the section that follows, the
mandible is described as moving from centric occlusion to

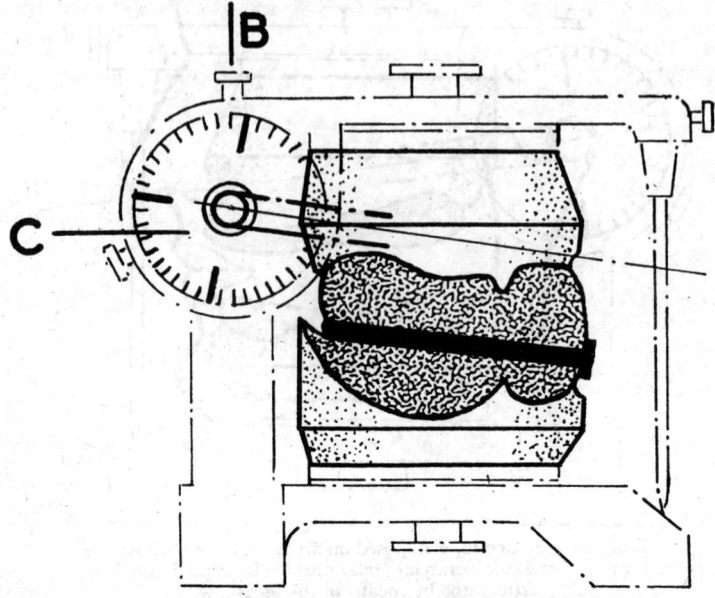

Fig. 219. – Setting the right condylar path of the articulator
by inserting the left lateral wax template between the record
blocks.

eccentric positions of occlusion with the occlusal surfaces of the
teeth in contact. During mastication, of course, the reverse
action actually occurs, the teeth occluding in an eccentric position and the lower teeth then moving in contact with the upper
teeth back into the centric position. However, provided the
records have been taken correctly, the articulator adjusted
properly and the teeth set to provide balance, it makes no
difference which way the mandible moves. Before the factors
influencing the position of the teeth can be formulated, and
before the articulator can be given the final adjustment
which will enable it to be used for setting-up, the factors,
influencing the movements of the mandible with the teeth in
contact, must be understood. Given a motive force, which is
the muscles, two factors influence these movements, they are:

(a) The condylar paths.
(b) The inclination of the contacting surfaces of the teeth.

During protrusion, with the teeth in contact, there must be a vertical drop equal to the depth of the anterior overbite, or to the depth of the posterior cuspal interdigitation, and this drop must be obtained during a forward movement equal to the overjet (*see* fig. 220). With the natural dentitions under consideration, the depth of the anterior overbite is greater than the posterior cusp depth, with the result that when the

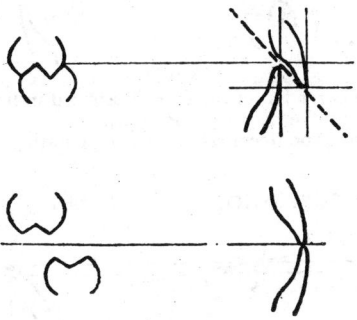

FIG 220. – Deep overbite leading to loss of contact of the posterior teeth when the mandible is protruded.

incisors are in edge-to-edge contact the posterior teeth are out of occlusion, This unbalanced articulation may be satisfactory for a time with the natural teeth supported in the bone, but it is a very unsatisfactory arrangement for artificial dentures; tipping and rocking of the denture is almost certain and the strains so imposed are apt to cause pain. excessive alveolar absorption and general instability.

This lack of balance can be corrected in dentures by increasing the steepness of the compensating curve, or by using posterior teeth with deeper cusps, or by a combination of both of these (*see* fig. 221). Only within narrow limits will these expedients prove satisfactory and beyond these limits the strains introduced will cause instability and pain.

Since the condylar control is a fixed factor which cannot be altered by the prosthetist, and the setting of the anterior teeth is capable of wide variation, it is obvious that the latter must be modified from the original when full dentures have to be constructed. This modification usually takes the form of a reduction

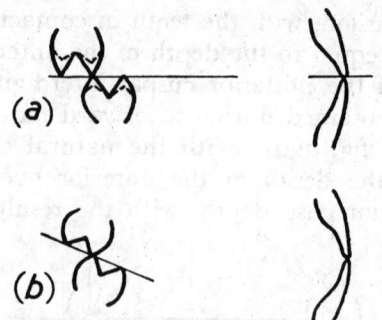

FIG. 221. – Correction of the fault illustrated in fig. 220 by –
(a) Increasing the height of the cusps.
(b) Increasing the steepness of the compensating curve.

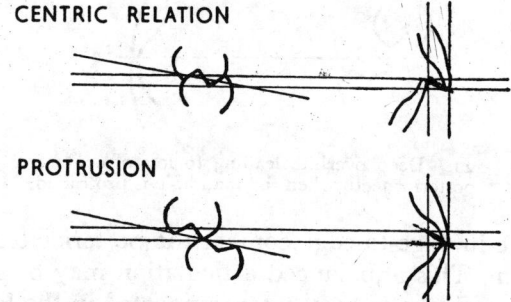

FIG. 222. – A reduction in the amount of overbite allows the
use of shallower cusps and a less extreme compensating curve.

in the amount of overbite, thus reducing the amount of vertical
opening necessary to bring the incisors edge to edge: this in
turn allows less deeply cusped teeth to be used and a less
extreme compensating curve (*see* fig. 222). The flatter the lower
ridge (i.e. the less it can resist lateral pressure), the less should
be the anterior overbite. It will be clear from a study of the
diagrams that a steepening of the anteroposterior compensating
curve will decrease the cusp angle, and vice versa.

Lateral Movements

The same lack of balance is found during lateral movements of
the mandible; the condyle on one side remains almost
stationary and therefore the posterior teeth on that side remain

in contact, with the lower cusps moving down the cusp inclines of the upper. On the opposite side, the head of the condyle moves downwards and forwards, thus tending to move the teeth on that side out of contact. The same conditions apply as for protrusion, i.e. that lack of lateral balance produces unsatisfactory dentures and that balance which is restored by very steep cusps, or a very steep compensating curve, will produce unstable dentures.

The Mandibular Path

In a protrusive movement with the teeth in contact, as has already been stated, the path of the mandible is directed at the back by the movements of the condyles down their respective paths, and in the front by the movement of the lower teeth against the inclines of the upper teeth.

In lateral movement the mandibular path is directed by the path of the moving condyle and the inclines of the teeth on the side towards which the mandible moves. To fix the movements of the mandible to certain well-defined channels, both the condylar angles and the slope of the tooth inclines must be known. We already know, and have transferred to the articulator, the slope of the condylar path but we do not know the cusp angles of the individual patient. Fortunately, however, we can fix these inclines within the limits set by the effect of the condylar paths, as we wish, and make the mandible follow our dictates.

The movement of the frame of the articulator is governed the three points, viz. posteriorly by the two condyles and anteriorly by the incisive guide pin which rests on the incisive guide table. Whilst each of these can be varied on the articulator, the condylar angles are determined by the patient and only the incisive angle is decided upon by the operator. Varying the angle of the incisive guide table will alter the angle which the path of the contacting surfaces of the anterior teeth makes with the horizontal, i.e. the incisive angle. The way in which one chooses the angle of the incisive guide table is explained later in the chapter.

It will be appreciated that there is no incisive guide table present in the mouth and when the dentures are inserted it is only the condyles and the teeth which govern lateral and protusive movements when the teeth are in contact. The incisive guide table is in fact merely a convenient substitute for the teeth prior to their insertion.

Figs. 223 and 224 illustrate the effect on the protrusive path of the mandible when the incisive guidance is altered while the condylar guidance remains the same. For any given setting of the condylar angles and incisive guide table the protrusive path followed by the mandible can be determined as follows:

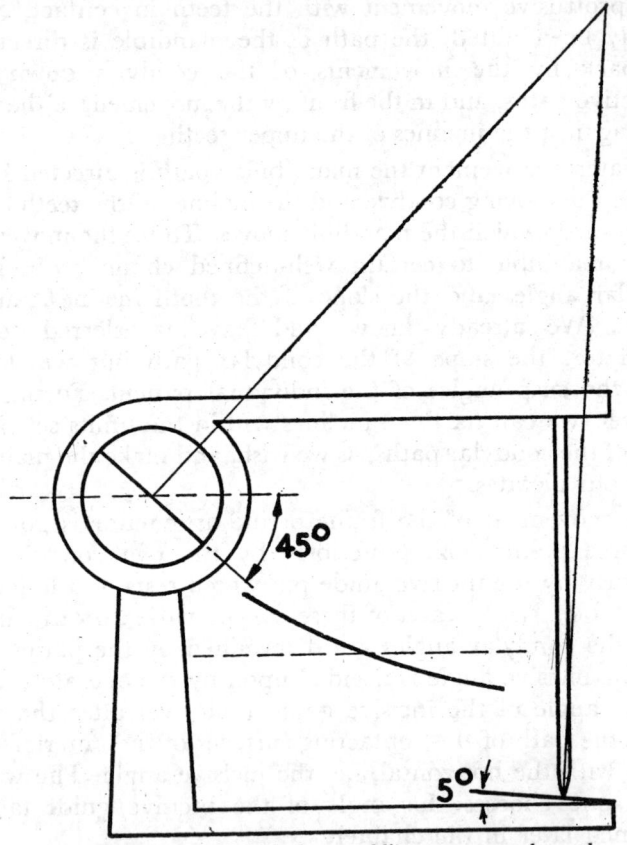

Fig. 223(a). – The thick black curved line represents the path of the mandible in protrusion with a condylar angle of 45° and an incisive angle of 5°. (A 45° condylar angle is never encountered in practice, but it simplifies the illustration.)

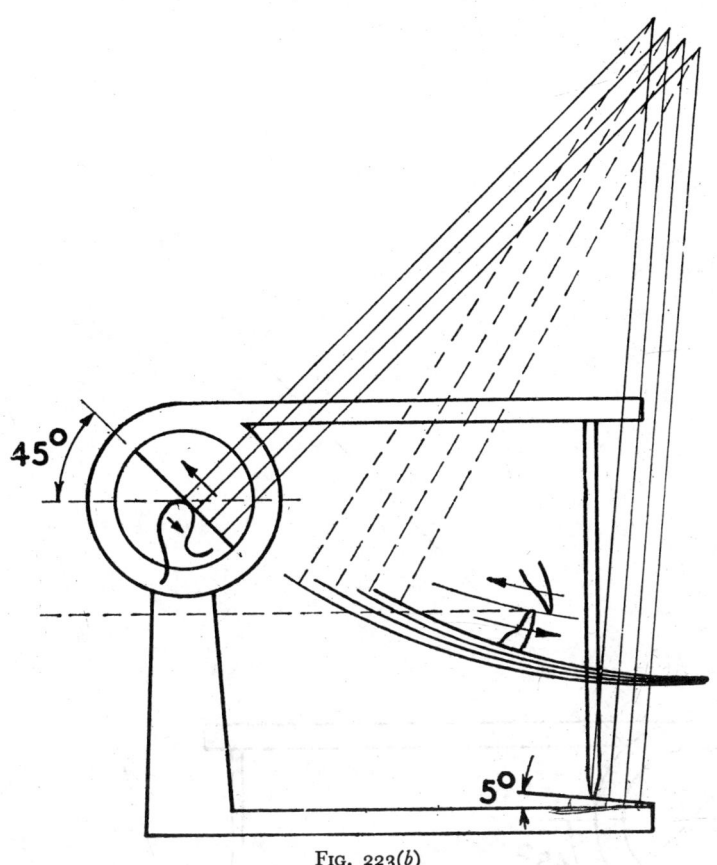

FIG. 223(b)

A line is drawn at right angles to the condylar path from the centre of the condyle, and another at right angles to the incisive guide table from the point of the incisive guide pin. The point where these lines meet is the rotation centre for the path of the mandible on that side (*see* figs. 223 and 224). It must be understood that the rotation centre is constantly changing as the mandible travels its path, but that, as the mandible moves, any given point on it moves with it and maintains the same relationship to each successive rotational centre. It may thus be stated that, for a given condylar path angle, the steeper the angle of the incisal guidance, the steeper

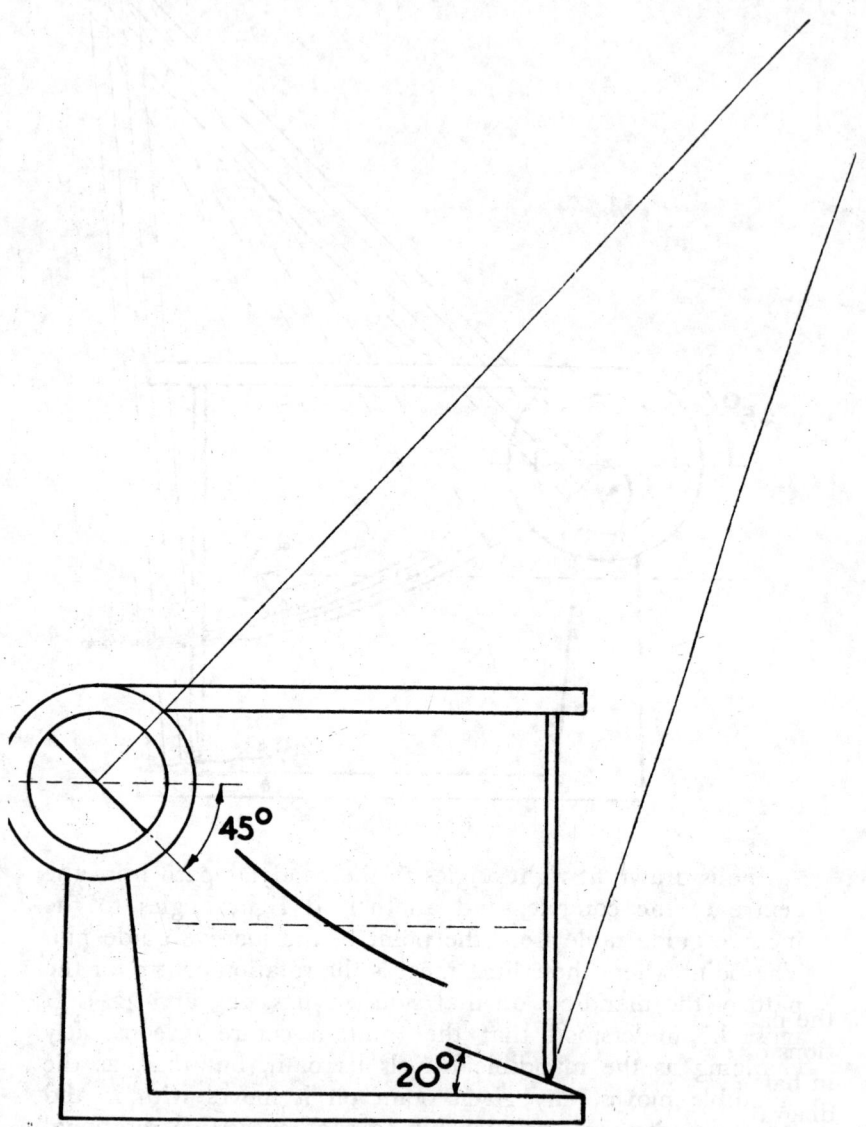

Fig. 224. – The thick black curved line represents the path
of the mandible in protrusion with a condylar angle of 45°
and an incisive angle of 20°. Compare with fig. 200a.

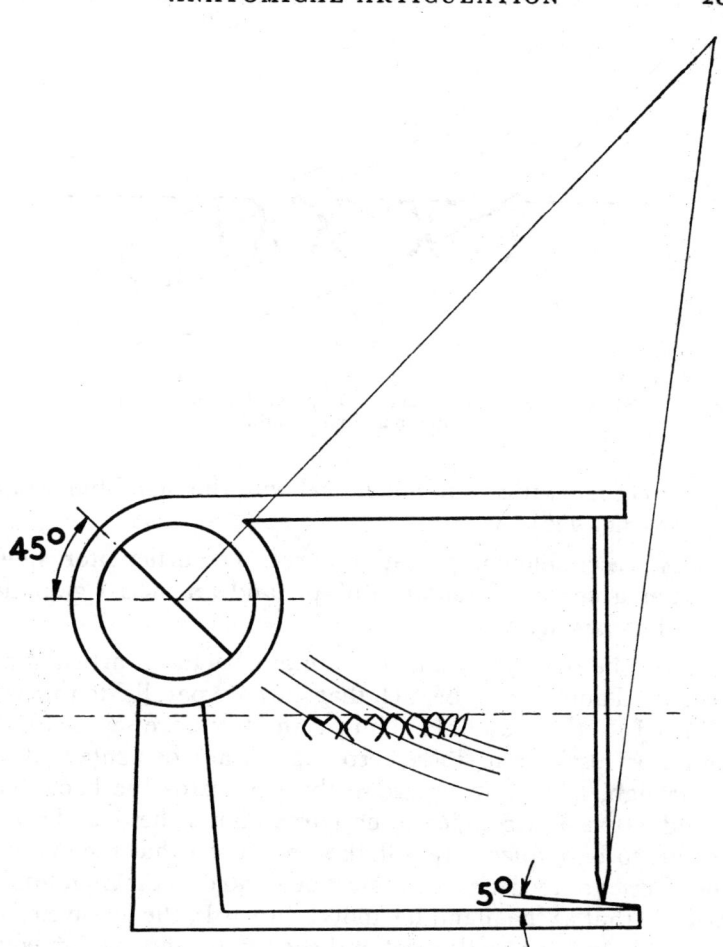

FIG. 225

(a) Illustrating the steepness of the cusps necessary when the teeth are set to a horizontal occlusal plane.

the path of the mandible, and vice versa The effect of variations of steepness of the mandibular path, on setting the teeth in balanced occlusion for protrusive movements, is best shown diagrammatically, and the following illustrations depict the variation in the cuspal angles of the teeth when they are set to:

(a) A horizontal occlusal plane (see fig. 225).

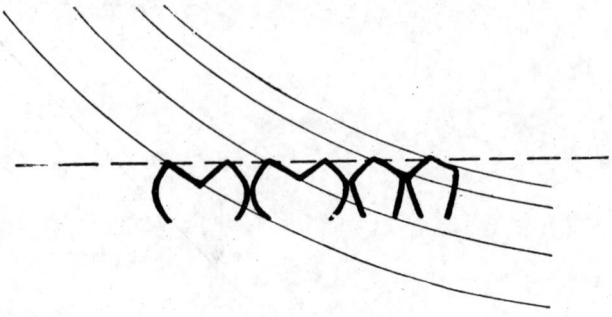

FIG. 225
(*b*) Enlargement of teeth to show parallelism of cusp angles
with the mandibular path.

(*b*) A compensating curve identical with the mandibular path
(*see* fig. 226).

(*c*) A reasonable compensating curve. The articulator shown
has a condylar guidance of 45° and an incisal guidance
of 5° (*see* fig. 227).

It will be observed that, to maintain balanced articulation,
the cuspal angles must be such that they are parallel to the path
followed by the mandible. Thus, if the teeth are set to a horizontal occlusal plane, these cusp angles must be acute and the
cusps high, becoming progressively so towards the back. The
introduction of a compensating curve allows these angles and
heights to be reduced. It will also be noticed that the overbite
and overjet of the front teeth must be related to the mandibular
path, so that as the mandible moves forwards, the incisive edges
of the lower front teeth meet and slide upon the incisive edges
of the upper front teeth (*see* fig. 228). This may be summed up
by saying that within the limits set by the path of the mandible
the greater the overbite, the greater must be the overjet, and
vice versa.

The rotational centres for the lateral movements are more
difficult to show diagrammatically, because they alter according to the part of the mandible being considered. Thus in the
molar region the condylar guidance is the stronger influence
and the incisive guidance is weak, whilst in the first premolar

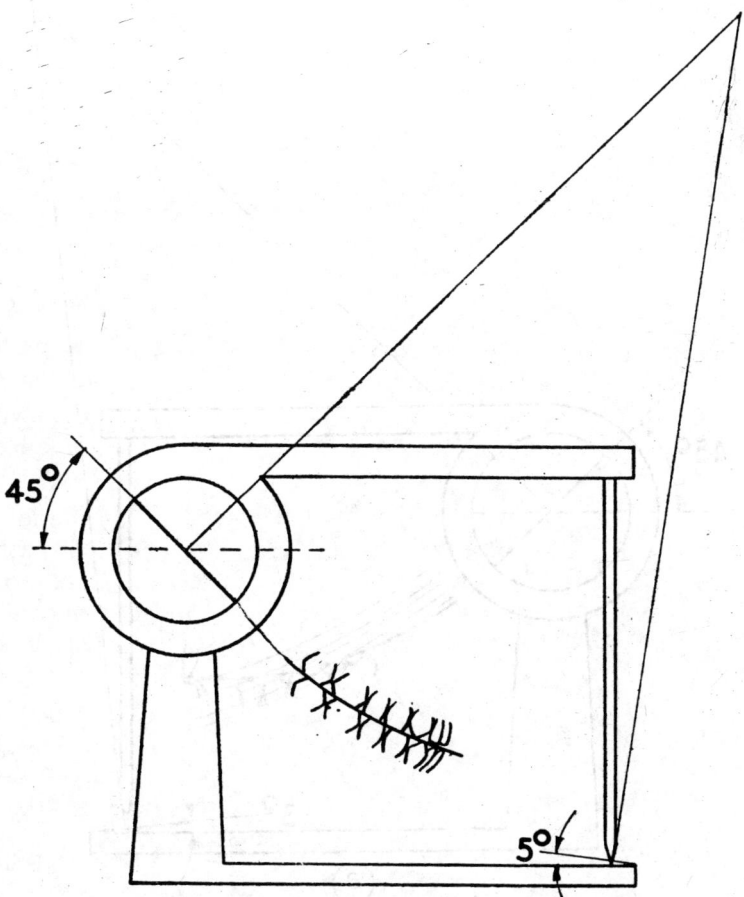

FIG. 226. – Teeth set to a compensating curve identical with the mandibular path. No cusp angle at all – flat-topped teeth.

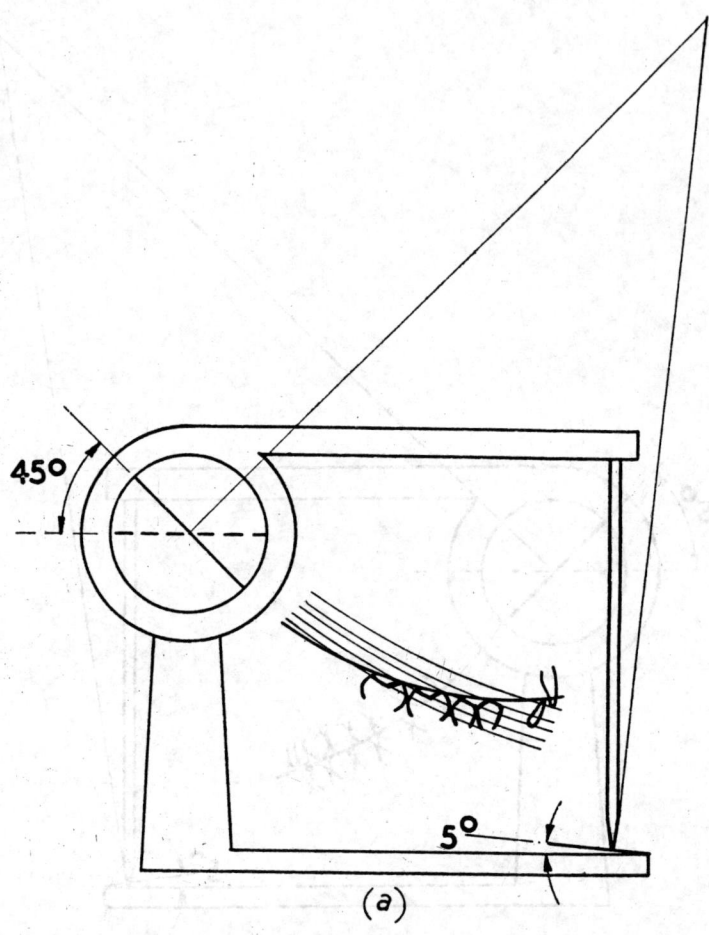

FIG. 227

(a) Teeth set to a reasonable compensating curve requiring cusps of normal height.

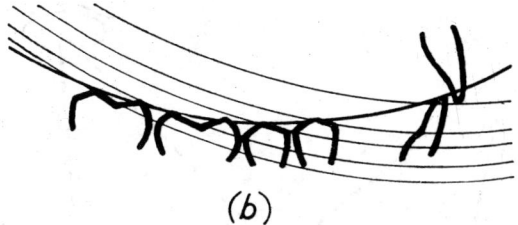

(b)

FIG. 227

(b) Enlargement of teeth to show how the parallelism of the cusp angles to the mandibular path is obtained by tilting the long axes of the teeth.

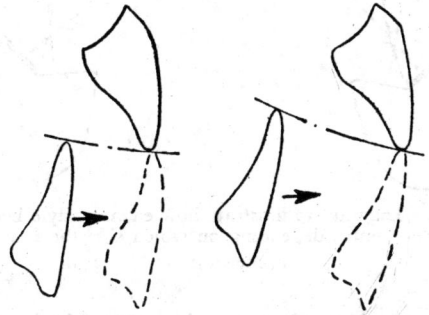

FIG. 228. – Illustrating how the overbite and overjet are related to the mandibular path.

region these conditions are reversed. Thus fig. 229 shows diagrammatically how each condyle becomes a rotational centre when it is on the working side. and fig. 230 shows the effect of an identical condylar and incisive guidance, i.e. both set to 30°, which gives an even lift to the moving frame of the articulator along the whole length of the balancing side. The side towards which the mandible moves is termed the working side, and the side from which it moves, the balancing side. On the working side the condylar guidance is nil, because that condyle does not move (except for the Bennett movement which is not allowed for in most articulators). Thus the only upward movement of the working side is controlled by the incisal guidance, which decreases in influence from before backwards.

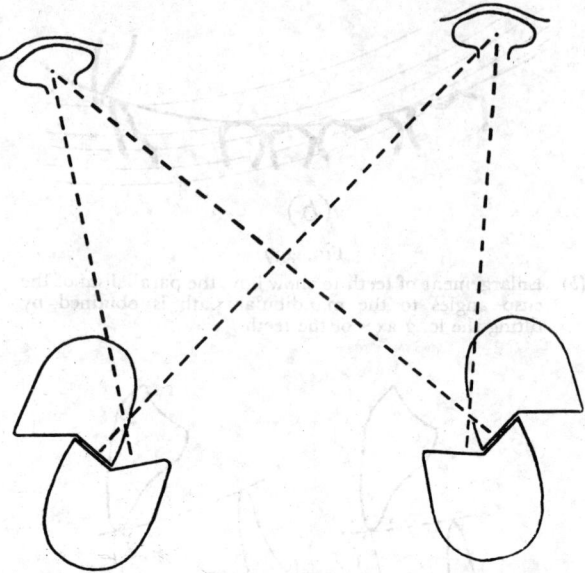

FIG. 229. – Diagram to illustrate how each condyle becomes
a rotational centre depending on which side the individual
is chewing.

Fig. 231 shows the effect on the mandibular path in the
regions of the various teeth, with a condylar guidance of 30°
and an incisive guidance of 5°. The angles of the path given are
rough approximations, but they enable a picture to be formed
of the influence on lateral mandibular movements of the condylar and incisal guidance, and show clearly how an alteration
of the incisal guidance alters the mandibular path.

Thus if a composite diagram is drawn showing the paths
followed in both right and left lateral movements, of a case
with both condylar guidances of 30° and the incisal guidance
5°, then AB is the path followed when the left side is the
balancing side and CB the path when it is the working side
(see fig. 231).

Thus in order that tne teeth shall maintain balance during
lateral mandibular movements, they must be set as shown in
fig. 232.

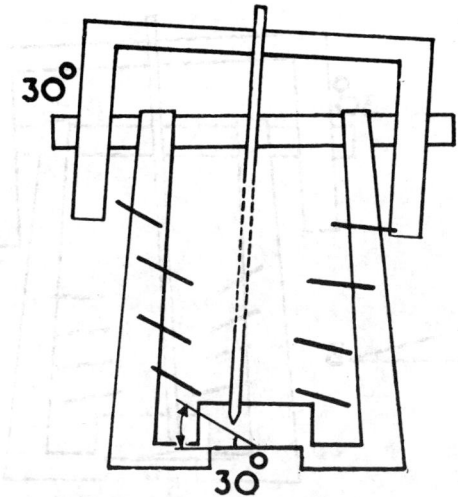

Fig. 230. – Diagrammatic representation of the paths of the posterior teeth during a lateral mandibular movement with a condylar and incisive guidance both of 30°. The paths represent in ascending order those of the 1st premolar, 2nd premolar, 1st molar, and 2nd molar teeth.

The left side in the diagram is the balancing side and the right the working side, because on the articulator it is the upper frame which moves.

Fig. 233 shows how they maintain balance when in balancing occlusion, and fig. 234 when in working occlusion.

The palatal inclines of the maxillary teeth, and the buccal inclines of the mandibular teeth, must be parallel to the path AB, and the buccal inclines of the maxillary teeth, and the lingual inclines of the mandibular teeth, must be parallel to the line CB.

Fig. 235 shows how cuspal interference will occur if teeth are set to a horizontal occlusal plane, and how the introduction of the lateral compensating curve corrects this.

Fig. 236 shows how cusp locking can also occur in a protrusive movement if the anteroposterior cuspal angles are not in harmony with the protrusive path of the mandible.

The Setting of the Incisal Guide Table

From the foregoing it will be realized that the angle of the incisal guide table will markedly affect the cusp angles,

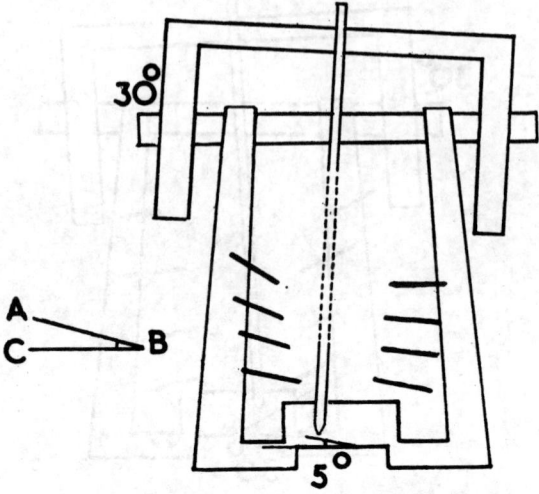

Fig. 231. – Diagrammatic representation of the paths of the posterior teeth during a lateral mandibular movement with a condylar guidance of 30° and an incisive guidance of 5°.
    AB represents the path followed by the 2nd premolar tooth when the left side, in the diagram, is acting as the balancing side, and CB represents the path followed by this tooth when the left side is acting as the working side.

cusp heights, the overbite and the overjet. The question, therefore, is how it is set for any given case. The way to do this is as follows:

Set up the upper and lower six front teeth to the required overbite and overjet, and then alter the incisal guidance table so that in protrusion, and right and left lateral movements, the incisive edges of the upper and lower teeth just slide upon one another. Remember, however, that the steeper the slope of the guidance table, the higher and steeper will need to be the cusps of the molar teeth, and even with balanced articulation high steep cusps are liable to cause instability. Therefore, when setting the teeth, make the overbite as small as possible.

This is particularly true when the mandible is flat and almost entirely ridgeless, where in extreme cases the posterior teeth must be virtually cuspless if functional stability is to be attained.

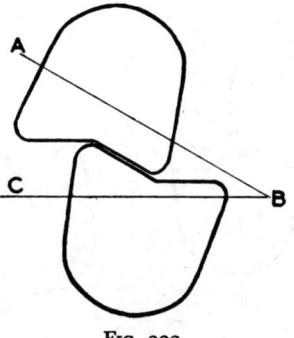

FIG. 232

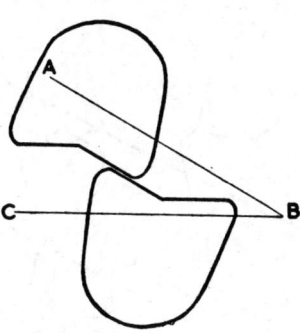

FIG. 233

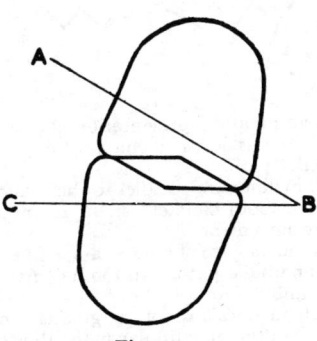

Fig. 234

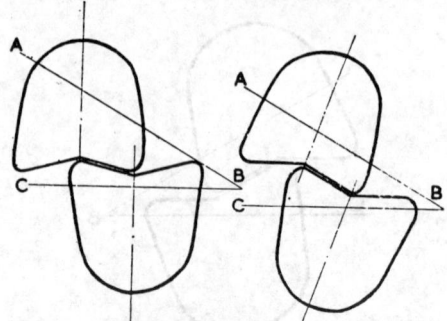

FIG. 235

(a) Teeth set with long axes vertical. Cuspal inclines not parallel to planes of movement.

(b) Long axes of teeth inclined to lateral compensating curve. Cuspal inclines are now parallel to planes of movement.

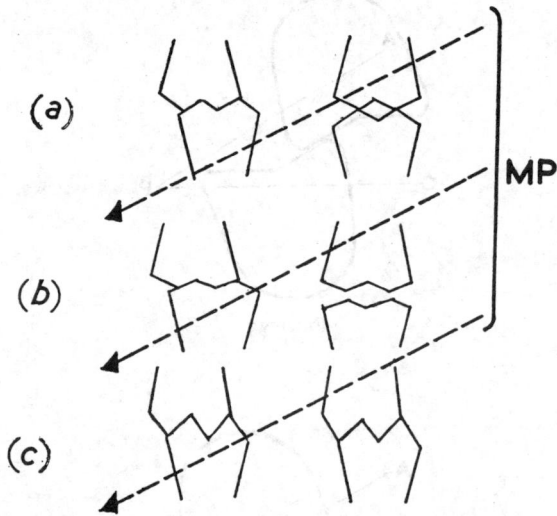

FIG. 236. – Diagrammatic representation of cusp locking and loss of cuspal contact.

MP = mandibular path.

(a) The cuspal inclines are parallel to the mandibular path and therefore tooth contact can be maintained during mandibular movement.

(b) The cuspal inclines are of a lesser angle to the horizontal than the mandibular path, thus tooth contact will be lost during mandibular movement.

(c) The cuspal inclines are of a greater angle to the horizontal than the mandibular path; thus cusp locking occurs if mandibular movement is attempted.

4. *Teeth for Anatomical Articulation*

Several varieties of teeth have been manufactured especially for use with anatomical articulators, and their cuspal angles are arranged to facilitate occlusal balance: in a few instances the angle which the cuspal plane makes with the horizontal plane is stated.

Cusped Teeth

A cusped posterior tooth should generally be used in preference to a cuspless one for two reasons:

(*a*) Greater efficiency.

(*b*) Balance is more easily obtained.

(*a*) *Greater Efficiency.* – A convex surface makes point contact with a flat or convex surface, and this point contact, moving under pressure, results in a cutting action. The cusps also produce a grinding action when moving through the inter-cuspal spaces which help to hold the food in position whilst it is being ground Provided that the cusps and sulci are correctly shaped, there is ample clearance space for the ground and cut particles to escape from the occlusal surfaces. Flat, cuspless teeth, whilst able to crush and grind food, cannot possibly cut vegetable or animal fibres, which must therefore be reduced to a length suitable for swallowing before being placed in the mouth.

(*b*) *Balance.* – With cusped teeth it is a simple matter to obtain a balanced articulation and to perfect it by grinding any points of contact where pressure may be slightly excessive. With cuspless teeth it is very difficult to obtain a balance and the most satisfactory way of doing so is to use a technique employing plaster of Paris and pumice record blocks which will shortly be described. Final adjustment of these cuspless surfaces is difficult, as the surface contacts are so broad.

Inverted Cusped Teeth

There are several makes of teeth, which are described as having 'inverted cusps' which are in effect flat-surfaced teeth with hollows ground into the occlusal surface. The claim is made for these teeth that food fibres are cut between the edges of the hollows, whilst the flat surfaces allow lateral movements without cuspal interference. With most teeth of this type the first claim is quite inaccurate as the hollows are not provided with escape grooves for the food, and consequently immediately become filled up and clogged. The second claim is correct in that they will avoid cuspal interference, but on the other hand it is difficult to grind these flat surfaces to give balanced articulation.

Plaster Record Rim Technique

The techniques which have been described so far have all left the degree of curvature of the compensating curves to the discretion of the technician, whilst the object of this technique is to obtain the individual curves of a given patient. Briefly, this is attained by inserting record blocks with friable rims and allowing the patient to grind them together until they are in balanced articulation.

1. Bases

Stability of the record blocks is essential for accuracy since there will be a considerable lateral and protrusive drag, owing to friction, during the process of grinding and, therefore, the bases should be made of acrylic resin.

2. Rims

These are made of a mixture of plaster of Paris and an abrasive, the latter being coarse carborundum, pumice or sand and a suitable mixture which is fairly strong, and quick cutting, is 60 per cent artificial stone with 40 per cent carborundum. The width should be approximately 1 cm. which is necessary to define the lateral curves and is also required for strength.

It is essential when employing this technique that the jaw relationship is first recorded using wax blocks and the blocks with abrasive rims are constructed to models mounted to the correct jaw relationship but with the vertical height opened by about 5 mm. to allow for the closure which will result from the grinding.

The plaster rims should be allowed to set for at least twenty-four hours before being used and should then be painted, except on the occlusal surfaces, with three coats of sandarac varnish. This varnishing helps to prevent crumbling of the rims during grinding, particularly on the edges of the occlusal surfaces.

Another method of constructing the rims is to make them of composition to within 6 mm. of the estimated correct height, to groove the composition for retention and then build up the plaster-pumice for a further 1 cm. (*see* fig. 237).

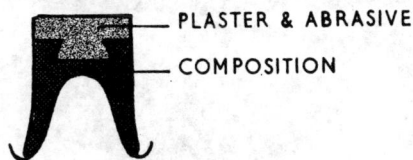

PLASTER & ABRASIVE

COMPOSITION

Fig. 237. – Details of the construction of a plaster bite rim.

3. *Grinding*

The patient is instructed to grind the blocks together with both lateral and protrusive movements but only to use the minimum pressure necessary to keep the blocks in contact. The necessity for using very light pressure must be emphasized since the high proportion of abrasive which is needed for rapid cutting very materially weakens the plaster which will crack or crumble if anything approaching full masticatory pressure is used.

Denture adhesive is useful to assist stability of the blocks, or the operator may support the blocks with his fingers to prevent any movements in the preliminary stages of grinding.

The patient should be instructed not to swallow the debris, and the record blocks must be removed from time to time for cleaning and inspection and to allow the patient to rinse his mouth and also to rest.

The grinding should be continued until the correct vertical height is obtained which will usually be accomplished within ten minutes. The occlusal surfaces of the rims now show correct balancing curves for that individual (*see* fig. 238) which are reproduced in the denture by mounting the lower teeth to occlude with the upper block and then the upper teeth to occlude with the lower ones (*see* fig. 239).

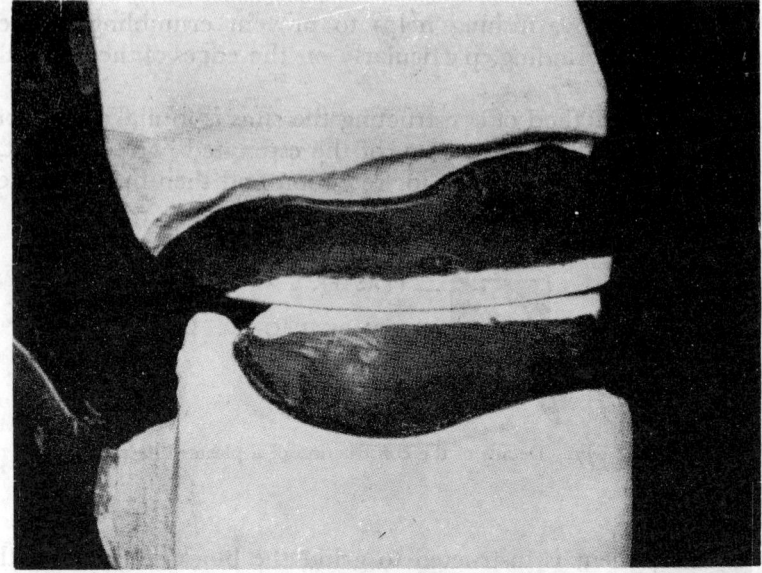

(a) From the side.

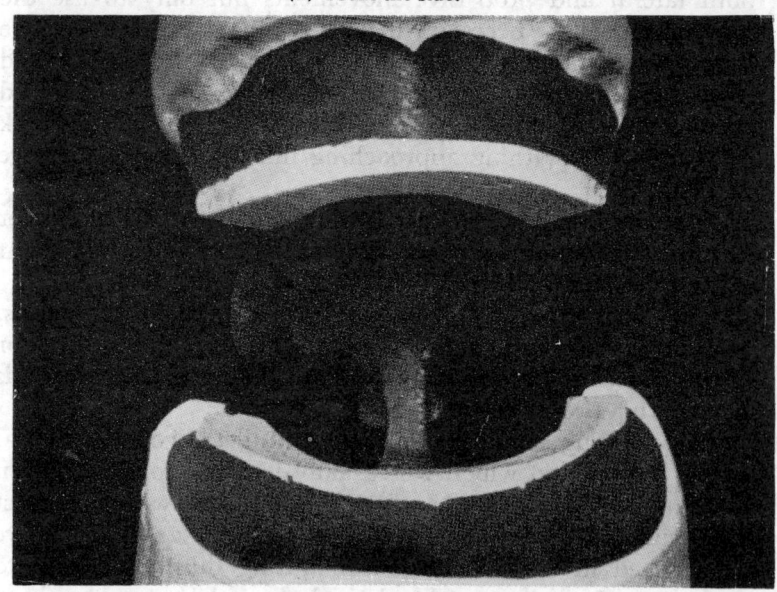

(b) From the front.
FIG. 238. – Plaster pumice blocks after having been ground in.

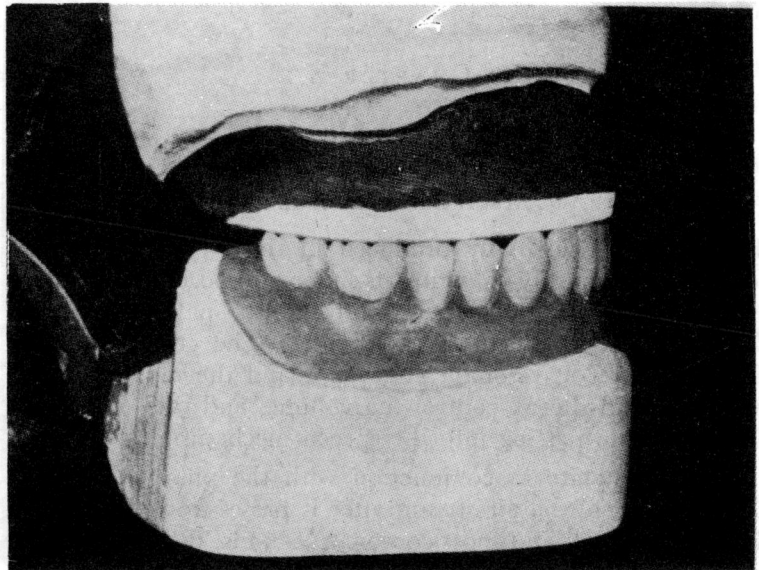

FIG. 239. – Lower teeth set to upper ground in block.

It should be appreciated that there are numerous balancing curves suitable for every individual and that curves obtained by this grinding technique under different conditions are not interchangeable. The form of curve will vary with the height of the occlusal surfaces and also with the original shape of the plaster-pumice blocks, whether flat or curved.

Chapter X

PHONETICS

Mechanism of Speech

The voice is principally produced in the larynx, whilst the tongue by constantly changing its shape and position of contact with the lips, teeth, alveoli and hard and soft palates, gives the sound form and influences its qualities. The oral cavity and the sinuses act as resonant chambers, and the muscles of the abdomen and thorax control the volume, and rate of flow, of the air stream passing into the speech mechanism.

The soft palate in conjunction with the pharynx controls the direction of the air stream after it passes from the larynx. In all the vowel, and most consonant sounds, the air stream is confined entirely to the oral cavity, but a few nasal sounds do occur, e.g. M, N, and NG, in which the air is expelled mainly through the nose. The former are produced by raising the soft palate into close contact with the pharynx, thus sealing off the nose and forcing the air to proceed through the mouth.

With the nasal sounds the soft palate is pressed downwards and forwards and the dorsum of the tongue humped up to meet it, thus sealing off the oral cavity and forcing the air stream to proceed through the nose. The vowel sounds A, E, I, O, U are formed by a continuous air flow, the alteration in size of the mouth and the change in shape and size of the lip opening giving the various sounds their characteristic form.

The consonant sounds are produced by the air stream being stopped in its passage through the mouth by the formation of complete or partial seals or stops. These are produced by the tongue pressing against the teeth or palate, or by the closing of the lips. The sudden breaking of the seal brought about by the withdrawal of the tongue, or the opening of the lips, produces the sound. In many sounds there is a build up of air

302

pressure behind the stop which when the seal is released produces an explosive effect. Examples of these are: the lip closure of the P and B sounds; the tongue and anterior hard palate contact in T and D sounds.

In some cases the seal or stop is not complete, but the channel through which the air stream must pass is made extremely narrow: an example of this is the production of an S, Z, or C soft sound, in which the tongue separates itself from the anterior aspect of the hard palate by about 1 mm., forming a thin slit-like channel through which the air stream hisses.

Speech, therefore, is largely a matter of the control of the size and shape of the mouth, which is chiefly governed by the position of the tongue and its contact with the teeth, alveoli and palate.

Fortunately for the prosthetist, the tongue possesses remarkable qualities of adaptability, and rapidly becomes accustomed to changes occurring in the mouth. After the extraction of teeth, or the insertion of a denture, some difference may be noticed in the quality of the speech, but improvement quickly follows as the tongue adjusts itself to the new conditions. In extreme cases, such as the edentulous state or when poorly designed complete dentures are worn, the previous tone and quality are not always re-established. The tongue's adaptability is illustrated by the number of individuals wearing dentures, designed with little regard to their effect on phonation, who exhibit no obviously apparent speech defects; the reason being that in the construction of those dentures the general principles of setting up were followed, coupled with due regard to the aesthetic requirements and the attainment of the correct vertical dimension. This has produced the occlusal plane at a level corresponding to that of the natural dentition, the anterior teeth in approximately the same position anteroposteriorly as the natural teeth, and the new dental arch conforming to that of the previous arch, thereby allowing the correct tongue space. Thus the artificial dentures replacing the lost tissues have conformed closely to the state which existed naturally, the main difference being the increase in bulk – a factor for which the tongue must compensate.

However, some knowledge of phonetics in relation to dentures is necessary, in order to correct the speech defects that may occur in denture wearers, and also to act as a guide for the more accurate construction of complete dentures.

The Factors in Denture Construction Affecting Phonation

The Vowel Sounds

These sounds are produced by a continuous air stream passing through the oral cavity which is in the form of a single chamber for the A, O, U sounds and a double chamber for the I and E sounds, the division occurring through the dorsum of the tongue touching the soft palate in the post-dam region. The tip of the tongue, in all the vowel sounds, lies on the floor of the mouth either in contact with or close to the lingual surfaces of the lower anterior teeth and gums. The application of this in denture construction is that the lower anterior teeth should be set so that they do not impede the tongue positioning for these sounds; that is, they should not be set lingual to the alveolar ridge. Since the vowels E and I necessitate contact between the tongue and soft palate, the upper denture base must be kept thin, and the posterior border should merge into the soft tissue in order to avoid irritating the dorsum of the tongue, which might occur if this surface of the denture was allowed to remain thick and square-ended.

The Consonant Sounds

For convenience, these sounds may be classified thus:

(a) *Labials*

Formed mainly by the lips (e.g. B, P, M).

(b) *Labiodentals*

Formed by the lips and teeth (e.g. F, V, Ph).

(c) *Linguodentals*

Formed by the tongue and teeth (e.g. Th).

(d) *Linguopalatals*

Formed by the tongue and palate.

(i) Tongue and anterior portion of the hard palate (e.g. D, T, C (soft), S, Z, R).

(ii) Tongue and portion of the hard palate posterior to that of (i) (e.g. J, CH, SH, L, R).

(iii) Tongue and soft palate (e.g. C (hard), K, G, NG).

(e) *Nasal* (e.g. M, N, NG – also belonging to the other groups).

Unless careful consideration is given to the following aspects of denture construction, speech defects will occur varying from the almost indiscernible to the unpleasantly obvious.

1. *Denture Thickness and Peripheral Outline*

The prosthetist's aim is to produce dentures which are mechanically functional, aesthetically pleasing and permit normal speech. The most satisfactory attainment of the first two requirements may cause slight defects in the patient's speech but this should not be allowed to happen and some compromise will often be required satisfactorily to balance these three aims. One of the reasons for loss of tone and incorrect phonation is the decrease of air volume and loss of tongue room in the oral cavity resulting from unduly thick denture bases. The periphery of the denture must not be overextended so as to encroach upon the movable tissues, since the depth of the sulci will vary with the movements of the tongue, lips and cheeks during the production of speech sounds. Any interference with the freedom of these movements may result in indistinct phonation, especially if the function of the lips is in any way hindered.

Most important is the thickness of the denture base covering the palate, for here no loss of natural tissue has occurred, and the base reduces the amount of tongue space and the oral air volume. The palate in this instance does not include that part forming the tooth-bearing area – artificial alveolus.

The production of the palatolingual group of sounds involves contact between the tongue, and either the palate, the alveolar process, or the teeth. With the consonants T and D, the tongue makes firm contact with the anterior part of the hard palate, and is suddenly drawn downwards, producing an explosive sound; any thickening of the denture base in this region may cause incorrect formation of these sounds. When producing the S, C (soft), Z, R and L consonant sounds, contact occurs between the tongue and the most anterior part of the hard palate, including the lingual surfaces of the upper and lower incisors to a slight degree. In the case of the S, C (soft), and Z sounds, a slit-like channel is formed between the tongue and palate through which the air hisses. If the artificial rugae are over-pronounced, or the denture base too thick in this area, the air channel will be obstructed and a noticeable lisp may occur as a result.

To produce the Ch and J sounds the tongue is pressed against a larger area of the hard palate, and in addition makes contact with the upper alveolar process, bringing about the explosive effect by rapidly breaking the seal thus formed. The Sh sound is similar in formation, but the air is allowed to escape between the tongue and palate without any explosive effect, and if the palate is too thick in the region of the rugae, it may impair the production of these consonants.

2. *Vertical Dimension*

The formation of the labials P, B and M require that the lips make contact to check the air stream. With P and B, the lips part quite forcibly so that the resultant sound is produced with an explosive effect, whereas in the M sound lip contact is passive. For this reason M can be used as an aid in obtaining the correct vertical height since a strained appearance during lip contact, or the inability to make contact, indicates that the bite blocks are occluding prematurely. With the C (soft), S and Z sounds the teeth come very close together, and more especially so in the case of Ch and J; if the vertical dimension is excessive, the dentures will actually make contact as these consonants are formed, and the patient will most likely complain of 'clicking teeth'.

3. *The Occlusal Plane*

The labiodentals, F, V and Ph, are produced by the air stream being stopped and explosively released when the lower lip breaks contact with the incisal edges of the upper anterior teeth. If the occlusal plane is set too high the correct positioning of the lower lip may be difficult, if on the other hand the plane is too low, the lip will overlap the labial surfaces of the upper teeth to a greater extent than is required for normal phonation and the sound might be affected.

4. *The Anteroposterior Position of the Incisors*

In setting the upper anterior teeth consideration of their labiopalatal position is necessary for the correct formation of the labiodental F, V and Ph. If they are placed too far palatally the contact of the lower lip with the incisal and labial surfaces may be difficult, as the lip will tend to pass outside the teeth: the appearance usually prevents the operator from setting these teeth forward of their natural position. If the anterior teeth are placed too far back some effect may be noticed on the quality of the palatolinguals, S, C (soft), and Z, in which the tip of the tongue makes slight contact with the upper and lower incisors: this will result in a lisp due to the tongue making contact with the teeth prematurely. The tongue will more readily accommodate itself to anteroposterior errors in the setting of the teeth than to vertical errors.

5. *The Post-dam Area*

Errors of construction in this region involve the vowels I and E and the palatolingual consonants K, NG, G and C (hard). In the latter group the air blast is checked by the base of the tongue being raised upwards and backwards to make contact with the soft palate. A denture which has a thick base in the post-dam area, or that edge finished square instead of tapering, will probably irritate the dorsum of the tongue, impeding speech and possibly producing a feeling of nausea. Indirectly the post-dam seal influences phonation, for if it is inadequate the denture may become unseated during the formation of those sounds having an explosive effect, requiring the sudden repositioning of the tongue to control and stabilize the denture; this applies particularly to singers. Incidentally, speech is usually of poor quality in those individuals whose upper denture has become so loose that it is held in position mainly by means of tongue pressure against the palate. Careful observation will show that the denture, in such cases, rises and falls with tongue movements during speech.

Before passing to the next factor it should be mentioned that the consonants M, N, NG also belong to the nasal group in which the air stream is allowed to escape into the nasal cavity through a slight channel formed by the incomplete approximation of the soft palate and pharynx.

6. *Width of Dental Arch*

If the teeth are set to an arch which is too narrow the tongue will be cramped, thus affecting the size and shape of the air channel; this results in faulty phonation of such consonants as T, D, S, M, N, K, C and H, where the lateral margins of the tongue make contact with the palatal surfaces of the upper posterior teeth. Every endeavour should be made, consistent with the general mechanical principles, to place the lingual and palatal surfaces of the artificial teeth in the position previously occupied by the natural dentition.

7. *Relationship of the Upper Anterior to the Lower Anterior Teeth*

The chief concern is that of the S sound which requires near contact of the upper and lower incisors so that the air stream is allowed to escape through a slight opening between the teeth. In abnormal protrusive and retrusive jaw relationships, some difficulty may be experienced in the formation of this sound, and it will probably necessitate adjustment of the upper and lower anterior teeth anteroposteriorly, so that approximation can be brought about successfully. The consonants Ch, J and Z require a similar air channel in their formation.

SUMMARY

To summarize, it will be seen that speech requirements call for dentures having a correct vertical dimension, an accurate periphery and an arch formation permitting natural tongue space, so that adequate freedom for movement is ensured. The position of the anterior teeth should be such that they follow that of the natural teeth, thus fixing the occlusal plane at the correct level and preventing the placing of the artificial teeth inside or outside the natural arch, which would require the tongue to adapt itself to new circumstances. Finally, denture bases should be fashioned suitably thin, but consistent with the other factors of denture construction, so that contact by the tongue takes place in as near a natural and normal manner as is possible.

CHAPTER XI

TRYING IN THE DENTURES

Having set-up the teeth according to the information secured at the record stage, it is necessary to try the waxed-up dentures in the patient's mouth before finishing them, so that they may be checked. Once the dentures have been processed it is laborious and difficult to effect any alterations, whereas in the waxed-up stage changes can easily be made. Since so many points require checking, it is sound practice to get into the habit of working to a definite plan, and the following order is suggested:

1. *The Lower Denture By Itself.*
Check –
    (*a*) Peripheral outline   (i) Buccal and labial.
                               (ii) Lingual.
                               (iii) Posterior extension.
    (*b*) Stability to occlusal stresses.
    (*c*) Tongue space.
    (*d*) Height of the occlusal plane.

2. *The Upper Denture By Itself.*
Check –
    (*a*) Peripheral outline   (i) Buccal and labial.
                               (ii) Posterior border.
    (*b*) Stability to occlusal stresses.

3. *Both Dentures Together.*
Check –
    (*a*) Position of occlusion   (i) Horizontal relationship.
                                 (ii) Vertical height.

(*b*) Evenness of occlusal pressure.

(*c*) Balanced occlusion (anatomical articulation only).

(*d*) Appearance   (i) Centre line.

(ii) Anterior plane.

(iii) Shape of the teeth.

(iv) Size of the teeth.

(v) Shade of the teeth.

(vi) Profile.

(vii) Amount of tooth visible.

(viii) Regularity of the teeth.

(*e*) Approval of appearance by the patient.

Before carrying out these checks, remove the dentures from the articulator and place them in a bowl of cold water. It is important that 'waxed-up' dentures should be frequently placed in cold water as wax softens appreciably at mouth temperature and, if left in the mouth too long, the teeth may be displaced. The method of carrying out these checks is as follows:

1. Trying in the Lower Denture By Itself

Place the denture in the mouth and seat it on the ridge.

(*a*) Check the Peripheral Outline

The entire periphery should be checked to ensure that it is not over, or under, extended.

(i) *The Buccal and Labial Periphery*. – Hold the denture in place with light pressure on the occlusal surfaces of the teeth, and move the cheek on one side gently, but firmly, upwards and inwards, thus simulating the motion it makes when chewing. Now relax the pressure on the teeth and observe if the denture rises from the ridge. If it does, trim the periphery where it is seen to be overextended until little or no movement occurs. Pay particular attention to the buccal fraena and ensure that they have adequate clearance. Repeat for the opposite side and for the lip. Note the bulk and shape of the buccal aspect of the denture. It should take the form of a gentle concavity looking outwards and upwards (*see* Chapter II). Such a contour will aid the retention of the denture as the cheek will tend to fit into the concavity and hold the denture down.

(ii) *The Lingual Periphery.* – Hold the denture in place with light pressure and ask the patient to protrude his tongue sufficiently to moisten his lips; if the denture lifts at the back, it is overextended in the region of the lingual pouch. Next, ask the patient to put the tip of his tongue as far back on his palate as possible; if the denture lifts in the front, it is overextended anteriorly, probably in the region of the lingual fraenum. Such overextension must be relieved, but care should be taken to avoid over-trimming, which is very easily done owing to the difficulty of seeing the functional depth of the lingual sulcus when the denture is in place. Final adjustments are more easily and more accurately made after the finished denture has been worn for a few days, when areas of slight inflammation will indicate the precise location of overextension.

(iii) *Posterior Extension.* – Ensure that the heels of the lower denture are extended as high up the ascending ramus of the mandible as is practicable. The purpose of this is to buttress the denture against the backward pressure of the lower lip (*see* fig. 240).

(iv) *Under Extension.* – Though of less common occurrence than over extension it is equally important that the periphery should not be under extended since dentures must cover the

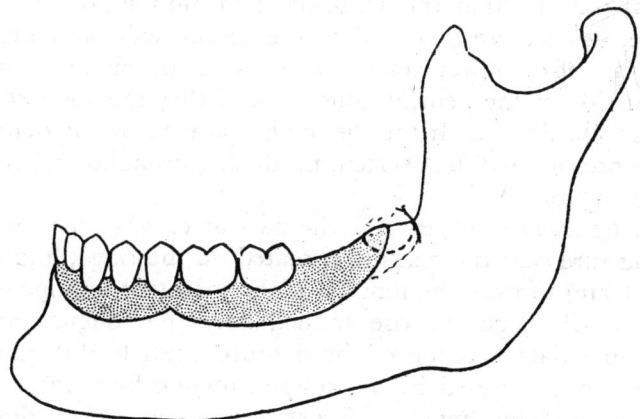

Fig. 240. – The back-edge of the lower denture should cross the retromolar pad. The retromolar pad is indicated by the dotted line.

greatest possible area if maximum retention and stability are to be obtained. If the denture is found to be under extended in any part of the periphery as shown by the presence of a gap between it and the functional position of the surrounding mucous membrane, replace the denture on the model and check whether the base has been carried to the full extent of the impression at this point. If it has, it implies an inaccuracy in the impression which must, therefore, be retaken before proceeding further.

(b) Check of Stability under Occlusal Stresses

This test is used to determine if occlusal stresses will be transmitted outside the ridge. Apply pressure with the ball of the finger in the premolar and molar regions of each side alternately: this pressure must be directed at right angles to the occlusal surface. If pressure on one side causes the denture to tilt and rise from the ridge on the other side, it indicates that the teeth on the side on which pressure is applied are outside the ridge.

(c) Tongue Space

Natural teeth occupy a position in the mouth where the inward pressure of the cheeks and lips is equalled by the outward pressure of the tongue, and it is into this zone of neutral pressure that the artificial teeth must be placed. The tongue, being more mobile than the cheeks, will cause greater instability of the lower denture if the teeth are mounted to the lingual side of the neutral zone than if they are mounted to the buccal side of it. If the tongue is cramped by the denture, lateral pressure will be exerted, producing instability when the tongue moves.

Test for cramped tongue: Ask the patient to relax the tongue, making sure that the denture is seated on the ridge, and then request him to raise the tongue. If the tongue is cramped, the denture will begin to rise immediately the tongue moves. This immediate reaction of the denture tends to differentiate the movement caused by a cramped tongue from the movement caused by lingual overextension; movement due to the latter cause does not occur until the tongue has risen some distance.

The causes of tongue cramping:

(i) Posterior teeth set inside the ridge.

(ii) Molar teeth which are too broad buccolingually. Such teeth should be replaced by smaller ones or their width reduced by grinding.

(iii) Molar teeth leaning inwards. This will not always cause cramping of the tongue but should never be allowed to occur as it interferes with the free vertical movements of the tongue. If this inward inclination is necessary to obtain occlusion, it is best to finish the denture and then grind away the lingual cusps (*see* fig. 241).

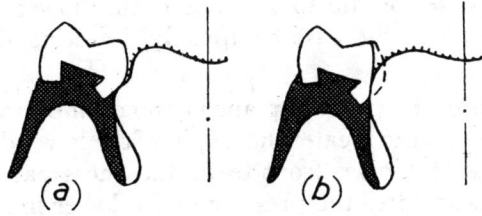

FIG. 241

(*a*) An overhanging lingual cusp allowing the tongue to get underneath and lift the denture.

(*b*) The cusp has been ground away.

(*d*) Height of the Occlusal Plane

To obtain maximum stability of a lower denture, the occlusal plane of the lower teeth should be very slightly below the bulk of the tongue, so that the tongue performs the majority of its movements above the denture and thus tends to keep the denture down (*see* fig. 242).

The denture must therefore be examined to see if the tongue, when relaxed, lies above or below the occlusal plane. Ask the patient to relax and place the tip of the tongue comfortably and without strain behind the lower front teeth, which is the normal relaxed position of the tongue, and then open his mouth without moving his tongue. If the height of the occlusal plane is correct, the tongue will be seen to lie on top of the lingual cusps.

If the lower denture still tends to rise unduly after the lingual periphery has been trimmed, and as much lateral

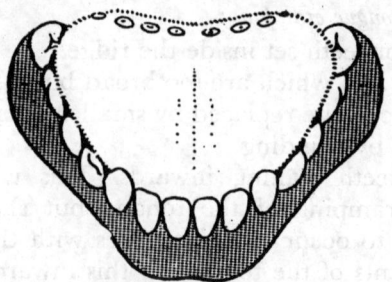

FIG. 242. – Low occlusal plane allows tongue to rest on
occlusal surface.

space as possible for the tongue has been allowed, it may be
necessary to re-set the case completely, lowering the occlusal
plane.

The height of the occlusal plane is also of importance for the
following reason: the greater the height of the lower denture, the
longer will be the lower front teeth and the greater therefore
the surface exposed to the pressure of the lower lip.

This concludes the examination of the lower denture alone,
and it should be removed from the mouth and placed in a
basin of cold water

2. TRYING IN THE UPPER DENTURE BY ITSELF

Place the upper denture in the mouth and examine as follows:

(a) *Check the Peripheral Outline*

(i) *The buccal and labial* periphery is checked as for the
lower denture.

(ii) *Position of Posterior Border.* – Verify carefully that the
posterior edge is correctly situated on the soft palate and
that the post-dam area on the model has been placed
correctly (*see* fig. 243).

(b) *Check the stability to occlusal stresses*, as for the lower denture,
but if the teeth have been set outside the ridge for reasons dictated by the occlusion or to enhance the appearance then this
test will obviously be omitted and reliance will be placed on the
positive retention of the finished denture to produce stability.

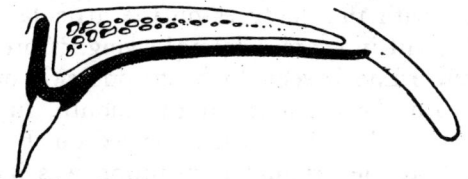

FIG. 243. – Showing posterior edge of upper denture correctly post-dammed.

3. BOTH DENTURES TOGETHER

Remove the upper denture from the mouth and chill in cold water for a few seconds, and then place both dentures in the mouth. If it is found necessary to improve the retention of the dentures when using a shellac type of base-plate, some adhesive powder may be sprinkled on their fitting surfaces.

(a) Position of Occlusion

(i) *Check the Anteroposterior Relation*. – Hold the lower denture in position on the ridge and ask the patient to relax, then to close the teeth together gently and maintain them in occlusion whilst the examination is carried out. If the bite registration was accurate, the teeth should interdigitate in the mouth in exactly the same manner as they do on the articulator, but if the registration was wrong, the teeth will not interdigitate correctly and may even occlude cusp to cusp on one or both sides. The operator must make quite certain that the occlusion he sees in the mouth is not due to movement of the dentures on the ridges, tilting of either denture or dropping of the upper denture. This is best tested by asking the patient to keep the teeth together and then trying to separate the posterior teeth by means of a thin spatula or knife; this test should be carried out on each side of the mouth alternately. The teeth should be brought into occlusion several times, using any of the registration aids which can be adopted at this stage, in order to make certain that the position of occlusion is correct or, if it is incorrect, to ascertain the type of error, i.e. whether the mandible can be retruded from the previously recorded jaw relationship or whether a lateral swing has occurred. Observation of the upper and lower centre lines in relation to each other, with the dentures on the articulator and then in the mouth, will indicate a lateral swing, if present. When the lower centre line is seen to be to one side of the upper centre line, with the dentures in the mouth, in contrast to the coincidence of these lines when viewed on the articulator, it is possible that the original registration was incorrect and that of a lateral position was recorded; this may be checked by the occlusion of the posterior teeth. If the original position was incorrect, the lower cusps will be slightly farther back on one side indicating a fuller retrusion of the condyle on that side. Should the lower cusps be slightly forward on one side, it indicates that the original recording of the occlusion was correct and the patient is now giving a lateral position (*see* fig. 244). Major errors in the position of occlusion are easily detected, but minor errors may pass unnoticed; therefore it is extremely important to watch for any slight movement of the dentures on their respective ridges from the time the teeth first make contact until they reach the position of complete inter-digitation, the reason being that the cusp inclines of the teeth guide the dentures into occlusion and will move the dentures

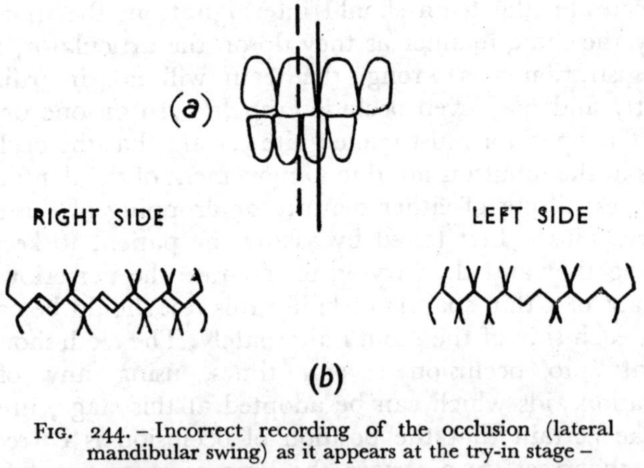

RIGHT SIDE LEFT SIDE

(b)

FIG. 244. – Incorrect recording of the occlusion (lateral mandibular swing) as it appears at the try-in stage –

(a) A right swing seen from the front – note lack of continuity of upper and lower centre lines.

(b) A right swing seen from the side. Posterior teeth on left side still interdigitate but have shifted laterally. Those on right do not interdigitate.

in relation to the ridges when only a slight error of jaw relationship exists from that which was obtained when taking the
records. Care is needed when holding the lower denture in
place on the ridge, to avoid pushing it backwards. When errors
of occlusion are noted at the try-in stage they must be corrected
by re-taking the position of occlusion.

Re-taking the anteroposterior position: The dentures are seated
on the models on the articulator and the posterior teeth
removed from one of the dentures and replaced by wax
blocks, which should be trimmed to occlude with the posterior
teeth of the other denture without altering the vertical dimension as set on the articulator (*see* fig. 245). In this way con-

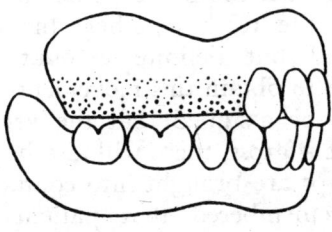

FIG. 245

siderable time may be saved in trimming the blocks in
the mouth, as then only minor adjustments are necessary to
produce evenness of occlusal pressure. The position of occlusion
is recorded by adding a little softened carding, or base-plate
wax to the chilled blocks, placing the dentures in the mouth
and asking the patient to close together, thus impressing the
cusps of the opposing teeth into the soft wax (*see* fig. 246).

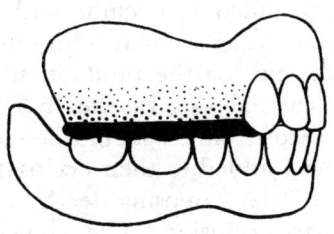

FIG. 246

The chilled wax blocks in occlusion with the opposing teeth will prevent any alteration in the vertical height. Care must be taken to see that the new position of occlusion gives the necessary correction. Points which may aid in this are – observations of overbite, overjet, and the relation of the centre lines. When correcting a lateral swing care must be taken to see that the lower anterior teeth do not impinge on the upper teeth, as this may cause the mandible to be guided into an incorrect position, or the dentures to tilt. If any contact of the anterior teeth occurs the offending lower teeth should be removed and the position re-taken.

(ii) *Check the Vertical Height.* – Ask the patient to relax with the lips closed. Watch the point of the chin and then ask the patient to · close the teeth together; the chin should move upwards a small but definite amount (*see* Chapter VI). If it is impossible to obtain this movement in spite of repeated attempts, it can be assumed that the vertical height is too great, and, if this is gross, there will also be a strained appearance when the lips are brought into contact with each other. It should be remembered that patients who are mouth breathers relax with their lips parted, and frequently have a large free-way space. An overclosed vertical height will be associated with an excessive free-way space, and when the teeth are in occlusion the lips will be seen to be pressed too firmly together with some loss of the vermilion border.

Correcting the vertical height: The posterior teeth are removed from one of the dentures and replaced by wax blocks. The articulator should be closed or opened approximately the amount required to establish a suitable free-way space, and the blocks then trimmed to occlude with the opposing teeth at the new vertical height. Final adjustments for evenness of occlusal pressure, and for the production of the correct free-way space, are carried out in the mouth. Once these are satisfactory, the record blocks should be chilled in cold water, and a little soft wax added to their occlusal surfaces to register the impressions of the opposing teeth when registering the position of centric occlusion. The chilled blocks resist the pressure of occlusion during this stage and prevent over-closure.

With cases set on an anatomical articulator the articulator may be closed or opened 2–3 mm. without taking a further occlusal registration, provided the face-bow and condylar records are correct; the reason being that the articulator reproduces the patient's individual jaw and temporo-mandibular joint relationships, and that a closure or opening of 2–3 mm., on the articulator, will produce no appreciable difference in the balance of the finished dentures, since such changes of vertical dimension occurring in the patient may be considered as a simple hinge-type movement.

(b) Evenness of Occlusal Pressure

Provided centric occlusion is correct, the evenness of the occlusion is next checked.

As the teeth close, they should occlude evenly and with equally distributed pressure all round. It frequently occurs that the teeth on one side of the mouth occlude slightly before those on the other, or the molars before the premolars. This may be due to:

(i) Pressure on the blocks being heavier on one side than the other when the records were taken.

(ii) A slight error in sealing the models in the blocks when articulating them.

(iii) Warpage of the base-plates.

Such errors may escape notice at the try-in stage because the waxed-up dentures will readily tilt because the retention of the base-plates is less than that of finished dentures, thus allowing the waxed-up teeth to be in occlusion when in fact they should not be in contact on the side on which the dentures have tilted (see fig. 247). Such irregularity of pressure may be slight or very considerable, but if it escapes notice at the try-in stage, when the dentures are finished the teeth will be held apart in the area of heavy pressure and may require excessive grinding to correct this: it may be so gross as to necessitate completely re-making one of the dentures. Teeth out of contact in the incisor and premolar region, due to the molars occluding too early, is frequently due to this cause (see fig. 248).

To test for evenness of occlusal pressure, proceed as follows:
Place two pieces of thin celluloid strip between the teeth in

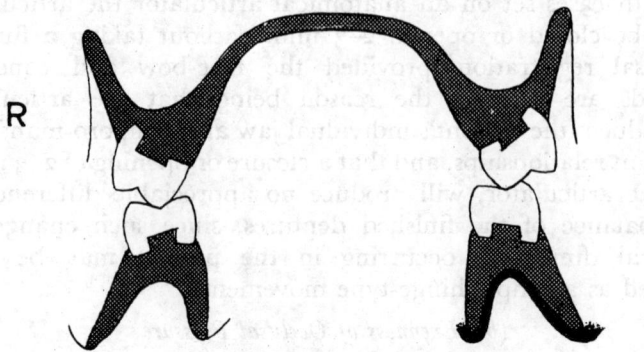

FIG. 247. – Section through a full upper and lower denture at the try-in stage. Inspection in the mouth would reveal apparently even contact between the molar teeth on both sides. What has actually occurred, however, is that heavy pressure on the right side has caused the lower denture to lift from the ridge on the left side until the teeth make contact. The use of celluloid strips to check occlusal pressures will reveal such an error.

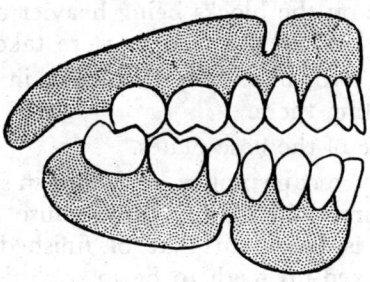

FIG. 248. – An anterior open 'bite' due to the molars occluding too early.

the molar region, one on each side. Request the patient to close and then endeavour to remove the celluloid strips simultaneously, holding one with each hand, by pulling them out between the closed teeth. Any difference in the force required to remove the strips will be readily appreciated, and if this force is interpreted in terms of occlusal pressure, an assessment may be made of whether or not it is even. Repeat the test in the premolar regions.

To test whether the front of the denture is rising slightly from the ridges when the back teeth are occluding, insert the point of a wax knife between the upper and lower incisor teeth and attempt to push the upper denture upwards and the lower denture downwards. Any appreciable movement may be interpreted as excessive pressure in the molar region.

Correcting unevenness of pressure: If it is slight, gently soften, with a pin-point flame, the wax supporting the teeth of one of the dentures on the offending side. Replace the dentures in the mouth and, holding the lower firmly in place, request the patient to close. The teeth on the side of heavy pressure will sink slightly into the softened wax until the occlusion of the teeth on the opposite side arrests them, thus evening the occlusal pressure. If the unevenness is more than slight, this technique will not serve, as the teeth will be forced out of place. Complete re-taking of the record of centric occlusion with built-up wax blocks is the only solution.

In cases in which difficulty is experienced with the position and evenness of occlusion it frequently simplifies the problem if the upper denture is finished first and then the waxed up lower denture is re-tryed against this denture. Small alterations in the occlusion can easily be made to the waxed up lower denture before it is finished, and with the closely fitting, well retained upper denture in place patients seem to find it simpler to produce a correct position of occlusion.

(c) Balanced Occlusion and Articulation
(anatomical articulation only)

The first check is for centric occlusion, which, if found to be incorrect, necessitates the removal of the lower posterior teeth and the recording of the correct position on the wax blocks replacing them. The lower model is then removed from the articulator and re-set according to the new position, thus keeping the upper model in the same position as it was set by means of the face-bow. When the centric position is found to be correct, the testing of the waxed-up denture continues in the following manner:

Check for evenness of occlusal pressure in the centric position with celluloid strips and then test for balance with gentle lateral and protrusive movements. With the teeth in a lateral position of occlusion, insert the point of a wax knife between the teeth on the balancing side, and attempt to separate them; if they do separate, it shows that the occlusion of the teeth on that side is apparent only and is resulting from the displacement of the denture bases from the ridges. The cause of this error may be due either to an incorrect face-bow reading, or to an incorrect condylar path registration. When the error is considerable, these registrations must be taken again, the models re-mounted on the articulator and the teeth re-set; but if the error is only slight, it may be corrected by grinding the occlusal surfaces of the teeth when the dentures are finished. Minor errors of cuspal interference may be eliminated at this stage, or when the dentures have been finished and fitted, by careful grinding of the teeth concerned.

(d) Appearance

This aspect of the try-in is a matter more for individual judgment and the patient's ideas than for set rules. Certain things require to be checked, however, as routine. They are:

(i) *Centre Line.* – Stand in front of the patient, some distance away; a wrong centre line will be obvious, but if in doubt any of the aids described in Chapter VI may be applied.

(ii) *Anterior Plane.* – This may be observed from the same position and any tendency for this plane to slope markedly up or down should be noted and corrected (*see* fig. 249).

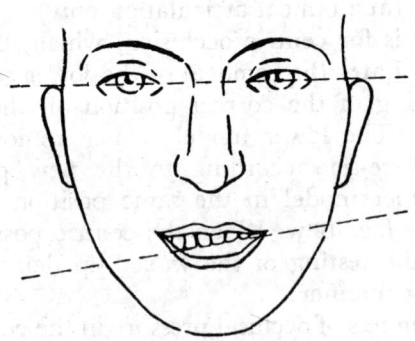

Fig. 249. – The plane of the anterior teeth is sloped.

(iii) *Shape of the Teeth*. – Ensure that the selected teeth conform with the patient's facial type (*see* Chapter VII), and invariably consult the patient, to whom a mirror has been handed.

(iv) *Size of the Teeth*. – Individual judgment must be relied on here together with the patient's opinion.

(v) *Shade of the Teeth* (*see* chapter on Tooth Selection).

(vi) *Profile*. – Observe the patient's profile and note if the lips are either excessively distended or unduly sunken. In the first case, remove some wax from the labial flange and try the dentures in again. If this produces insufficient improvement, examine the denture to see if the teeth can be set farther in, or if smaller teeth can be used. If this is not possible, the six front teeth may need to be set to the gum. If the lips are sunken, build up wax on the labial flange, especially in the canine and premolar regions, until the profile is correct, and in some cases set the anterior teeth further forward.

(vii) *Amount of Tooth Visible*. – Ask the patient to say 'Yes', and smile, and note how much tooth shows. Consider whether you like it or not. In this connexion remember that a smiling person usually only shows the upper teeth; if much of the lower incisors are visible, or only the lowers show, examine the amount of overbite and, if excessive, reduce it by lowering the mandibular teeth. If this does not effect an improvement, the height of the occlusal plane may require to be altered.

(viii) *Regularity of the Teeth*. – Few natural dentitions exhibit perfection, and to perfect a set-up in the incisor region, especially in persons of middle age, tends to emphasize that the teeth are artificial, therefore a little irregularity is usually desirable. Some common types of irregular set-up are illustrated in the following diagrams (*see* figs. 250, 251 and 252). If the patient already has dentures and likes the appearance of them, copy them, since it is always inadvisable to alter a patient's appearance radically, without his consent.

(e) Approval of Appearance by the Patient

It is always wise for the operator to obtain the patients' approval of the appearance of the waxed-up dentures before

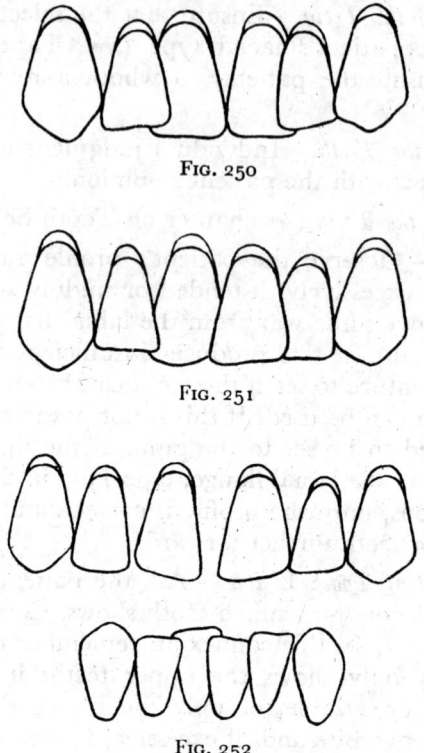

Fig. 250

Fig. 251

Fig. 252

they are passed to the technician for completion, as this enables the operator to make necessary adjustments. Some patients are quite prepared to leave the question of appearance to the operator, whilst others are extremely fussy over the smallest detail. When dealing with the former class, the operator should insist that they consider the matter of their appearance, otherwise when the dentures are finished they may react unfavourably. In the case of the fussy patient, much time and trouble must be spent on getting the shade, shape and set-up of the teeth just as the patient wishes. (It is very important to obtain his final approval before finishing the case.) In this connexion the operator often needs to use his restraining influence to avoid extremely bad errors of aesthetics, and a waste of time. It should be remembered that other people will see more of a patient's dentures than he will, and if they are not aesthetically pleasing in the opinion of his relations and friends he will usually become dissatisfied with them. It is, therefore, advisable to ask the patient to bring a relation or candid friend with him at the time of trying-in the dentures, and the approval or criticism of this second individual should be sought as well as that of the patient himself.

Chapter XII

FITTING THE FINISHED DENTURES

Examination of the Finished Dentures

Before fitting the dentures they should be inspected to ensure that they have been correctly finished by the technician, the following points being most important:

1. The fitting surface must show no irregularities which are not present in the mouth. The commonest defects arise from a cut or scratch on the model, or air bubbles present in the plaster model. Both faults result in an excrescence on the fitting surface which should have been removed by the technician.

2. The entire periphery should be rounded and highly polished except the back-edge of the upper denture and the posterior lingual flange of the lower which should be thinned down almost to a knife-edge; but perfectly smooth and not sharp.

3. The edges of the relief area should be rounded and not left square and sharp (*see* fig. 253).

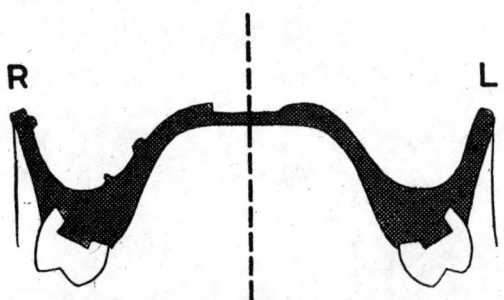

Fig. 253. – Illustrating the correct and incorrect finish of a denture. On the left side the edge of the relief chamber has been chamfered, the periphery of the denture rounded and polished, and small nodules of acrylic on the fitting surface removed.

On the right side the denture is shown before the finishing described above has been carried out.

Place the dentures, which have previously lain in tepid water, in the mouth and examine them as for the try-in. Test the retention of the upper by placing a finger behind the incisor teeth bringing pressure to bear in an outward and upward direction. If the back-edge of the denture has been correctly placed, considerable force should be needed to break the peripheral seal. The retention will increase after the patient has worn the dentures for a few days, due to the adaptation of the soft tissues to the denture.

CHECKING THE OCCLUSION

If the try-in has been done carefully, the occlusion should be almost perfect. Slight unevenness often occurs, however, due to processing errors, and so the occlusion should be checked with articulating paper; this is paper impregnated with a blue dye. Place a piece between the teeth and ask the patient to chew up and down in centric occlusion. Remove the dentures from the mouth and examine them. The occlusal surfaces will exhibit areas of blue coloration where the cusps and fossae of the opposing teeth have been in contact. These blue areas should be evenly spread over the occlusal surface, and the coloration of them should be uniform. Areas of hard or uneven pressure will show up as darker, and broader, blue spots; areas of low pressure, or no contact at all, as very lightly coloured spots, or not coloured at all. To equalize the pressure, the high spots should be lightly ground with a carborundum stone. The denture should then be washed to remove the dye and a further test with articulating paper made, and so on until occlusal balance is obtained.

The Use of Wax Templates

Articulating paper has the disadvantage that it will colour a tooth even if it only rubs lightly against it, and thus areas which are not in occlusion are frequently marked. If this possibility is borne in mind, articulating paper can be very successfully used to adjust the occlusion of finished dentures.

A more satisfactory way of adjusting the occlusion is by using wax templates. The technique of this is as follows: Two strips of pink wax 6 mm. wide, of either single or double thickness, are softened and laid one on either side of the lower denture on the occlusal surfaces of the posterior teeth. The denture is then inserted in the mouth and the patient instructed to chew up and down on the wax with slow deliberate movements. The lower denture is removed from the mouth, and the wax templates chilled in cold water and gently removed from the denture. If these templates are then viewed by transmitted light, those areas where the occlusion is hard will be seen as thinned, completely transparent wax; or even as a hole right through the wax. Replacement of the template on the denture will enable the exact area of the tooth which requires grinding to be observed.

Another advantage of the templates is that, by fitting the upper and lower dentures into their correct positions in one template, the actual position of occlusion on the opposite side of the dentures, as it exists in the mouth, may be observed, and gross errors readily seen.

It requires to be emphasized that the even adjustment of the occlusion is most important to the success of the dentures, as uneven occlusion may cause soreness on the ridge, or in the sulcus, in its immediate vicinity. This should not be overlooked if a patient returns complaining of pain, because frequently the periphery of a denture is blamed for what is in reality a fault of occlusion.

Uneven occlusion will also increase the patient's difficulties when attempting to eat with the new dentures because they will feel uneven and uncomfortable when in occlusion.

To achieve perfection of occlusion a check record should be taken, the dentures remounted on the articulator and the cclusion ground in as described in Chapter XIII.

FITTING ANATOMICALLY ARTICULATED DENTURES

Check as for the try in. Test the articulation in centric, lateral, and protrusive relations with articulating paper and carry out a check record.

At the second visit, when the dentures have had time to settle, the teeth should be ground in, in the mouth, using a carborundum powder in wax, or carborundum powder mixed with tooth-paste. Place a strip of carborundum wax between the teeth and ask the patient to chew, until satisfied that the articulation is even. Although the wax holds the carborundum powder firmly, it is important to caution your patient not to swallow when grinding in the dentures as carborundum powder in the stomach is an irritant. This is specially important if tooth-paste is used as the vehicle.

FINISHED DENTURES EXHIBITING AN INCORRECT CENTRIC OCCLUSION

If the centric occlusion is discovered to be incorrect at the finished stage, as will occasionally occur in spite of the greatest care being taken at the try-in stage, it may be due to a slight retrusion of the mandible, i.e. the dentures have been made to a slightly forward position. If this is not more than a ¼ cusp it may be corrected by means of a check record (*see* Chapter XIII). When the error is gross it will require the removal of all the osterior teeth from the lower denture as follows:

Gently flame the posterior teeth of the lower denture, playing the flame actually on to the porcelain and not the acrylic base; conduction of the heat through the porcelain softens the acrylic without burning it, and the teeth may be prised off the denture. Wax blocks are then built to replace the teeth, trimmed to the correct height by trial, and the centric occlusion re-taken. The dentures are then re-articulated, and the back teeth re-set. If the over-jet resulting from the new record is abnormal, the lower front teeth must also be removed from the denture and re-set. If acrylic posterior teeth were used they are merely ground down and replaced with wax blocks for the new registration. In most cases of gross error the denture needs to be completely re-made.

ATTRITION OF THE FRONT TEETH TO IMPROVE THE APPEARANCE

When the upper and lower incisors erupt, the incisal edges present three small tubercles as shown in fig. 254. As the teeth some into use for incising, these tubercles are gradually worn away by the grinding of the lower teeth against the upper. This attrition results, firstly, in the formation of an even incisive edge, then, as age advances, this edge becomes irregular, due to

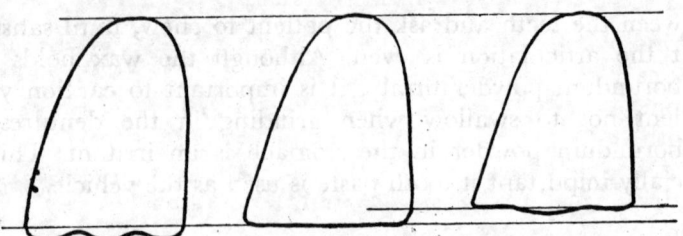

(A)   Illustrating the alteration which occurs in the form of
of the incisive edge of an upper central incisoras the
years advance.

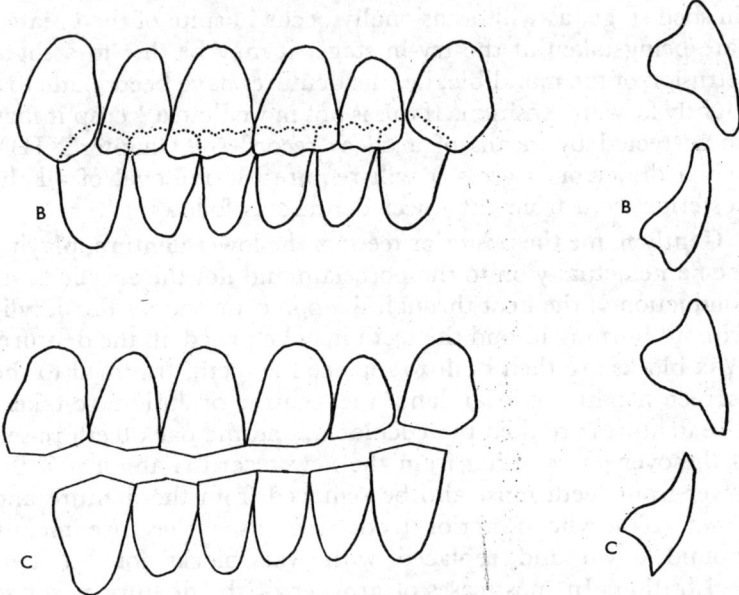

(B)   Illustrates the shape of the incisive edges of the newly
erupted front teeth and

(C)   shows how they wear by attrition. Close study will
reveal how the pattern develops.

FIG. 254.

uneven wear, and sometimes assumes a chisel-like form when
viewed from the side.

Many artificial teeth, as supplied, present a regular, even
edge and if no attempt is made to simulate the wear of the
natural teeth they appear obviously false. A little judicious

grinding of the incisive edges of the teeth with a carborundum stone makes a remarkable difference and enhances the natural appearance of the dentures. This should only be done, however, with the patient's approval.

The older the patient the greater will be the effects of attrition – therefore the attrition seen in a man of 70 should not be copied on dentures for a girl of 21. The observation of people who possess their own teeth will disclose much about the wear of the incisive edge and the irregularity of the appearance.

While on the subject of appearance, a few words on the reflection of light from the labial surface of the teeth may be useful. Examination of the labial surface of a natural incisor will disclose that two vertical grooves separate three ridges: the canines usually have one ridge separating two depressions. The rest of the surface, although smooth, is not regularly contoured, being built up from a large number of facets.

All these irregularities result in the incident rays of light which strike the tooth surface being, in the main, scattered as they are reflected, and only one or two of the more prominent ridges reflect light evenly as highspots.

If artificial teeth are to appear natural therefore, they must scatter the incident rays, and here again the brea ing up of the surface of the tooth by judicious grinding, followed by gentle polishing, can considerably enhance the appearance.

Instructions to the Patient

Many patients will have had experience with full dentures and may thus not require an explanation of the points about to be considered, but those patients having dentures fitted for the first time will need, and benefit by, information concerning the following:

1. *Wearing Dentures at Night*

Dentures invariably occupy more space in the mouth than did the natural teeth which they replace, and to begin with, the patient will be extremely conscious of their presence. Therefore, in order to reduce this period of discomfort to a minimum, it should be suggested that the dentures be worn at night. thus allowing the tongue, cheeks and lips to become accustomed to the bulk during the hours of sleep. Once the patient has become accustomed to the dentures it is no longer necessary for them to be worn at night, but the final decision should be left to the individual who may have personal reasons for wishing to continue the practice. From the point of view of the health of the tissues, it is preferable for the dentures to be removed at night, although in some cases there appears to be no difference, clinically, between the mouths of patients who wear their dentures continuously and those who remove them at night.

Symptoms of over-closure, due to a patient sleeping without dentures, may be relieved by advising him to wear his denture continuously. Generally, however, patients should be instructed to remove their dentures at night in order to rest the tissues which support them.

2. Cleaning

Whenever possible dentures should be removed after every meal and food debris washed away, particular attention being given to the fitting surface so that no food particles remain to stagnate and so irritate the tissues. At least once a day the dentures should be thoroughly cleaned with a soft brush and soap, or any recognized brand of denture cleaner. If not worn at night, they should be placed in water, or a mild antiseptic solution. In the case of acrylic bases and teeth, solutions containing phenol must be avoided as they are liable to craze the surface of a denture: also the patient should be warned against using harsh abrasive materials and hard bristle brushes, since both will wear away the surface detail of the teeth and denture base. Finally, with regard to this material, it is important to remember that hot water may cause warpage.

As a precaution against chipping teeth, or fracturing a denture, it should be advised that the hand basin be half-filled with water, during the cleaning operation, to act as a cushion if the denture slips from the fingers.

3. Eating

All full denture wearers have to pass through a period of learning before they can eat with comfort, since mandibular movements are generally much more restricted, and the tongue has to control the lower denture as well as the food. The following suggestions may be of some help during the tedious period of learning to eat.

(a) The food should be cut into small pieces and only a little placed in the mouth at a time.

(b) Commence by chewing in the premolar region on one or both sides; the latter causing the least instability.

(c) The soft and non-sticky foods are easier to eat than the more fibrous types.

(d) Chewing with the posterior teeth should be mastered before any attempt is made to bite with the incisors.

4. *Talking*

People who have been edentulous for a considerable period will have adapted themselves to the prevailing conditions, and probably will have corrected any speech defects arising from the loss of the teeth. With the insertion of dentures, the conditions are suddenly changed and the tongue is conscious of the reduction of space, and may be cramped temporarily by the bulk of the lingual flange of the lower denture. This may lead to difficulty in forming some of the speech sounds until the tongue has had sufficient time to adapt itself. Patients who are likely to experience speech difficulties should be advised to read aloud, and practise any word which causes trouble. A few hours spent in this manner will enable most patients to speak naturally and with complete ease.

EASING THE DENTURES

With the fitting of correctly constructed dentures, and instructions to the patient, the prosthetist's part in the rehabilitation is almost complete for, except for minor adjustments of the peripheries and occlusion, it is now the patient's perseverance and ability to learn to use the dentures which decide the final success of the case. The patient should be asked to attend for examination forty-eight hours after the insertion of the dentures so that the prosthetist may carry out any necessary adjustments. Soreness may occur in that time due to the fact that functional trimming of the peripheries at the impression stage rarely reproduces all the functional movements, and when the dentures are first worn there is probably slight overextension somewhere. The flange of the denture is thus too deep and presses into the tissues of the sulcus, forming first an angry red line, which later breaks down into an ulcer, the depth and extent of which depends on the degree of over-extension of the denture base. Also, in that time, the dentures will have settled with possible slight changes in the evenness of occlusion. The overextended flange must be trimmed and the occlusion ground in. A further visit may be necessary for final corrections, as it is never wise to remove too much of the periphery at one stage, since over-easing may lead to a leak in the peripheral seal. Other causes of soreness, and the complaints made by patients, are dealt with in the next chapter.

If, after being worn for a short time, the dentures hurt, they should not be discarded immediately, unless the pain is severe, since perseverance will often overcome slight soreness. If the dentures have to be left out because of pain, they should be worn for a few hours immediately before visiting the dental surgeon because, unless this is done, there probably will be no mark in the mouth to indicate where the denture is over-extended.

The technique of easing: It is essential to locate exactly which area of the denture base is overextended. Sometimes this can be done visually, but frequently the ulcer cannot be seen when the denture is in place. In these instances a mark must be made on the tissues, which will transfer itself to the denture base in the vicinity of the ulcer. Such a mark can be made with either zinc oxide paste, tooth-paste, or indelible pencil. The tissues are dried, a little paste is placed on the sore area with a probe, or a mark is made with a wet indelible pencil, the denture is then inserted and pressed gently but firmly into place. When it is removed the paste, or some of the indelible material, will have transferred itself to the denture base. A better method, and one which can be employed even before an ulcer has developed, if, when fitting the denture one suspects that it is overextended anywhere, is to coat the area of the periphery or fitting surface in question with a paste of equal parts of zinc oxide, starch and lanoline, so thickly that the acrylic cannot be seen through the paste and then insert the denture. The patient is then instructed to chew, swallow and move the lips and cheeks because pressure points frequently develop only in function.

The denture is then removed and if overextension exists it will be readily visible as an area of acrylic completely uncovered by the paste (*see* fig. 255). This area of the denture is

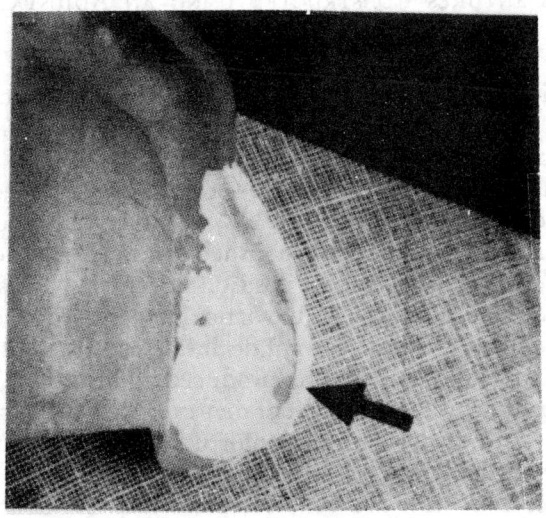

FIG. 255. – Area of overextension has been coated with easing paste and this has been squeezed away in area of hard pressure (arrowed).

then trimmed with a stone or file, highly polished and the denture reinserted. In cases of gross overextension resulting in severe ulceration, the patient should be instructed to leave the denture out for twenty-four hours in order to allow the swelling to subside, otherwise the denture will require to be over-trimmed and this may reduce its retention.

When easing it should always be remembered that soreness and ulceration of the tissues is frequently caused by unbalanced occlusion, or cuspal interference, causing excessive pressure to be applied to the tissues under the denture base. It is therefore sound practice always to check the occlusion when easing a denture.

CHAPTER XIII

CHECK RECORDS FOR COMPLETED DENTURES

A. DENTURES CONSTRUCTED USING AN ADJUSTABLE TYPE ARTICULATOR

The efficiency and comfort that a patient experiences when using full dentures depends to a large extent on the harmony of the occlusion.

A suitable impression technique, carefully carried out, will result in dentures which are stable provided that there is no overextension and that the polished surfaces are correctly shaped. With care the correct position of centric occlusion may be obtained and if an adjustable articulator is used in conjunction with a face-bow and lateral occlusal records a satisfactory balanced articulation will be produced. This, then, should result in comfortable and efficient dentures with an harmonious occlusion and articulation; unfortunately, however, faults occur during the construction of dentures which result in errors in the occlusion that are indetectable when the dentures are examined in the mouth (fig. 256). These faults may be clearly seen however when the dentures are mounted in an articulator after centric check records have been taken (fig. 257).

Such dentures may cause discomfort to the wearer and result in reduced efficiency unless the faults of occlusion are rectified. The errors which occur are due to one, or a combination of the following:

(1) Incorrect registration of centric occlusion.
(2) Irregularities in setting the teeth.
(3) Tooth movement when flas ing and packing.
(4) Incomplete flask closure.
(5) Wear in moving parts of the articulator.

(1) *Incorrect Registration of Centric Occlusion.* – This is probably the most common cause of error in the occlusion of finished dentures. When registering the position of centric occlusion considerable

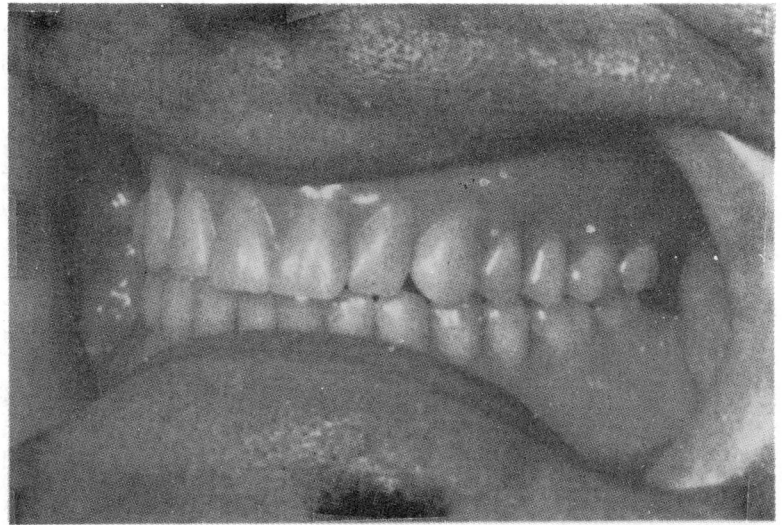

(a)

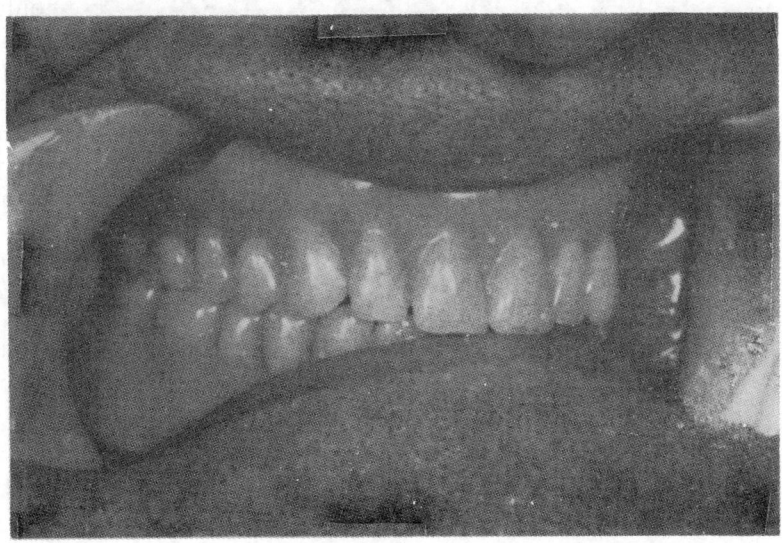

(b)

FIG. 256 (*a*) and (*b*). – Completed dentures showing apparent
even occlusion on both right and left molar regions. Compare
with fig. 257.

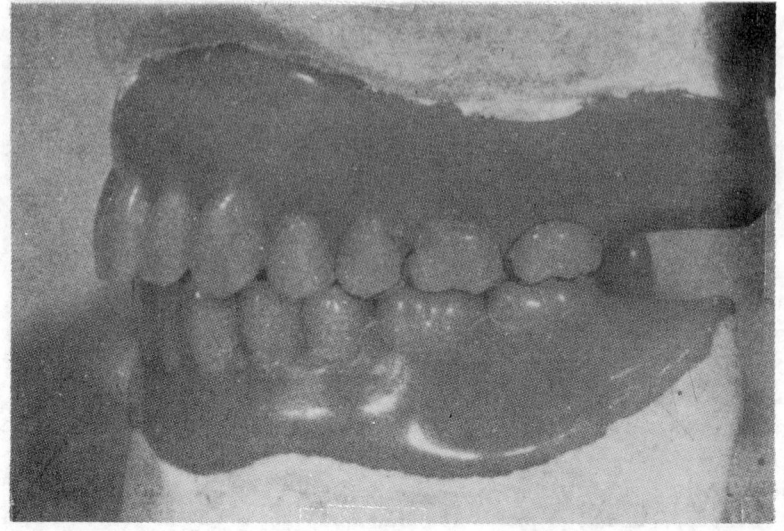

(a)

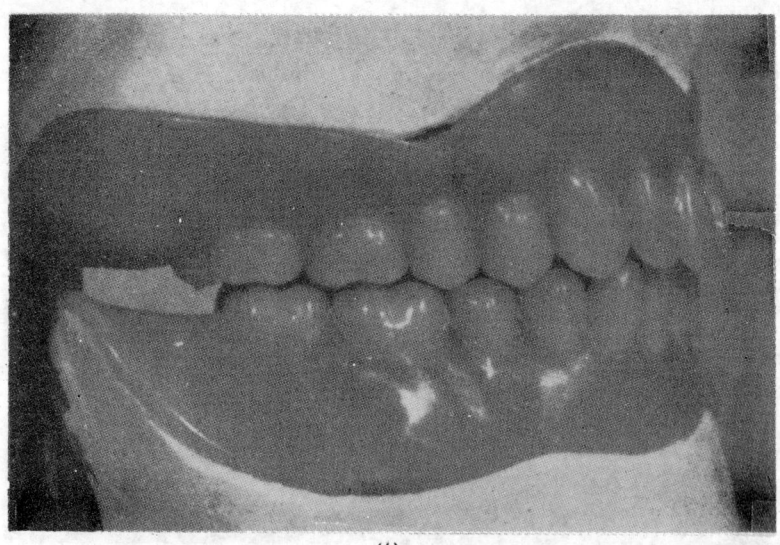

(b)

FIG. 257(a) and (b). – The dentures seen in fig. 256 mounted in an adjustable type articulator following centric check records.   The left side shows contact between the opposing teeth, the right side being out of occlusion.

care is taken to obtain a correct vertical dimension and the physiological fully retruded position of the mandible, but often the record rims when brought together exert uneven pressure on their respective supporting alveolar ridges, and this condition passes unnoticed. The uneven pressure may be due to premature contact of the record rims on one side of the mouth, in the second molar region of both sides, or in the incisor region. This causes uneven compression of the mucosa supporting the record blocks and often displaces them from the ridges in areas away from the region of premature contact. When the plaster models are placed in the record blocks obviously no such compression or displacement occurs and therefore the occlusion as registered in the articulator differs from that registered in the mouth. Thus an error in occlusion has been established which possibly may be passed over at the try-in stage due to the poor fit of the trial denture bases allowing movement to take place. On finishing the denture the teeth are found to occlude only in the area where the premature contact of the record rims occurred, the remainder of the teeth being slightly out of contact (see fig. 257). The degree of separation will be related to the degree of premature contact occurring between the record rims. This will vary from the almost indiscernible (see fig. 256) to a stage when a wax knife blade may be inserted between the un-occluding teeth.

Another fault causing errors in the occlusion of the finished dentures results from slight movement of record blocks on the ridges during centric registration due to their imperfect fit and inadequate retention. The position of centric occlusion of the finished dentures will be slightly inaccurate for this reason and the dentures will tend to move on the ridges as the cuspal inclines of the teeth guide the dentures into their slightly inaccurate position of occlusion when the mandible assumes its correct centric relationship with the maxilla. This continual denture movement during mastication causes soreness of the ridge; usually the lower since this denture is the more unstable of the two.

Finally, an error of occlusion may result from the manner in which the models and record blocks are set in the articulator. The models may not be placed accurately in the blocks, or the articulator may not be handled with due care when the models are being attached with plaster.

All the forementioned errors may be of a minor nature and can usually be avoided by using an accurately fitting acrylic base in preference to the shellac type of base which invariably warps slightly. The minor errors only cause slight discrepancies in the occlusion of the teeth and will probably pass unnoticed at the try-in stage, and often in the finished denture stage, and are observed only when carrying out a centric check record (*see* figs. 256 and 257).

(2) *Irregularities In Setting the Teeth.* – The technician when setting up teeth is unlikely to produce a perfectly even contact in centric and lateral occlusions, some teeth will be in good occlusion whilst others will be slightly out of occlusion, thus producing areas of heavy pressure. Also, when setting and testing the occlusion for lateral slide the teeth being held in wax, which exhibits a certain amount of resiliency, permits tooth movement to occur when hard occlusal contact areas are encountered. This cannot happen when the teeth are held firmly in the final denture base material and results in areas of premature tooth contact in the occlusion and articulation of the finished dentures.

In waxing up following the setting of teeth it is possible for them to move slightly due to the contraction of the wax on cooling, causing irregularities in the articulation and occlusion of completed dentures.

These possibilities point to the need for a final adjustment of occlusion once the dentures are finished.

(3) *Tooth Movement when Flasking and Packing.* – Movement of the teeth may occur at the time of boiling out the wax trial base after the dentures have been flasked and if such teeth are not correctly repositioned they will cause minor occlusal irregularities. Also, when packing, teeth may be driven into the enveloping plaster, particularly when packing follows soon after investing and the plaster is in the 'green state'. The possibility of such an error occurring is increased when the methyl methacrylate is used in a slightly advanced stage of dough, and when the posterior teeth have been ground to fit

close to the ridge. Rapid closure of the flask in the press will add to the hazard.

(4) *Incomplete Flask Closure.* – Such an occurrence not only causes an increase of vertical dimension but also results in an upset of balanced occlusion.

(5) *Articulator Wear.* – All articulators are subject to wear and the older and more worn the articulator the greater will be the errors in occlusion and articulation. Every piece of mechanical apparatus exhibits some play in its moving parts and when this becomes easily detectable the bearing should be replaced.

It can be appreciated that even with care on the part of the surgeon and technician slight errors may occur which influence the final occlusion and articulation of finished dentures. These errors in some instances may be corrected by careful use of articulating paper at the chairside but such correction is often proved false when check bites are taken for confirmation. It is far more satisfactory and often less time consuming, clinically, to register the position of centric occlusion again, this time using the finished dentures as the bite blocks; take a face-bow reading and lateral records, set the finished dentures in an adjustable type of articulator and grind-in the occlusion. The following are details of the procedure:

(1) *Registration of Centric Relationship without Tooth Contact.* – The upper denture is seated in position in the mouth. A sheet of pink wax is thoroughly softened in the bunsen flame and two half-inch wide strips of double thickness, and of sufficient length to cover the premolar and molar teeth of both sides, are laid on the occlusal surface of the lower denture (fig. 258). Whilst the wax is still very soft the denture is seated in the mouth and the patient requested to close in the retruded position (Chapter VI) until the teeth are almost in occlusion. This can be judged by observing the separation of upper and lower incisors (fig. 259). The wax templates are chilled in the mouth with a cold water jet and removed and placed on one side whilst a second registration is carried out. It is advisable to take two sets of templates so that one may be used as a check of the other when the dentures have been set in the articulator.

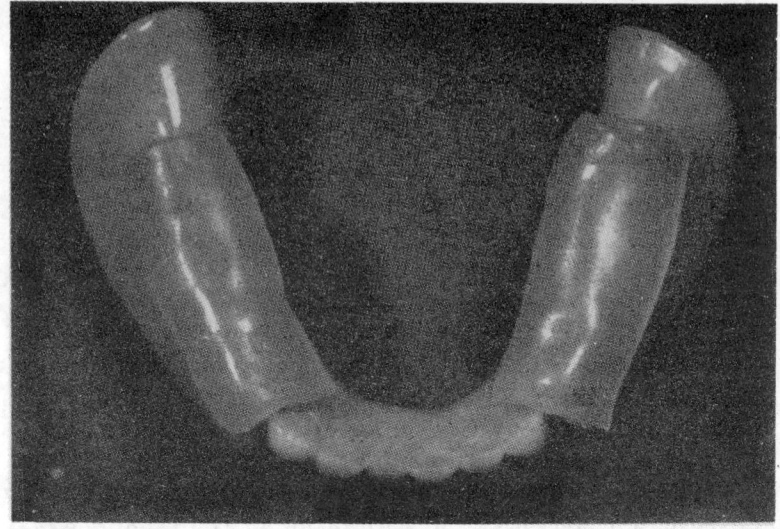

FIG. 258. – Soft wax strips placed on the occlusal surfaces
of the posterior teeth.

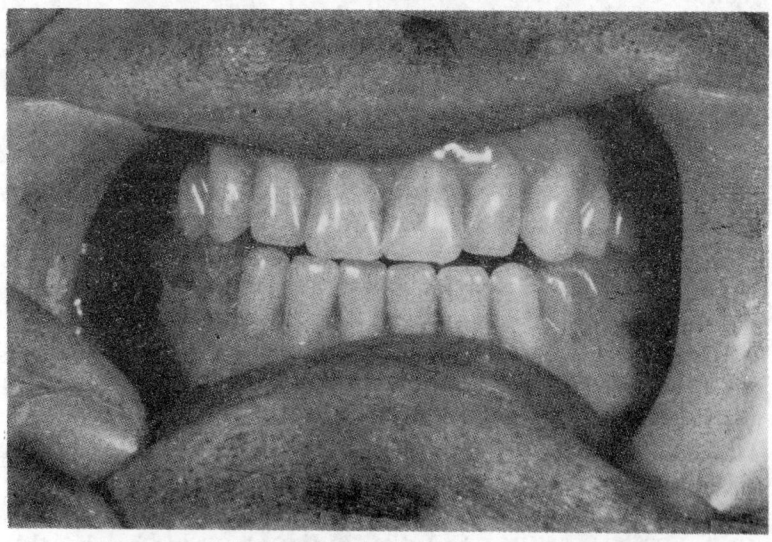

FIG. 259. – Centric relationship recorded using very soft wax.
Mandibular closure is stopped before posterior tooth contact
occurs; this position must fall within the limits of the free-way
space.

Any discrepancy between the two sets of templates necessitates further centric readings.

The wax should be as soft as possible when the lower denture is placed in the mouth in order to minimize compression of the mucosa supporting the dentures. Plaster of Paris may be used as an alternative to wax.

It is extremely important when securing this position of centric relation between the mandible and maxilla that the teeth are not allowed to make contact, for if tooth contact does occur the lower cusps by moving along the cuspal inclines of the upper teeth may guide the mandible into the position of occlusion to which the dentures were constricted and thus, if an error exists, prevent the desired correction of maxillo-mandibular relationship.

(2) *Lateral or Protrusive Records.* – A strip of softened wax of double thickness is placed on the occlusal surface of the lower denture, the denture placed in the mouth and the mandible moved to the right lateral position and closed almost to tooth contact. A second template records the left lateral position (Chapter IX). If the patient experiences difficulty in making lateral movements then a single protrusive record should be taken with the mandible protruded approximately $\frac{1}{4}$ in. These records are used to set the condylar guide paths of the adjustable articulator.

(3) *Face-bow Registration.* — A treble thickness of softened pink wax is moulded around the prongs of the face-bow fork and the fork placed between the occlusal surfaces of the teeth with the arm of the fork projecting straight out but set to one side of the mid-line. The patient closes into the soft wax and holds the fork firmly in position whilst the face-bow is attached to the fork and related to the condylar heads (fig. 260).

The reason for taking the face-bow record is that it enables the technician to set the upper denture in the articulator frame in the same relationship to the hinge-axis of the articulator as the denture, when in the patient's mouth, bears to the condylar axis of the mandible when the condyles are in the physiologically fully retruded position in the fossæ.

By using the wax template recording the centric relation,

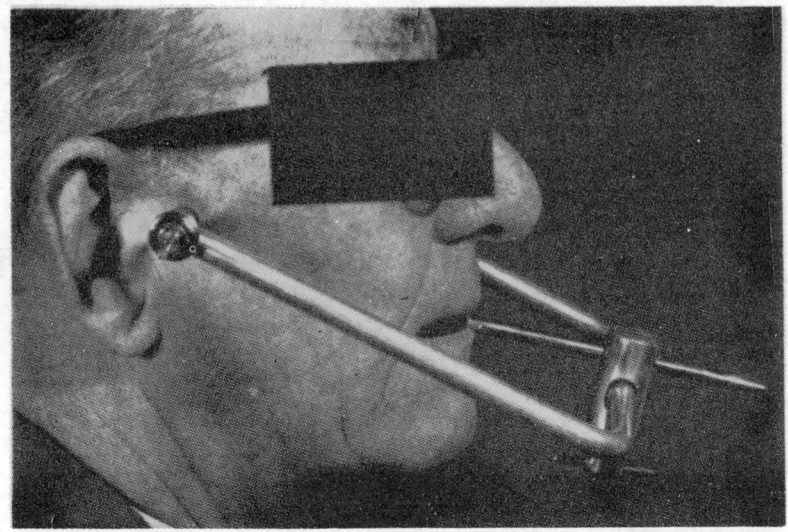

(a)

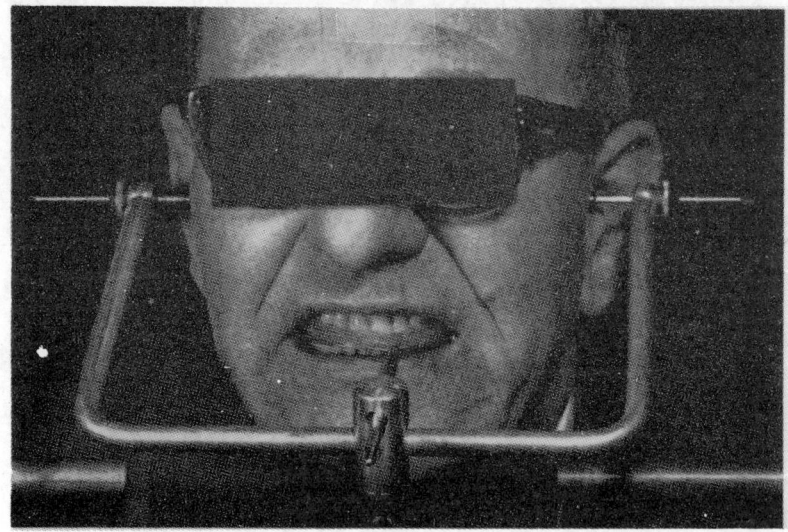

(b)

FIG. 260

(a) Lateral view of face-bow. The condylar cups are positioned on a line from the outer canthus of the eye to the top of the external auditory meatus and 1 cm. in front of the latter.

(b) Front view. The fork of the face-bow positioned to one side of the midline to facilitate mounting in the articulator.

previously taken, the lower denture can also be positioned in
the articulator frame in a relationship to the hinge axis of the
articulator which is identical to the lower denture's relationship to the condylar axis when the denture is in the mouth.
The relationship of the upper and lower dentures to the hinge
axis, both human and mechanical, are thus identical. Therefore, provided that it is accepted that movement through the
free-way space is a pure hinge type movement it is now
possible to close the articulator frame, within the limits of the
free-way space, with the knowledge that both the paths of
closure of the articulator and the mandible will be the same.
If the thickness of the wax template recording centric relation
is not in excess of the free-way space then it can be removed
from between the dentures when in the articulator and the
teeth closed together to show their true relationship since the
human and mechanical paths of closure will be the same in
each case.

(4) *Mounting the Dentures in an Adjustable Articulator.* – The face-
bow, with the upper denture secured to the fork, is adjusted on
the articulator (Chapter IX) and the denture attached to the
upper arm of the articulator with plaster of Paris; the undercuts of the fitting surface of the denture having previously been
blocked out with wax or plasticine (fig. 261).

After the face-bow has been removed the lower denture is
attached to the upper denture by means of one set of wax templates recording the centric relation and in this position the
lower denture is secured to the lower arm of the articulator
(fig. 262). When the plaster has set the wax templates are
removed from the dentures and the wax templates recording
the lateral, or protrusive, positions of the mandible substituted
in order to set the condylar guides of the articulator (Chapter
IX).

Once the condylar guidance has been set the wax template
of centric relation is repositioned between the teeth and the
locking nut of the incisal guide pin tightened, after which
the template can be removed and the teeth examined to
ascertain whether or not there is contact between the upper
and lower teeth which would indicate that the patient had

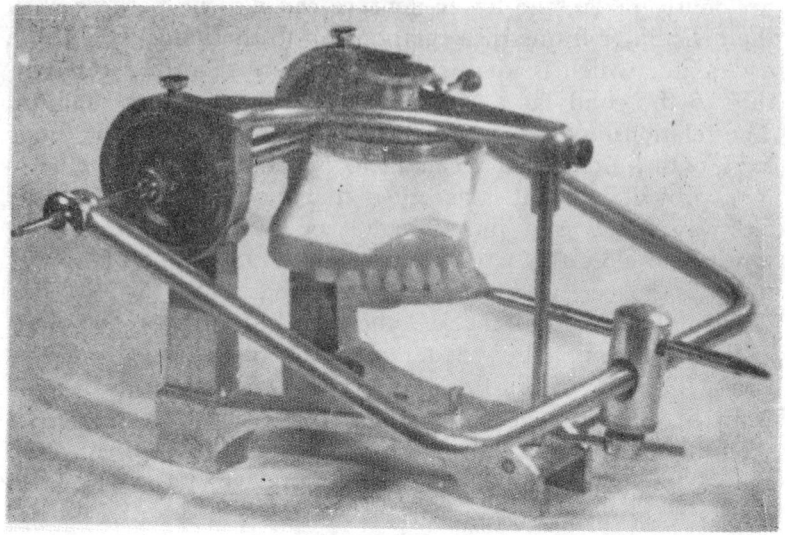

(a)

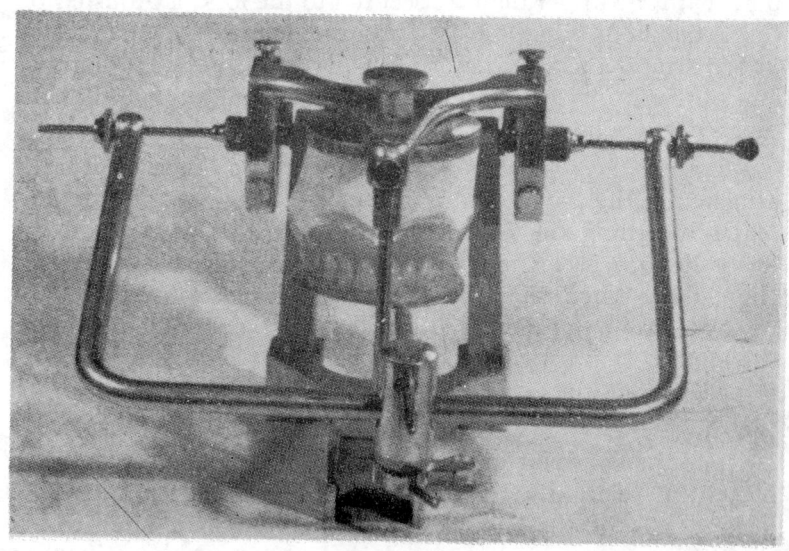

(b)

FIG. 261(a) and (b). – Upper denture mounted in the
articulator by means of the face-bow.

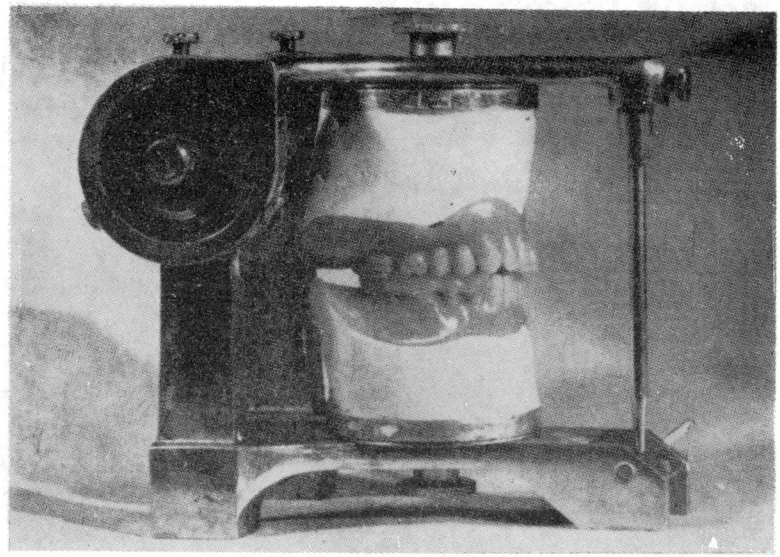

FIG. 262. – Centric relationship record used to mount the lower denture in the articulator.

closed too firmly into the wax template during the recording of the centric relation (fig. 263). If the wax record is satisfactory and no tooth contact occurs then the incisal guide pin may be removed and the articulator closed until the teeth occlude and the occlusion studied for points of premature contact or change in maxillo-mandibular relationship (fig. 264).

Figs. 265 and 266 illustrate two cases of corrected centric relationships associated with areas of premature tooth contact obtained by check records, and their appearance after grinding-in the occlusion.

(5) *Correcting the Occlusion by Spot Grinding.* – In order to produce a satisfactory result it is important to carry out the grinding systematically to ensure that:

A. The vertical dimension is maintained.

B. An even distribution of occlusal stress is obtained in centric occlusion.

C. An even distribution of stress is maintained in lateral positions.

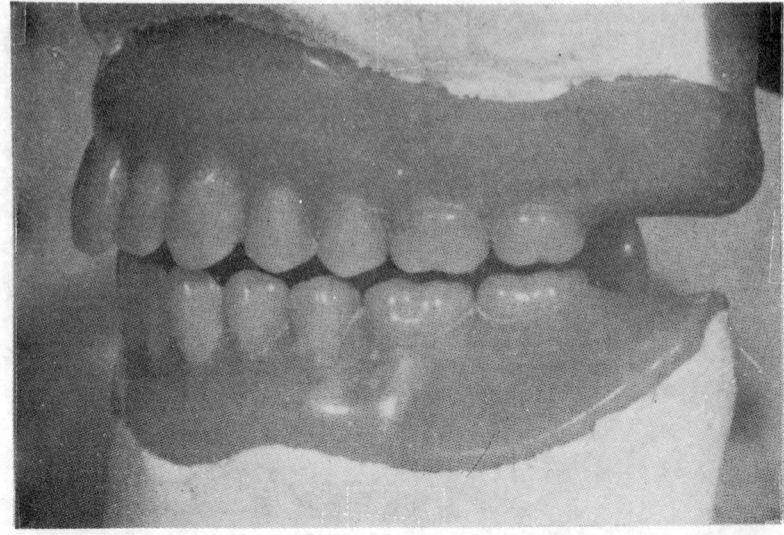

(a)

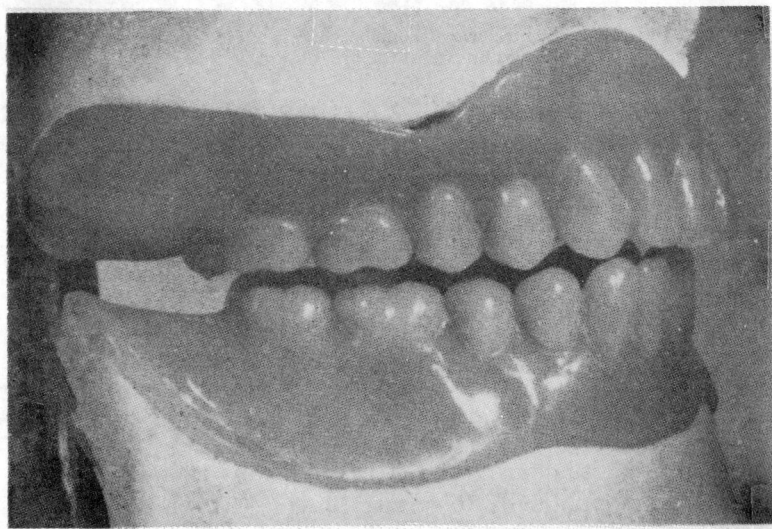

(b)

FIG. 263(*a*) and (*b*). – The centric relationship record has been removed, after locking the incisal guide pin, to show the relation between the upper and lower dentures. Note that no occlusal contact was made during the centric check record registration, and that there appears to be greater separation between the upper and lower teeth on the right side than on the left. Also on the left side there appears to be slight retrusion of the mandible judged by the cuspal relationship of the opposing teeth.

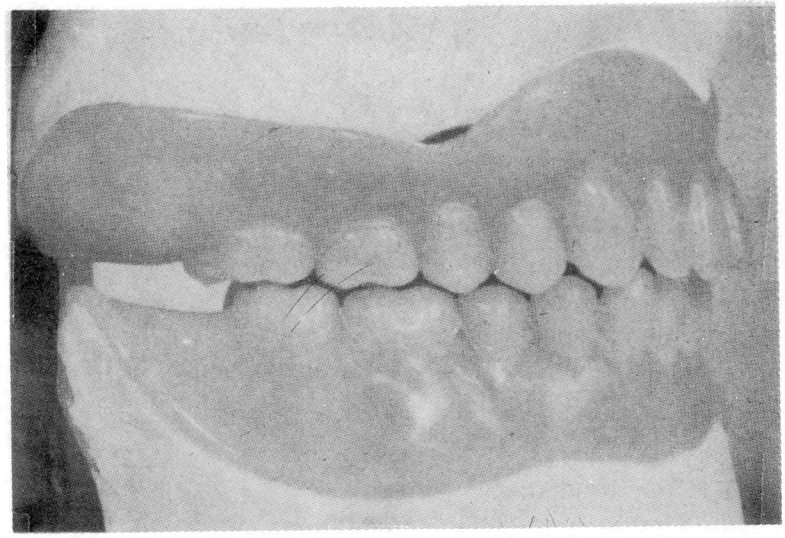

Fig. 264(a)

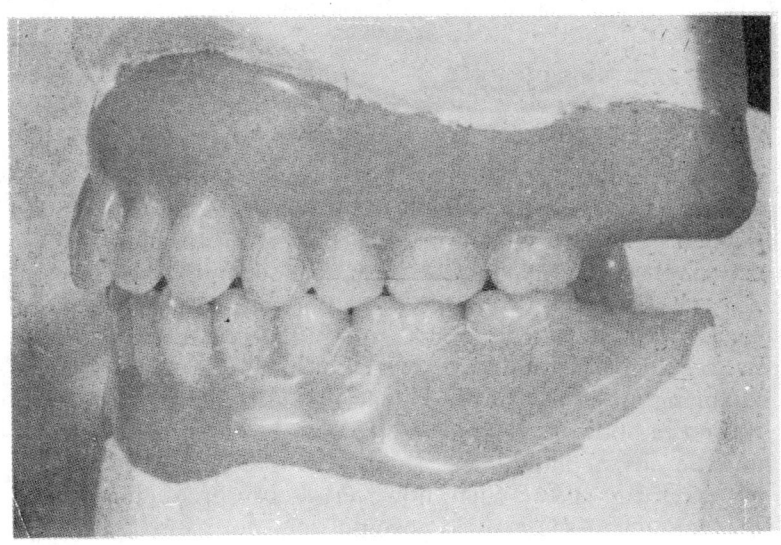

Fig. 264(b)

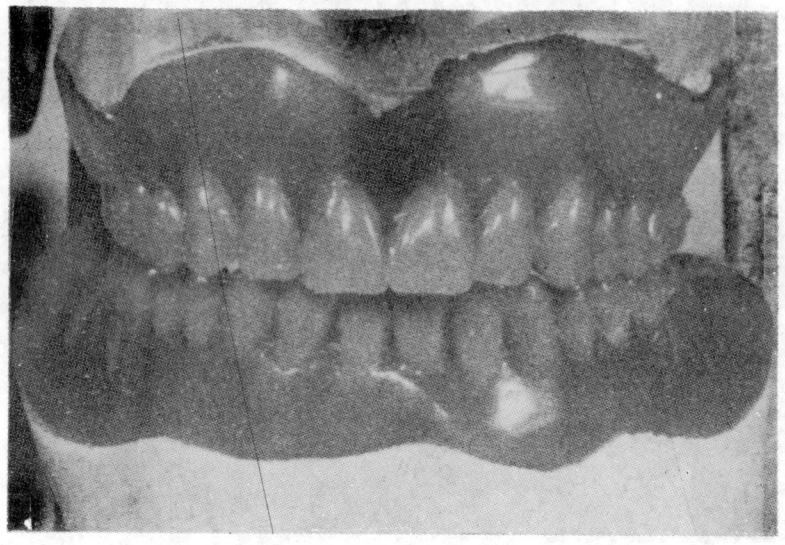

(c)

FIG. 264. – The incisal guide pin has been removed and the articulator closed to give tooth contact. Right and left side, and front views are shown. Tooth contact occurs on the left side whilst the right side shows lack of contact.

The vertical dimension is controlled by the lower buccal cusps and the upper palatal, cusps and their opposing fossae, therefore it is essential that these zones must receive careful consideration when establishing centric and lateral occlusions.

Grinding in to Centric Occlusion. – Place thin blue articulating paper on the occlusal surface of the lower teeth and close the articulator with sufficient pressure to record just the first contact areas (fig. 267). Observe the prominent cusp or cusps and decide whether the cusp or its opposing fossa should be ground by checking this cusp in its lateral working position and then its balancing position. If the offending cusp makes premature contact in both centric and lateral positions then the cusp, and not the fossa, should be ground to produce even centric occlusion (fig. 268). When, however, a cusp producing premature contact in the centric position does not cause premature contact when in working and balancing positions then the

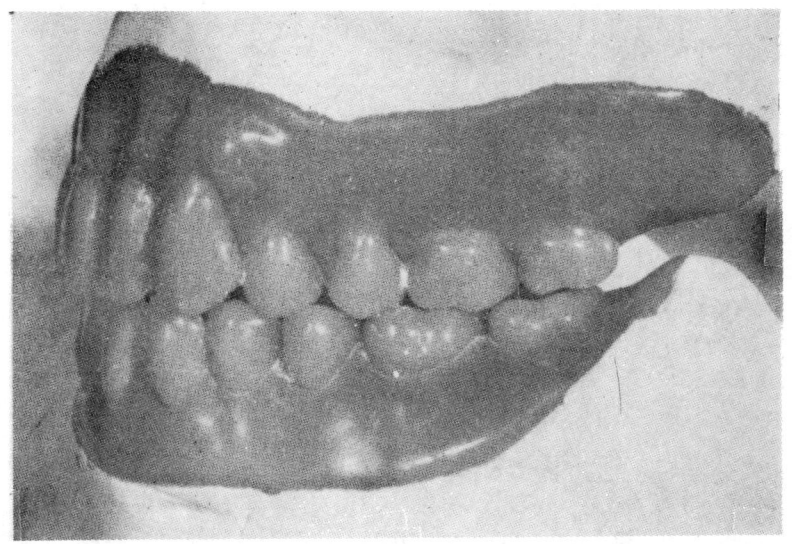

FIG. 265(a)

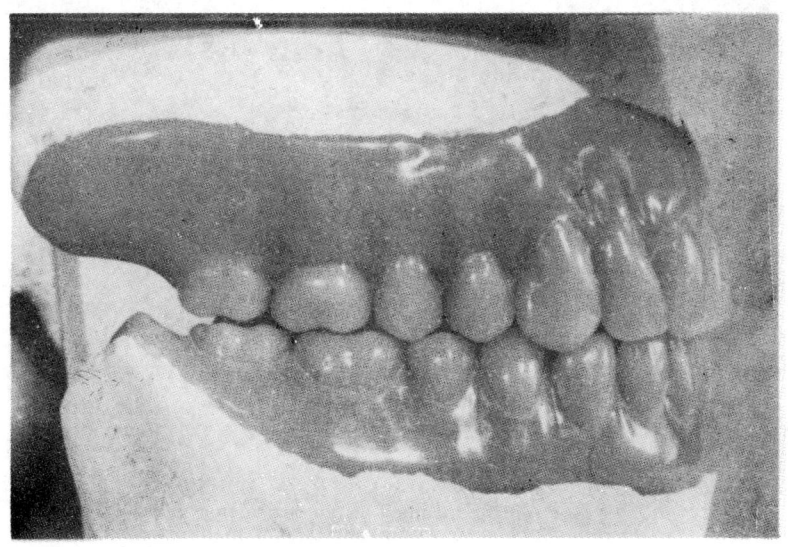

FIG. 265(b)

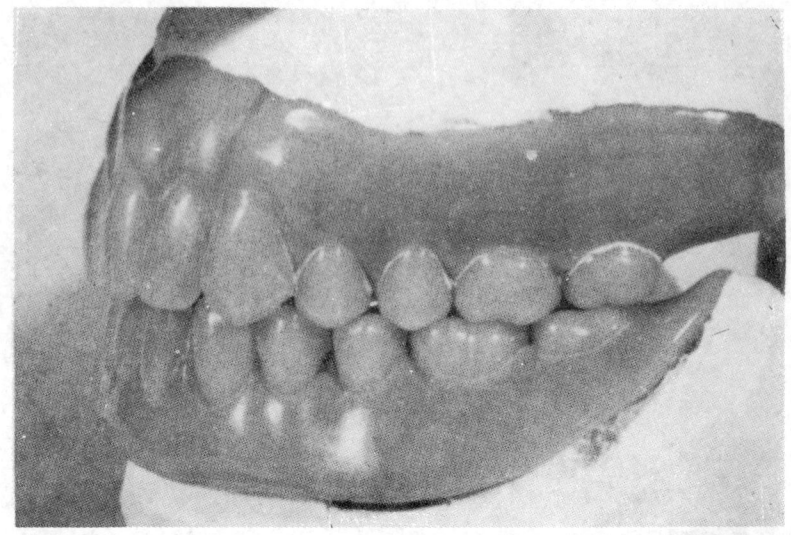

(c)

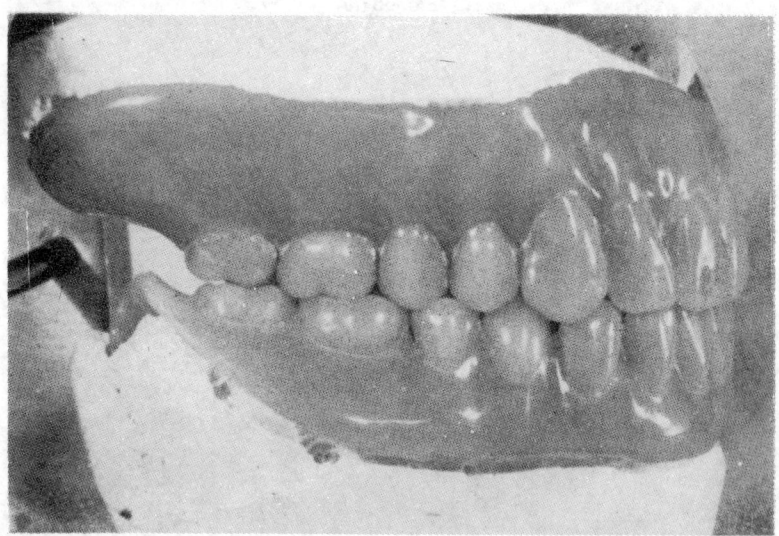

(d)

FIG. 265. – This case, mounted in an articulator following
check records, shows premature contact points in the premolar
area of both sides with slight retrusion of the mandible (a)
and (b). By careful grinding an even occlusion is obtained
(c) and (d).

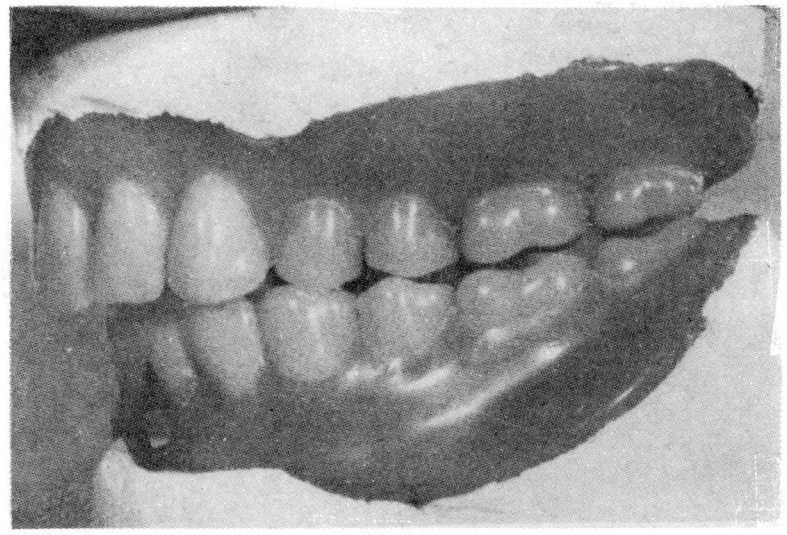

FIG. 266(a)

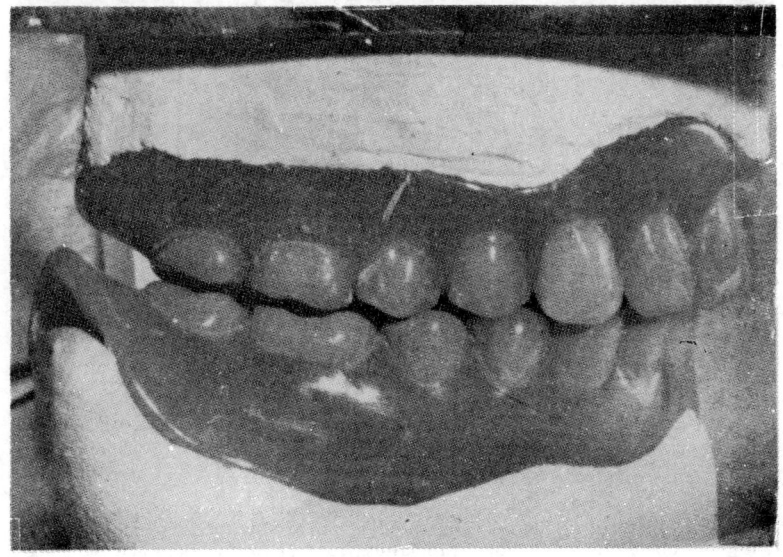

FIG. 266(b)

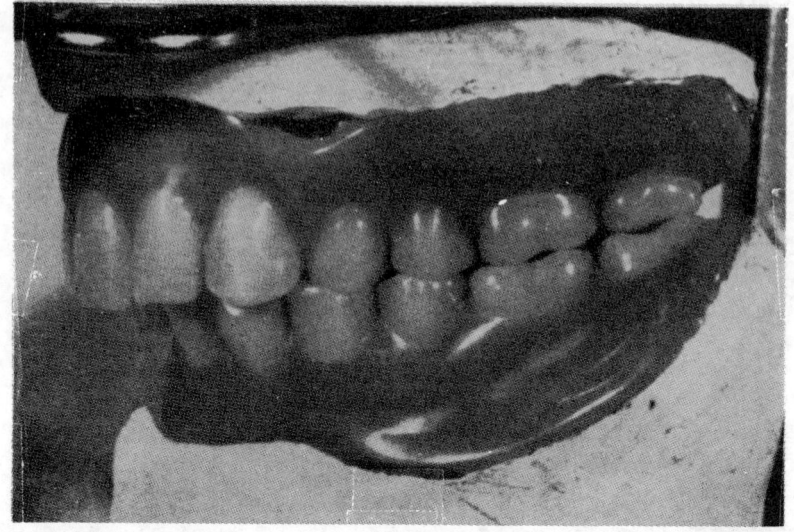

(c)

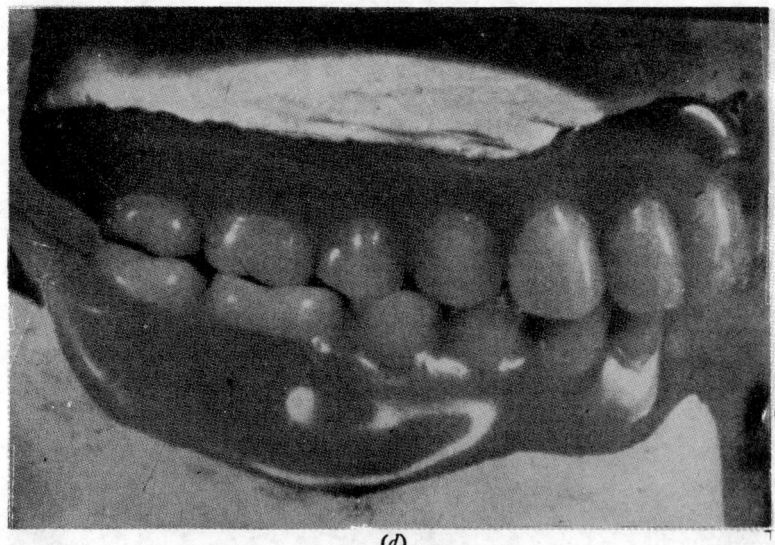

(d)

FIG. 266. – This case, mounted in an articulator following check records, shows premature contact in the premolar region of both sides with marked retrusion of the mandible (a) and (b). Grinding produces an even centric occlusion (c) and (d). Extreme cases such as this are usually observed and corrected at the try-in stage.

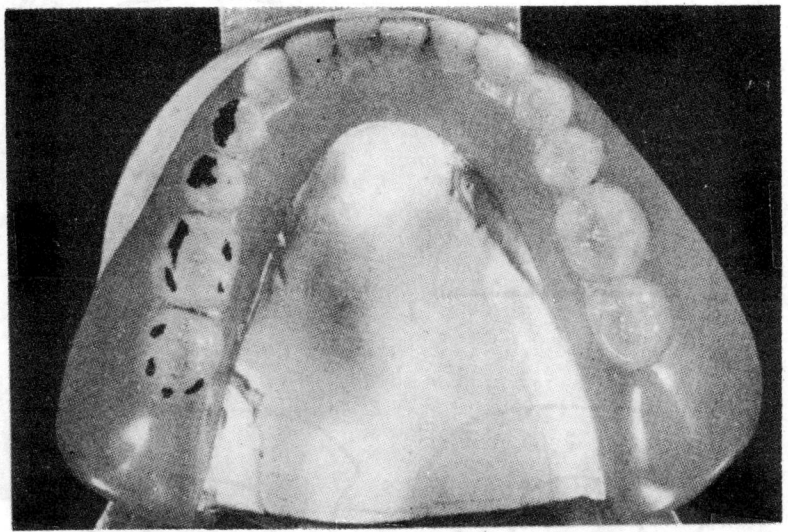

FIG. 267. – Areas of premature contact recorded with articulating paper. Note heavy occlusion in /45 area and the complete lack of contact on the opposite side.

fossa is ground to accommodate the cusp (fig. 269). (The lateral contacts can be marked with red articulating paper for purposes of differentiation.) This principle is followed until an even centric occlusion is obtained throughout the dentition.

Grinding-in for Lateral Excursions. – To enhance the retention and stability of the dentures and to reduce the stress applied to the alveolar ridges as the mandible moves laterally it is most important to provide a free sliding lateral articulation and elimination of cusp lock.

Red articulating paper is placed between the occlusal surfaces of the teeth, and the dentures moved with light pressure from centric occlusion into right lateral occlusion. If the upper and lower buccal cusps make premature contact and the balancing side is out of occlusion then the upper buccal cusp is ground (fig. 270) as the lower buccal cusp is required to maintain vertical dimension and even pressure in centric occlusion.

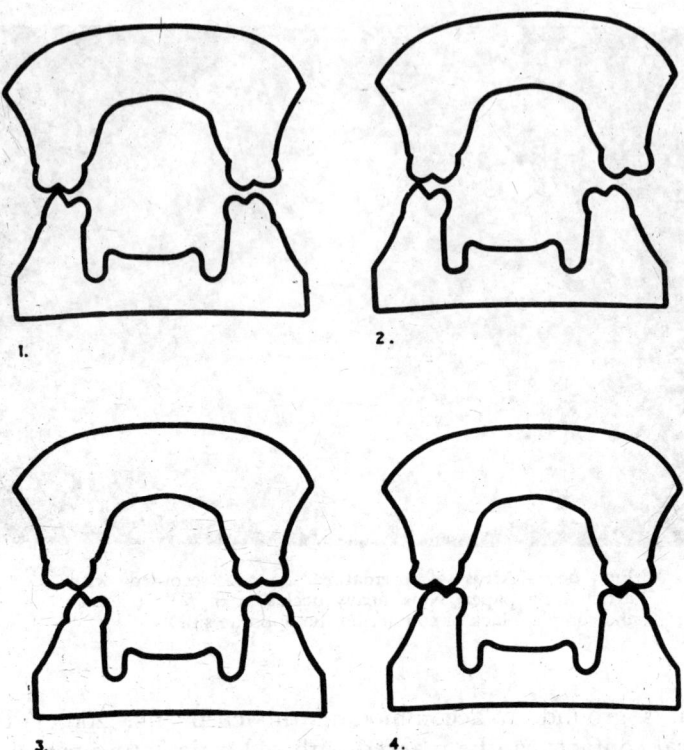

FIG. 268. – 1. The lower right buccal cusp occludes prematurely in centric occlusion. 2. When tested as a working side contact it is found to be in premature occlusion, as is the case, also, when tested as a balancing side contact. 3. Therefore the lower buccal cusp is ground to produce even contact in centric occlusion. 4. Compare with fig. 269.

When the lower lingual and upper palatal cusps occlude prematurely in this lateral position the lower lingual cusp is ground to produce balance of both sides of the denture (fig. 271); the upper palatal cusp being required for the maintenance of vertical dimension in centric occlusion. The grinding of the Buccal Upper and Lingual Lower cusps to produce balance in lateral movements is often referred to as grinding to the BULL rule.

Should the balancing side exhibit premature occlusion between the lower buccal cusp and the palatal upper cusp it

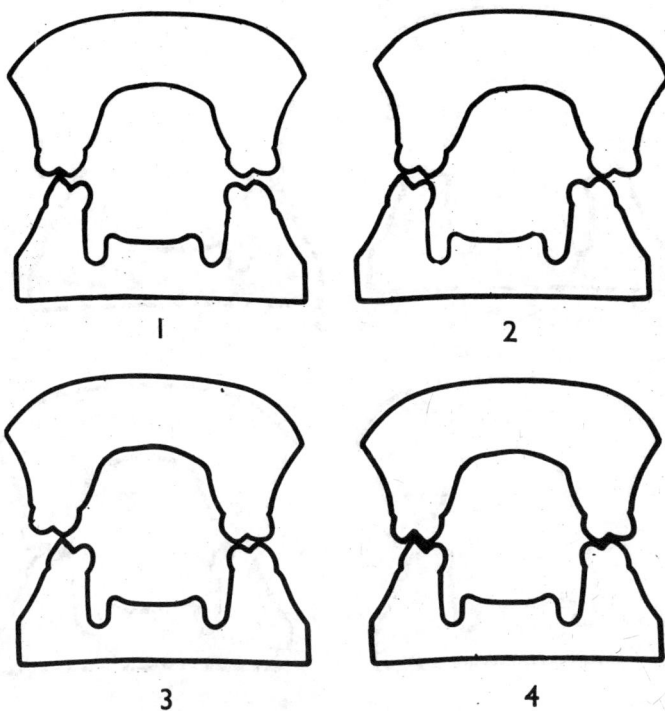

Fig. 269. – 1. The lower right buccal cusp occludes prematurely in centric occlusion. 2. When tested as a working side contact occlusion of the teeth on the balancing side occurs. 3. If the lower right buccal cusp is checked in its balancing side contact it would be observed that the working side (left) also shows tooth contact. Therefore the fossa of the upper right tooth should be deepened to produce even contact in centric occlusion. 4. Contrast with fig. 268. The checking and grinding is carried out in stages and it may be necessary to grind tooth fossa and cusp in order to produce the desired balance in centric and eccentric occlusions.

will be necessary to grind the palatal upper cusp and not the lower buccal cusp since this cusp is required to maintain vertical dimension and even pressure in centric occlusion and contact in the working lateral position.

The procedure having been completed for the right lateral position it is then repeated for the left lateral excursion.

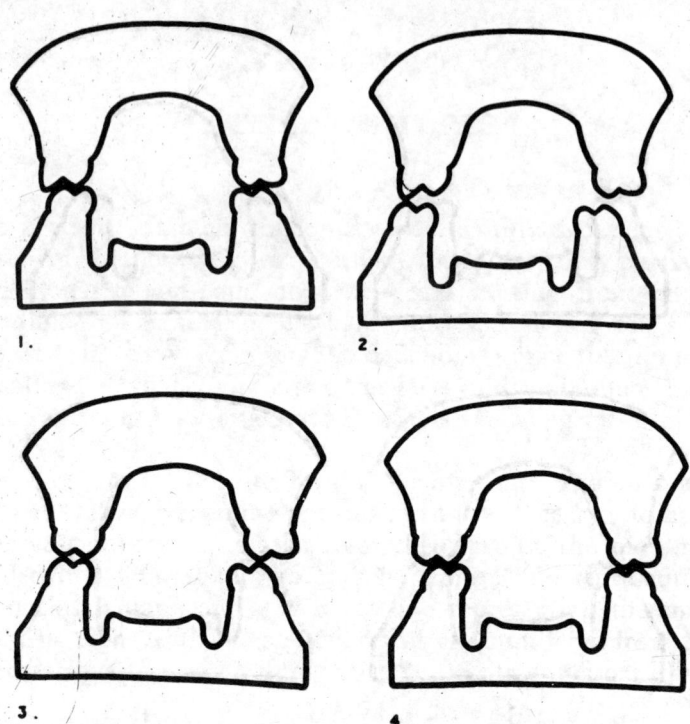

Fig. 270. – 2. The upper right buccal cusp is seen to be in premature contact when the right side is acting as the working side. 3. The upper buccal cusp is reduced to bring the teeth on the balancing side into occlusion. 3. This does not alter the evenness of centric occlusion, 1 and 4.

Having established a free lateral sliding movement of the occlusion of the protrusive contacts are studied.

Correction of Premature Contacts in Protrusion. – As we are dealing with an artificial dentition, and are not concerned with the possible over-eruption of teeth as may occur with a natural dentition, most of the grinding for correction of premature contacts of incisal edges of anterior teeth, when in protrusive occlusion, can be carried out at the expense of the lower incisors (fig. 272). A limited amount of grinding, however, of the upper anterior teeth to simulate attrition, related to the patient's age, can enhance the appearance of the dentures.

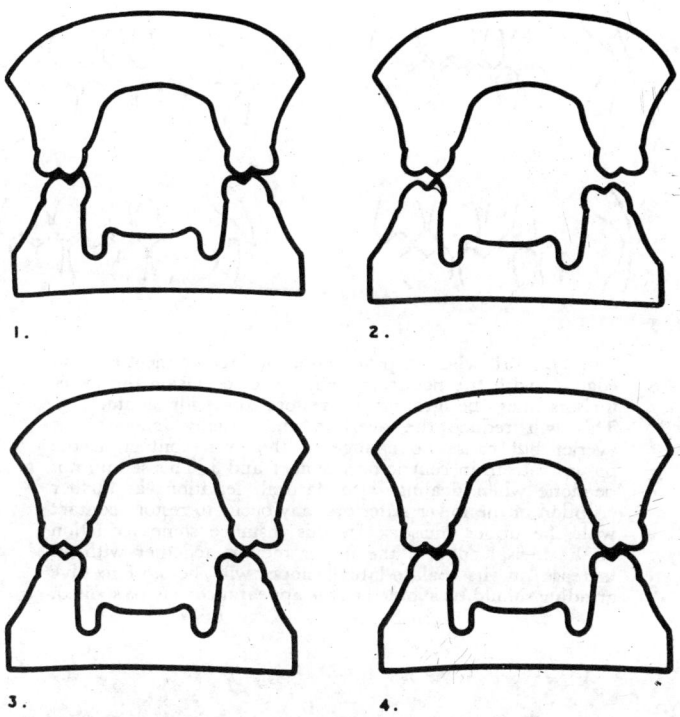

1.   2.

3.   4.

Fig. 271.-2. The lingual cusp of the lower right tooth occludes prematurely when the right side becomes the working side. In order to produce contact on the balancing side the lingual cusp must be reduced, 3, and not the upper palatal cusp which is required to maintain even centric occlusion, 1 and 4.

(6) *Perfecting Articulation with Grinding-in Paste.* – The main correction of occlusal irregularities must be carried out with small mounted abrasive stones in a hand-piece so that the vertical dimension is kept under control. The amount of adjustment made with grinding-in paste must be small as this will reduce all occluding surfaces and if excessive will result in loss of vertical dimension. A paste of coarse grit carborundum powder mixed with vaseline or tooth paste is used first, followed by one of fine grit carborundum to smooth the previously ground tooth surfaces and produce a perfectly even occlusion

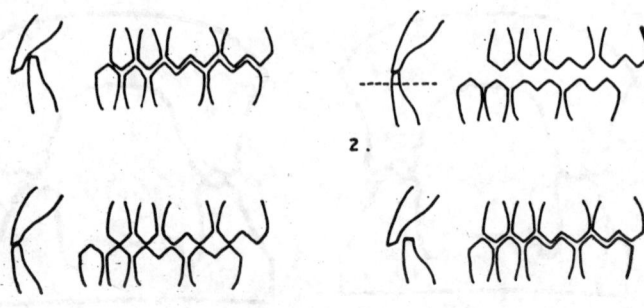

Fig. 272. – If, when in protrusion, the incisors meet edge to edge, 2, with the posterior teeth out of occlusion the lower incisors may be ground to restore posterior contact, 3. This will reduce the overbite and usually increase the overjet but cause no change in the even contact of the posterior teeth in centric occlusion, 1 and 4. This should not be done when dealing with natural dentitions as further eruption of the lower anteriors may occur to restore contact with the upper incisors. In this instance some reduction of the incisal edge of the upper incisors together with an increase in its palato-labial slope will help. Excessive grinding should be avoided as the appearance may be spoiled.

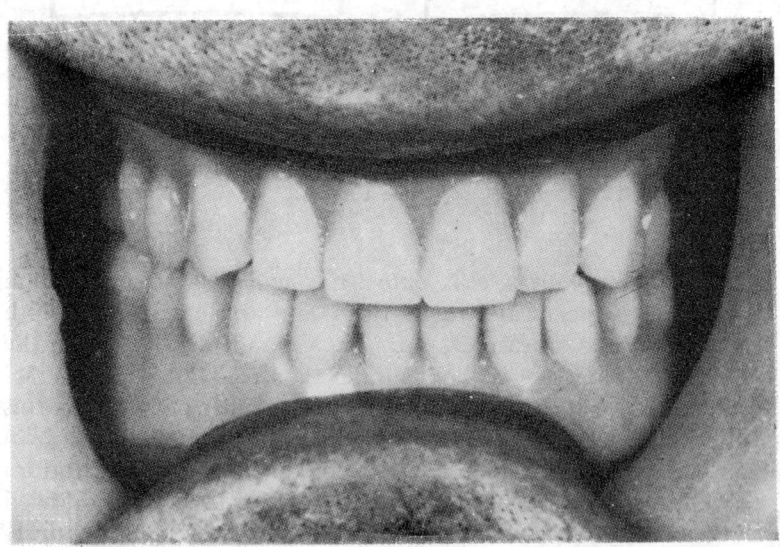

Fig. 273(a)

(fig. 273(a) and (b)). A final grinding-in of the occlusion may take place in the mouth when the dentures are returned to the patient if it is considered desirable, but if carried out it should be for a very limited period as the patient may make lateral excursions with some degree of protrusion which will disturb the previously arranged articulation, and long periods of grinding will close the vertical dimension further. When using the paste, either with the articulator or in the mouth, it is placed on the occlusal surface of the lower denture and lateral movements are made with the teeth maintaining contact. Movement is continued until such time as a free sliding articulation results.

A warning must be given to the patient not to swallow whilst the carborundum paste is in the mouth, rest periods must be given to allow accumulated saliva to be rinsed away.

(7) *Reduction of Sharp Edges of Ground Teeth.* – On the completion of all grinding, sharp edges occurring buccally and lingually must be rounded to prevent tongue and cheek irritation. Rubber wheels, Water of Ayr stone, and finally pumice paste used with polishing brushes will produce a smooth finish.

The patient now has harmonious occlusion and articulation (fig. 273 (c), (d) and (e)).

B. DENTURES CONSTRUCTED IN A PLANE LINE ARTICULATOR

The same check record technique should be used with dentures set in a plane line articulator and although it is not possible in every case to produce a completely free sliding occlusion in the anterior region, excellent results are obtained for a very large majority of patients. The depth of overbite, however, in a few cases restricts the free sliding movement and can only be eliminated by the mutilation of the appearance. Nevertheless, if, when the teeth are being set up, a minimum overbite of the anterior teeth is employed with an equal overjet, and compensating curves are introduced there should be no difficulty in establishing a sliding articulation free from cusp lock.

Even where the depth of overbite restricts lateral movements it is possible to provide a reduction of cusp lock posteriorly and the technique has the considerable advantage of permitting correction of minor errors in centric occlusion and the estab-

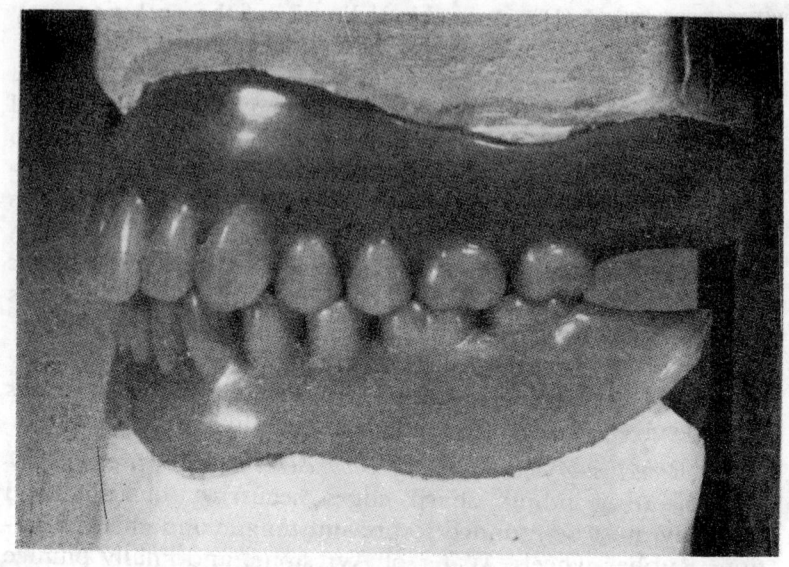

FIG. 273(b)

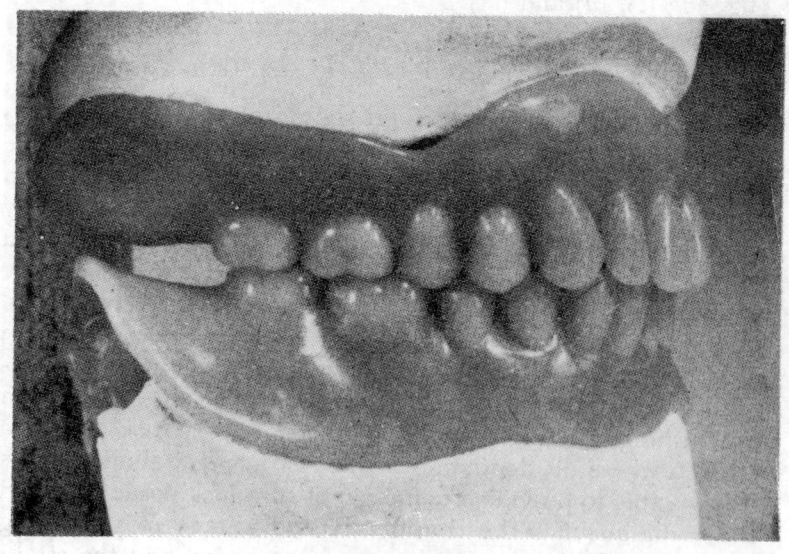

FIG. 273(c)

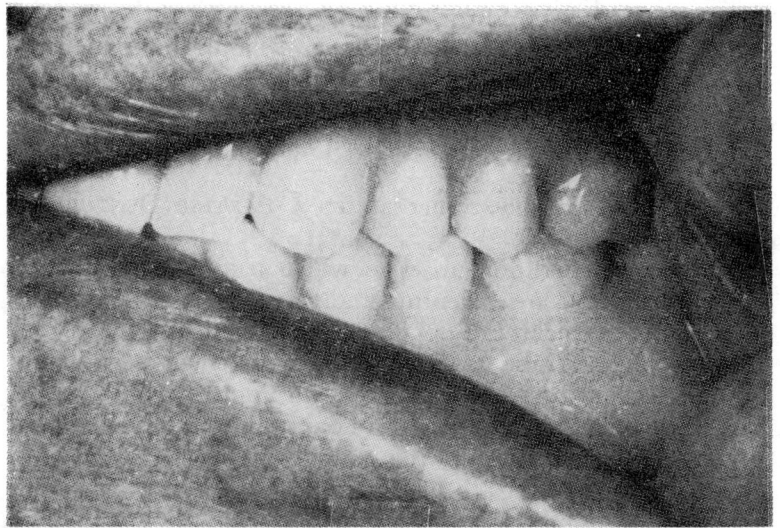

FIG. 273(d)

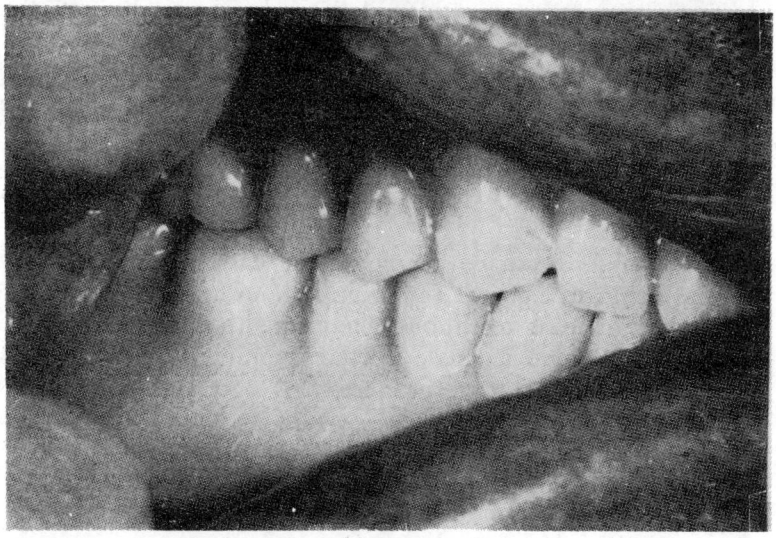

(e)

FIG. 273. – The dentures, seen in figs. 256 and 257 have been ground-in to produce an even occlusal contact. The dentures seen in fig. 273 (b) and (c) have been returned to the patient and the right and left views show even contact in centric occlusion. The front view illustrates the slight amount of grinding carried out on the upper incisors to simulate attrition. Compare with fig. 286.

lishment of even pressure in centric and eccentric occlusions, excluding protrusion and for this reason should be carried out for all cases mounted in plane line articulators. Increased comfort of the denture and improved masticatory ability follow the check record adjustments.

C. Full Dentures Opposed to a Partial Denture

Frequently a condition arises in which a full upper denture opposes a partial lower denture and natural teeth, or occasionally a full lower denture opposes a partial upper denture and natural teeth. These cases can be approached in a similar manner to the previous cases, the variations to be borne in mind are the necessity of obtaining an impression of the lower partial denture in situ and the limited grinding of any natural teeth. When casting the impression the denture must be retained in it, and it is preferable to flow low fusing metal into the impression area of the natural teeth to give strength and surface hardness to withstand lateral movements of the articulator. If it is necessary to grind the represented natural teeth a note of the areas ground must be made so that a similar adjustment can be carried out to the natural teeth when the dentures are returned to the patient.

D. Partial Upper and Lower Dentures

The technique can be employed in cases involving large partial dentures e.g., where the upper and lower anteriors are the only remaining teeth, but where small partial dentures are opposed or where a single partial denture occludes with a natural dentition it may be necessary to correct the natural occlusion from the point of view of a locked articulation before proceeding with the denture construction.

CHAPTER XIV

COMPLAINTS

It is manifestly impossible to discuss every complaint which may be made by a patient, but the following are the most common and will give a comprehensive outline of how the prosthetist may diagnose their causes and how they should be treated.

Most complaints will fall under one of the following headings though frequently a patient will have more than one complaint:

1. Pain.
2. Appearance.
3. Inefficiency.
4. Poor retention.
5. Instability.
6. Chattering teeth.
7. Nausea.
8. Discomfort.
9. Altered speech.
10. Biting the cheek and tongue.
11. Food under the denture.

Each heading will now be considered at greater length.

1. PAIN

(a) Overextension of the Periphery

This is by far the most common cause of pain with new dentures. It is due to incorrect moulding of the impression or incorrect outlining of the denture on the model and is visible in the mouth as an area of hyperaemia, an angry red line or an ulcer, depending upon how continuously the denture has been worn, or how gross the overextension.

Treatment: Mark with an indelible pencil on the denture the exact position and extent of the area or use easing paste and reduce the periphery at that spot. Except in cases of severe ulceration this will give immediate relief.

If the denture is an old one, the overextension may be due

to alveolar absorption and the slow, chronic irritation may have caused a local hyperplasia

In this case cut the denture away freely and when the hyperplasia has absorbed, or been removed surgically, construct a new denture, as the ridge absorption which caused this condition will have also altered the vertical height and articulation, as well as universally destroying the fit.

(b) Poor Fit

Easily detected by the poor retention, rocking, tilting and inability accurately to seat the denture in any position. The movement of the denture rubbing the mucous membrane causes pain, and patches of redness are sometimes visible.

Treatment: New dentures, but the old ones can be worn in the meantime with a lining of zinc oxide paste.

(c) Insufficient Relief

The denture will usually rock on the hard area causing pain. The painful area is red and possibly ulcerated.

Treatment: Apply a very thin coating of easing paste or white tooth-paste, to the area which requires relief, insert the denture and on removal the area will be clearly marked; bur away this part of the fitting surface until adequate relief is obtained.

(d) Incorrect Centric Occlusion

This may be any one of the following faults, or a combination of them.

(i) Wrong Anteroposterior Relationship

When the teeth are in centric occlusion the mandible will not be fully retracted. Attempts to retrude it fully will drag the dentures against the mucous membrane as they are locked together by the interdigitation of the teeth. This is often difficult to diagnose and can only be seen by watching the occlusal plane very closely whilst the patient slowly approximates the teeth and increases the pressure to the maximum. At some stage in these movements the lower denture will be seen to move. This is often associated with a slight over-closure.

Treatment: If only slight it can be cured by a check record and grinding of the dentures; if gross, new dentures will be required.

(ii) *Uneven Pressure*

This may be the result of faulty setting-up of the teeth and, if so, is usually very slight. More commonly it is the result of an undetected tilting of the record blocks, which was again undetected at the try-in. Pain may be due to trauma caused by the heavy one-sided pressure and is then confined to the crest of the lower alveolar ridge on that side; sometimes small white areas 4 mm. to 6 mm. in diameter are to be seen, as in an opened vertical height. Pain may also be due to tilting of either denture, more usually the lower, and is then situated near the buccal periphery on the side of excessive pressure and near the lingual periphery on the opposite side. Diagnosis can be made by trying to insert a thin spatula between the molar teeth, first on one side, and then on the other, with the teeth in firm contact. Lesser degrees of error can be detected by inserting a thin celluloid strip on either side between the occlusal surfaces of the posterior teeth, while the patient closes just sufficiently to hold them in place. The strip on the side of the heavy pressure will be immovable while that on the opposite side can be easily withdrawn.

Treatment: If detectable with a spatula, a new lower denture must be constructed, but, if it can only be found with celluloid strips, then spot-grinding, using articulating paper, or better still a full check record technique will usually effect a cure.

(iii) *Over Open*

This is due to an error in record taking and is almost always due to increasing the vertical height beyond normal, very rarely indeed except in old people, to restoring the height to normal. Pain is associated with the lower pressure-resisting area, as distinct from the lateral surfaces of the ridge, and one or more small white patches are to be seen in the painful area. Relief of the denture over these white patches usually gives immediate relief from pain, but within a few days the patient returns with the same condition but differently situated. In nearly all cases of excessive opening the patient also complains that the teeth jar, clatter, are 'in the way' or 'too high' when eating, and sometimes when talking.

Treatment: New lower denture to a slightly decreased vertical dimension, if the occlusal plane of the upper is judged to be correct, otherwise, new upper and lower dentures.

(iv) *Over-closed*

Pain from this cause is rarely associated with new dentures, it is almost always the result of loss of vertical height through lower alveolar absorption. The pain is often indefinite in locality and frequently resembles neuralgia of the cheek on one or both sides.

Costen's Syndrome. – This is said to be the result of prolonged over-closure though rarely is the complete syndrome encountered. It consists of:

1. Mild, catarrhal deafness and dizzy spells which are relieved by inflation of the eustachian tubes.
2. Tinnitus, or at times a snapping noise in the joint which is experienced while chewing. Painful, limited or excessive movements of the affected joint.
3. Tenderness to palpation over the temporo-mandibular joint or dull pains in the ear.
4. Various neuralgic symptoms, such as burning or prickling sensation of the tongue, throat and side of the nose. Various forms of atypical head pain, particularly that referred to the temporal region or the base of the skull.
5. Dryness of the mouth due to disturbed salivary gland function.

Treatment: New dentures with the vertical dimension increased by a few millimetres. This will not always relieve the symptoms known as Costen's syndrome.

(e) *Cuspal Interference*

A dragging action will be exerted on both upper and lower dentures during all lateral and protrusive movements with the teeth in contact if cusped posterior teeth are used:

(a) with a plane line articulator,
(b) with an anatomical articulator if care has not been taken to obtain balanced articulation.

The same effect may be obtained with an excessive overbite or an incorrect incisive angle.

This dragging will cause pain with well-fitting dentures and also instability with those having poorer retention. The pain is usually widely distributed and often only experienced when attempting to eat. Sore areas may sometimes be found, usually on the labial or buccal surfaces of the alveolar ridges, less frequently on the lingual surfaces of the lower ridge. This condition can easily be detected by asking the patient to grind the teeth with plenty of movement, when shifting of the dentures can be seen. Another simple method of diagnosing this fault is to hold the upper denture gently in place between the fingers and thumb which are placed above the canine teeth, asking the patient to grind the teeth and the dragging can easily be felt.

Treatment: If the cuspal interference is slight, or confined to only one or two teeth, it can be corrected by the careful use of articulating paper and grinding, or in cases where it is very slight, by covering the occlusal surfaces of the teeth with a grinding-in paste and letting the patient himself wear down the offending high spots. The taking of a check record and grinding the occlusal surfaces in on the articulator is the most accurate method of correcting this error. If the interference is gross, correctly articulated new dentures will be required.

(f) Teeth Off the Ridge

Pain from this cause is confined chiefly to the upper buccal sulci and maxillary tuberosities. It is usually the result of setting the upper teeth too far buccally in an attempt to overcome marked discrepancies between the size of the upper arch and that of the lower. During mastication the upper denture tilts, digging the periphery of the denture into the mucous membrane on the working side, and pulling it down over the tuberosity, or other undercut area, on the opposite side. The actual tilting can be seen if the patient bites on a wooden spatula placed on the posterior teeth, first on one side and then the other.

Treatment: New dentures, or sometimes only a new upper

denture, with the teeth correctly placed and, if necessary, tilted or mounted to a crossed bite.

(g) Retained Root or Unerupted Tooth

Pain may be caused by direct pressure on an area which is already tender and will be felt very soon after inserting new dentures. It may also be caused by a well-fitting denture preventing drainage from an undetected sinus and so causing increased pressure within the bone. Well-fitting, functional dentures appear in some cases to stimulate the eruption of unerupted teeth. The painful area will usually be localized and often close inspection will reveal a small sinus or, if an unerupted tooth, a hard swelling. Diagnosis should be confirmed by X-ray

Treatment: Extraction of the root or tooth followed by re-lining of that part of the denture. If for some reason extraction is contra-indicated, then relief may be given by easing the denture freely over that area.

(h) V-shaped Ridge

More usually associated with the lower, and caused by the pressure during mastication pressing the mucous membrane against a sharp ridge of bone. The pain is worst on the side habitually used for eating, but it may be all round the ridge; it is most severe during, and immediately following, a meal, and is increased by perseverance on the part of the patient.

Treatment: In the lower, alveolectomy followed by re-lining the denture. In the upper, relief over the crest of the alveolus is often sufficient since the palate can usually resist the masticatory stresses, the exception being the V-shaped palate.

(i) Mental Foramen

Under normal conditions the mental foramen is situated on the buccal surface of the mandible below the lower alveolar ridge and is thus outside the denture bearing area. If, however, gross absorption of the alveolar and basal bone has taken place, the foramen may come to lie under the denture (*see* fig. 274) and so be subject to pressure from it. When a new denture is constructed to these altered conditions, adequate relief should be given for the mental nerve, otherwise there is every likelihood

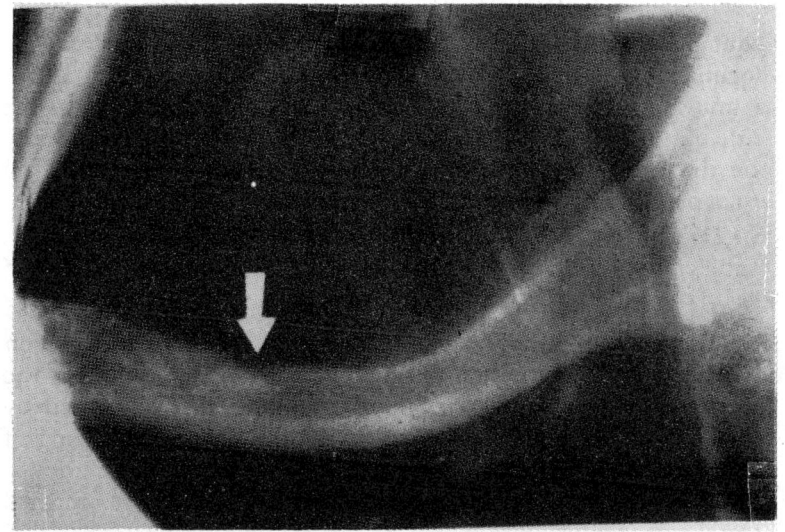

(a)

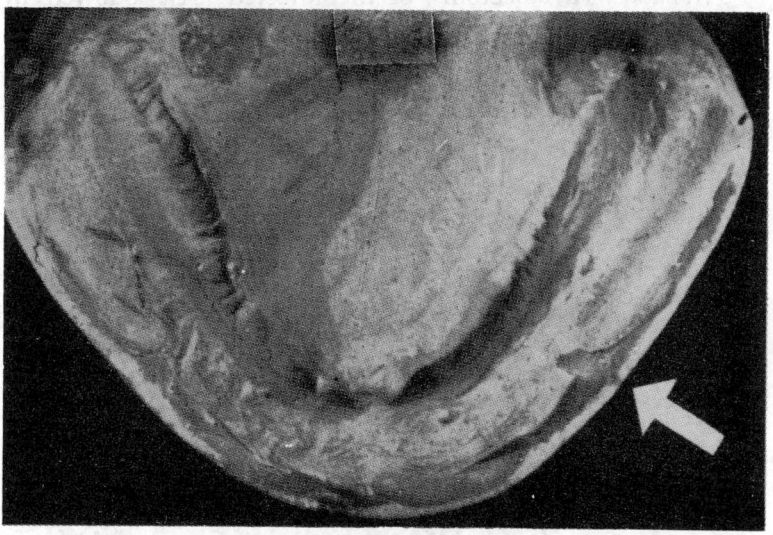

(b)

Fig. 274.

(a) X-ray photograph through grossly absorbed mandible showing mental nerve on surface of ridge (arrowed).

(b) Model of surface of mandibular ridge from implant impression. Arrow shows mental nerve on surface of ridge.

that pain will be caused by pressure on it. The pain may be localized to the immediate vicinity of the mental foramen, or it may be referred, and is then felt as a neuralgic pain in the side of the face or, more rarely, in the lips or chin. It can usually be diagnosed by locating the mental foramen and applying firm pressure in that area which will cause the same type of pain.

Treatment: Relieve the denture so that the nerve cannot be subjected to pressure.

(j) Irregular Absorption

Sometimes during alveolar absorption an area is formed which is rough, with a number of sharp spicules of bone, and if the mucous membrane covering it is thin, pain will be caused by pressure on it. This is very similar to the pain complained of with V-shaped ridges except that it is localized. The uneven alveolus can be detected by gentle palpation and confirmed by X-ray (*see* fig. 275).

Treatment: Alveolectomy of the affected area followed by re-lining that part of the denture, if necessary with a soft lining.

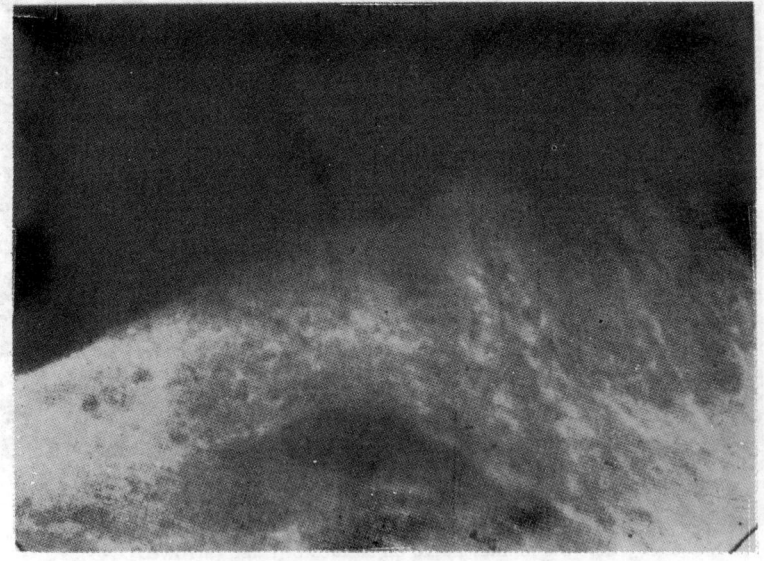

Fig. 275. – Rough irregular surface of alveolar ridge in 4321/ area.

(k) Pathological Conditions

These will usually have been diagnosed and treated before the construction of new dentures is undertaken, but, of course, they may also arise under old dentures. For the diagnosis and treatment of these conditions the reader must refer to a textbook on oral pathology.

(l) Allergy

In certain rare cases a patient will be found to be allergic to the plastic material of which the denture is made. The metals used in denture construction do not appear to produce this effect, but it has been proved in the case of vulcanite and is suspected with methyl methacrylate (*see* fig. 276); the latter can undoubtedly cause severe irritation if worn in a state of incomplete polymerization. The patient complains of a burning sensation in the mouth whilst wearing the dentures and, sometimes, for some hours afterwards. The mucous membrane, in contact

FIG. 276. – Result of patch test for acrylic sensitivity. Test is performed by strapping some filings from the suspected denture under gauze to the skin. This test is positive, note the cluster of vesicles.

with the dentures, appears slightly inflamed and bright red in colour. In most cases the irritation is confined to the tissues in contact with the unpolished surfaces of the dentures, though occasionally it also affects the cheeks, lips and tongue to a lesser degree. It may only affect the upper denture area, and is always less marked under the lower denture, owing to the thicker layer of intervening saliva.

Treatment: New dentures must be constructed in another material. Fortunately there do not appear to be any recorded cases of an individual being allergic to both vulcanite and methyl methacrylate.

(m) Rough Fitting Surface

If a denture has been processed on a poorly poured model, small pimples will be found on the fitting surface where the material has been forced into the small air bubbles of the model. Normally these pimples are removed by the technician, but if they are overlooked the patient will complain of pain under pressure and a local area of angry red irritation can be seen, usually in the palate.

Treatment: Remove the offending roughness from the denture.

(n) Infection with Monilia albicans

The area of the palate which is damaged traumatically by the rough fitting surface of a denture frequently becomes second-arily infected, usually by one of the fungi – *Monilia Albicans* whose presence can be vertified by culturing a swab from the tissues. Especially is this so if the patient lives on a low protein and vitamin diet and also wears the dentures at night or has had long continued anti-biotic therapy. The appearance of the palate is of an acute red inflammation terminating sharply at the borders of the denture. The mucous membrane will be swollen and smooth in early cases but in those of long standing will present a granular type of hyperplasia (*see* fig. 277).

The treatment is to polish the fitting surface of the denture and instruct the patient to apply daily to the fitting surface for 01 days a fungicide such as Nystatin ointment or Fuchsonium. In severe cases Nystatin may be given systemically. The patient should also be instructed to remove the denture at

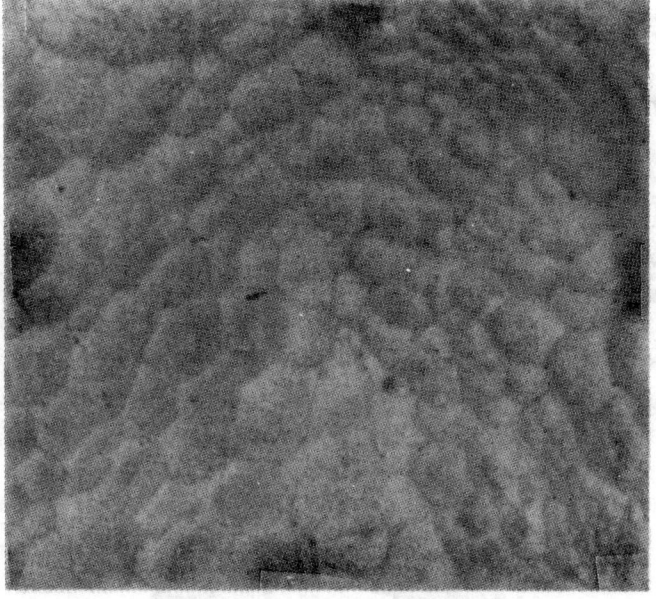

FIG. 277. – Close up of hyperplasia of palate: compare with
fig. 53.

night without fail and place it in a dilute solution of hypochlorite such as Milton. During the acute phase the denture
should not be worn during the day more than necessary. A
hypochlorite mouthwash as hot as tolerable should also be
used two or three times a day, the hot fluid being held in contact with the inflamed tissues as long as possible. The protein
and vitamin content of the diet should be increased and the
carbohydrate content reduced.

This condition is difficult to treat, but perseverance with
the above routine will, in several weeks, usually produce a
very marked improvement.

This condition is becoming common these days, probably as
a result of the increasing use of alginate impression materials
which copy on the model all the small surface details of the
palatal tissues (see fig. 278). If such impression materials are
used the palatal surface of the model should be covered with

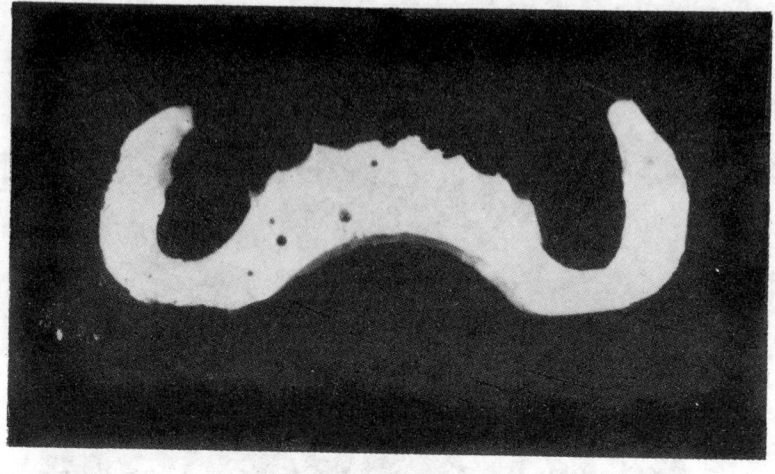

(a)

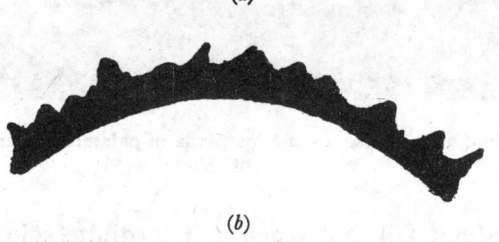

(b)

FIG. 278.

(a) Coronal section through alginate impression showing the sharp detail of the palate which it produces.
(b) Silhouette of fitting surface of denture made to a model cast from such an impression.

thin tinfoil before the denture is processed so as to reduce its roughness.

(o) Swallowing and Sore Throat

These two complaints are listed together as they are merely different ways of describing pain arising from a common cause, which is invariably the overextension of a well-fitting denture. The cause in the upper is extension on to the soft palate with firm pressure and good retention, or excessive pressure in the hamular notches, whilst in the lower it is over-extension distally in the lingual pouch. The pain ceases if the offending denture is left out, and starts again very soon after its reinsertion.

Treatment: The patient will usually know which denture is at fault and examination of the regions described will show a slight redness. Reduction of the overextension is all that is required.

(*p*) *Undercuts*

Sometimes an operator will make use of an undercut area which in his judgment is unlikely to cause pain, and although the new denture was inserted with comfort, the patient returns with the complaint that inserting and removing the denture is getting increasingly painful. The maximum bulge of the alveolus in this area is found to be red and painful, and in some cases ulcerated.

Treatment: It may be possible to insert this side of the denture first, quite painlessly, and then the opposite side, removing it in reverse order. If this manoeuvring is not successful the fitting surface must be cut away until the denture can be inserted comfortably but the periphery must not be reduced in height. Often the flange will be too thin to allow sufficient to be removed from the fitting surface and if this is so the flange must be thickened by the addition of more material. Should this easing ruin the retention, as is likely to be the case if much has to be cut away, an alveolectomy will be necessary followed by a new buccal or labial flange. This may cause warpage with an acrylic denture in which case a completely new denture will be the only remedy.

2. APPEARANCE

In spite of the greatest care on the part of the operator to obtain the patient's full approval of his appearance at the 'try-in' stage, there will always be some patients who are dissatisfied with their appearance when wearing the finished dentures. The patient should not be condemned too severely for this inconsistency, as it is difficult to form a considered opinion on all details of facial appearance when sitting in a strange chair, under strange surroundings, with strange and bulky apparatus in the mouth, and being asked to criticize the work of a professional man. The number of patients who are dissatisfied with their appearance with the final dentures can be much reduced if the operator insists on a relation or candid friend being present at the try-in stage. The number can be reduced even further if the patient is allowed to take the set-up dentures home for the criticism of his immediate circle of relations and friends. The risk of damage to these waxed-up dentures will only be slight with the averagely intelligent individual, if it is explained to him that the teeth are only mounted in wax, which will soften if worn in the mouth for more than three minutes without removal and hardening in cold water, and that nothing can be eaten or drunk whilst wearing them without their complete destruction. A man will quite often express his complete satisfaction with the finished dentures only to return rather sheepishly a few days later with the remark: 'My wife says she does not like them, in fact she says they look dreadful.'

The following examples of complaints about appearance are by no means comprehensive but will be found to cover the main points.

(a) Nose and Chin Approximating

This complaint may be made of new dentures, or of old ones, and is due to a so-called closed 'bite,' which term is synonymous with excessive free-way space.

Treatment: As previously described for over closure.

(b) Cheeks and Lips Falling In

This is a condition which only arises after a patient has been edentulous for a number of years, and is due partly to the lack of tone of the facial muscles, and partly to the lack of support of them by the teeth and alveolar ridges. This support is mainly maxillary, where unfortunately the greatest alveolar absorption is buccal and labial.

Treatment: This consists of building out the upper denture, frequently to a greater extent than the original tissues, to compensate for the loss of muscular tone. This 'plumping' should be placed in the canine and premolar area, i.e. the region of the modiolus and not in the anterior region (*see* fig. 279). In cases where the retention is really excellent, the teeth may be set-up outside the ridge, but this must not be excessive. Care must be taken when making these additions to the denture to retain a concavity directed outwards and downwards, to that the buccinators can support the denture upwards and inwards, otherwise the extra bulk will merely supply a ledge which will enable these muscles to pull the denture down.

(c) Angular Cheilitis or Soreness of the Corners of the Mouth

As described previously this is frequently the result of loss of vertical dimension and muscle tone and the corners of the mouth fall in and become bathed in saliva and develop fissures. Frequently however, as with traumatic damage to the palate, a secondary infection with *Monilia albicans* supervenes, especially if such an infection already exists in the mouth. In these cases treatment, such as that outlined on pages 373 and 374, should be instituted and at the same time the vertical dimension should be restored (but never opened) and the upper denture 'plumped' to help restore the muscle tone.

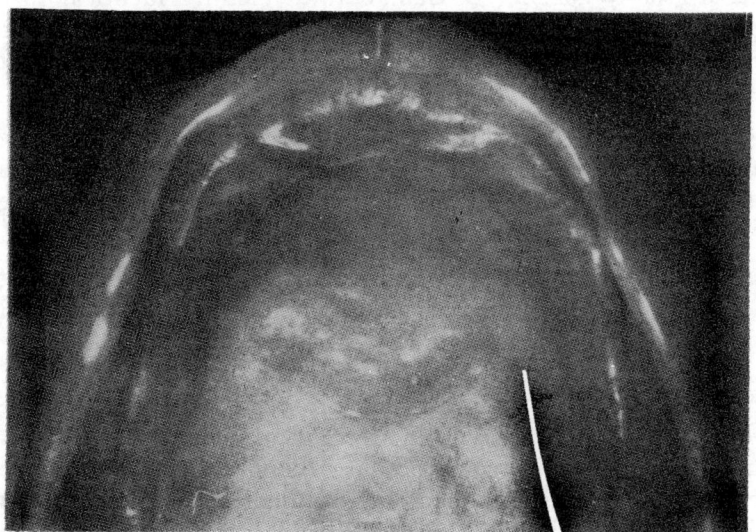

FIG. 279. –'Plumped' upper denture seen from fitti\g surface.

(d) Colour, Shape and Position of Anterior Teeth

Colour: This complaint is almost invariably that the teeth are too dark or too yellow, but before changing them it must be explained to the patient that natural teeth darken with age and that very light-shaded teeth look more artificial than darker ones.

Treatment: Comply if possible with the patient's request for lighter teeth, usually by a compromise between the shade chosen by the operator and that chosen by the patient. If the operator feels that a patient is insisting on such an unreasonably light shade that the dentures will look absurd, he may be well advised to refuse to replace the teeth by others which will damage his reputation as an artistic prosthetist.

Shape: Few people are sufficiently observant to be able to describe the shape of their lost teeth and are likely to say vaguely, when referring to their dentures, that 'they don't look right'. This question of shape is closely bound up in that of apparent size, and a different make of tooth of the same basic shape and size may well look more natural. Artificial teeth usually look larger than natural teeth of identical size, probably because their mesial and distal surfaces are not so rounded, and so the eye is able to focus on their width more accurately.

Treatment: Remove the teeth complained of and replace them with others mounted in wax, until by a process of trial and error mutually suitable ones are obtained, which are then permanently attached.

Position: Irregularities of individual teeth which the patient wishes to have reproduced in his dentures will have been described at, or before, the try-in stage, and the complaint under consideration is that the teeth are too far back in the mouth, or are too far forward, more often the former. If the setting-up is left entirely to the technician without any instructions he will, quite rightly, place them as nearly over the remaining ridge as he can, but if the patient has been edentulous for some time the labial absorption of the upper alveolus makes this the wrong position for the anterior teeth. A fear is sometimes expressed that moving the teeth anterior to the ridge, into the position the natural teeth occupied, will affect the stability of the denture, but this is not so. Stability will be jeopardized much more by encroaching on the tongue, than by setting the teeth in the neutral zone where pressures of tongue and lip are equalized. A further point to be remembered is, that a patient who has been edentulous for a sufficient length of time for this degree of absorption to have taken place, will almost certainly have been wearing dentures, and will have acquired a considerable degree of muscular control.

Treatment: New dentures will almost certainly have to be made. If only the anterior teeth of the existing denture are moved forward, larger ones will be required if proximal contact is to be maintained, and this is contra-indicated if the teeth originally chosen were correct; if the teeth are to be moved back the converse is equally true.

(e) Amount of Tooth Showing

This complaint is nearly always with regard to the upper anteriors, and will be that either too much or too little tooth is showing. It must be remembered that the upper natural teeth show less in old age than in youth, owing to attrition and laxity of the lips.

Treatment: Usually the dentures should be entirely re-made with the occlusal plane raised or lowered as the case may be, with longer or shorter anterior teeth if necessary. If the complaint is that too much tooth is showing, there is a temptation to grind away the offending portion, but this will ruin a balanced articulation since the patient will be unable to obtain incisive contact.

(f) General Dissatisfaction

One of the most difficult cases with which a prosthetist may have to deal is that of the patient, fitted with new dentures, who returns a few days later with the vague remark that he 'does not like them'. He can specify no particular complaint and it will be found on questioning that comfort, retention, stability and efficiency are not at fault, so the conclusion, which is invariably right, is that it is a question of appearance.

It may be due to diffidence on the part of the patient who is unwilling to make a specific complaint which would appear to criticize the operator's skill. If the prosthetist is fortunate enough to have a spare room, and the right type of sympathetic surgery assistant, he is well advised to leave it to her: rarely will she fail to find out what is really in the patient's mind, although it may take a considerable time. Sometimes the patient will bring a photograph to illustrate what he used to look like and what he was expecting the prosthetist to reproduce. These photographs are almost entirely useless, whether studio portraits or snapshots, as they were invariably taken many years previously, often thirty or more. If the complaint can be pinned down to one particular point it can, of course, be remedied, at least partially, but if it is a psychological longing for lost youth it will take much tact to satisfy the patient that the colour of the hair, the complexion and the tone of the muscles have all altered, and that the teeth alone cannot produce the desired effect. These patients are almost all women and the vast majority are middle-aged spinsters often at the menopausal period; impatience or harshness will only antagonize them but with tact, kindness and genuine sympathy they can almost always be brought to see the matter in its true proportions, and thereafter are among the operator's most enthusiastic practice builders.

3. INEFFICIENCY
(a) Inability to Eat Anything
This complaint is mainly confined to patients who are wearing full upper and lower dentures for the first time, and are impatient at the time which must be spent in acquiring new habits of eating. Careful attention by the operator to the psychological approach to denture wearing, as described in Chapter III, will eliminate this complaint except in rare cases, and these must be persuaded to persevere, so that they will either learn anew how to eat, or will define some specific complaint which can then be remedied.
(b) Inability to Eat Meat
This is a complaint which may be made of new-dentures,

never old ones, though the wearer may have had previous full dentures for many years. It may be due to·

(i) *Flattening of the Cusps* of the posterior teeth by over-enthusiastic spot-grinding to correct an unbalanced denture.

(ii) *The Use of Cuspless Posterior Teeth.*

(iii) *Overclosure* with its decreased muscular efficiency.

(iv) *The Use of Acrylic Posterior Teeth* due to their resilience and softness.

(v) *Unbalanced Articulation* which will not allow the teeth on the balancing side to remain in contact during the lateral movements necessary to shear through food fibres.

(vi) *Cuspal Interference* preventing free lateral movements, under which heading is included, too great an overjet for the degree of overbite, or an incorrect incisive angle.

(vii) *Inexperience* on the part of a patient wearing his first full dentures, when none of the foregoing faults are present.

Treatment: Having discovered which of these faults is the cause of the complaint, the remedy is sufficiently obvious to require no further mention.

(c) Dentures Dislodged by Eating

This is applicable to either or both dentures and the common causes are:

(i) *Cuspal Interference,* which has already been discussed as has also

(ii) *Unbalanced Articulation.*

(iii) *Upper Teeth Outside the Ridge,* which may cause the denture to tilt down on the non-working side. This is particularly liable to happen if the upper ridge is narrow bucco-palatally, if the maxillary tuberosities are very small, if the buccal sulcus is very shallow, or in cases with mandibular protrusion.

Treatment: Re-make the dentures, if necessary, with a crossed occlusion.

(iv) *Insufficient Tongue Space* will often cause the lower denture to be moved about during the process of eating, though it may be stable under other conditions.

Treatment: Re-make, allowing more tongue space, using narrower posterior teeth if necessary.

(v) *Periphery Overextended.* – It is quite possible for a denture to be slightly overextended and yet to be stable during speech and swallowing. This is because movements during eating are more extensive than those employed when trimming the periphery. The commonest place for them to occur is in the region of the posterior lingual pouch. It is frequently difficult in these cases to locate the exact area of overextension, since the tissue contact with it is too intermittent to cause pain or hyperaemia. Intelligent observation by the patient of the exact movement which causes the instability will eventually enable the operator to locate the overextension.

Treatment:. Cut away the excess.

(vi) *Inexperience.* – The posterior natural teeth are often lost some time before the anterior ones, with the result that a habit is formed of eating on the anterior teeth. When full dentures are being worn for the first time, it is only natural that the wearer should try to continue his previous eating habits in these cases with bad results. Most experienced wearers of full dentures have such excellent, though unconscious, control of them that they can bite into an apple, or eat corn off the cob, with little difficulty, but this automatic skill can only be acquired with time and patience. Biting, which is the function of the anterior teeth, as opposed to chewing, which is the function of the posterior ones, is the last thing which the new denture wearer should attempt. When he has mastered this he has learnt denture control.

Treatment: Careful explanation to the patient, followed by perseverance on his part.

(vii) *Eating Causes Pain.* – This has already been described under the heading of pain to which reference should be made.

4. POOR RETENTION
(a) *When Opening the Mouth*

Patients more often complain that the lower denture lifts than that the upper one drops. If this lifting only occurs when the mouth is widely opened, as in yawning, it should be explained that this is normal. The following are the usual causes:

(i) *Overextension*

This has already been discussed under the heading of pain, the difference in these cases being that the overextension is so slight that the tissues do not make constant contact with it, and consequently soreness does not arise. The treatment is identical.

(ii) *Tight Lips*

These can be a most potent source of trouble when in conjunction with a flat, ridgeless lower. The inward pressure from these tight lips will seat the upper denture more firmly in position but will push the lower denture backwards and upwards.

Treatment: Re-make with the lower anterior teeth set more lingually, with a definite labial concavity on the denture, and with the maximum extension in the region of the retromolar pads. Alternatively gum-fit the lower anterior teeth.

(iii) *Tongue Cramped*

There are two causes for this complaint, one is that the lower posterior teeth are tilted lingually producing an undercut area into which the wide middle-third of the tongue will press, when movements of the tongue will lift the denture. The second cause is setting the lower posterior teeth too far lingually, possibly to avoid a crossed occlusion, so that any movement of the cramped tongue will cause a tilting of the lower denture.

Treatment: Re-make the dentures allowing more tongue space, if necessary by crossing the occlusion or by using teeth which are narrower buccolingually.

(iv) *Underextension*

This fault is by no means uncommon, and its effect on the retention of the denture is most marked. Maximum retention cannot be obtained without covering the greatest possible denture-bearing area. Some very careful operators produce this fault by placing excessive tension on the soft tissues during the peripheral moulding of the impression, through their desire to avoid overextension. Where this cause is suspected of being the fault, it can be checked by using tracing composition round the periphery, moulding it carefully and noting the result.

Treatment: Moulded tracing composition replaced by denture-base material.

(v) *Lack of Peripheral Seal*

Retention will have been poor when the dentures were first inserted, and the operator may have persuaded the patient to wear them for a few days in the hope that they would "bed-in".

Treatment: Tracing composition round the periphery, followed by a wash impression with zinc oxide paste, and re-lining.

(vi) *Lack of saliva* or a very thin watery saliva.

There is no specific treatment for this condition but perseverance will give a certain degree of muscular control. This cause only applies to the upper denture.

(b) When Coughing or Sneezing

Occasionally a new denture wearer will complain that his upper denture falls and his lower denture lifts, whenever he coughs or sneezes violently.

Treatment: It must be explained to the patient that when coughing or sneezing there is a moment when the pressure of air in the mouth is greater than atmospheric pressure, so that the peripheral seal of the upper denture is broken and it is able to fall: also there is unusual muscular movement which will cause the lower denture to lift. There is no way of preventing these movements of the dentures, but they are a very minor inconvenience.

5. INSTABILITY

This question has already been discussed in relation to its two main causes:

(a) *When Eating:*

Under the heading of inefficiency.

(b) *When Talking:*

In Chapter X on phonetics.

(c) *The Defensive Tongue:*

Some individuals have what may best be described as a defensive tongue. It is primarily concerned with preventing any foreign body other than food reaching the pharynx or remaining in the mouth. When dentures are fitted it subconsciously but positively ejects them and the patient finds it difficult or impossible to train a tongue of this type to control the dentures. Such a tongue is illustrated in fig. 280. Note how it is withdrawn into the mouth and is under the denture instead of on top of it.

Treatment: Persuasion to develop correct tongue habits. If this does not succeed, springs.

6. CLATTERING TEETH

The noise appears to be considerable to the patient and it is, in fact, frequently audible to his fellow diners. There are two main causes for this complaint of which the first mentioned is the most common.

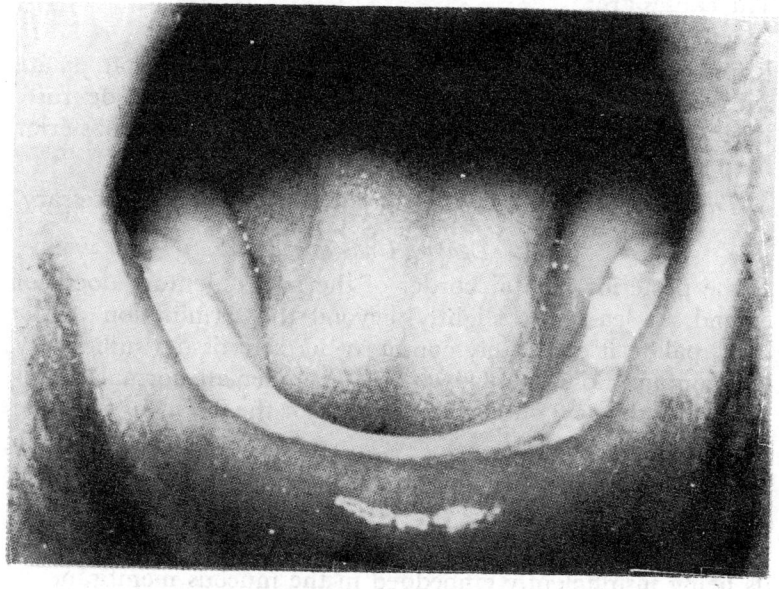

FIG. 280. – The defensive tongue

(a) Too Great a Vertical Height

This will cause the teeth to come into contact sooner than expected and therefore noisily.

Treatment: Reduce the height.

(b) Gross Cuspal Interference

Complaints from this cause are rarely met without the accompanying complaint of instability, but in either case it is easily distinguished from too great a vertical height.

Treatment: This is as already described under the heading of pain.

7. NAUSEA

Although this subject has been discussed from the point of view of impression taking, there are some essential differences when considering nausea in relation to wearing a full upper denture. The cause of the sickness is the same in both cases, light or intermittent contact on the soft palate or back of the tongue, and the patient's complaint is almost invariably 'that the upper denture goes too far back and makes me feel sick'. The causes are:

(a) Denture Slightly Overextended

Rare, but, if it does exist, the movements of the soft palate will cause it to make intermittent contact with the denture. Easily diagnosed by observing the relation of the posterior border to the vibrating line.

Treatment: Remove the excess and re-post-dam if necessary.

(b) Denture Underextended

If the posterior palatal border of the upper denture does not extend, at least very slightly, beyond the termination of the hard palate it can rarely compress the soft tissues sufficiently to maintain close contact with them under all normal conditions, and this will often cause nausea for the following reasons:

(i) *Intermittent Contact*

The denture moves owing to an inadequate air-seal.

(ii) *A Palpable Edge*

The edge is detected by the dorsum of the tongue, owing to its being insufficiently embedded in the mucous membrane.

Treatment: Extend the denture almost to the vibrating line and post-dam adequately.

(c) Thick Posterior Border

This is a very common cause of nausea resulting from the dorsum of the tongue being irritated by the thick edge. The palatal edge of the upper denture should be thin, and slightly embedded in the compressed mucous membrane, so that the tongue is unable to detect any definite junction of denture and mucosa.

Treatment: Thin down the posterior border of the denture.

8. DISCOMFORT

Patients sometimes complain that new dentures are not comfortable but can give no specific cause for complaint. These cases are difficult to diagnose since they are not accompanied by pain, and retention appears to be satisfactory, but as the patient has nearly always previously worn dentures a careful comparison of the new with the old will generally give a clue to the cause. The causes may be:

(a) Cramped Tongue Space

This is the most common reason for this complaint, the teeth on the new upper denture having been set-up on the centre of alveolar ridges which have absorbed considerably since the older denture was made. Since the absorption is greatest on the buccal aspect of the upper ridge, the teeth are now mounted nearer to the mid-line, so decreasing the tongue space.

(b) Altered Vertical Height

It is more probable that this is extremely slight and is an unintentional opening of 1 mm. or 2 mm., but it may be sufficient for a sensitive patient to notice a difference, particularly if the original dentures were made with a very small free-way space.

(c) Altered Occlusal Plane

Again, as in the case of an altered vertical height, the height of the occlusal plane is unlikely to have been changed by more than 1 mm. but even this slight alteration will require some adjustment of automatic muscular movement.

Treatment: Unless any of the above-mentioned factors are gross the patient should be encouraged to persevere for several weeks, by which time, in most cases, the discomfort will have disappeared; but if it has not, then nothing remains but to make new dentures, accurately copying the old ones.

9. ALTERED SPEECH

Reference should be made to the chapter on phonetics. When full dentures are first worn there is always some temporary alteration in speech owing to the thickness of the denture covering the palate, necessitating slightly altered positions of the tongue. Commonly this is only a temporary inconvenience, most rapidly overcome by reading aloud; when there is an altered position of the upper incisors, a change in their palatal shape, or any reduction of tongue space, adaptation may be very difficult even with perseverance.

Treatment: The dentures must be re-made paying particular attention to the principles laid down in Chapter X.

10. BITING THE CHEEK AND TONGUE

Cheek Biting

Two common causes for this condition exist:

(i) *Insufficient Overjet*

The normal occlusal relationship of the posterior teeth is with the buccal cusps of the upper teeth outside those of the lower teeth ; this arrangement normally prevents the cheeks getting caught between the teeth and bitten. If for any reason this arrangement has been altered, or if a patient has very lax cheeks, cheek biting may occur.

Treatment: Increase the buccal overjet and plump the denture; in some cases it may be necessary to remove the last molar teeth or grind the buccal surfaces of the lower posterior teeth so that the lingual cusps only will make contact with the upper teeth.

(ii) *Reduced Vertical Height*

If the vertical occlusal dimension is grossly reduced, the

resultant bunching of the cheeks allows of their being caught between the occlusal surfaces of the teeth as they occlude.

Treatment: Restore the vertical dimension or, if this is impossible, grind off the buccal cusps of the lower teeth.

Biting the Tongue

This is almost invariably due to a decrease in the tongue space occurring when fitting new dentures for patients already wearing dentures.

11. Food Under the Denture

This complaint is usually made by patients wearing dentures for the first time and who have not yet learnt how best to control the food. Undoubtedly a perfect peripheral seal will prevent the ingress of food beneath the denture but perfection is rarely attained and, owing to alveolar absorption, never maintained. Scraping a groove in the model, along and near the entire periphery of the denture, is sometimes carried out but this food-line, as it is termed, usually causes some inflammation and ulceration until it is finally established as a groove in the mucous membrane; it is rarely completely successful.

Treatment: This usually consists of covering the maximum possible area and obtaining an adequate peripheral seal; thereafter, only perseverance by the patient can bring about any improvement.

At the conclusion of this chapter it may be worth stressing that in the experience of the authors the six commonest causes of dentures failing are:

(1) Incorrect antero-posterior relationship of the mandible to the maxilla.
(2) Uneven and locked occlusion – this is always present unless a careful check record has been carried out.
(3) Open vertical dimension – not necessarily gross but sufficient to deprive the patient of a freeway space.
(4) A cramped tongue.
(5) Poor retention – due to incorrect outline – usually underextension of the periphery.
(6) Failure to copy existing dentures when making new ones for an experienced denture wearer.

Chapter XV

RE-LINING, RESILIENT LININGS, AIDS TO RETENTION AND REPAIRS

The term re-lining is used to denote the production of a new fitting surface in an existing denture.

REASONS FOR RE-LINING

Owing to the fact that alveolar absorption is a continuous process, though varying in degree, the comfort, efficiency, stability, retention and appearance of dentures are all liable to become impaired with the passage of time. Thus the reasons for re-lining a denture are:

1. *To Improve Retention and Stability*

Loss of fit will make the maintenance of peripheral seal impossible and will greatly impair the retentive effects of adhesion and cohesion. It may also permit a rocking or tilting of the denture during function and, in extreme cases in the lower, a lateral movement.

2. *To Improve the Appearance*

One effect of alveolar absorption in the mandible is that the lower denture sinks below the original occlusal plane, and thus the patient has to close beyond the original vertical dimension in order to occlude the teeth. This over-closure is frequently noticed by the patient as a protrusion of the mandible and an undue approximation of the nose and chin, giving an appearance of age. Absorption of the upper alveolar ridge will not have so marked an effect on the vertical dimension because the hard palate does not materially alter. The original vertical dimension can often be restored by re-lining the lower denture alone.

3. *To Restore the Vertical Dimension*

If the vertical dimension to which a denture was made is reduced, masticatory efficiency is impaired, but the previous efficiency can usually be restored by re-lining.

4. *To Restore the Evenness of Occlusal Pressure*

With any alteration in the fit of the dentures there will be some alteration of the pressure transmitted to the tissues when the teeth are brought into occlusion. This can be corrected, if of small degree, by careful grinding of the teeth, but if the balance is grossly disturbed re-lining the dentures is the simplest means of restoring the original conditions.

5. *To Alleviate Pain*

If a denture has been worn with comfort and then becomes painful, it is usually due to the fact that the supporting tissues have altered allowing the dentures to tilt. rock or move, and thus transmit undue pressure to one area. Re-lining will alleviate pain arising from this cause.

IMPRESSION MATERIALS FOR RE-LINING

Those in general use for the purposes of re-lining are:

(1) Zinc oxide-eugenol paste.

(2) Composition or black gutta percha.

(3) Plaster of Paris containing starch.

(4) Cold cure acrylic.

Ordinary plaster of Paris or sodium alginate may be used as re-lining impression materials, but they have the disadvantage of breaking and flaking away from the fitting surface of the denture as it is being removed from the mouth.

TECHNIQUE OF RE-LINING

The periphery of the existing denture should be carefully examined for its relationship to the functional position of the sulci. If the denture border was positioned accurately when the denture was originally constructed, it will probably now appear slightly overextended, due to alveolar absorption. This excess denture flange must be trimmed away until the periphery is a fraction short of the functional level of the sulci.

In addition, flanges which fit into undercut areas must be relieved so that the impression, within the denture, can be readily removed from the plaster cast, without fear of fracturing the ridge. A further point to consider is whether or not any substantial increase of the vertical dimension is desired, as this influences the quantity of material used for the impression, and the manner in which the latter is obtained.

When improved retention is the only consideration, a very thin layer of zinc oxide-eugenol paste is spread evenly over the entire fitting surface of the denture, which is then seated in position in the mouth and the teeth brought together in centric occlusion; a slight pressure is maintained until the material hardens. About 30 seconds after the insertion of the impression, the periphery is trimmed by suitable lip and cheek movements to record their functional positions. Lingual excess should be trimmed by the usual tongue movements, before the teeth are brought into occlusion.

In cases where the vertical dimension has to be re-established in addition to the fit, the layer of impression material used must be of greater thickness, and since zinc oxide-eugenol paste flows somewhat readily it will be found unsuitable (as the sole impression material) for use in cases which require a restoration of 3 to 4 mm. In such cases the lower denture should first be lined with composition and an impression taken with the teeth in occlusion. The thickness of composition used should be such that it almost restores the desired vertical dimension. The composition is then chilled, dried, and the final impression to the correct height taken with a film of zinc oxide paste.

If the vertical dimension is being increased beyond 3 to 4 mm., and both dentures are being re-lined, the question arises which denture should accommodate the greater part of this opening. The lower ridge, in the majority of cases, will have absorbed more than the upper, and the hard palate not at all. As a general guide, the incisal level of the upper anterior teeth should be studied in relation to the lip line, and the upper impression should be taken first, with sufficient thickness of material to bring the upper incisors into the desired position.

Although there is no apparent absorption of the hard palate, it will frequently be found that incisors, which originally showed to the extent of 1 to 2 mm. below the lip, have completely disappeared when the lip is at rest. This effect is caused by:

(1) Upper alveolar absorption allowing the denture to tilt and rise anteriorly.

(2) Some loss of muscular tone of the upper lip which thus tends to droop slightly lower than previously,

The operation is completed by lining the lower denture with impression material of sufficient thickness to complete the increase in vertical dimension.

Alternatively the complete impression may be carried out with composition alone. Whenever composition is being used, it is an advantage to grind away about 2 mm. from the fitting surface of the lower denture, except in cases of flat lower ridges, in order to allow for a greater thickness of material. It will be found that if there is only a wafer of composition it is very difficult to keep it in a soft, workable condition when inserting it into the mouth as it cools too rapidly; the greater thickness overcomes this difficulty,

Black gutta percha, unlike composition, possesses the ability to flow for a long time after it has been softened, and can therefore produce a thin accurate reline.

A strip is cut from the sheet of gutta percha, placed in boiling water for a few minutes, dried and laid on the dry fitting surface of the denture and then inserted in the mouth. As the patient occludes, the gutta percha flows until the denture is fully and accurately seated. Peripheral movements are also accurately reproduced by gutta percha and the patient may even wear it for some days to allow complete functional adaptation before the gutta percha is replaced with acrylic.

Should the upper denture need a thick layer of impression material to adjust the occlusal plane in relation to the lip line, or to eliminate excessive rock across the torus, the seating of the denture can be more accurately effected if some impression of the anterior and posterior ridges are obtained first in composition or softened wax. The stops so formed will

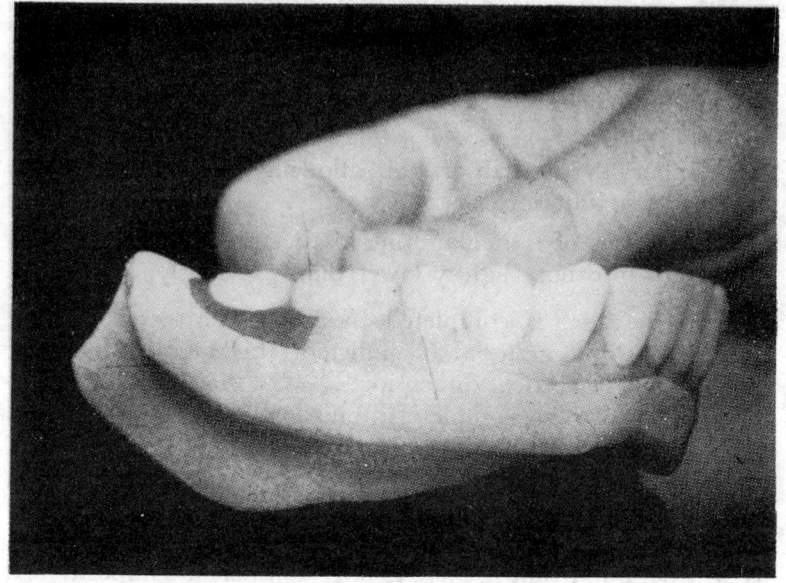

FIG. 281. – Soft lining. Note thickness of lining. Thin linings
are useless to relieve pressure pain.

prevent loss of vertical height when the teeth are brought into
centric occlusion during the zinc oxide-eugenol impression
stage.

Improved retention and stability are obtained, when re-
lining a denture, if the periphery is carefully adapted to the
functional level of the sulci with tracing compound. The areas
of soft tissue, including the retromolar pads, which have been
selected for post-damming, should be adequately compressed
with the same material.

Cold cure acrylic resin has been suggested as a material
for re-lining dentures since it avoids any laboratory technique
and the inconvenience caused to the patient by being temporarily deprived of his dentures. The procedure involves lining
the dried denture with a thin layer of this acrylic dough and
placing it in position in the mouth, the mucous membrane
having previously been smeared with vaseline. The dough is
allowed to polymerize in the mouth for a period of four

minutes, but no longer. The denture is then removed and polymerization completed in a warm water bath of approximately 40° C., the time required being about ten minutes. The denture borders must be trimmed and polished.

A serious disadvantage to the use of this material is the fact that acrylic dough often causes considerable and painful irritation of the mucous membrane.

RESILIENT LININGS (*see* fig. 281)

When other causes have been eliminated and pain under the lower denture is considered to be due to the type of ridge formation and the susceptibility of the mucosa to bruising, which cannot withstand the transmitted pressure of mastication, some relief of the symptoms may be obtained by re-lining the denture with a resilient material. The clinical procedure calls for a thin zinc oxide-eugenol paste wash in the existing denture; the remainder of the technique being carried out in the laboratory. This may involve reconstructing the denture in vulcanite incorporating velum rubber as a lining. Alternatively, sufficient material may be removed from the fitting surface of the denture, to allow for a thickness of 2 to 3 mm. of gutta-percha to be substituted and impressed on the ridge under occlusal stress; subsequently the periphery is moulded to the functional position of the sulci. This lining is of a temporary nature as it has to be replaced about every six months owing to its distortion in use. This technique is used only in cases where all other methods have failed.

Polyvinyl chloride is a soft plastic which has been used as a resilient lining but which has been found to be unsatisfactory as the plasticizer leaches out and the material then becomes hard.

At the present time a large number of proprietary resilient linings are available, many of them based on the synthetic rubbers. Some of these materials are very satisfactory and produce a comfortable denture. The life of the most resilient linings is limited to a year or two at the most and then they require renewal, but if the patient is comfortable then frequent renewal is well worth while.

If the resilient lining is thick and is attached to an acrylic denture, the latter will soon fracture as a result of flexion unless a thick cast metal strengthener is incorporated on the lingual side of the denture.

In the laboratory the re-lining of a denture may be carried out by merely replacing the impression material with the denture base material, after suitable means of retention have been prepared for it. Alternatively part, or the whole, of the denture base may be replaced, using the existing teeth, or new teeth.

The use of such confusing terms as re-base, re-model and re-make have been avoided as they are merely variations of re-lining methods. Techniques in which trays are used for impression taking, followed by the usual stages of denture construction, except that the teeth of existing dentures are removed and used again, are virtually new dentures and should be considered in that category. The terms re-base and re-make are apt to confuse the layman and to suggest the idea of something inferior.

REPAIRS

Unfortunately there is a tendency to regard denture repairs as a constant evil, without any necessity to find out the cause of the breakage, with the result that many dentures are mended only to break again shortly afterwards, when they should be either re-lined or new dentures constructed. It cannot be too strongly emphasized that no denture which breaks in the mouth should be repaired without the cause of the breakage being ascertained.

Before considering the principal causes of breakage it should be pointed out that quite a number of dentures which are brought by patients as having cracked in the mouth, have in fact been dropped. The crack which was started by the accident has passed unobserved, and the stresses of mastication have completed the fracture. These cases are often impossible to diagnose as patients will rarely, either through forgetfulness or untruthfulness, admit that they have ever dropped the denture.

Fractured dentures, whenever possible, should be united with sticky wax and strengthened with wire, and tried in the mouth for perfection of fit before being repaired. Where the fit is found to be deficient it will be necessary to re-line the denture after it has been repaired, or otherwise a further fracture will occur in a very short time.

Warpage resulting from one repair frequently causes a second fracture. Dentures made of methyl methacrylate will warp to a certain extent each time they are re-cured and very rarely is the fit of an acrylic denture satisfactory if it has been repaired more than twice, the resultant bad fit being a common cause of further breakage.

Breakage of a denture in the mouth almost invariably starts with a small crack, spreading across the denture rather as though it were being torn instead of broken. Often the first thing to be noticed by the patient is the sensation of the feel of a hair on the denture – a hair which cannot be moved – and a very close inspection is often required to see the small crack at this stage.

Breakages are of two main kinds:

(1) Fracture of the denture base.

(2) Fracture of a tooth or teeth on the denture.

FRACTURE OF THE DENTURE BASE
1. *Poor Fit*

Causes.

This is a very wide term and can more readily be described under separate headings:

(*a*) *Alveolar Absorption*

This will be found to be the cause of breakage in dentures which have been worn for some considerable time, or which were made shortly after the extraction of the teeth. The alveolar absorption will cause the denture to be unevenly supported and is a common cause of fracture.

(*b*) *Warpage*

Warpage, as a cause of fracture, is almost entirely confined to the acrylic resins and is also a very common cause of further fractures of a denture which has already been repaired. Vulcanite may also warp if incorrectly treated – for example, cooled too rapidly on removal from the vulcanizer or revulcanized many times. Metal dentures also are capable of distortion with faulty handling either in soldering, heat treating, or welding.

(c) *Inadequate Relief*

Unless a self-relieving impression technique has been employed, such as a compression impression, or adequate ampirical relief has been provided, in mouths exhibiting gross veriations in the thickness of the mucous membrane, the denture will flex over the hard areas of the palate and fracture

(d) *Excessive Relief*

This will sometimes account for a broken denture by reducing in the mid-line of the palate the thickness of the base beyond the limit of safety, and should have been prevented by adding to the polished surface an amount equal to that removed from the fitting surface.

(e) *Inaccurate Impression*

If the impression on which the denture was constructed was not accurate, considerable stresses will be induced in the denture base during mastication owing to the unevenness of its support, and eventually the base will give way. The length of time before this happens depends on the stresses induced and also on the physical properties and thickness of the material used. The following list of materials most commonly used for denture bases is given in the order of their susceptibility to breakage from fatigue:

(i) Methyl methacrylate.

(ii) Vulcanite.

(iii) Cast gold alloys.

(iv) Wrought gold alloys.

(v) Stainless steel and cobalt chrome.

2. *Upper Teeth Set Outside the Ridge*

When the upper teeth are set outside the ridge the force of mastication is applied outside the axis of the ridge, the ridge itself becoming a fulcrum point, causing a large component force to be transmitted to the mid-line of the denture. This will frequently result in a mid-line fracture (*see* fig. 282).

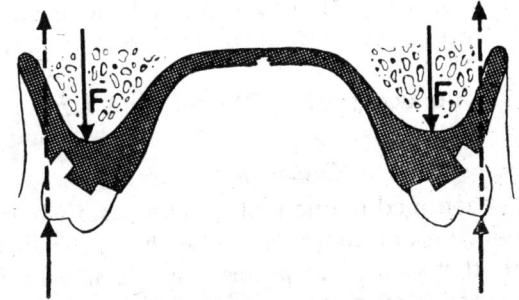

FIG. 282. – Illustrating a common cause of a mid-line fracture. The long partially broken arrows represent the forces of mastication applied outside the ridge, which is itself acting as a fulcrum, F.

In cases of continued fracture the only satisfactory treatment is to provide a chrome cobalt palate which is carried right up the palatal surfaces of the anterior teeth (*see* fig. 283). This prevents the initial fracture which invariably occurs between

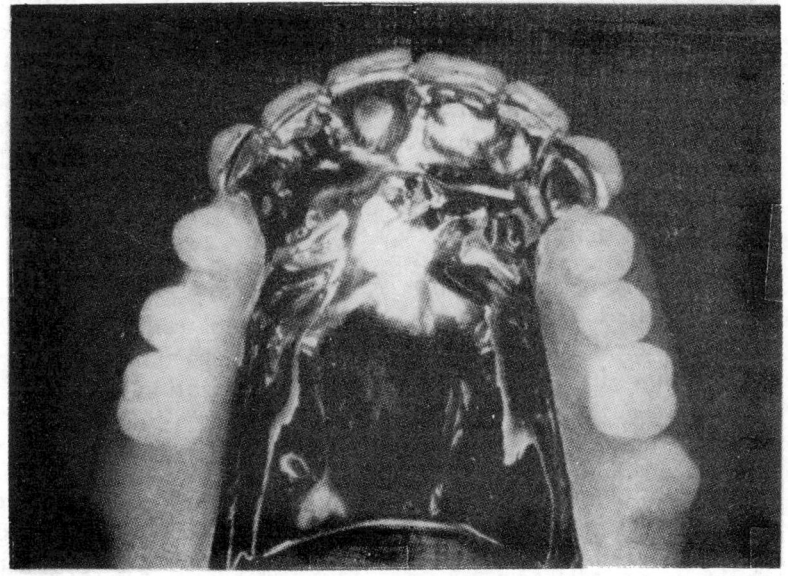

FIG. 283. – A chrome cobalt palate carried up the palatal aspects of the anterior teeth.

the upper incisor teeth. If a conventional metal palate is used the acrylic uniting the front teeth to it still cracks.

BREAKAGE OF A TOOTH OR TEETH

Causes

1. *Cuspal Interference*

Where this is confined to one tooth, or in cases where the pressure is heavier on one tooth than elsewhere, it will frequently cause the tooth to split. An anterior tooth may be broken off if there is excessive overbite with insufficient overjet.

2. *Faulty Tooth*

This is almost entirely confined to anterior porcelain pin teeth and is very rare when one considers the number of these teeth in use. An undetected flaw in the porcelain usually results in the tooth breaking across the line of the pins.

3. *Deterioration of Retention*

A common accident is for a porcelain pin tooth to be bitten off unbroken and this is really a case of faulty retention. This poor retention is brought about by the denture base covering the pins being worn away until the pin is exposed. The gold covering on the pins is extremely thin and it is soon worn away leaving the base-metal core exposed and this, in time, corrodes and the tooth breaks off. This corrosion of a base-metal pin is considerably accelerated by the use of sodium hypochlorite for cleaning the denture.

4. *Contraction of Acrylic Resin*

This may be a cause of fracture in porcelain teeth set in an acrylic base. It is due to the large and uneven contraction of the acrylic resin which occurs during polymerization, inducing excessive stresses in the porcelain teeth, although it is doubtful whether these stresses will cause a fracture to occur unless a flaw was originally present in the tooth.

5. *Excessive Grinding of a Tooth*

Excessive grinding of either the occlusal or ridge surface of a porcelain posterior tooth to facilitate setting up will frequently so weaken it as to cause its fracture in use.

Aids to Retention

There are certain devices which aid in holding full dentures in place but their permanent use should only be employed as a last resort.

The following list does not include every device which has been tried or suggested, but it includes those in everyday use.

1. *Springs*

These are made of coiled stainless steel or gold-plated base metal and have their ends attached to swivels in the premolar areas on both sides of the upper and lower dentures. The dentures are thus permanently attached to each other and are held in occlusion for insertion into the mouth: as soon as they are released the dentures are forced apart by the action of the springs and held in place (*see* fig. 284).

Recently nylon springs of continental origin have become available (*see* fig. 285). These have the advantage of being thin and not collecting food. Their life is limited to about six months,

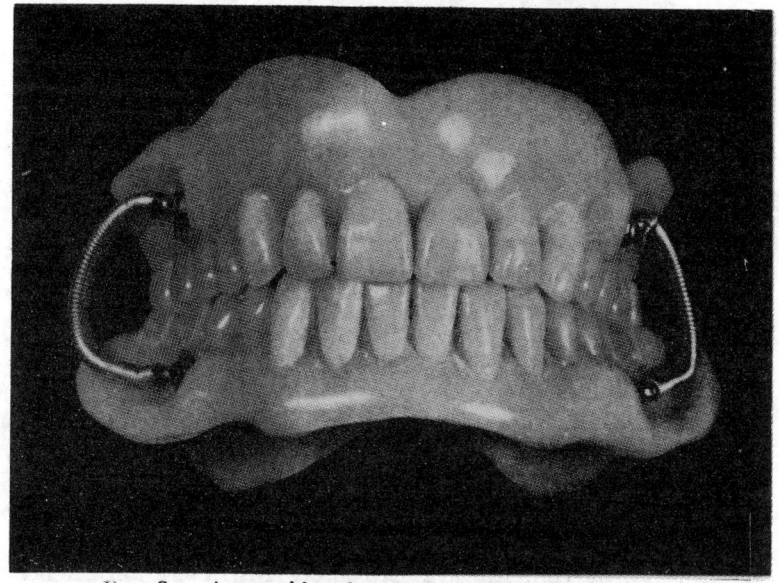

Fig. 284. – A case with springs fitted – springs protruding too far buccally on left side. Right side correct.

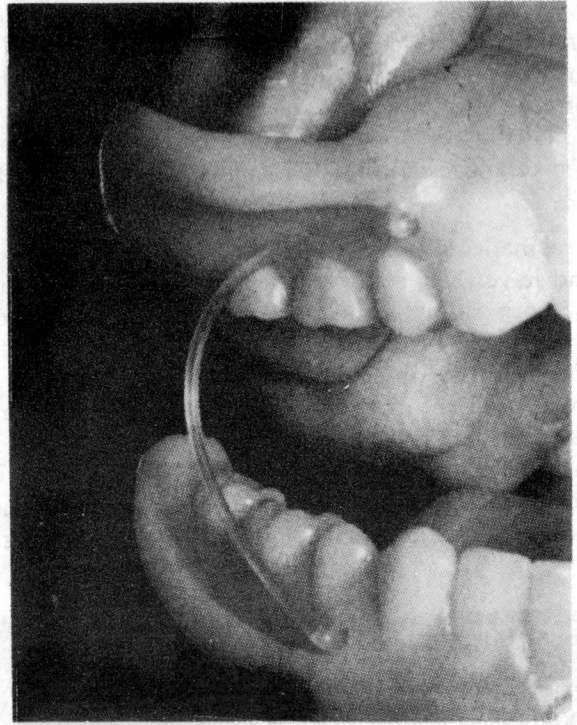

FIG. 285. – Nylon Spring.

and the method of their attachment to the denture, which is a nylon ball and socket joint, is not very efficient. If this were improved they would be very satisfactory.

Disadvantages

(*a*) The constant pressure may cause excessive alveolar absorption.

(*b*) In some cases the mucous membrane will not tolerate the constant pressure.

(*c*) The inner surfaces of the cheeks frequently become sore from frictional contact with the springs.

(*d*) Lateral movements are extremely restricted and hence the efficiency of the dentures is impaired.

(*e*) They are unhygienic. When in the mouth, the coils of the springs are separated enough to allow small particles of food to pass between them into the hollow centre: Out of the mouth the coils are in close contact and so are very difficult to clean.

2. *Gum Tragacanth*

This is used in powder form and is sprinkled on the moist, fitting surface of the denture which will then usually stick in place for several hours. Gradually the sticky jelly is pressed from under the denture or washed away by the saliva and for this latter reason is rarely of any use for holding lower dentures. Even with prolonged use it does not appear to affect the mucous membrane.

Uses

(*a*) To hold the upper record block in position when securing intra-oral records.

(*b*) To prolong the usefulness, for a short time, of an immediate upper denture which is becoming loose through alveolar absorption.

(*c*) To enable a patient to wear an old, ill-fitting upper denture whilst a denture in normal use is being repaired.

(*d*) Sometimes used, unnecessarily, by public speakers, such as actors or clergymen, to give them mental comfort from the assurance that the upper denture will not move whilst they are addressing their audiences.

Disadvantages

(*a*) It has an unpleasant feel as soon as it is pressed out from beneath the denture.

(*b*) It is only a temporary expedient and the less accurate the fit of the denture the more rapidly is the gum washed away.

(*c*) It is of little use for retaining lower dentures.

(*d*) Its constant use is said to cause constipation.

3. *Suction Chambers*

These often resemble relief areas in shape but differ from them in having a clearly defined outline instead of merging into the surrounding surface (*see* fig. 286). When the denture is inserted the patient creates a partial vacuum in this chamber by sucking

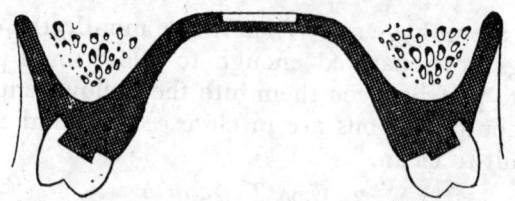

FIG. 286. – Cross section of an upper denture with a suction
chamber. Note the square edges in contact with the palate.

and swallowing and this small area of reduced pressure helps
to keep the denture in place. The mucous membrane in this
area of reduced pressure will proliferate, and in time will fill
the whole suction chamber, thus limiting the usefulness of this
device and at the same time limiting the amount of damage
(hyperplasia) which it can cause.

Uses

(*a*) To prolong the usefulness of immediate dentures.
(*b*) To assist in the retention of the dentures in difficult cases
whilst the patient is acquiring muscular control.
(*c*) Deliberately to raise a stud of hypertrophied tissue in the
palate to assist in lateral stability in cases with a very flat
palate and very small sulci.

Disadvantages

They only function for a few months before they are filled
with proliferated tissue.

4. *Rubber Suction Discs*

Although these are still used they are only included in this
list in order to condemn them. They consist of a rubber disc
which is buttoned on to a stud sunk into the fitting surface of
a denture. The partial vacuum created within the perimeter
of this disc holds the upper denture suspended from the hard
palate. They cause a constant irritation and no operator who
has had the misfortune to see a case of epithelioma resulting
from the use of one of these discs would dare to use one (*see*
fig. 287).

Disadvantages

(*a*) Due to the swelling and spreading of the rubber disc they

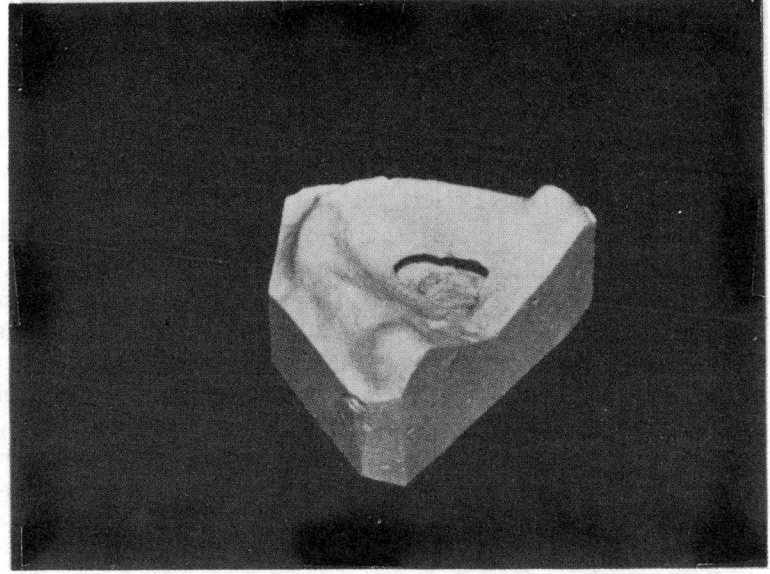

FIG. 267. – Perforation of the palate resulting from an epithelioma caused by the prolonged use of a suction disc.

are not self-limiting in action as is the case with a suction chamber. Cases have been reported where the constant irritation has caused, not only a perforation of the hard palate, but in some cases a malignant tumour (epithelioma).

(*b*) They are unhygienic. The soft rubber disc is porous and it soon perishes, swells and becomes very foul.

5. *Magnets*

From time to time the use of small steel magnets embedded beneath the molar and premolar teeth and arranged with similar poles opposite each other, has been advocated. In theory the repulsion effect will keep both dentures in place but in practice it will be found that owing to magnetic force being inversely proportional to the square of the distance and also the small size of the magnets which it is possible to fit, that the repulsive effect is undetectable when the dentures are separated by more than one or two millimetres.

CHAPTER XVI

OUTLINE OF TECHNIQUES SUITABLE FOR OVER-COMING DIFFICULTIES ENCOUNTERED IN FULL DENTURE PROSTHESIS

From the facts obtained during the mouth examination and case history recording, the prosthetist should be in a position to anticipate difficulties, and, by selecting suitable materials and operative techniques, be able to overcome them. A list follows of conditions which may cause varying degrees of difficulty, with suggested methods for obtaining a satisfactory result. The points are discussed elsewhere in the book but are presented here in tabulated form for the reader's convenience.

The causes of the difficulties are:

1. V-SHAPED PALATE

Reason for the Difficulty. – Retention by adhesion is diminished because the palate, having sloping sides, offers only a small area which is horizontal to a vertical displacing force. Also, plastic denture bases tend to warp during curing, and the imperfect fit at the sharp angle of the palate further reduces the forces of adhesion and cohesion.

Treatment. – An impression technique involving careful peripheral trimming, and which includes compression of the soft tissues of the denture-bearing surface. A cast metal palate produces a more accurate fit.

Prognosis. – Satisfactory results will depend on the excellence of the peripheral seal obtained in the impression technique, because the main retentive factor in these cases is atmospheric pressure.

2. FLAT PALATE WITH SHALLOW RIDGES

Reason for the Difficulty. – The denture may easily be displaced during mastication through lack of ridge support; the shallow sulci adversely influence peripheral seal.

Treatment. – An impression technique incorporating careful peripheral adaptation. An anatomical bite registration and set up, or the use of cuspless teeth, to reduce the lateral drag from cuspal interference.

Prognosis. – Very good results are obtained provided the periphery is adequately sealed and is free from interference by the adjacent musculature. The flat palate allows excellent retention by adhesion, and an anatomical articulation prevents displacement by cuspal interference.

3. Undercut Ridges

Reason for the Difficulty. – Retention will be reduced as the denture will have to be trimmed, during fitting, in order that it may pass over the bulbous areas of the ridge, thus causing loss of peripheral seal.

Treatment. – (*a*) An alveolectomy to reduce the undercut; or (*b*) Careful blocking out of the undercut areas on the model. This eliminates the possibility of over trimming which might occur when the denture is being fitted. A hydrocolloid impression may be necessary to avoid the discomfort caused by, and the fracture of, a plaster impression.

Prognosis. – The most satisfactory result is obtained when alveolectomy is carried out, as the operator is then able to construct a denture having the maximum peripheral seal. When a denture is trimmed, or the undercuts blocked out on the model, some reduction in peripheral seal is inevitable.

4. Knife-like Lower Ridge

Reason for the Difficulty. – The patient with a ridge of this type frequently complains of pain during mastication as the pressure exerted on the mandible via the denture compresses the soft tissue between the fitting surface and the knife-like process forming the crest of the alveolar ridge.

Treatment. – (*a*) Alveolectomy to reduce the sharp process; or (*b*) A relief for the knife-like ridge area formed by swaging No. 4 gauge tin foil on to that area on the model; or (*c*) Construct a denture having a resilient lining; or (*d*) An implant.

Reducing the vertical dimension in such cases may be advantageous as this reduces the force applied during mastication.

Prognosis. – Usually the most satisfactory results are obtained after an alveolectomy since this removes the cause. However, when surgical treatment is contra-indicated some reduction in the pain and discomfort experienced by the patient may be obtained by relieving the ridge area, thereby placing the greater proportion of the occlusal stress on the lateral borders of the ridge; but this, occasionally, can be as painful as the previous condition. A denture constructed with a resilient lining, forming a cushion, usually reduces the symptoms, but the lining has to be replaced periodically as it hardens, and, also it tends to become foul because of its absorbent nature.

5. Flat Lower Ridge

Reasons for the Difficulty. – The shape of the ridge provides no resistance to lateral movements of the denture; also, interference from adjacent musculature is pronounced.

Treatment. – (*a*) A peripherally adapted impression having adequate extension on to the retromolar pads, and the teeth set up to produce balanced articulation. If a plane-line articulator is used cuspless or shallow cusped teeth should be selected for the set-up; (*b*) Dentures fitted with springs; (*c*) An implant.

Prognosis. – A satisfactory result can be obtained if the maximum denture-bearing surface is used provided it is free from muscle interference. The balanced articulation ensures the minimum displacement during masticatory function, as cusp-locking, with resulting drag, is eliminated. Springs produce a very satisfactory result in those patients who will persevere and learn to use this type of prosthesis.

6. Lower Ridge Considerably Higher in the Incisor Region than Elsewhere

Reasons for the Difficulty. – Anterior teeth of normal length would in this case present a large surface area for the lip to press against.

Treatment. – (*a*) Short incisor teeth to reduce the area which the lip can press against; (*b*) Alveolectomy.

Prognosis. – A more stable denture is obtained if the anterior teeth are short as lip pressure is limited to a smaller area and the denture is not so readily displaced backwards. The appearance is not unduly spoilt as it is seldom that the lower teeth are exposed to any great extent in normal function. Alveolectomy may permit normal-sized teeth to be used anteriorly but it may result in a loss of very necessary ridge support.

7. LARGE TORUS PALATINUS

Reasons for the Difficulty. – The denture may rock across the mid-line and eventually fracture; retention may be reduced, as an under-relieved torus prevents the denture bedding into the soft tissue.

Treatment. – (*a*) A compression impression technique; or (*b*) Adequate relief of the denture in the area of the torus. A metal palate will withstand strain from fatigue better than a plastic denture base.

Prognosis. – Both (*a*) and (*b*) produce dentures which do not exhibit any rock across the mid-line, and if a metal palate is incorporated in the denture it will withstand any slight rock that occurs, due to later alveolar absorption, far better than a plastic base.

8. LARGE TUBEROSITIES

Reason for the Difficulty. – Fitting the finished denture requires considerable trimming with loss of peripheral seal.

Treatment. – (*a*) Surgical removal of part of the tuberosity; or (*b*) Undercut area blocked out on the model; or (*c*) Denture flange carried only slightly into the undercut area.

Prognosis. – The most satisfactory denture is produced if the undercut is eliminated by surgical means as the operator can then achieve the maximum peripheral seal. If the undercut is only blocked out a space will exist, allowing the ingress of air and food between the denture and the tissue in that area, which will have an adverse effect on retention. If the flange is carried only slightly into the undercut area intimate contact between the denture and tissue is maintained but since the flange does not extend into the full depth of the sulcus the peripheral seal is reduced.

9. SHALLOW SULCI

Reason for the Difficulty. – The denture tends to tilt and move readily due to lack of ridge support and peripheral seal is thus easily broken.

Treatment. – A peripherally trimmed impression technique and the teeth set up to give balanced articulation.

Prognosis. – Improved retention and stability due to well-developed peripheral seal and freedom from cuspal interference.

10. ABNORMAL FRAENA

Reason for the Difficulty. – The denture is more easily displaced when fraena are attached near to the crest of the ridge.

Treatment. – Division of the fraena surgically before, or at, the time of insertion of the denture.

Prognosis. – Increase in denture stability during function and increased peripheral seal.

11. VARIATION IN TISSUE COMPRESSIBILITY FROM AREA TO AREA

Reason for the Difficulty. – (a) The air seal is broken due to the denture moving during mastication; (b) The denture may fracture because the occlusal pressure transmitted, through the tissue to the supporting bone, is uneven.

Treatment. – Compression impression technique and balanced articulation when setting up the teeth.

Prognosis. – Equalization of the pressure exerted on the bony support reduces denture fatigue and therefore the tendency to fracture. A balanced articulation reduces denture movement during mastication and thereby assists in maintaining the peripheral seal.

12. FLABBY RIDGE

Reason for the Difficulty. – Flabby tissue compressed during mastication causes the denture to be tilted and the seal thus broken.

Treatment. – (*a*) Compression impression technique when flabbiness is not excessive, otherwise a plaster of Paris impression; or (*b*) Partial excision of fibrous tissue; and (*c*) Balanced articulation.

Prognosis. – The maximum seal obtained in a carefully adapted compression impression technique increases retention and together with the incorporation of balanced articulation produces dentures which exhibit the minimum displacement during mastication. Where excessively flabby tissue is encountered it is advisable to avoid compression impressions and rely on balanced articulation to minimize the tilting effect caused by the flabbiness. If surgical removal of part of the tissue is contemplated moderation in the amount removed should be exercised otherwise complete loss of the ridge may present even greater difficulties than the previous flabbiness.

13. TIGHT LOWER LIP

Reason for the Difficulty. – Instability of the lower denture due to the backward displacement caused by lip pressure, and vertical lift occurring in the premolar and canine region from the pressure of the modioli.

Treatment. – (*a*) Keep the occlusal plane low thus reducing the contact area with the lip; (*b*) Adequate extension on to the retromolar pads to counteract the lip pressure; (*c*) Keep the denture narrow across the premolar area; (*d*) Upper canines and premolars should be prominent to resist the modioli pressure on the lower denture.

Prognosis. – The combination of as many of the above points as possible will considerably aid lower denture stability and should enable the patient to use the prosthesis satisfactorily.

14. LARGE TONGUE

Reason for the Difficulty. – If the tongue is cramped, or the teeth set up so that they overhang it, the denture will be moved during function.

Treatment. – (*a*) Keep the occlusal plane low; (*b*) Provide the maximum intermolar distance by using narrow teeth or grinding away the lingual cusps; (*c*) Anterior teeth should be set up slightly forward of the ridge; (d) Peripherally trimmed impression technique.

Prognosis. – A satisfactory denture can only be produced provided the tongue can move freely and be brought to rest easily on the occlusal surface of the lower teeth.

15. ABNORMAL JAW RELATIONSHIPS

(a) *Close Bite*

Reason for the Difficulty. – Lack of interalveolar space.

Treatment. – Acrylic posterior teeth.

Prognosis. – A satisfactory denture is obtained as the probable fracture of ground porcelain posterior teeth is avoided.

(b) *Superior Protrusion*

Reason for the Difficulty. – Narrow and retrusive lower arch in relationship to a normal-size upper arch.

Treatment. – (a) Maintain the natural overjet which will be large; (b) Peripherally adapted impression technique.

Prognosis. – Little difficulty is encountered if nature's arrangement is followed but trouble should be anticipated if extensive aesthetic corrections are contemplated.

(c) *Inferior Protrusion*

Reason for the Difficulty. – Large and wide lower arch in comparison to the upper arch, leading to an unstable upper denture.

Treatment. – (a) Peripherally adapted impression technique; (b) Metal palate; (c) Balanced occlusion; (d) Posterior cross bite; (e) Anterior edge-to-edge bite.

Prognosis. – A metal palate incorporated in a denture having the maximum peripheral seal enables the technician to set the upper posterior teeth outside the ridge, and the balanced articulation ensures that the denture remains stable during mastication, thus producing the most satisfactory result. Excessive difference in the size and protrusive relationship of the lower jaw to the upper usually necessitate a posterior crossed occlusion and an anterior edge-to-edge occlusion, or the upper anteriors set distal to the lower anteriors. This involves some loss of stability as it is impossible to maintain balanced articulation.

16. LENGTH OF TIME THE PATIENT HAS BEEN EDENTULOUS

Reason for the Difficulty. – Individuals without teeth, or having anterior teeth only for many months, develop a habit of protrusive chewing which causes difficulty when recording the position of occlusion.

Treatment. – Patience, tolerance and perseverance, and the use of the aids given in Chapter VI. In the most difficult cases a Gothic arch tracing may obtain the desired result.

Prognosis. – The Gothic arch tracing, provided it is carried out on stable bases, is probably the most certain method of obtaining the true position of centric occlusion.

17. RETCHING AND NAUSEA

Reason for the Difficulty. – Apprehension and sensitivity.

Treatment. – (*a*) Zinc-oxide-eugenol paste impression in a base-plate tray; (*b*) 1 : 80 phenol mouthwash. (*c*) A Benzocaine tablet to suck; (*d*) A thin acrylic base-plate worn by the patient until tolerance is gained.

Prognosis. – It is seldom that impressions cannot be obtained provided that the minimum bulk of impression tray and material is used. However, when this does not succeed a phenol mouthwash or a Benzocaine tablet to suck prior to the taking of the impression may assist in mild cases of nausea and retching. Severer cases require that an acrylic base-plate be constructed and worn by the patient until sufficient tolerance has been gained, when the impression taking should proceed without difficulty.

18. RETCHING AND NAUSEA IN DENTURE WEARERS

Reason for the Difficulty. – (*a*) A thick back-edge to the palate of the upper denture; (*b*) Insufficient post-dam seal, often placed in the wrong position.

Treatment. – (*a*) Thin down the back-edge; (*b*) Re-post-dam on the soft compressible tissue of the soft palate anterior to the vibrating line. Trace, and readapt, the periphery of the denture and re-line for better retention.

Prognosis. – The distressing symptoms can usually be relieved by correctly placing, and keeping suitably thin, the posterior border of the upper denture.

19. PROMINENT PREMAXILLA

Reason for the Difficulty. – Causes excessive prominence of the upper lip when a denture possessing a labial flange is fitted.

Treatment. – (*a*) Set the anterior teeth to the gum without a labial flange; (*b*) Severe cases require alveolectomy.

Prognosis. – Gum-fitted anterior teeth lead to some loss of retention varying in degree according to the support given by the posterior ridges and other factors of retention. Alveolectomy produces a satisfactory result as a labial flange can be utilized thus providing maximum peripheral seal.

20. OCCUPATIONS

Singers and Public Speakers

Reason for the Difficulty. – The sudden loss of retention due to the air seal being broken in the vocal effort.

Treatment. – A peripherally trimmed impression technique and the correct positioning, with adequate seal, of the posterior border of the palate. Singers require a very thin metal palate.

Prognosis. – Satisfactory retention can generally be achieved provided the maximum peripheral seal has been obtained.

21. BURNING SENSATION OF THE PALATE AND MOUTH WHEN WEARING DENTURES

Reason for the Difficulty. – (*a*) Allergy to a particular denture base. Treatment: New dentures using a different denture base; (*b*) Pressure on nerves and blood vessels leaving the palatal or mental foraminae. Treatment: Relief of those areas. (*c*) Mal occlusion with or without open vertical dimension. Treatment: provide an adequate freeway space and a balanced occlusion and articulator. (*d*) Cause unknown. Treatment: Refer to a physician for an opinion.

Prognosis. -- These symptoms are often difficult to eradicate in some patients, others will respond readily to new dentures of a different material, with or without foramina relief.

This condition is frequently manifested by female patients at the menopause and disappears of its own accord when this change is completed.

Chapter XVII

APPEARANCE*

A great deal has been written in journals and textbooks on the techniques of impression taking and bite registration, but little space has been devoted to that aspect of denture construction which embraces the harmonious appearance of the denture when in the patient's mouth. This can be attributed to the fact that artistic appreciation is a personal appraisement and reaction. What the writer considers to be a pleasing result when full dentures are fitted, the reader may readily find unattractive, and for this reason it is difficult to set out rules and principles in association with appearance.

Our aim should be to produce dentures which blend in with the patient's facial and general characteristics and which are an unobtrusive part of the general facial appearance. A denture in which the lateral incisors are set to the same occlusal level as the centrals and canines with the teeth positioned in a perfectly vertical manner, and their colour that of the lightest possible hue will result in an effect which appears obviously artificial, except in one or two isolated instances (*see* figs. 288 and 289).

Operators having an artistic temperament will have little difficulty in producing a pleasing result, but unfortunately we are not all so endowed and some may even experience difficulty in judging the horizontal from the angulated line. In order to aid those who may find the question of appearance perplexing a certain number of points will be discussed which, with individual interpretation, should help the student to produce dentures which are not conspicuously artificial.

1. *Selection of Tooth Mould*

The most important teeth from the point of view of appearance are the central incisors, they are generally the teeth most

*The material of this Chapter is based to a large extent on the published work of Frush and Fisher (*see Reference in Bibliography*).

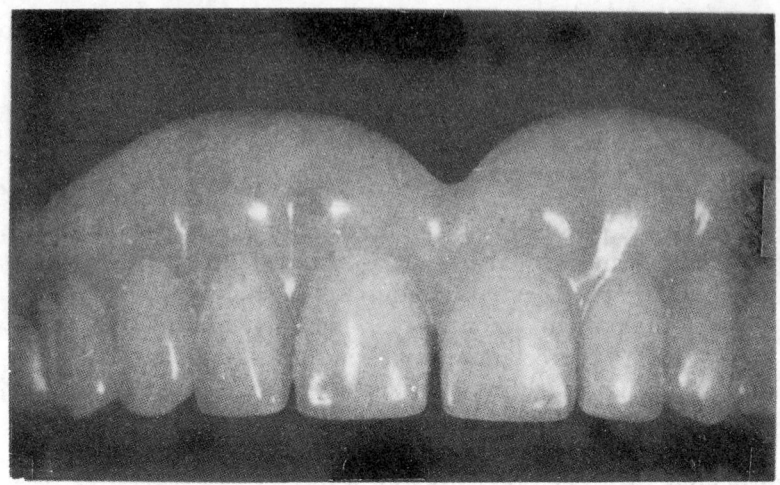

FIG. 288. – Acrylic denture with acrylic anteriors.

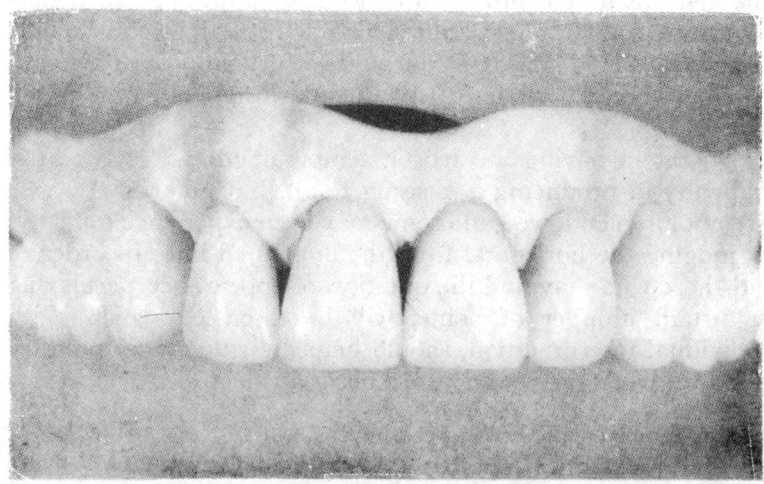

FIG. 289. – Vulcanite denture with porcelain teeth, made about 1935. Both dentures are typical of the 'artificial look' having a vertical arrangement of the anterior teeth, which are also all set with the incisal edges at the same level.

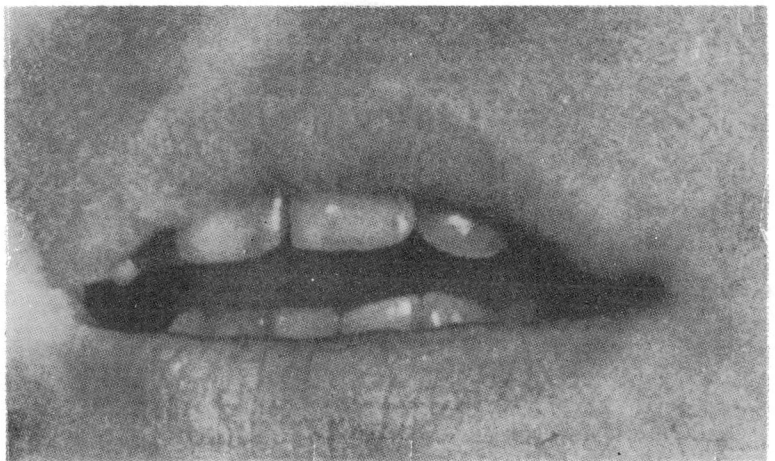

FIG. 290. – During conversation the central incisor is usually
the most exposed tooth, the lateral incisors just show and
the canine is seldom seen.

exposed during conversation and usually the focus of attention
when an individual smiles or laughs (fig. 290), and therefore
the selection of the right mould of central incisor is important.
There are two main points to be considered in its selection,
firstly the sex, and secondly, the personality of the patient.
One associates the female form with curves whilst the male form
presents angles and straight lines (figs. 291, 292). If this is trans-
lated into tooth mould then a central incisor selected for a female
should have a basically curved outline with rounded mesial
and distal corners; such an outline is often referred to as the
ovoid mould. The basic mould for an incisor for the male
should be a straighter sided tooth with moderately sharp
mesial and distal corners; the tapering or square mould
(fig. 293). This does not mean that all women must have
ovoid teeth and all men square or tapering teeth. Obviously
the Venus de Milo type represents the group of individuals
who would probably be most suited to a truly ovoid tooth, but
the athletic, manly and more angular female, although
basically requiring teeth with curved outlines would not want
these accentuated, and square and tapering type teeth with

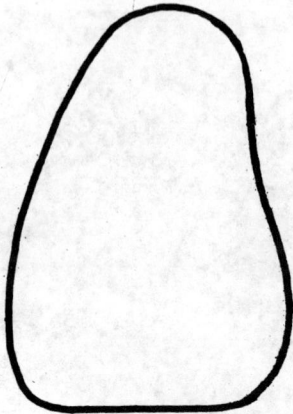

FIG. 291. – The outline of the female figure tends to be a
series of curves and the basic tooth form should be of the
curved sided or ovoid type.

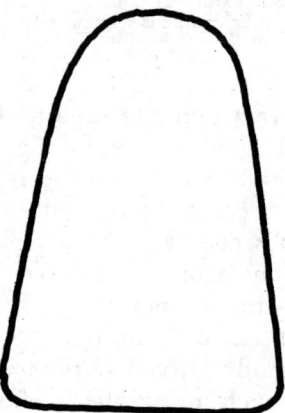

FIG. 292. – The outline of the male figure is more straight
lined and angular in contrast to the female form and the
basic tooth form should be tapering or square.

rounded mesial and distal corners could be most effective.
The male on the other hand, may not always produce the
angular and straight outline and a slightly curved tooth may be
acceptable provided the mesial and distal corners are not over
round. Thus, basically, we have curved outlines and curved
corners for the female, and straight lines and sharp corners
for the male (see figs. 291, 292).

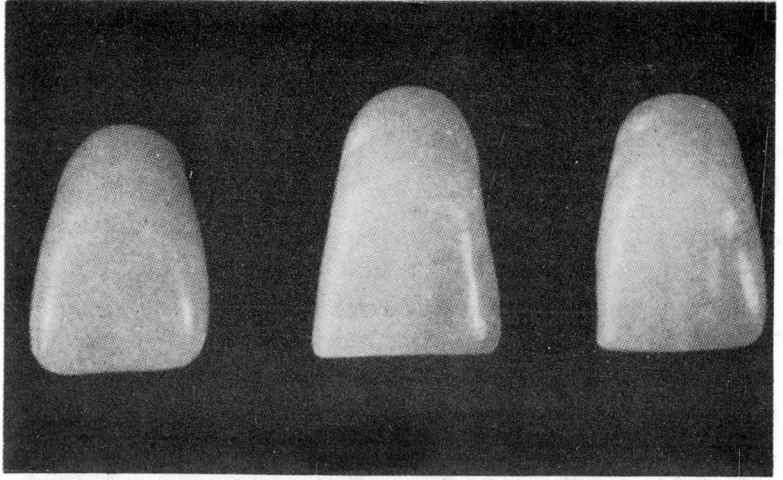

Fig. 293. – Left: Curved tooth form suitable to the female patient. Centre and right: Tapering and square tooth forms having sharp angled mesial and distal corners, suitable to the male patient.

The second point, that of personality, should be considered carefully when making the choice of tooth mould. Personality for this purpose is considered from the aspect of the physical and temperamental impression created by the patient. It cannot have a very precise bearing on the tooth selection, but nevertheless may prevent the choice of a wrong mould. There are two extremes of individuals to be considered, those who fall into the category of healthy, manly, muscular and active types, classed as a vigorous group and those who fall into the category of frail, timid, inactive individuals, classed as a delicate group. Ranging between these two groups will be those persons belonging to the average group. The greater proportion of individuals in the delicate group will be female whilst those in the vigorous group will be male. There will, however, be females ranging from the average group towards the vigorous group, such as some business executives and the committee-lady-chairman types, and to a lesser degree males ranging from the average group to the delicate group, for example, the effeminate or small-boned or debilitated types. Obviously the average group will be by far the largest and the vigorous group will be greater than the delicate group. Mould selection based on this grouping means that on the one extreme the tooth should be soft in its outline with curves and no sharp angles and a smooth labial surface – the delicate group, and on the other extreme the tooth should be bold, angular and show pronounced surface detail labially (ridges and grooves) – the vigorous group. If the personality is considered in conjunction with sex then the vigorous male would be suited best by a bold tapering tooth with sharp angular corners and a prominently contoured labial surface, whilst a delicate female might best be suited by a thin ovoid, smooth surface tooth (fig. 294). Square

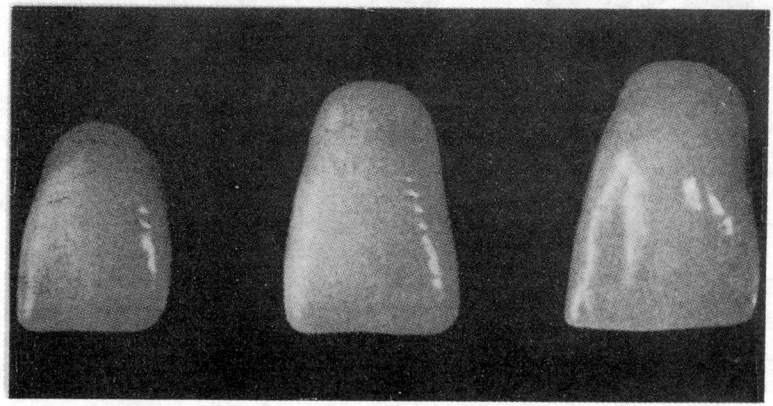

FIG. 294. – Right: Bold tapering tooth suitable to the vigorous male. Left: Small, delicate curved tooth suitable to the delicate female. Centre: An average size and mould of tooth suitable to the average group of individuals.

teeth are considered to be less vigorous than tapering ones but more vigorous than the ovoid type.

The lateral incisors aid considerably in creating the effect of vigour or delicacy and range from a long, tapering, square cornered tooth to a small narrow, round cornered tooth respectively, the lateral of average length and width and with a rounded distal corner suiting the average group of individuals (fig. 295).

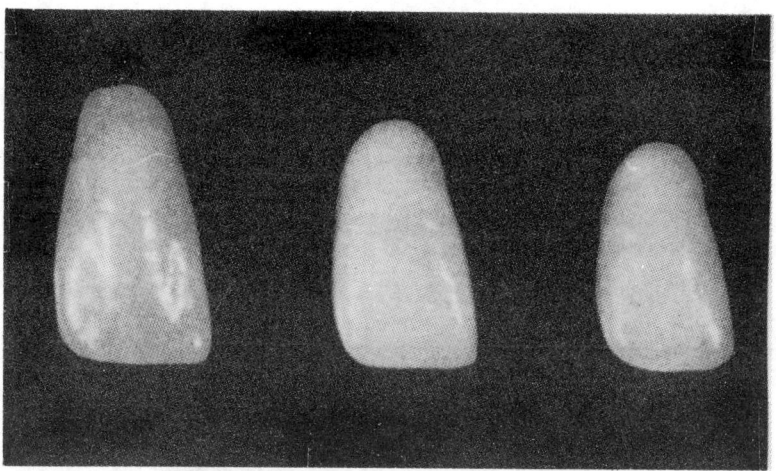

FIG. 295. – Left: A vigorous lateral incisor. Centre: An average lateral incisor. Right: A delicate lateral incisor.

2. *Tooth Size*

This will be governed partly by the sex and personality and partly by the physical build and lip mobility of the patient. With the natural dentition there are instances of slightly built individuals having large teeth and heavily built people having small teeth. This is often a conspicuous feature of the person and attracts attention. For this reason, since it is desirable that dentures should be an unobtrusive feature of the patient, it is advisable to select a size of tooth which blends with the general height and build of the patient, disregarding obvious obesity, and not necessarily related to the size of the patient's head. However, the length to breadth ratio of the selected tooth should bear a very close relationship to the length to breadth ratio of the person's head (fig. 296 *a, b, c*). One important factor which must be borne in mind when deciding the size of tooth, and also the level of the incisal edge relation to the lip, is the mobility of the upper lip. Obviously it is desirable to expose as little denture base material as possible when smiling and laughing and therefore a balance often has to be struck between tooth length and incisal edge level in order that the general tooth size may be kept in proportion with the patient's

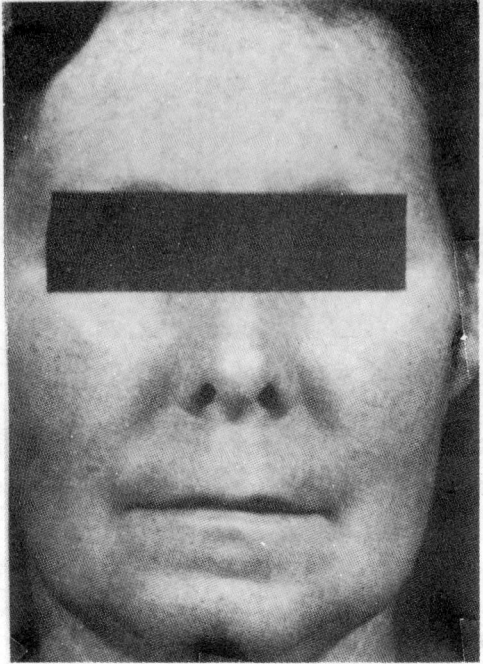

FIG. 296(a)

build. A slightly built patient with a very mobile lip may have to have the incisal edge, which would normally have been set 2 to 3 mm. below the lip, raised to lip level or slightly higher in order that a tooth of balanced length may be used instead of an overlong tooth.

Provided the tooth maintains proportions suitable to the individual the appearance will be best if the tooth fills, or very nearly fills, the space between the rest and smiling positions of the upper lip.

The size of the mouth will control the width of the tooth to a certain extent. It is obviously undesirable to select narrow teeth for a person with a very broad smile which exposes the molar teeth, but it is equally undesirable to select very broad teeth – which will also be proportionate in length – if the sex, personality and physical build of the individual indicates a

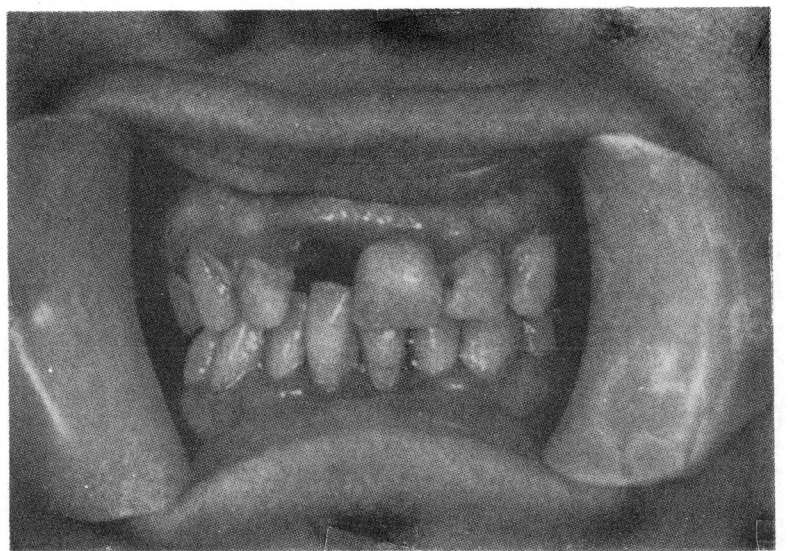

(b)

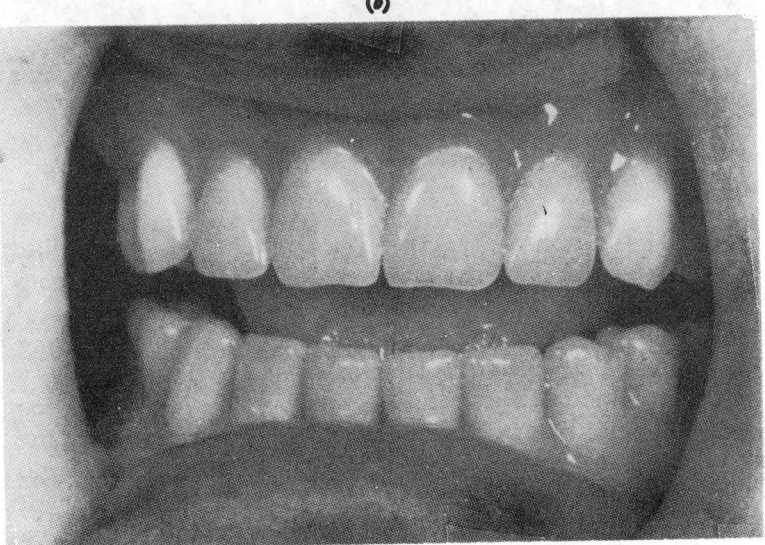

(c)

Fig. 296. – Comparison of tooth proportions to face proportions. Facial measurements are taken across the zygomatic
process on each side, and from the supra-orbital ridge line
to the inferior border of the chin.

(a) Patient before extraction of teeth.
(b) Natural dentition.
(c) Full dentures.

small mould of tooth. The alternative is to select the appropriate size of tooth to match the sex, personality and build of the patient and then to space the teeth when setting up, without producing an unpleasant appearance, to obtain the maximum width from canine to canine.

Generally, large people require large teeth and small people small teeth. Women usually require smaller teeth than men for relative builds (fig. 297). It is as well to remember that

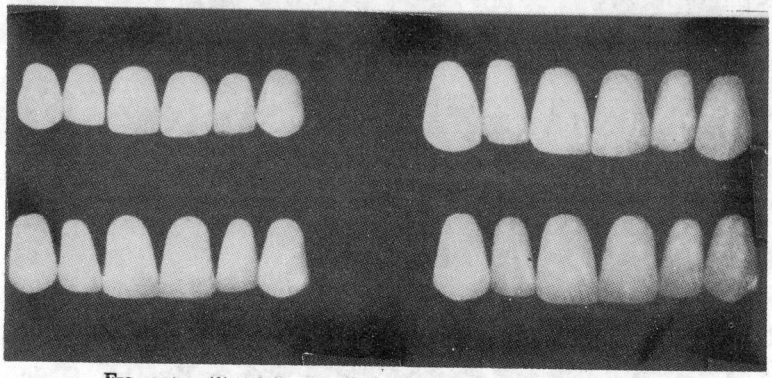

FIG. 297. – Top left: Small sized teeth – small, female form.
Lower left: Medium sized teeth – average male form.
Top right: Medium/large sized teeth – male or female of
more than average body size.
Lower right: Large sized teeth – large male form.

the size of the natural teeth does not change throughout life, excluding the effect of attrition but the body often undergoes considerable alteration in weight and therefore the dimensional changes sometimes occurring in middle age may be misleading when considering the size of teeth.

It is a common failing to select artificial teeth which are too small and this frequently results from the patient influencing the operator in his choice. Patients often imagine their natural teeth to have been smaller than was actually the case but it must be pointed out that there is an element of risk in pressing one's own choice of size and mould too vigorously. A compromise is sometimes necessary between that which the operator considers suitable and that which the patient desires, which with some elderly ladies may be small, white teeth.

3. Shade of Teeth

There is no rule which can be applied to the selection of the correct shade of tooth for an individual. Generally it is a question of trial and error, taking a tooth of one colour from a shade range, placing it in position behind the upper lip and assessing its colour tones in relation to the facial colour tones of the patient. This operation is repeated with different shades until one is found which most satisfactorily blends with the patient's general colouring. Blondes with light blue or grey eyes are usually best suited by a light ivory-yellow shade of tooth bordering on the white range. Darker eye colouring may require a slightly darker shade of tooth. Brown hair and medium coloured eyes call for the mid range of the biscuit yellow shade, and the darker hair and eye tones will require a darker shade of the biscuit yellow range. Occasionally a grey basic tone blends well with the elderly or pale debilitated individual, but its selection requires careful consideration, or the effect when the patient smiles is to accentuate the debility. Age has an important bearing on colour choice. Natural teeth tend to darken with age and the colour selected for a person of 25 years of age would be too light when that person was 50. For instance in the Peridon shade range 65 is found to blend well with the larger proportion of young adults whereas the shade 79 suits a larger proportion of those of 50 years and over. Both these shades are basically a biscuit yellow. The best advice for the student is to note the shades of teeth used in partial denture work and to categorize them according to the age and colour tone of the individual and relate this information to full denture construction. Selection of colour should always be made from a wet tooth under the shadow of the upper lip, the position which it will occupy and never from a dry tooth held in the hand.

4. The Position of the Teeth

Since our chief aim is to produce a denture which harmonizes with the person's appearance, presents a pleasant effect when smiling or laughing and is not conspicuously artificial, the question of tooth position is also important. Basically there are two considerations. Firstly, the person, male or female, who has classical features requires a normal arrangement of tooth position, otherwise their classical qualities will be diminished (fig. 298 *a*, *b*, 299). These will be very few indeed. Secondly, the very rugged type of individual requires irregularity in the positioning of the teeth as otherwise a perfectly normal arrangement of the teeth would contrast with the rugged features and therefore bring the focus of attention on to the denture, which is not desirable (figs. 300, 301 *a*, *b*). Most patients will be placed somewhere between these two extremes and many variations from the normal position of the individual anterior teeth will be found. Once again it is helpful to consider tooth position in relation to the personality and sex of the patient. There is, however, a third factor – that of age which also influences the arrangement of the anterior teeth. This latter point will be discussed under heading 5.

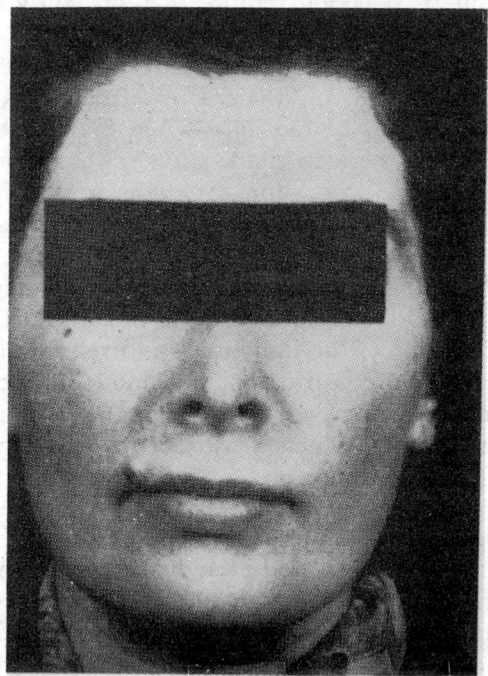

Fig. 298(*a*)

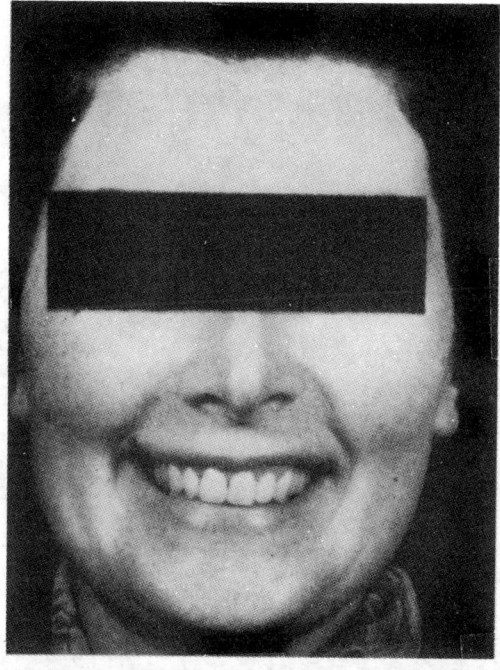

(*b*)

FIG. 298. – Well proportioned and attractive facial features
requiring a fairly regular setting of the anterior teeth.
(*a*) Ovoid facial type.
(*b*) Regular appearance of the natural teeth.

Apart from their ability to incise food and aid speech the
anterior teeth form the main feature of the smile and largely
influence facial expression. In order that they should fulfil
these latter two functions satisfactorily it is important that the
teeth should be placed in relation to the alveolar ridge in
such a manner that adequate support is given to the lip during
a smile (fig. 302), and that the lip is supported in its natural
forward position when the lip is at rest. Too often artificial
upper anterior teeth are set back underneath the ridge (fig.
303 *a*, *b*, *c*, *d*) and the lip hangs down vertically or may even
fall inwards. If fig. 304 is studied, which is a sagittal section of a
maxilla and full upper immediate denture three months after

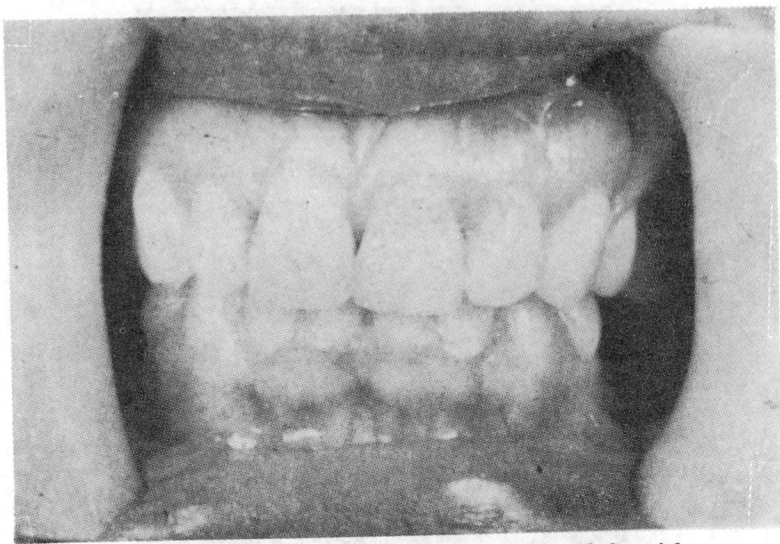

FIG. 299. – Note curve-sided central incisors, rounded mesial angles of lateral incisors, attrition of incisal edges of the centrals and canines, and the stippling of the gingival tissues.

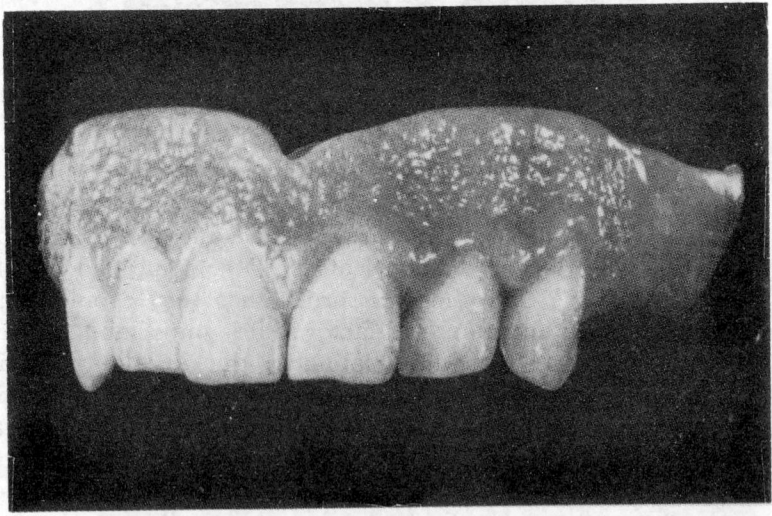

FIG. 300. – An arrangement of the teeth suited to the robust male type. Note, palatally rotated laterals, attrition of the incisal edges and increased details of the labial surfaces of the teeth.

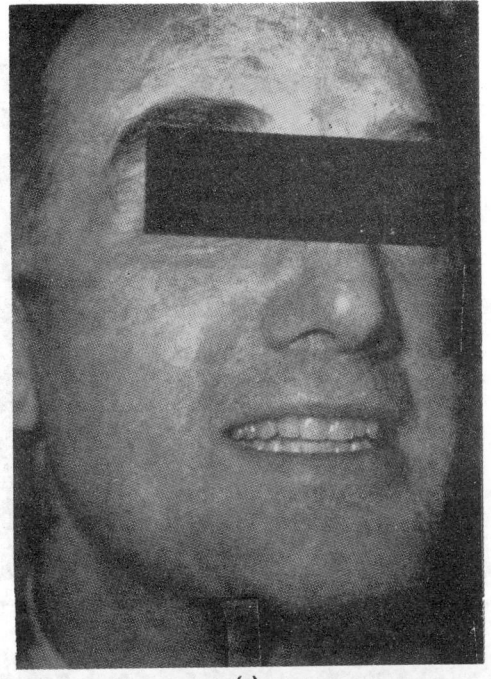

(a)

(b)
FIG. 301 (*a* and *b*). – Vigorous setting of the anterior teeth
used to emphasise male characteristics.

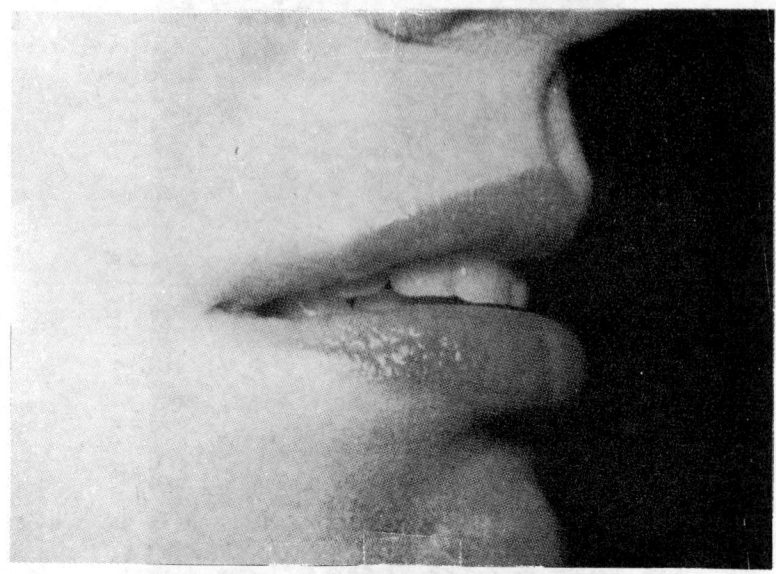

FIG. 302. – Lip support obtained from the correct forward placement of the upper anterior teeth.

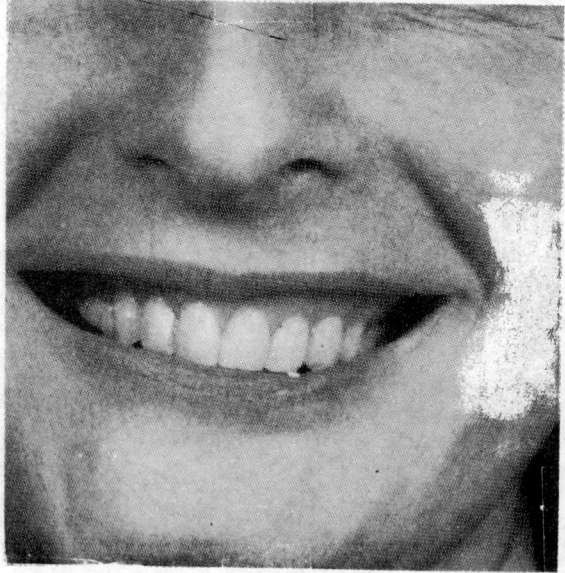

FIG. 303(a)

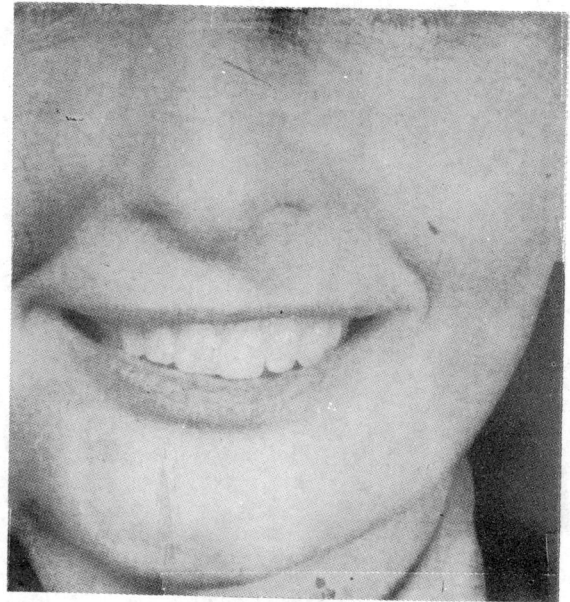

Fig. 303(b)

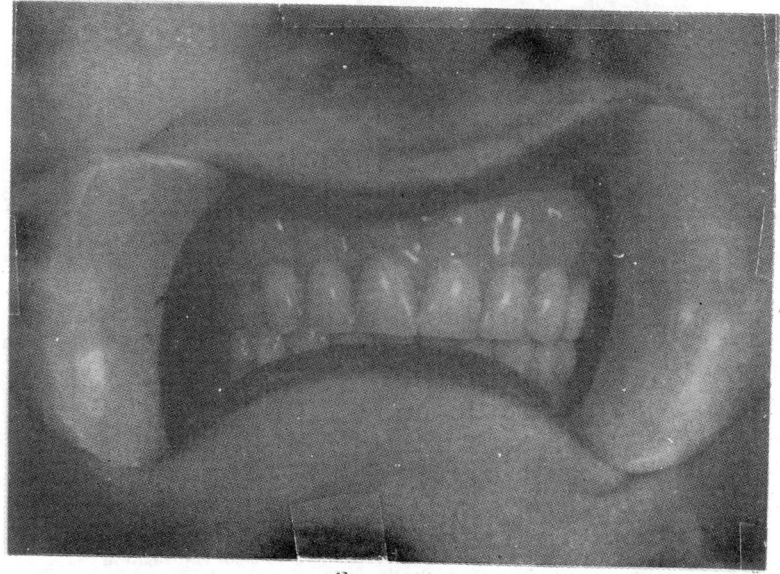

Fig. 303(c)

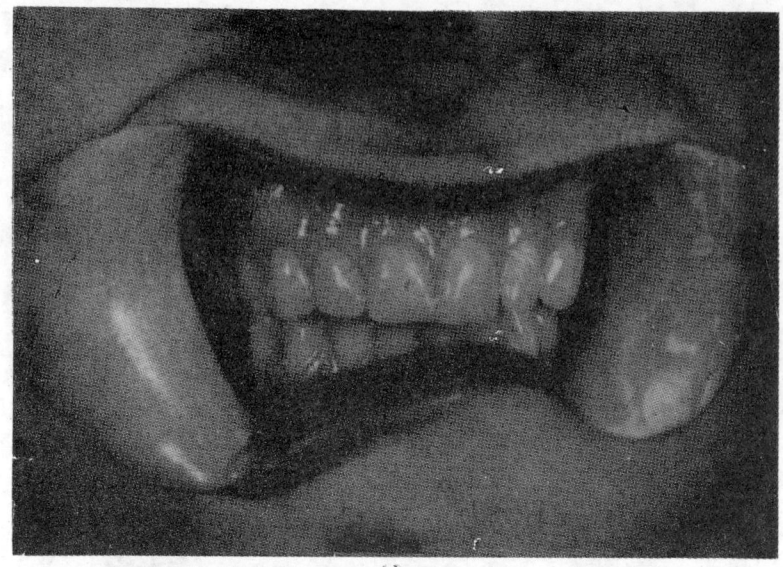

(d)

FIG. 303.

(a) Appearance with previous denture.
(b) Appearance with new dentures.
(c) Mould and arrangement of teeth of the previous denture.
(d) Mould and arrangement of teeth of the new denture.
    Note: The more oval type of tooth selected for the new
    denture in which the /1 has been rotated and set forward
    in the arch and slightly overlapping the 1/. The /2 is
    rotated and slightly spaced in relation to /1. The
    denture base has been contoured and stippled.

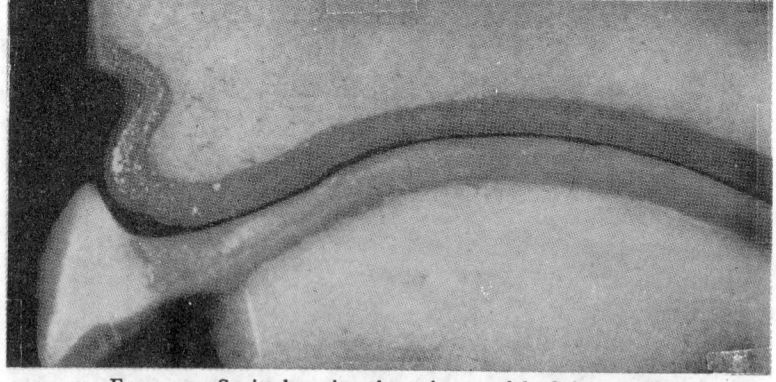

FIG. 304. – Sagittal section through a model of the maxilla
and an immediate denture three months after its insertion.
Note the upward and backward resorption of the alveolar
ridge; the upper incisor was 'socketed' initially.

insertion, it will be seen that alveolar absorption of the anterior
ridge has been upwards and backwards and that the necks of
the anterior teeth are positioned forward of the ridge and the
relationship of the whole tooth is somewhat forward of the
ridge. These teeth would be supplying the correct lip support
since they are an identical replacement of the patient's natural
teeth. This indicates the necessity for setting anterior teeth in a
forward relationship to the ridge in almost all cases. The degree
of this forward placement is related, obviously, to the extent
of absorption which has occurred anteriorly and to factors of
mechanics and retention associated generally with the construction of the dentures. The aim should be to restore correct
lip support and with this point established, the individual
positions of the teeth can be considered with a view to producing a harmonious appearance.

The Central Incisor. – Keeping both incisors in identically
correct positions indicates perfection and would probably only
suit those with classical features. If one incisor is moved forward
of the other at its incisal edge then a somewhat harsh appearance is created which would be suitable to a few male persons.
On the other hand if we start from the correct positions of the
centrals and move one out cervically leaving the incisal edges
in line a softer irregularity is created suitable for use with the
female patient. A more vigorous effect can be obtained by
bringing one central bodily forward of the other – the vigorous
male type. Further effects of softness or hardness may be
brought about by rotating or inclining laterally one or both
incisors (fig. 305 *a*, *b*). Overlapping can be effective particularly
in the female where the canine to canine distance requires to be
small but the tooth size average. In most instances the variations of position of the central incisors are acceptable to both
sexes. It is usually a matter of degree of irregularity which needs
consideration in relation to the sex and personality of the
patient.

The Lateral Incisor. – Although this is a comparatively small
tooth and less apparent than the central it does however play
an important part in establishing the sex and personality
factors associated with the general composition of the anterior

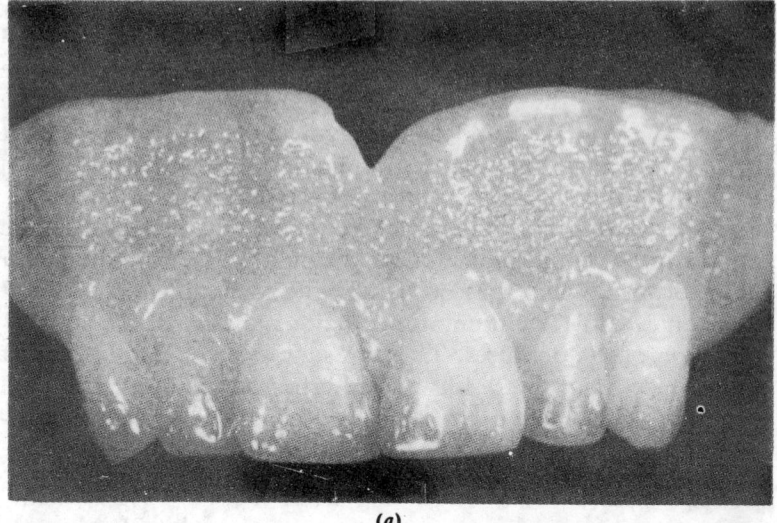

(a)

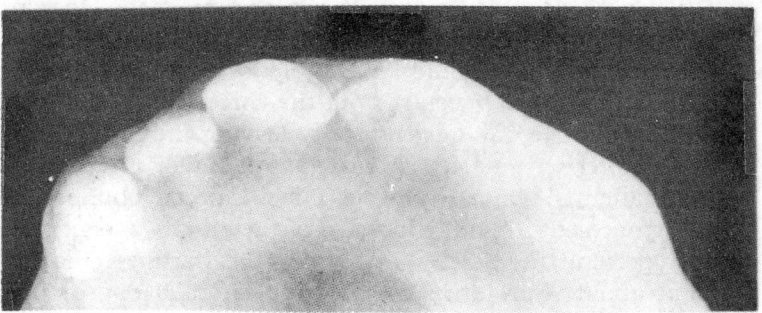

(b)

FIG. 305 (a) and (b). – Illustrate the rotation of central
incisors to break up an otherwise regular setting of the
anterior teeth. Acceptable to both male and female depending
on the degree of rotation.

teeth. If the lateral incisor is rotated so that the mesial surface
is brought forward then the effect of the smile is one of softness;
the tooth may overlap the central. By depressing the mesial
edge towards the palate the effect of hardness is obtained.
Lateral inclination from the normal vertical axis is an additional variation (figs. 306 a, b, 307 a, b).

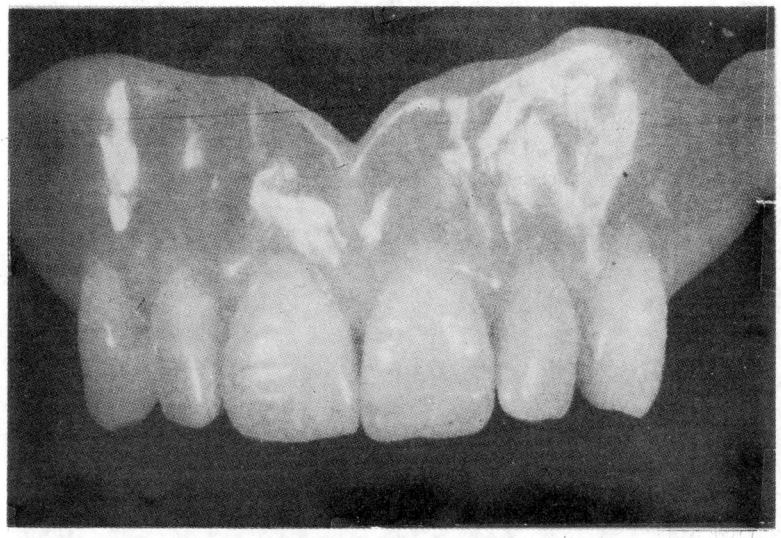

(a)

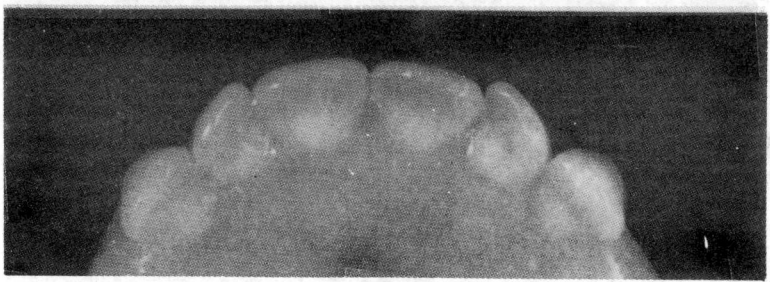

(b)

Fig. 306 (*a*) and (*b*). – Illustrate the use of labial rotation of the incisal tips of the lateral incisors to accentuate curvature of the anterior arch when producing a feminine effect.

The Canine. – This tooth should be set with the neck more prominent than the incisal tip and its long axis vertical. The more prominent the position of the canine and its cervical edge in the arch the more vigorous the smile becomes. Similarly the larger the tooth and the more marked the labial surface detail the greater the effect of masculinity.

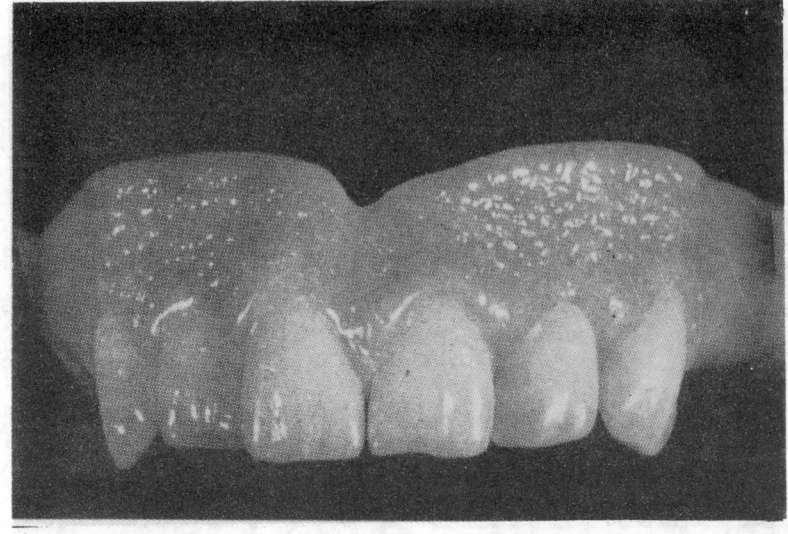

(a)

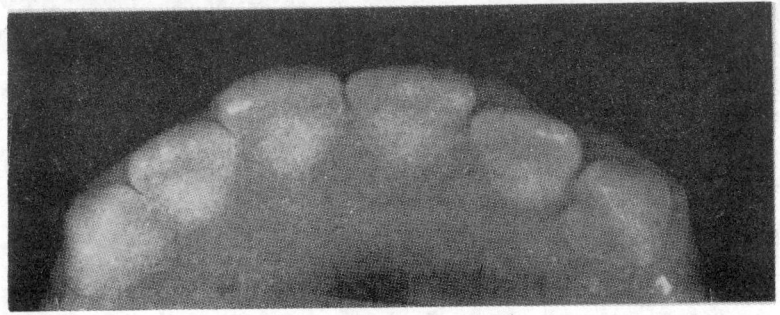

(b)

FIG. 307 (a) and (b). – Illustrates the use of palatal rotation of the mesial tips of the lateral incisors to harden the appearance by producing a more straight-line effect of the anterior arch; used when producing a masculine effect.

Feminity can be accentuated by setting the anterior teeth with a curvature running from the tips of the central incisors upwards to the canines (fig. 308). This imparts a sense of roundness to the smile.

Symmetry should be avoided when producing irregularities

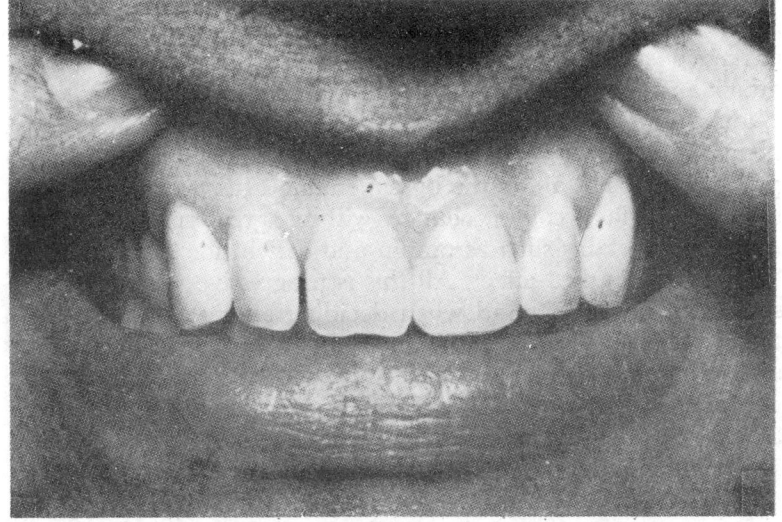

Fig. 308. – Femininity accentuated by the upward curvature
of the setting of the incisal edges, the central incisal line
sweeps up to the laterals and continues upwards to the
canine tips. Note the contouring of the labial flange and its
stippling.

as they frequently increase the appearance of artificiality. On
the other hand over accentuation of an irregularity is often
necessary to be effective and a tooth arrangement which
appears somewhat grotesque when set in the articulator
becomes pleasantly acceptable when the denture is fitted in
the mouth.

5. *Age*

Age in relation to appearance must be considered from two
aspects. One, chronological age and two, the physiological age
of the patient. People vary considerably in the effect of age on
their physical appearance, some young middle-aged people
appear very much older than their chronological age, whilst
some chronologically old people appear young and virile.
Tooth selection and arrangement should fit in chiefly with the
physiological age of the patient.

A person at the age of 18 years would probably have teeth of
a uniform colour and would still retain the bluish tint of the

incisal enamel but twenty-five years later these same teeth are likely to have undergone certain changes. They will have darkened slightly, areas of stain will have appeared, caries attack and subsequent fillings will have caused localized colour change, gingival recession will have exposed cementum and attrition of the incisal edges will have removed the greater proportion, if not all, of the incisal enamel. It is to be expected that the surface colour change will be greatest in smokers though food stains such as tannin and caffein for example will also have a marked effect. All this is progressive with age and should be borne in mind when deciding on the colour of the teeth selected for an individual. In certain circumstances effective results can be obtained by varying the shade of one or two of the anterior teeth and also by staining and simulating fillings in individual teeth, alternatively the dental manufacturing companies produce such teeth, which are referred to as naturalized or characterized teeth. Even if such desirable procedures are not adopted the standard set of anterior teeth can be made more balanced to the person's age by judicious grinding of the incisal edges, and a study of the attrition of natural incisors will indicate the type of wear which occurs from person to person. Fig. 309 shows the expected appearance of a canine tooth at three stages of life. Attrition will obviously affect the posterior teeth as well as the anterior teeth so that if a patient of middle or advance age is likely to show the premolar teeth when smiling or laughing a more natural effect can be created if the cusps of the premolars are suitably ground and not left in the form of a newly erupted tooth.

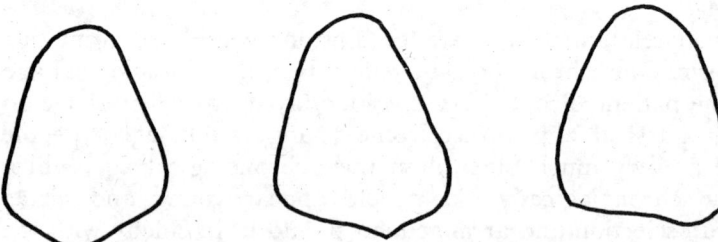

FIG. 309. – Left: Canine in the young person showing no attrition. Middle: Extent of attrition often seen in middle age. Right: Degree of attrition in old age.

Age also has a bearing on the position of the anterior teeth. Throughout life natural teeth are usually being lost for one reason or another and this means that the contact points of the remaining teeth become less firm or even lost, particularly if a partial denture is not fitted (fig. 310). It is not an uncommon state in the middle-aged person, where some posterior teeth have been lost, to find that the contact points of the

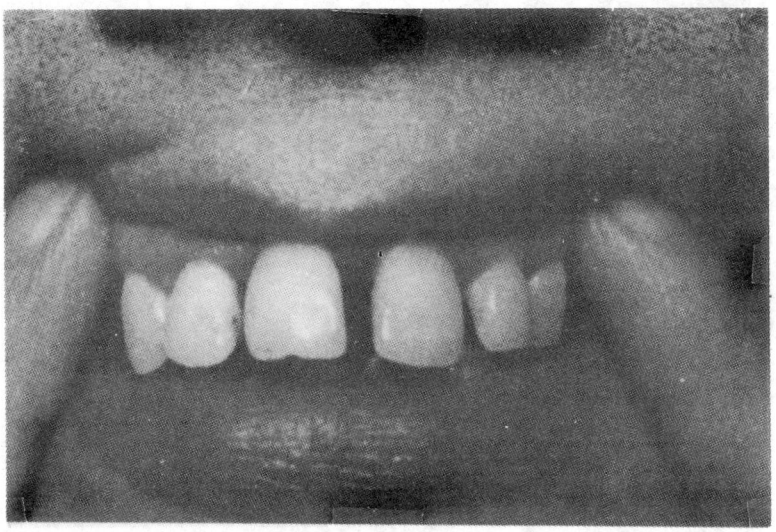

FIG. 310. – Spacing of natural teeth due to loss of posterior teeth (patient age 29).

anterior teeth have parted to the extent that the point of a probe can be passed freely between them, and this fact needs to be considered in relation to the setting up of the anterior teeth. Frequently the appearance of a full upper denture constructed for the 50–60-year-old patient is spoiled by having the teeth set with very tight contact between each tooth, producing an effect which is generally associated with youth. Varying degrees of spacing with either all or one or two of the anterior teeth aids in establishing a natural appearance in relation to age (fig. 311 a, b, c). A slight diastema between the centrals is a common occurrence but caution is necessary in reproducing

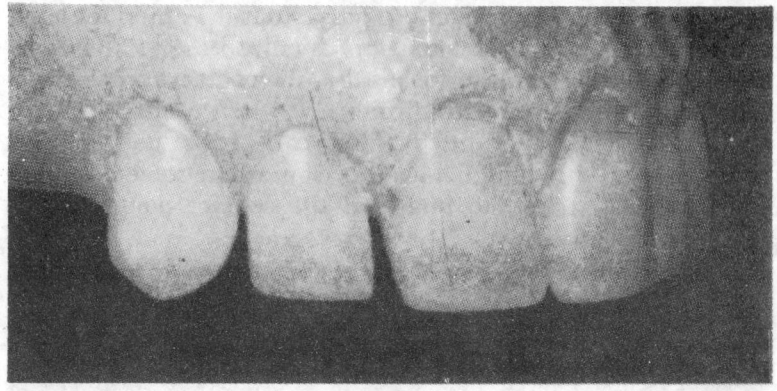

(a)

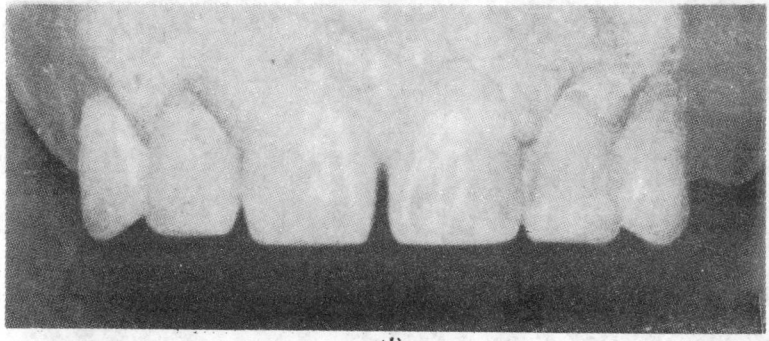

(b)

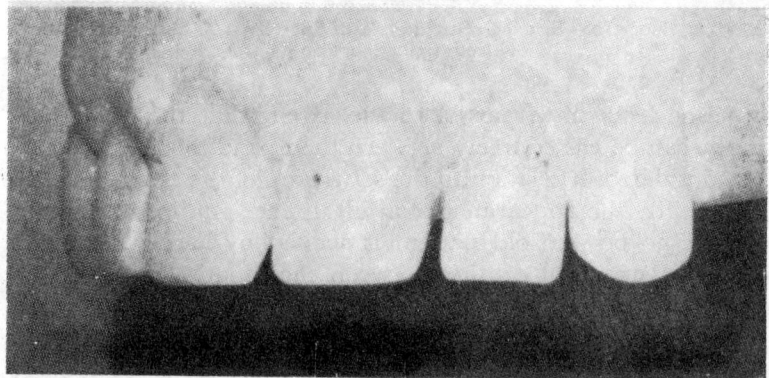

(c)

FIG. 311. – Spacing and the use of characterized teeth to
simulate a middle-aged appearance.

this state as it is possible that if exaggerated it may appear unpleasant and become a source of amusement to the observer: it may also be an embarrassing food-trap. The gingival contouring of a denture should also be related to the age of the patient and is the next consideration.

Just as tightly contacting teeth are predominantly associated with youth so are normal, triangular, sharp-pointed interdental papillae indicative of the young person (fig. 312). Greater

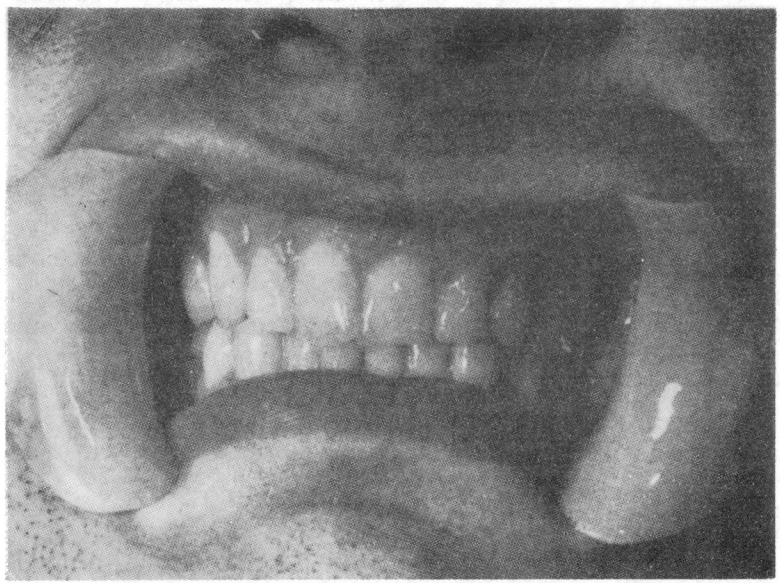

Fig. 312. – Natural gingival margins of youthful appearance: narrow, sharp pointed interdental papillae, stippled gingival tissue.

harmony in the appearance can be obtained by simulation of some of the changes which may occur throughout life in the shape and colour of the interdental papillae and gingival margins. Variation from the normal type papilla suitable to the youngish patient must be made with care, and spaces such as occur between teeth in advanced periodontal lesions should be avoided. However, the copying of some of the less advanced conditions in which the point of the papilla is rounded instead of pointed and the base is widened to overlap the labial and cervical areas of the tooth to a greater extent than normal can be most effective, especially if the gingival margin is thickened to form a slight rolled effect (figs. 313, 314, 315, 316). Denture base materials having reddish fibres or granules incorporated in them improve the general effect in some instances. A study of natural conditions which are not unpleasant in their appearance will be of considerable help to the student. Fig. 317 shows age changes which may be associated with the interdental papilla.

In the production of such interdental papillae, certain points need remembering.

(1) There should be a variation in the individual length and the degree of simulated change in the health of the tissue from papilla to papilla.

(2) They must be related to the age of the patient.

(3) They must be convex in all directions to avoid food being trapped about them.

(4) They should extend to the contact points of the teeth and fill the interdental space so that no areas exist for food accumulation.

This necessitates care in the selection of the tooth mould in order to avoid those moulds having low contact point areas which would mean overlong papillae.

6. *The Gingival Margin and Labial Surface Contour*

As previously stated, the gingival margins can be blended to suit the age by thickening or rolling the gingival margin of all or some teeth. In youth the margin is thin and pale pink in colour, in middle age an average appearance would be a slight rolling of the margin with increased red tint in the pink colour and the papillae would be blunter and thicker, whilst in advanced age the gingival tissue would give a characteristic thickened appearance and a deeper red tint, the papillae being broad based with very rounded apices (*see* figs. 313–316). The gingival level of the individual anterior teeth should vary, the central incisal gingivae normally being higher than those of the lateral incisors, but lower than those of the canine (fig. 318). Again symmetry needs to be avoided and variation in the

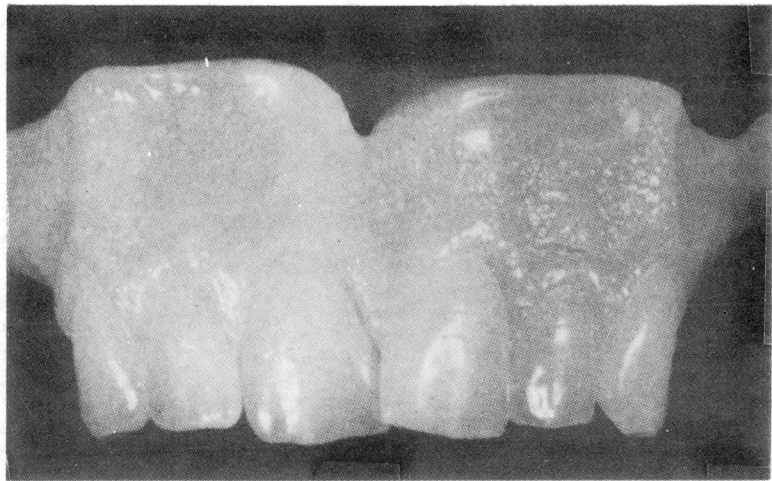

FIG. 313. – Youthful appearance of the interdental papillae
showing slight thickening of the gingival margins. Note the
use of overlap with the central incisors and the broadening
of the base of their interdental papillae.

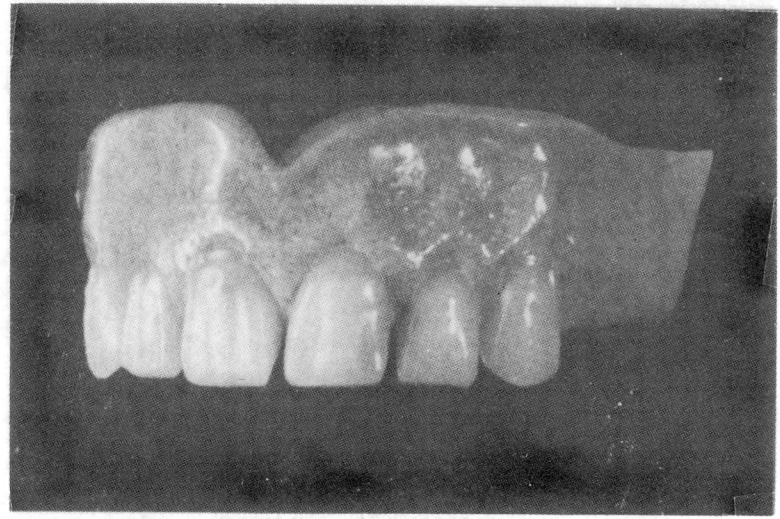

FIG. 314. – Illustrates a short, rounded and blunt papilla
between /12 which are also spaced.

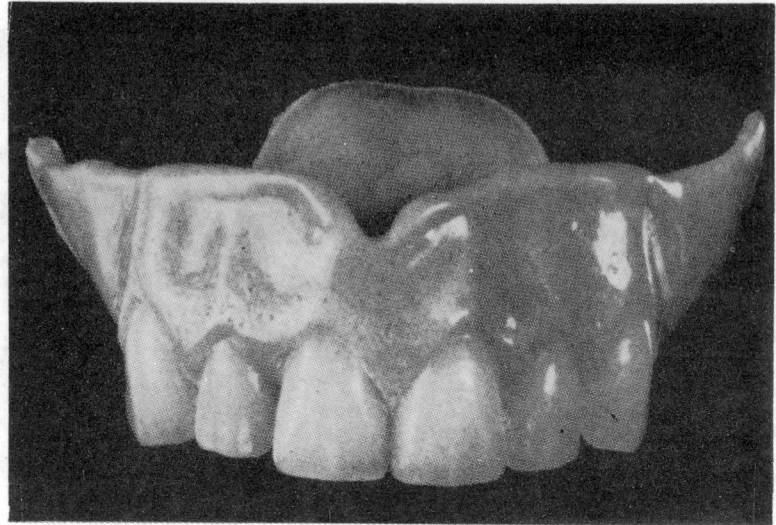

FIG. 315. – A very broad based papilla between 1/1 having the effect of tapering an otherwise square mould of tooth.

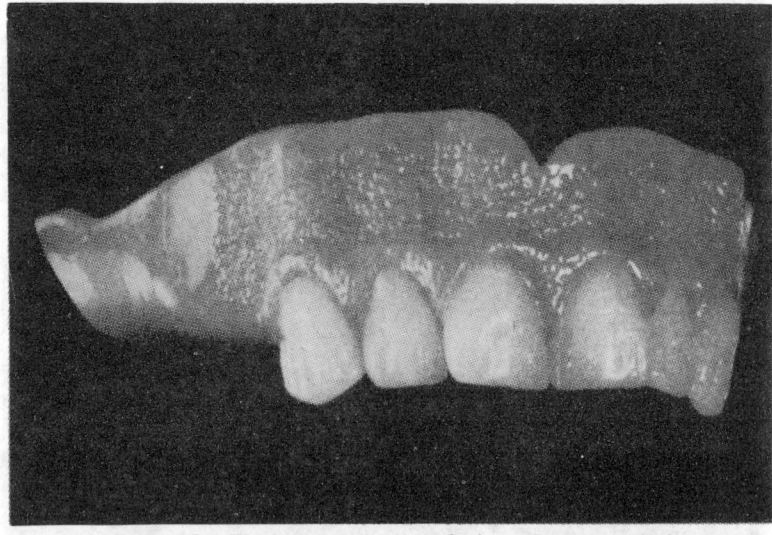

FIG. 316. – Thickening and broadening of the gingival margins and papillae respectively in an attempt to create a middle to advanced age appearance in the composition of the matrix of the denture.

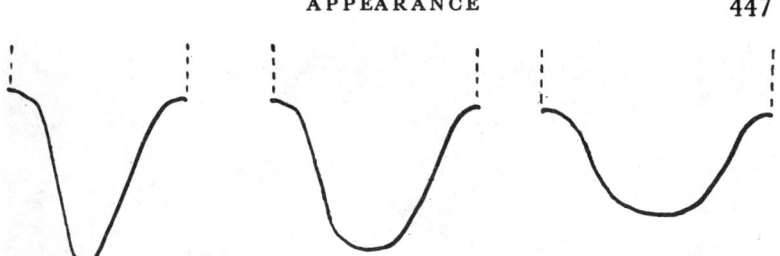

FIG. 317. – Illustrates the shortening and rounding of the apex of interdental papilla and the widening of its base from youth (left) to advanced age (right).

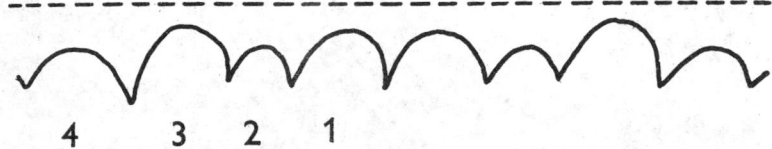

FIG. 318. – Variation in the gingival margin level of the anterior teeth. (The broken line is intended only for purposes of comparison.)

gingival levels should be followed. The premolar and molar gingival level should also vary if a broad smile exists, the first premolar level being below that of the canine, the others being variations of that level. A denture having the gingival margins uniformly shaped and all at the same level with all the teeth set vertically and level with the occlusal plane creates the impression of a row of fence palings, thereby making the denture look artificial.

Another reason for dentures appearing artificial is the manner in which the labial flange is shaped. Often this flange is a continuous arc from premolar to premolar and when light falls upon it during a smile or laugh it gives a flat reflection devoid of highlights and shadows (fig. 319), which is not the usual occurrence with natural tissues. By contouring the labial flange highlights and shadow effect can be obtained, breaking up the flat reflection of the light falling on the denture (fig. 313). To do this, the labial area should be contoured to simulate the prominences caused by the roots of natural teeth. The canine roots are usually the most prominent and plumping in that

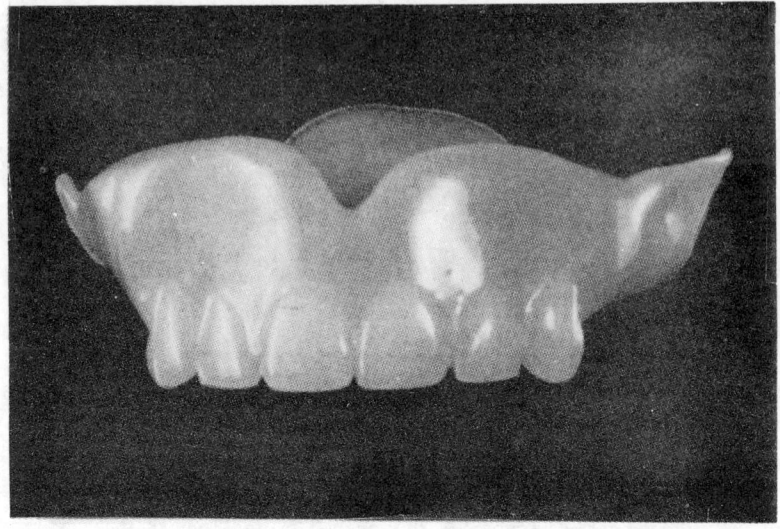

FIG. 319. - The smooth, flat, glossy surface of some dentures is
the cause, very often, of the artificial appearance of a denture
and is due to the type of light reflection which occurs from
such a surface.

region which follows the long axis of the crown of the tooth and
the anatomical shape of a root enables the canine to be set
prominently thus supporting the corner of the mouth and lip,
thereby diminishing the extent of the naso-labial crease which
often is so obvious in the edentulous patient. The root of the
central incisor will be less prominent than the canine and the
lateral the least of all. When contouring the roots of the teeth
the long axes of the crowns must always be followed and
anatomical detail copied realistically. Models taken from
natural dentitions as patterns are useful to have at hand when
shaping the labial flange. The finished denture should be
stippled, that is the reproduction of the minute creases and pits
occurring in natural gum tissue which gives it that orange peel
appearance, to break up further any large zones of light
reflection (*see* fig. 313). The area covered by the contouring and
stippling should be limited to the labial region and that part
only of the buccal region likely to be exposed when the patient
laughs. The reason for this being that a rough and uneven

surface tends to collect food particles, whereas a smooth, polished surface is more self cleansing. The inference here is that stippling and gingival contouring should be diminished or possibly avoided in those cases where oral hygiene is poor.

7. *The Smile Line and Arch Form*

The smile line related to the setting of the anterior teeth is a curve running through the incisal edges of the central incisors, sweeping upwards to the lateral teeth and thence to the tips of the canines. This arc is determined by the age of the patient, the more accentuated arc occurs in the young person since there is little attrition of the central incisors (figs. 320 and 321). As age

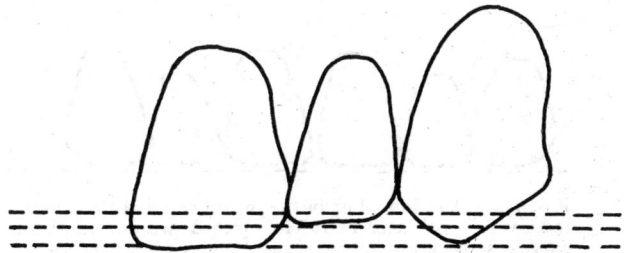

FIG. 320. – Illustrates attrition associated with varying age levels. (A) Youth. Little or no attrition. (B) Middle age. Attrition beginning to involve the lateral. (C) Old age. Marked attrition of all teeth.

and attrition progresses the arc flattens until in old age it is almost a flat plane. This smile line can also be related to the sex of the patient bearing in mind the basic curved form associated with femininity.

The amount of tooth showing during serious conversation is considered to be: In the young adult 2 mm. In middle age $1\frac{1}{2}$ mm. In old age 0 to − 1 mm.

It is sometimes an advantage to show a little more tooth in the female than in the male at the various age levels to enhance the quality of femininity.

The arch form of the anterior teeth should not necessarily be made to coincide with the resorbed alveolar ridge outline as this may have undergone considerable change, the features of the face should be studied and the arch made to harmonize

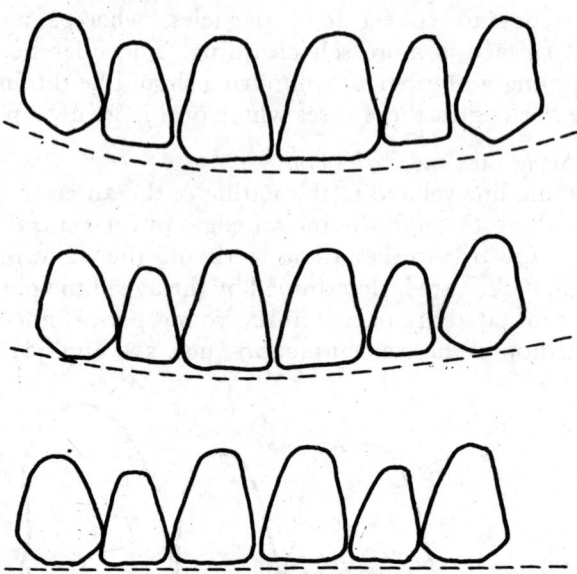

Fig. 321. – The smile-line of the incisal edges of the anterior teeth varies with age. Top: The upward sweep of smile line curve is seen mostly in youth where no attrition has occurred in the incisor region. Middle: In middle age the wear of the incisal edges flattens this curve. Lower: In old age this curve may be reduced to a flat plane by marked attrition.

with them. Generally it will be found that flat-faced individuals would be best suited by a flat arch and the pointed or sharp featured person suited to a tapering arch In between will be the moderate arch curve adopted for the majority of individuals. A tapering arch is most adaptable to the overlapping of teeth in the production of irregularities.

8. *The Vertical Dimension*

The restoration of the facial appearance of the edentulous patient requires attention to three points. First, the correct placing of the upper anterior teeth; second, the restoration, by the correct thickness and positioning of the denture flanges, of the tissue lost during extraction and alveolar absorption; and thirdly, the establishment of the correct vertical dimension of the jaw relationship for the individual. Vertical dimension from the point of view of appearance is important as it is

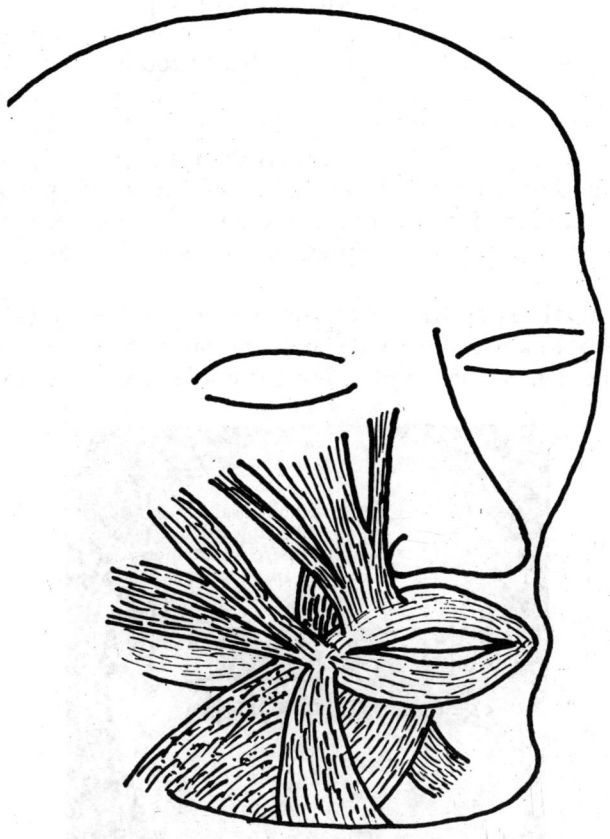

Fig. 322. – Diagrammatic illustration of the facial musculature.

If the upper anterior teeth are set too far back under the ridge, thereby reducing the distance between the origins and insertions of the more horizontal muscles associated with the upper lip, the naso-labial fold is often accentuated; also such setting of the teeth allows the corners of the mouth to fall in, which may lead to angular cheilitis.

Over-closure of the vertical dimension similarly reduces the distance between the origins and insertions of the more vertically running muscles, thereby causing a compression of the facial musculature giving the patient the appearance of old age (see fig. 323). It may be a cause of angular cheilitis.

related to the establishment of the correct separation of the origins and insertions of the muscles of the facial musculature. If these insertions are brought too close together the muscles will tend to sag and bunch, conversely, if they are too far apart the muscles will be stretched producing a strained appearance. For the muscles to be in their normal relationship the anterior teeth must be correctly positioned and the vertical dimension correct. The modiolus is then in its correct position and this tendinous node can effectively serve its purpose of acting as an anchor during contractions of certain of the facial muscles associated with expression and speech (figs. 322 and 323).

The final assessment of an appearance at the trial denture stage should always be made with the operator standing away from the dental chair and judgment made at varying distances

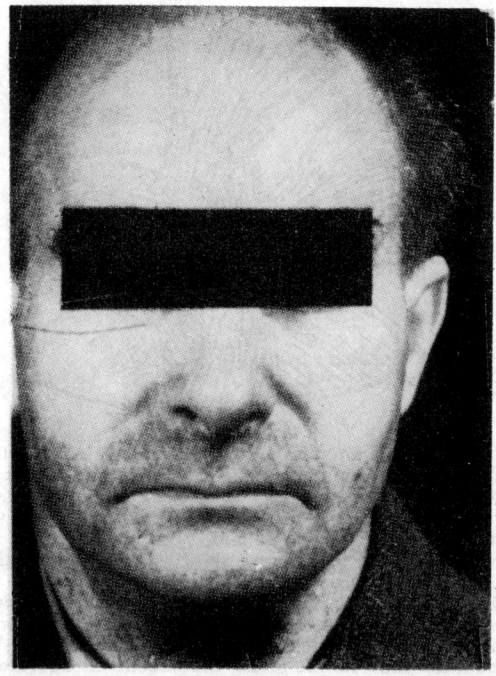

Fig. 323. – Facial appearance of an overclosed vertical dimension.

to obtain the overall effect. Furthermore, a relative or close friend should, if possible, attend at this stage to give their considered opinion. This often saves argument and ill-feeling between the operator and the patient after dentures have been worn for a few days and criticized by the family and close friends.

Most people dread the thought of losing their teeth and having to be fitted with dentures, one of the reasons being the fear of having an artificial appearance with dentures. Such people will appreciate the care and thought given to producing a natural appearance and it is therefore a wise plan to have available examples and photographs of the types of naturalized effects and their appearance when in the mouth. If the patient does not discuss the question of appearance then this question should be raised by the operator before any naturalized effects are introduced in the construction of a denture. Some people have a profound desire for their own conception of a perfect set of teeth, even though they carry the label 'artificial'.

Chapter XVIII

PARTIAL DENTURES

Assessment of the Partial Denture

The previous chapters concerned the edentulous patient and those which follow deal with individuals who are only partially edentulous, having one or more teeth missing from either mandible or maxilla or both. Dentures designed for such patients will vary considerably depending upon the number of natural teeth missing from the jaws and will range from those replacing only one tooth to others replacing all but one tooth.

In order to be able to record missing teeth and to make reference to the remaining natural teeth it is necessary to have some easy means of notation. For this purpose the mouth is divided into four quadrants by a horizontal line representing the occlusal plane and a vertical line representing the midline. The eight teeth in each quadrant are numbered from the front backwards, commencing with the central incisors, thus:

$$\text{Patient's right} \quad \frac{87654321}{87654321} \bigg| \frac{12345678}{12345678} \quad \text{Patient's left}$$

A similar plan is used to denote the deciduous teeth, but in this instance letters are used in place of numbers:

$$\frac{edcba}{edcba} \bigg| \frac{abcde}{abcde}$$

To denote individual teeth this chart is abbreviated by drawing only that quadrant in which the tooth or teeth to be recorded are situated; the upper left second premolar is noted thus $|5$, the lower right first molar $6|$, the upper right lateral and upper left canine $2|3$, and so on.

It does not follow that every individual who loses a natural tooth requires its replacements by means of a partial denture, sometimes a bridge is a better alternative and also there are instances in which the replacement of lost teeth is considered inadvisable. Therefore the treatment for the patient who has

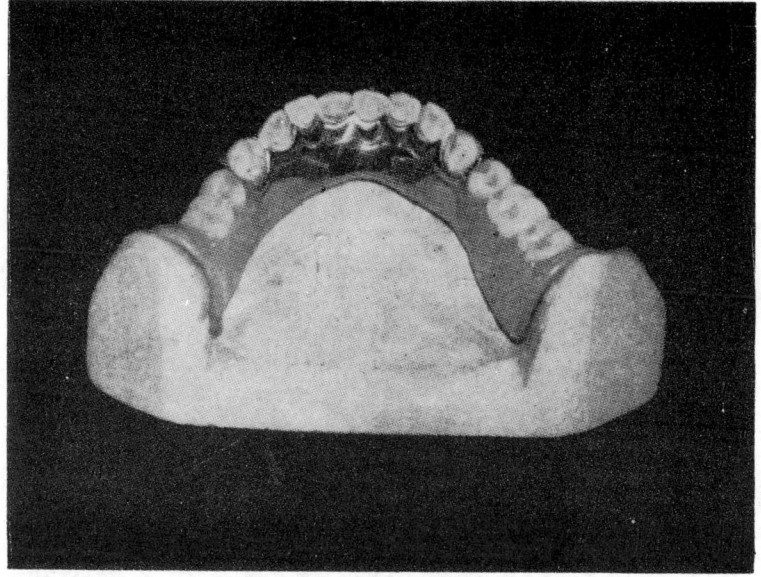

FIG. 324. – A partial denture.

lost one or more natural teeth can be effected in one of three ways:

(1) By fitting a partial denture.
(2) By fitting a bridge.
(3) By leaving the mouth as it is.

DEFINITION OF A PARTIAL DENTURE

A partial denture is an appliance, removable by the wearer, for the replacement of one or more natural teeth in the mandible or maxilla in which one or more natural teeth remain. It occupies more space than did the natural teeth which it replaces and is retained by its intimate contact with the mucosa and remaining natural teeth (fig. 324).

DEFINITION OF A BRIDGE

A bridge is an appliance which is fitted to two or more natural teeth prepared for, and restored by, inlays or crowns. It occupies no more space than did the natural teeth it replaces and it may be either permanently fixed in position or removable by the wearer (fig. 325).

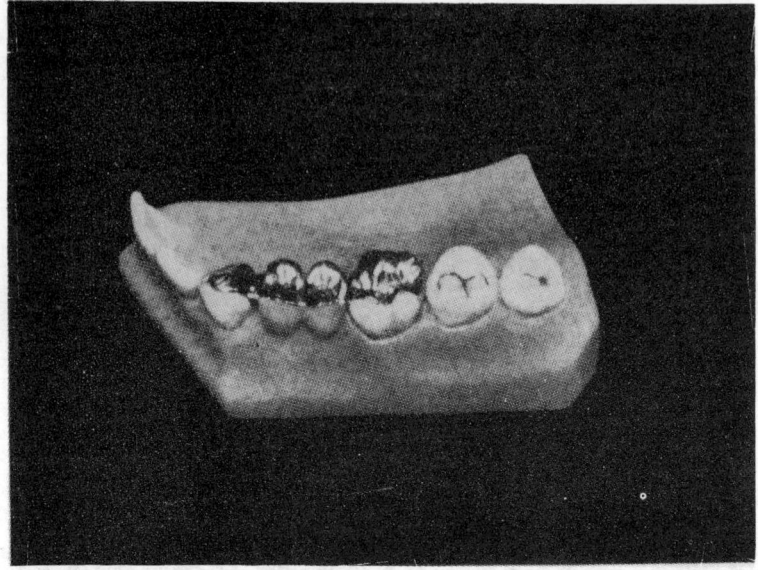

Fig. 325. – A bridge (constructed by Mr. E. Rosenstiel).

It must be pointed out that these definitions do not apply to American dental literature and skeleton dentures in England are frequently called removable bridges in the U.S.A.

THE FUNCTIONS OF A PARTIAL PROSTHESIS

When a mouth is examined in which some natural teeth are missing a decision has to be reached as to whether the replacement of the lost teeth by artificial substitutes, be it a partial denture or a bridge, will benefit the patient and if so what will be the most suitable type of restoration. To find the answer to each individual case it is necessary carefully to assess the advantages of a partial prosthesis against the disadvantages. A partial prosthesis functions in one, or more, of three ways.

(1) It restores masticatory efficiency.

Whilst it is an accepted fact that with the more highly civilized healthy peoples, living as they do on soft cooked foods, teeth are not necessary to maintain life, nevertheless most people consider it essential to have sufficient teeth to be able to masticate normal food with ease. The effect of long-continued inefficient mastication on a healthy alimentary system is difficult to assess but in individuals already suffering from digestive troubles, or other debilitating conditions, masticatory efficiency assumes great importance and its restoration may become a vital matter.

(2) It restores appearance and speech.

The commonest reason for a request by a patient for a partial denture is that of restoration of appearance. Many people will ignore the loss of the majority of their posterior teeth but demand the immediate replacement of a lost upper incisor.

Speech is often affected by the loss of the upper incisor teeth so that the labio-dental and linguo-dental sounds, particularly, undergo loss in quality (*see* Chapter X).

(3) It prevents collapse of the dental arch and over-eruption of teeth.

When a tooth is extracted from a normal dental arch the teeth adjacent to it, unless prevented from so doing by the occlusion, tend to drift towards each other, thus reducing the width of the gap made by the extraction. This causes these teeth to lose contact with the teeth adjacent to them and food can then pack between them with consequent damage to the gums and increased liability to caries (*see* fig. 326). Loss of occlusion will often cause over-eruption and this, if gross, may mean the loss of that tooth (*see* figs. 327–331). Thus two or three teeth extracted from different parts of the mouth, if not replaced with a prosthesis, may in a few years lead to complete collapse of the dental arch which rapidly leads to further loss of teeth. One point which cannot be emphasized too strongly when dealing with arch collapse concerns patients of school-age. Immediate replacement of lost incisors is imperative as otherwise lengthy orthodontic treatment (often 1–2 years) will be needed to regain the lost space. A delay of a few days in fitting a denture or space-maintainer after the loss of an incisor may result in appreciable loss of space.

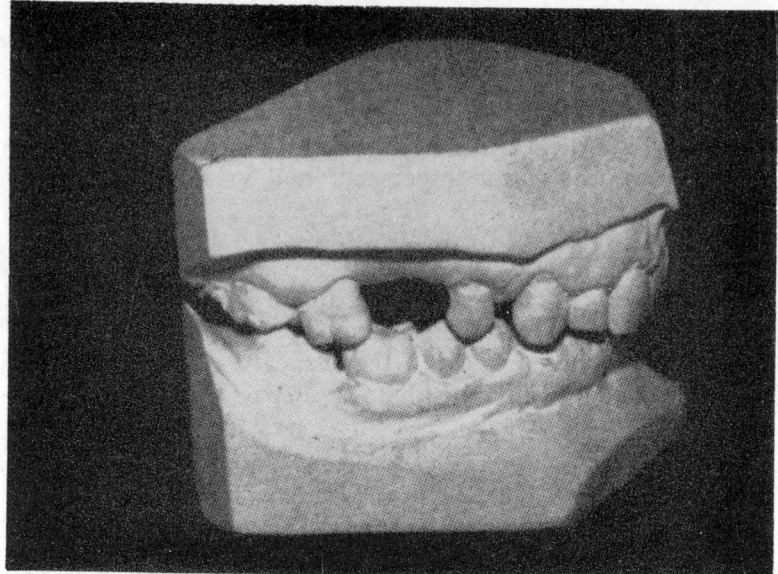

FIG. 326. – 4| has drifted backwards as a result of the failure to replace 65| with a denture.

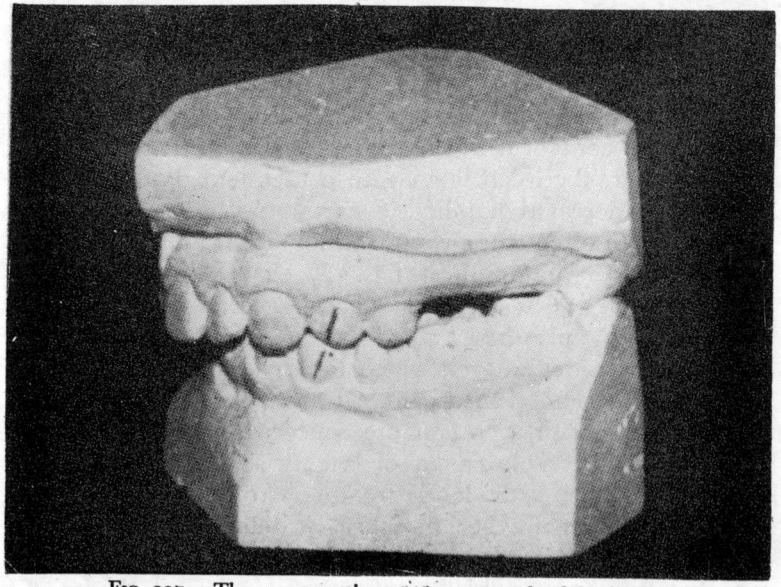

FIG. 327. – The over-eruption of |67 as a result of the failure to replace |67 with a denture.

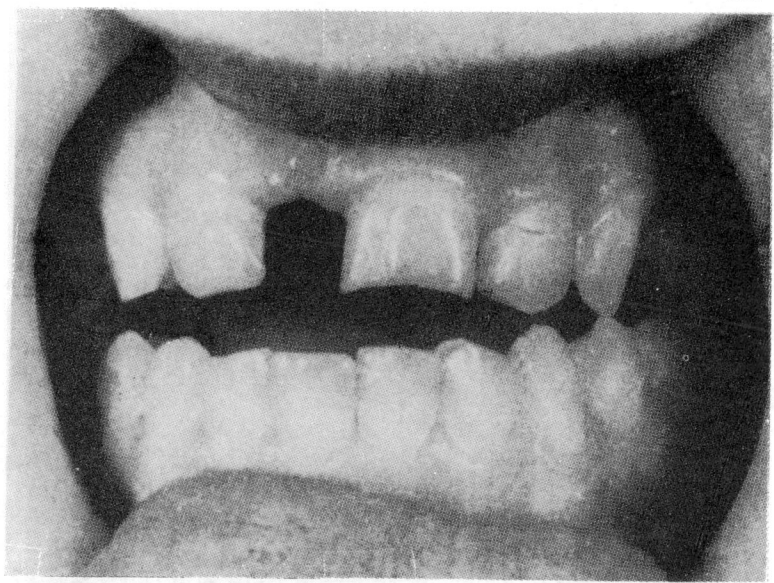

FIG. 328. – Closure of space in four weeks resulting from loss of 1/.

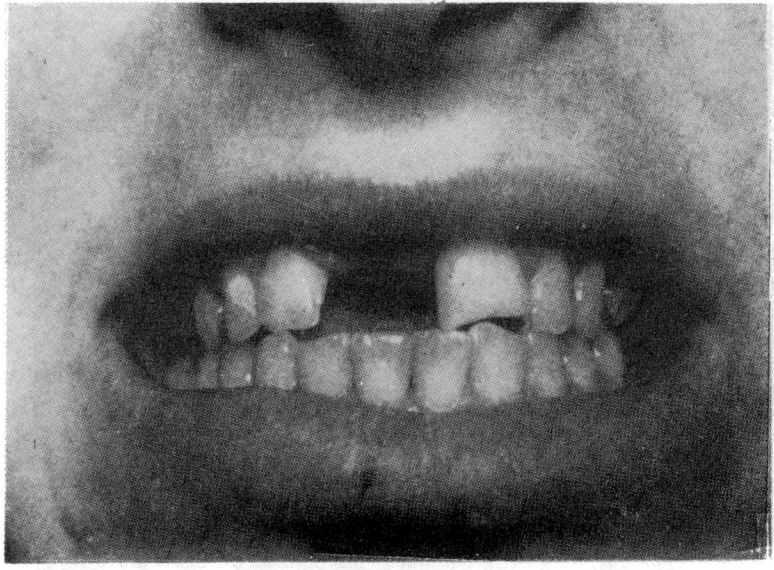

FIG. 329. – Space slightly over-restored by orthodontic treatment.

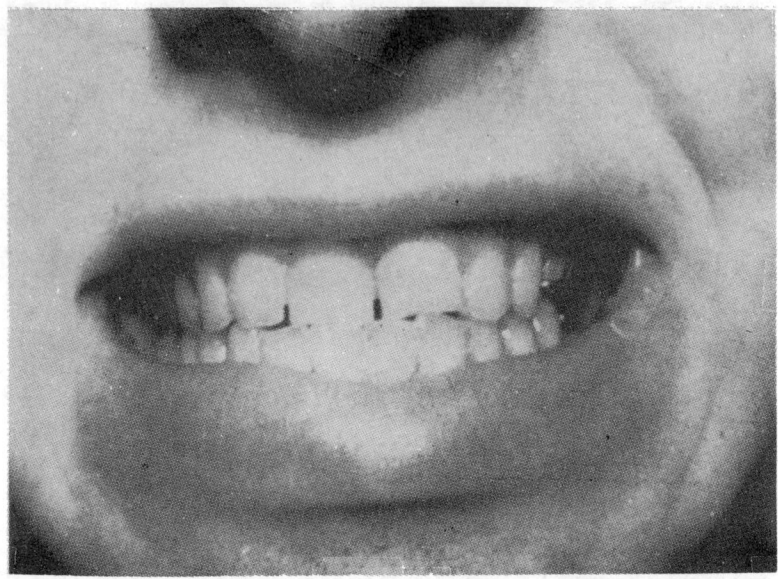

FIG. 330. – Denture replacing 1/ fitted and /1 allowed to return to correct position.

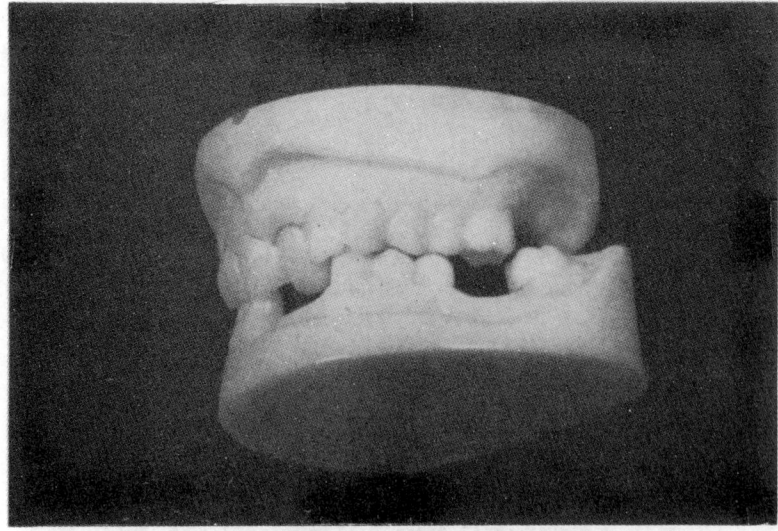

FIG. 331. – /12 extracted and /1 has been pulled backwards and downwards into space by powerful lower lip (six weeks after extraction).

The Disadvantages of a Partial Denture

(1) It can cause caries.

By harbouring food debris in close contact with the natural teeth a partial denture may promote caries. This will depend on several factors, chief of which are:

(a) The age of the patient. Up to the age of 25 years caries susceptibility is greatest, thereafter it tends to decrease.

(b) The habits of the patient. If the patient is very assiduous in cleaning his teeth and denture then less damage is likely to ensue.

(c) The design of the denture. This is all important because well designed dentures will cause far less damage to the mouth than those of thoughtless design (see Principles of Partial Denture Design). The caries which may result from denture wearing can be reduced by regular dental attention and partial denture wearers should always be advised of the necessity of regular dental inspection.

(2) It can damage the supporting tissues of the teeth.

In a healthy mouth the gum margins fit closely round the necks of the teeth, rising to a pointed crest between them; they are firm in texture and pink in colour. Their integrity is usually maintained in a well developed dentition because:

(a) Adjacent teeth are firmly in contact mesially and distally and, therefore, food cannot pack down between them and apply trauma to the gingival margins.

(b) The buccal, labial, lingual and palatal surfaces of the teeth are convex so that food passing over these surfaces strikes the gum below their free margin (see fig. 332). Any alteration in

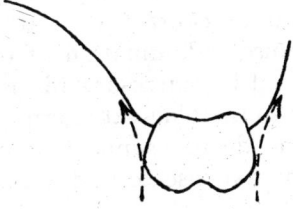

Fig. 332. – The arrows indicate the direction which the food takes as a result of the bulbous form of a tooth.

this arrangement which causes force to be applied directly to the free gum margins will tend to push the margin away from its contact with the tooth and thereby damage it.

Partial dentures may cause damage to the gum margins by:

(a) Fitting too closely into the gingival trough and causing mechanical injury to it (see figs. 333–336).

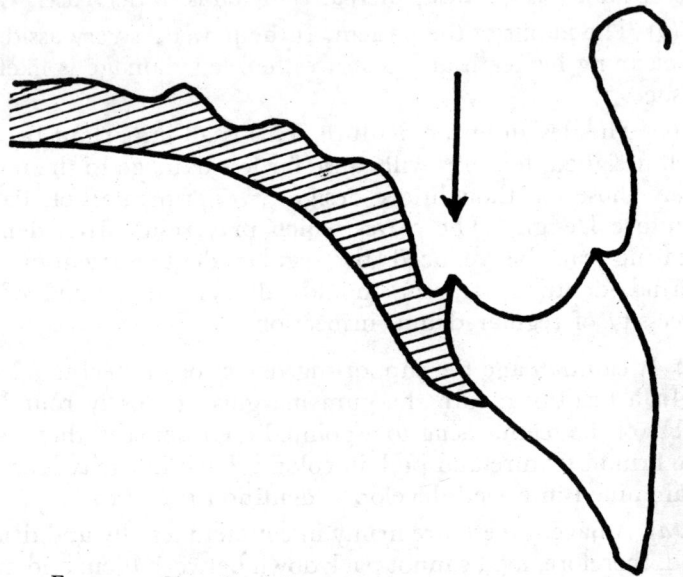

FIG. 333. – Close fit of denture base into gingival margin. Very traumatic.

(b) Allowing food to pack down between the denture and the teeth. Food packed under pressure against the gingival margins will force them away from the teeth (see fig. 337) and will also, if allowed to remain in contact with the gingivae for any appreciable time, cause inflammation of the tissues resulting from the toxins formed by micro-organisms incubating in this nidus. Such damage to the gingival margins, if untreated, progresses to involve the deeper supporting tissues of the teeth giving rise to periodontal disease and ending with the loss of the teeth.

(3) It may loosen the natural teeth by leverage.

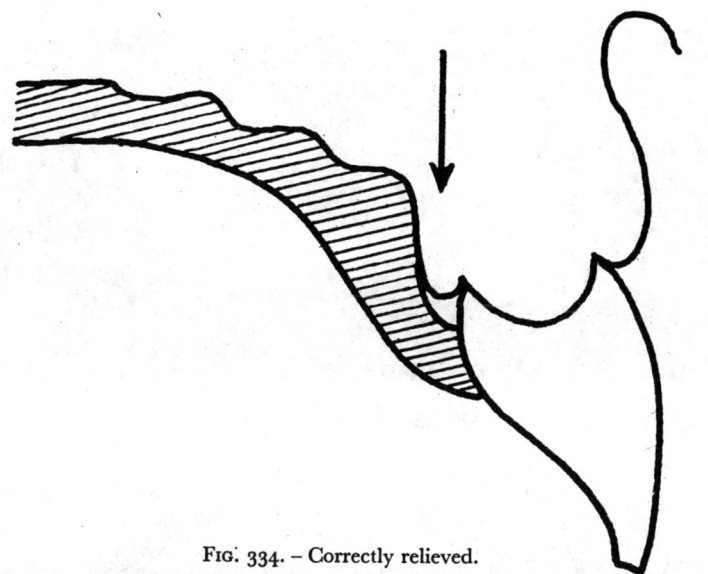

FIG. 334. – Correctly relieved.

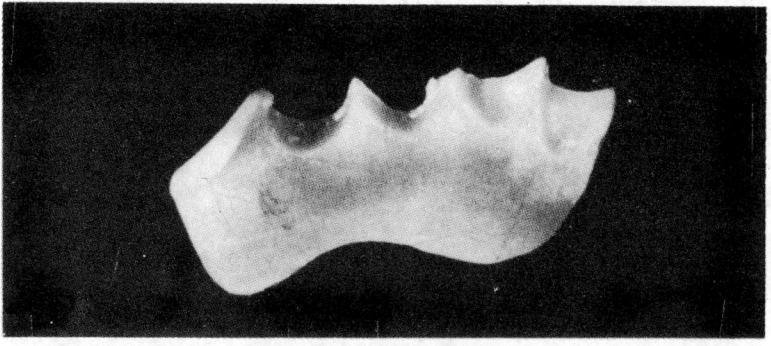

FIG. 335. – Sharp margin.

Clasps which grip the teeth too tightly or indirect retainers
(*see* Chapter XXI) which are badly placed may cause excessive
stresses to be induced in the natural teeth. This will be discussed at greater length in the section on design.

(4) It can cause traumatic damage to the palate as described
for full dentures on page 374 *et seq.*

All the types of damage which can be inflicted by a partial
denture are shown in figs. 338, 339.

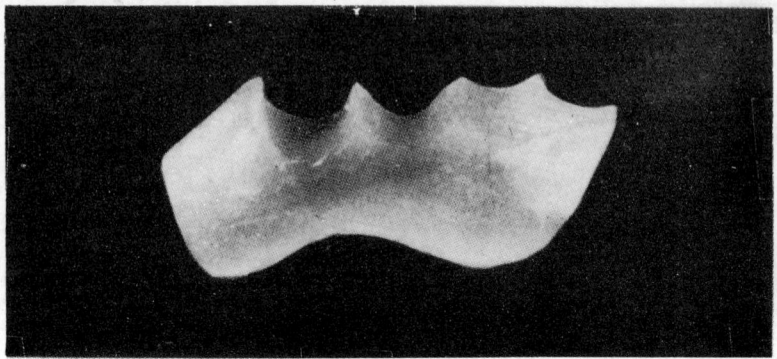

FIG. 336. – Correctly relieved.

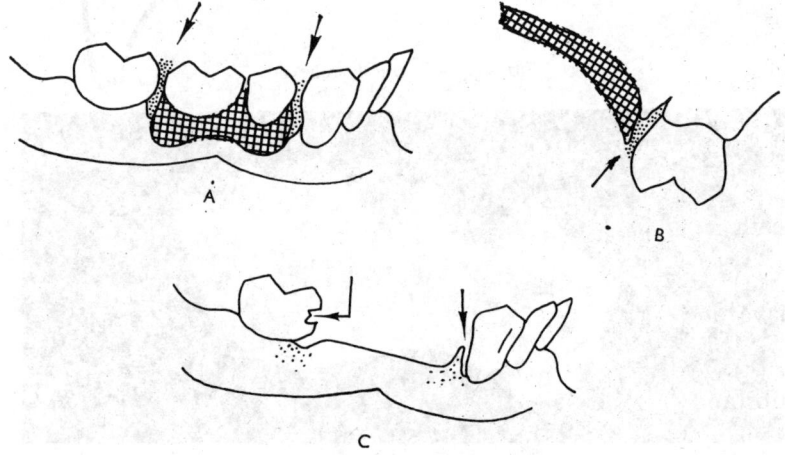

FIG. 337. – (a) and (b) food packing
(c) results of food packing

The advantages of dentures over bridges are:

(1) They can be constructed for any case, whilst bridges are confined to short spans bounded by healthy teeth and with a fairly normal occlusion.

(2) They can be constructed of plastic material and therefore more cheaply.

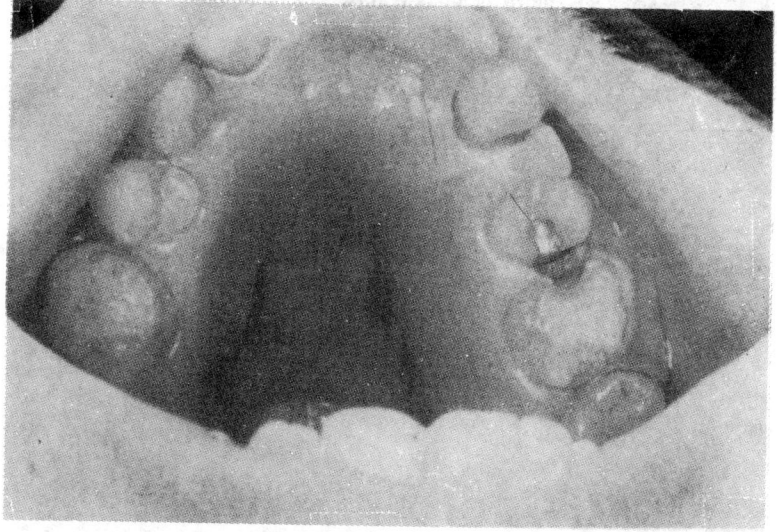

FIG. 337(d). – Gaps between teeth and denture allow food packing.

(3) They are more easily cleaned as are also the natural teeth in contact with them.

(4) They are more easily repaired and in many cases can have additions made to them.

(5) They do not normally involve the loss of natural tooth substance.

THE ADVANTAGES OF BRIDGES

The selection of the most suitable type of restoration for any given case cannot be fully discussed in a textbook on dentures. Instances occur in the following chapters in which a bridge would be preferable to a partial denture but in order to avoid confusion such a possible line of treatment is not discussed. However, the following advantages and disadvantages of bridgework need consideration when deciding upon the treatment for any case requiring a prosthesis.

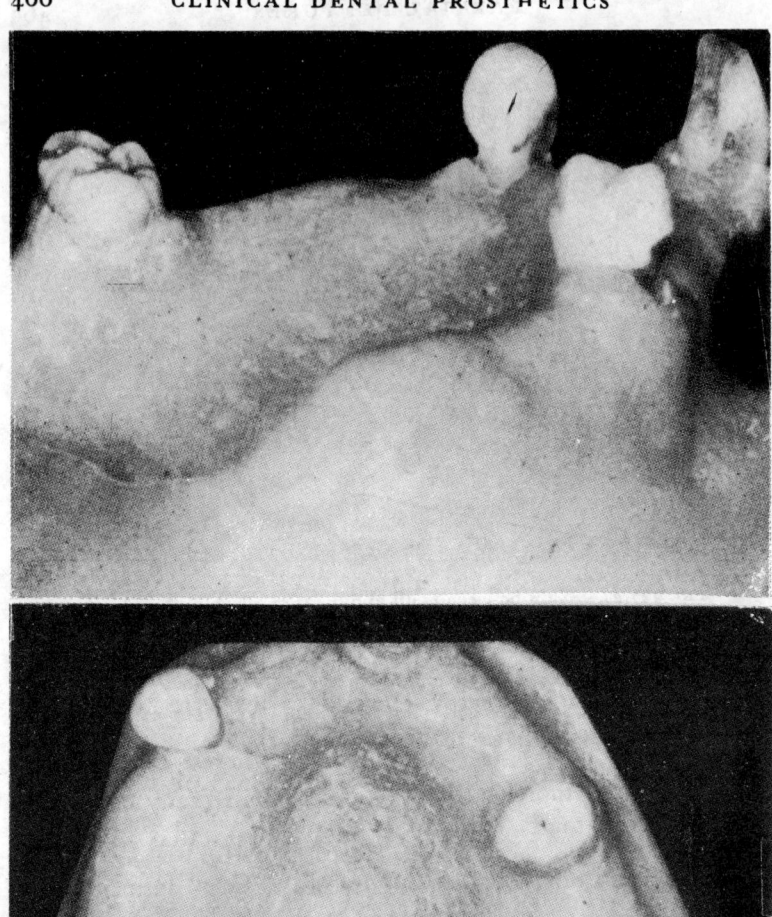

FIGS. 338 and 339. — The types of damage which partial dentures can inflict. Note: stripped gingival margins round 7 3/; granular hyperplasia of palate; hyperplastic ridge at back of palate; caries /4 caused by ill-fitting clasp.

The Advantages of Bridges over Partial Dentures are:

(*a*) They require no support from the mucous membrane and in fact in many instances they are not even in contact with it.

(*b*) They only occupy the same space as the natural teeth which they replace (with the sole exception of the 'Cantilever' bridge), and therefore feel more natural in the mouth.

(*c*) They will withstand greater masticatory loading than dentures, except when the latter are tooth-borne (Chapter XIX).

(*d*) Under no conditions is the wearer conscious of movement nor can he produce it with his tongue and thus habits of playing with the bridge are not induced.

As a result of the above advantages they feel more natural in the mouth and the wearer more readily becomes accustomed to them.

The Disadvantages of Bridges over Partial Dentures

(*a*) They are confined to short spans bounded by healthy teeth in good positions and alignment whilst dentures can be constructed for any case.

(*b*) Their construction is time consuming, requiring great precision, and is therefore expensive compared with the simpler construction of a plastic partial denture which is therefore less expensive.

(*c*) Since the majority are fixed in the mouth they are not so easily cleaned. Food debris tends to lodge between the bridge and the abutment teeth encouraging caries and periodontal disease.

(*d*) If damaged their repair is often difficult and costly.

(*e*) Frequently sound natural teeth have to be prepared for inlays or crowns to act as supports for the bridge.

(*f*) A natural tooth, lost at a later date, may often be replaced by a simple addition to a partial denture. A bridge can seldom if ever be adapted in this manner.

Cases Best Left Without Dentures

The decision not to fit a prosthesis when natural teeth are missing is usually a difficult one to make. If such a course is contemplated it is advisable to make a periodical examination of the mouth to ensure that no harmful effects result from the decision not to restore missing teeth.

As a general guide, the following questions should be answered and if these are mainly in the *negative* then the probability is that the patient will be better off without a denture.

(1) Is mastication inefficient with the remaining natural teeth?

(2) Is appearance and speech adversely affected?

(3) Is the occlusion of the teeth such that there is a possibility of over-eruption or tooth drift occurring?

(4) Will the benefits of a prosthesis outweigh the possible damage it may cause to the tissues?

(5) Does the patient maintain a careful oral hygiene, or is he likely to follow hygiene instruction?

(6) Are temporo-mandibular joint symptoms likely to develop as a result of a disturbed occlusion following the loss of teeth? (Chapter XXVI.)

(7) Is the patient's mental attitude to dentures satisfactory?

(8) Does the patient's medical history support the fitting of a partial prosthesis?

The answer to this last question may be the sole deciding factor regarding the fitting of a partial denture. (A prosthesis may be contra-indicated by a history of frequent and severe epileptic attacks).

Often one is confronted by a patient who has lost one or two posterior teeth in different parts of the mouth some time previously, adjacent teeth have drifted into the resultant spaces and there may have been some over-eruption. The question that arises is not, 'can damage be prevented', since it has already occurred, but one has to decide whether the damage will get worse if partial dentures are not constructed.

There are not many occasions when a partial denture is not necessary but the final conclusion can be obtained only after carefully weighing up the advantages and disadvantages in each individual case.

Chapter XIX

CLASSIFICATION OF PARTIAL DENTURES

Before proceeding to the principles of design of partial dentures it is necessary to know the various types of denture which can be constructed so that a correct choice may be made from the information obtained from the clinical examination and case history.

One method of dividing partial dentures into basic types is to consider the manner in which the pressure applied to the occlusal surfaces of the artificial teeth is transmitted to the body of the mandible and maxilla respectively. The masticatory loads which are ultimately taken up by the mandible and maxilla when the natural teeth are standing is through the medium of the natural teeth, periodontal membrane and alveolar bone. In the case of some partial dentures these structures may still transmit the masticatory loads and the denture is then termed tooth-borne. It is a type which has small projections called occlusal rests, which are placed on the occlusal surfaces of the natural teeth (Chapter XXI) so that the vertical masticatory loading is transmitted via the teeth bearing the rests and not via the mucosa underlying the denture (fig. 340). A second way in which the masticatory loading can be transmitted to the bone is through the interposed layer of mucosa A denture supported in this manner is termed tissue-borne and is one in which the vertical load is received directly by the mucosa without any assistance from the natural teeth (fig. 341). It may be braced against lateral loads by the standing teeth, which may also be fitted with clasps to aid in the retention of the denture. The vertical loading may also be transmitted partly by the teeth and partly by the mucosa, such a denture is referred to as tooth and tissue borne (fig. 342). Therefore, a very broad simple division of partial dentures can

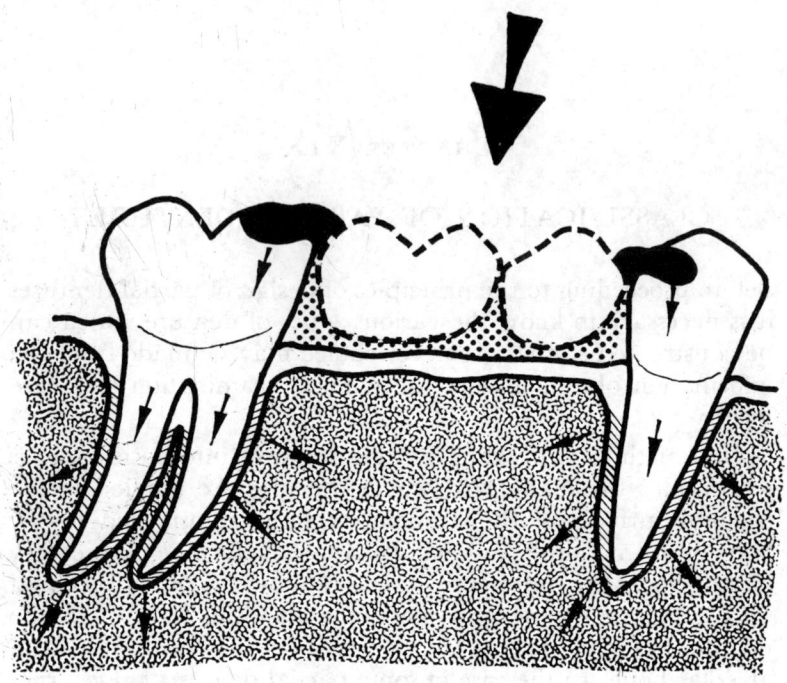

FIG. 340. – Occlusal load being transmitted to the bone via the rests and the teeth.

be based on the tissues which first receive the vertical load of mastication and they can be classified as:

(1) Tooth-borne.
(2) Tissue-borne
(3) Tooth and tissue borne.

The following should be considered when deciding upon the basic type of denture suitable for a given case.

(1) A tooth-borne denture can carry loads equal to those normally imposed on the natural teeth.

(2) Sound natural teeth or a tooth-borne denture will impose a greater load on the opposing teeth during mastication than a tissue-borne denture, due to the pain threshold of the mucosa compressed between the hard surfaces of the bone on one side and the denture base on the other side.

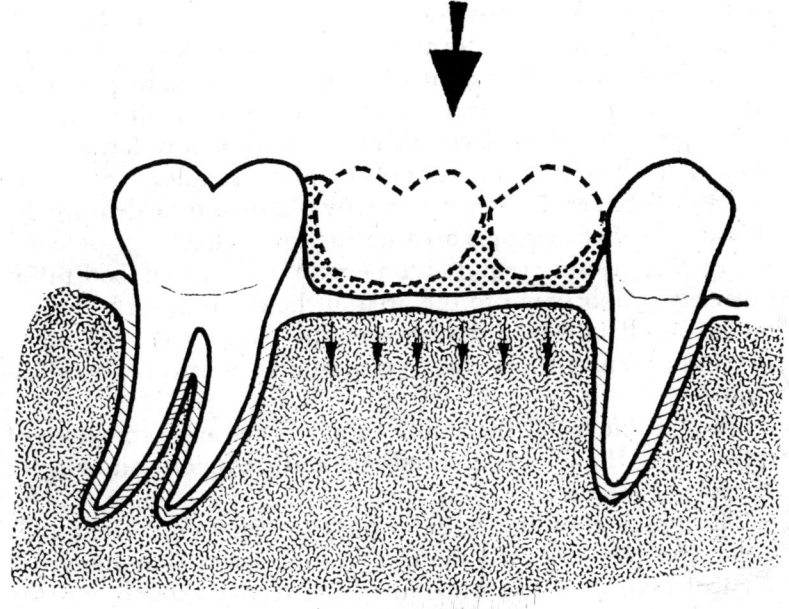

FIG. 341. – Occlusal load being transmitted to the bone via the mucous membrane.

(3) Occlusal rests must be strong enough to withstand the load applied to the denture but they must never prevent the even occlusion of the teeth.

It will frequently be necessary to create a special seating in the supporting tooth or to grind the opposing cusp, or both, in order to satisfy these two requirements (*see* figs. 412 and 413).

(4) Only premolar and molar teeth are suitable from their shape to carry occlusal rests. If a canine or incisor tooth is to be equally efficient, considerable operative work must be performed on it, even in some cases to the extent of crowning, in order to provide an adequate seat for the rest to resist vertical loading.

(5) Canines and incisors may sometimes be used to assist in resisting vertical loads particularly if taken together as a group of three or more teeth.

(6) If the resistance is to be through the mucous membrane, only the saddle areas are effective with a lower denture. The

lingual portion joining the saddles is nearly always too nearly vertical and so transmits very little of the vertical loading.

(7) An upper tissue-borne denture can usually spread the vertical load by covering at least some of the hard palate. A tissue-borne upper denture which only occludes with a tissue-borne lower denture does not need to cover any larger area than that covered by the sum of the lower saddles.

(8) The larger the area covered by a tissue-borne denture the smaller the load per unit area for any given load.

(9) The pressure required to penetrate any given foodstuff is inversely proportional to the area of the occlusal surface. This means in effect, that the narrower the teeth, bucco-lingually, the less muscular effort will be required to penetrate any given food.

The problem of the tooth and tissue-borne method of transferring the load is a vexed one and frequently the subject of misconception.

The opinion of the authors on this question is that it is impossible to construct a denture in such a way that any given vertical load is evenly distributed between the teeth and the mucous membrane. Further, where such an attempt is made an increasing load is placed on the teeth with the passage of time owing to alveolar absorption.

Consider the case of the saddle in fig. 342. In order to obtain an equal resistance to pressure by the mucous membrane as by the teeth the former must be compressed and distorted until further alteration in bulk and shape ceases and it will then act like a hard tissue and transmit any further load directly to the underlying bone. To obtain this result, a pressure of x lb. per inch will be required. At this exact pressure the occlusal rests must be seated on their respective teeth and thereafter any increased pressure will be evenly distributed, but at anything less than this exact pressure the denture will be entirely tissue-borne. If the occlusal rests are in contact with the teeth before this exact pressure is reached then the teeth are bearing more of the load than the mucous membrane, a condition which will inevitably arise when the supporting alveolar bone resorbs to the slightest extent. It is extremely unlikely that mucous membrane will tolerate this degree of pressure before the

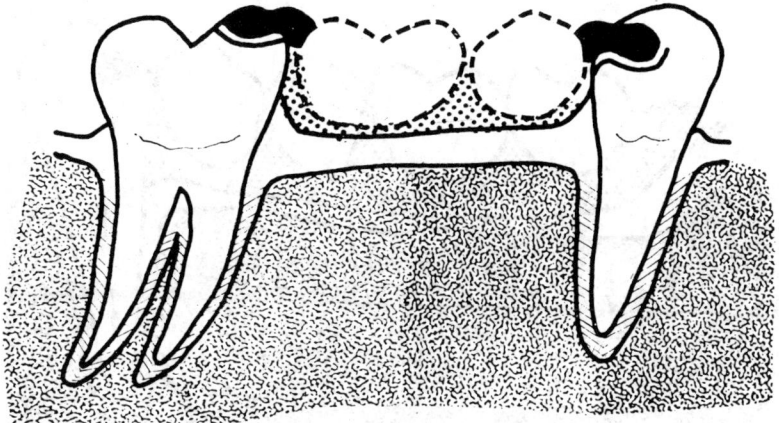

Fig. 342. – In this diagram the fitting surface of the denture saddle is in contact with the mucous membrane and the fitting surface of the occlusal rests are away from their seats in the teeth. When a load is applied to the denture the rests should be fully in place in their seats when the mucous membrane is compressed fully.

threshold of pain is reached so that the best that can be achieved is that the pressure is to some extent shared by the mucosa and this share is constantly diminishing in amount. Masticatory load is constantly varying and until this load equals that empirically chosen by the operator the denture will be entirely tissue borne and the more it exceeds this chosen load the greater the proportion which will be taken by the teeth till the denture becomes virtually tooth-borne.

The few advocates of tooth and tissue-borne dentures have never been able to suggest any method by which the optimum pressure for any given case may be assessed nor does it appear possible that such a method could be evolved.

This type of uneven loading is not infrequently seen when an attempt is made to make a free-end saddle tooth and tissue borne. If fig. 343 is observed it will be appreciated that the rest in the distal fossa of the first premolar will support the load of the saddle anteriorly whilst the mucous membrane in the third molar region must support the load at the other end of the saddle, thus leaving the mucous membrane along the main length of the saddle with a diminishing load to

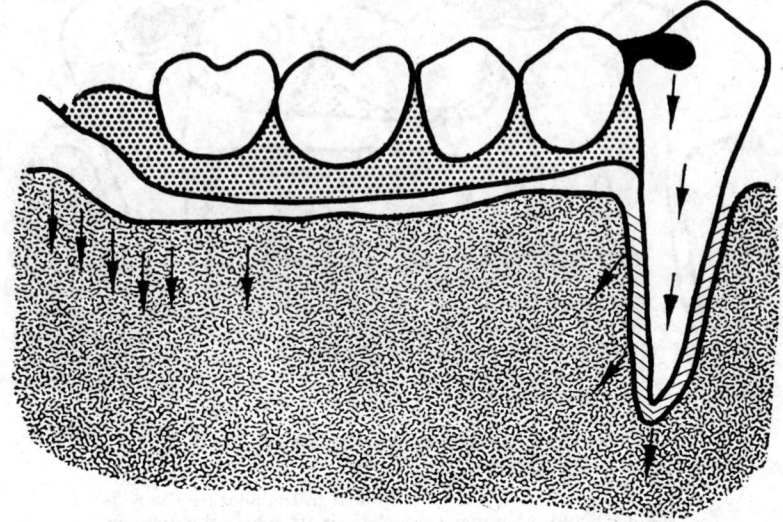

Fig. 343. – When a free end saddle is fitted with an occlusal rest – the arrows show where the concentrations of stress develop.

support. Such a state of affairs will overload the attachment of the premolar to the bone and probably lead to the early loss of this tooth and at the same time cause rapid absorption of the alveolar ridge at the distal end of the saddle. Fuller consideration is given to this problem in the appropriate section on actual design.

KENNEDY CLASSIFICATION

A further classification of partial dentures in general acceptance in this country is that devised by Kennedy, and, when used in conjunction with the forementioned classification, enables a fairly clear picture to be formed in the mind of the type of denture under consideration during a discussion on partial dentures.

The Kennedy classification is based on the relationship of the saddles to the standing teeth and has four main groups with subdivisions where necessary.

Class I.   Bilateral free-end saddles posterior to the standing teeth (figs. 344 and 345).

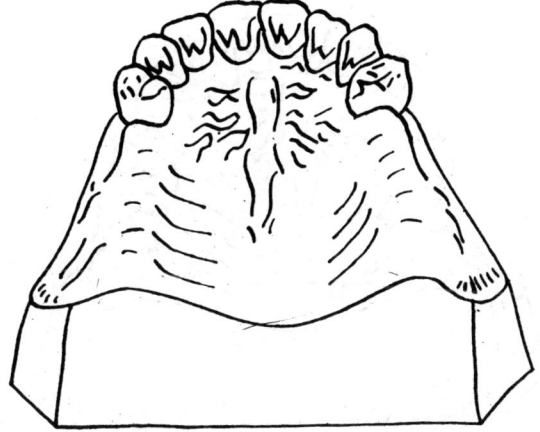

Fig. 344. - Kennedy Class I upper.

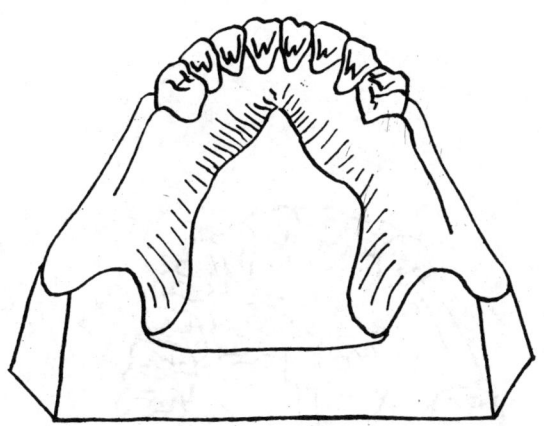

Fig. 345. - Kennedy Class I lower.

Class II.   Unilateral free-end saddle posterior to the standing teeth (fig. 346).

Class III. A bounded unilateral saddle having standing teeth either end (fig. 347).

Class IV.   A saddle anterior to the standing teeth (fig. 348).

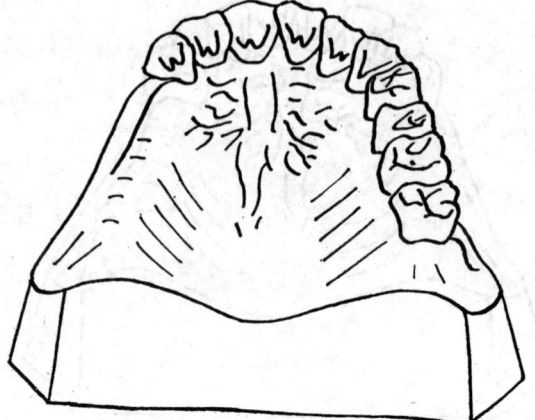

FIG. 346. – Kennedy Class II.

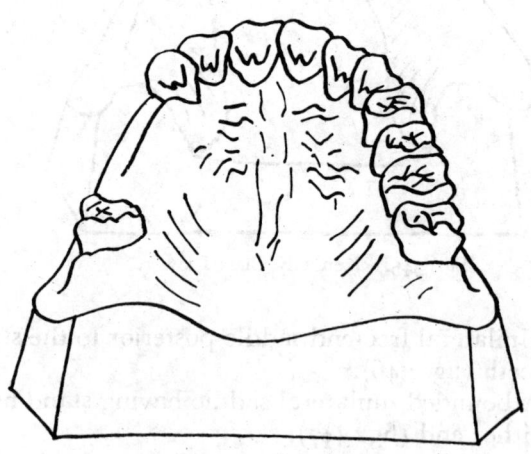

FIG. 347. – Kennedy Class III.

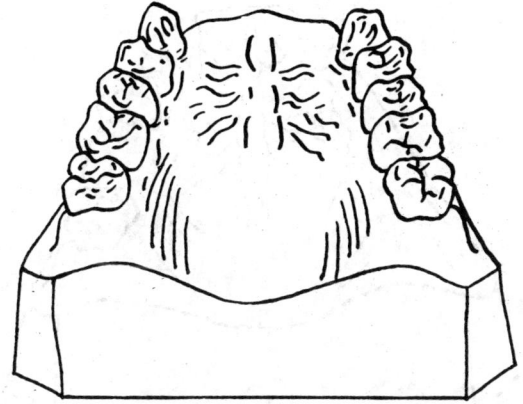

FIG. 348. – Kennedy Class IV.

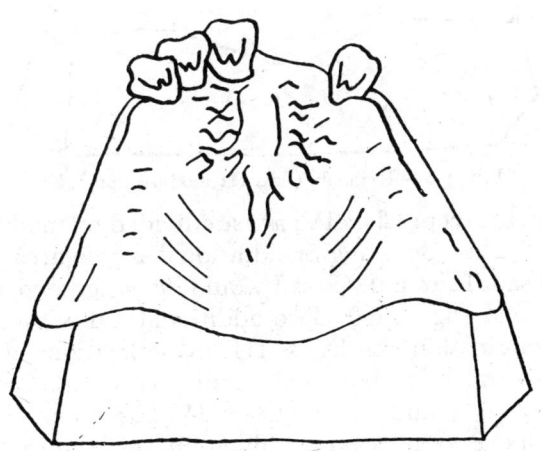

FIG. 349(a). – Kennedy Class I modification I.

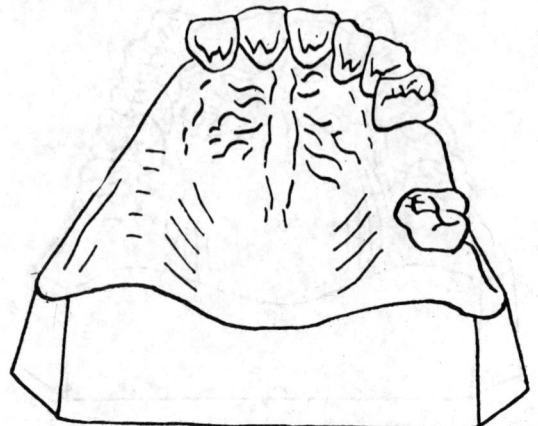

FIG. 349(*b*) – Kennedy Class II modification I.

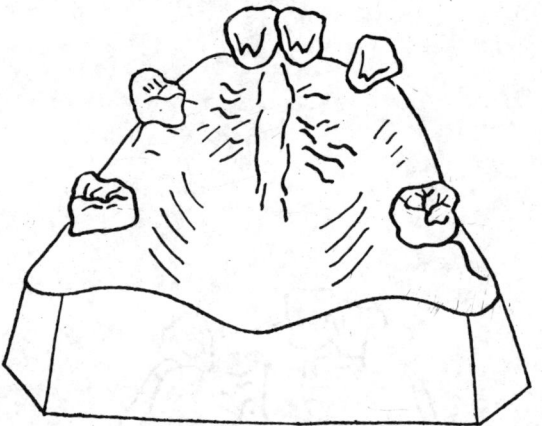

FIG. 350. – Kennedy Class III modification III.

All Classes, except Class IV, are subdivided by modifications, each modification denoting an additional saddle area. Thus an additional saddle area in Class I would be designated as Class I Modification I (fig. 349*a*). Two additional saddles would constitute Modification II Class III, Modification III would be a basic unilateral bounded saddle with three additional saddles, fig. 350, and so on. Class IV has no modifications since if such occurred then it would fall basically into one of the other Classes.

Chapter XX

THE COMPONENT PARTS OF A PARTIAL DENTURE

In order to be able to design a partial denture it is necessary to know the parts from which it is built and the function of each. These parts are:

(1) Saddles.
(2) Connectors.
(3) Direct Retainer (Clasps) (page 488).
(4) Indirect Retainers (page 525).
(5) Occlusal and Incisal Rests (page 530).

I. SADDLES

A saddle is that part of a denture which carries the artificial teeth. It can be either tooth or tissue-borne, as also can separate saddles in the same denture (*see* fig. 351).

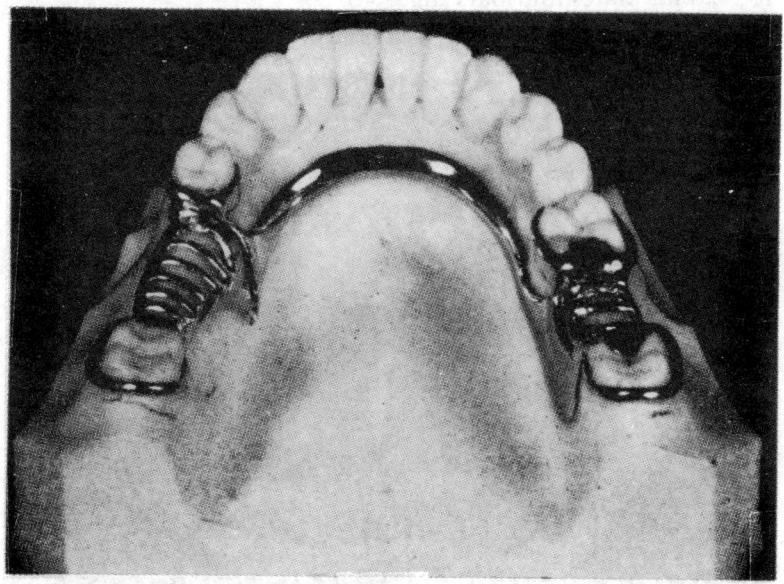

Fig. 351. – Partial lower denture tooth-borne on one side, tissue-borne on the other.

479

Dentures with tooth-borne saddles are generally made in metal since a strong material is necessary for the construction of occlusal rests and the metal should be capable of being cast so that an accurate fit of the occlusal rest to its seating can be obtained.

Dentures with tissue-borne saddles may be constructed either of metal or acrylic resin, but generally the latter for reasons of economy.

The periphery of the denture in the saddle regions should always reach to the functional depth of the sulcus and should be modified only in relation to the appearance when in the mouth.

2.   CONNECTORS

A connector is that part of a denture which joins one saddle to another, or, a clasp or indirect retainer to a saddle, and may be classified as follows:

(a) Palatal plates and bars, figs. 352 and 353.
(b) Lingual plates and bars, figs. 354 and 355.
(c) Labial plates and bars, fig. 356.
(d) Buccal plates and bars.

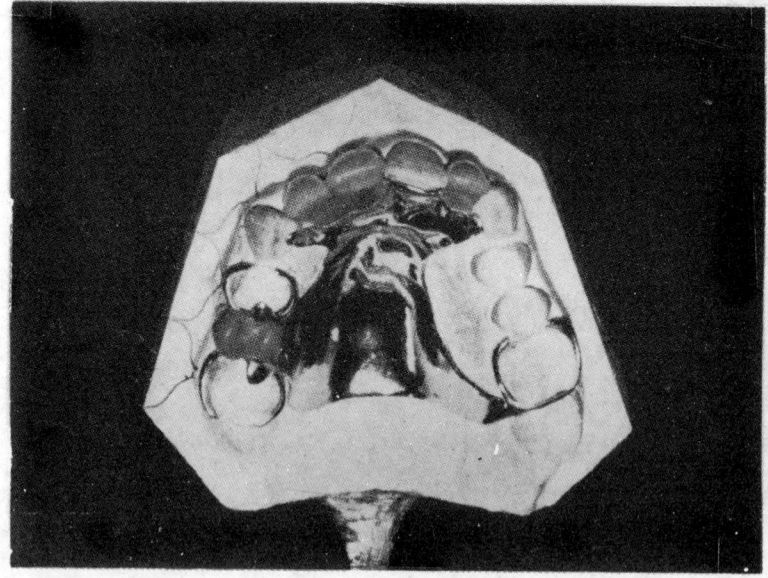

Fig. 352. – A palatal plate.

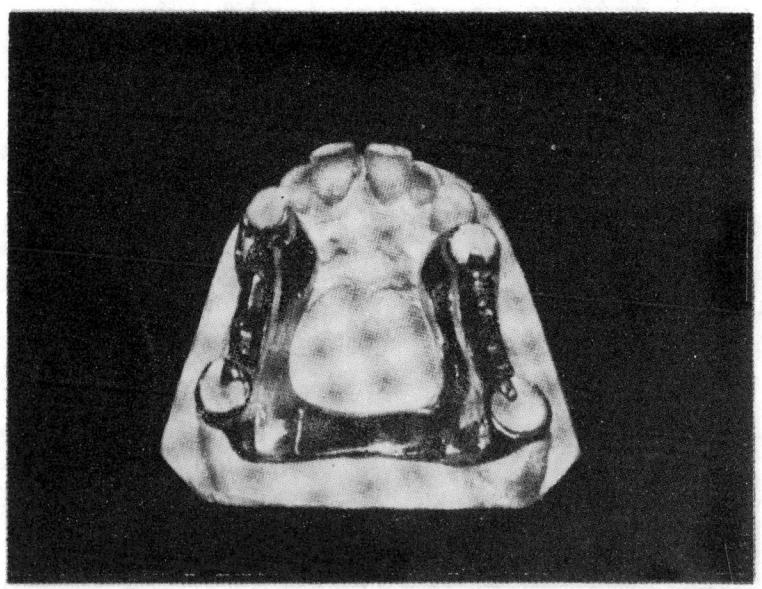

Fig. 353. – A palatal bar.

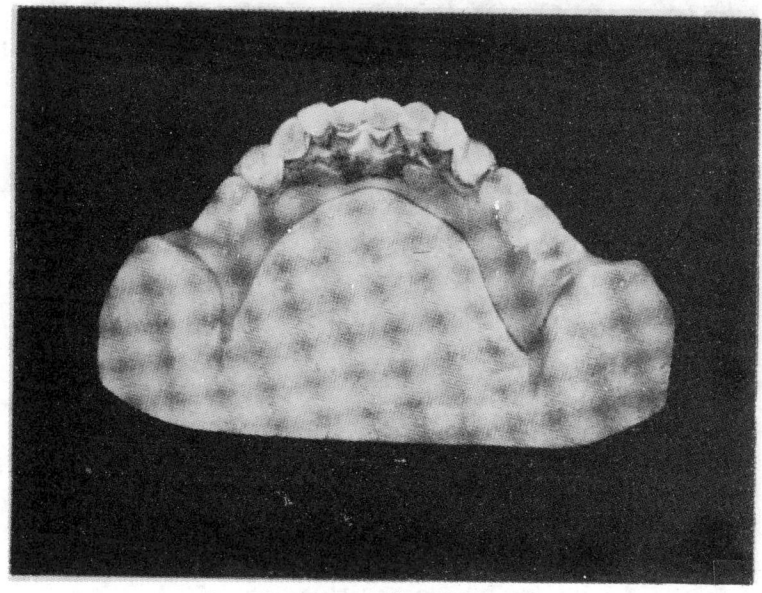

Fig. 354. – A lingual plate.

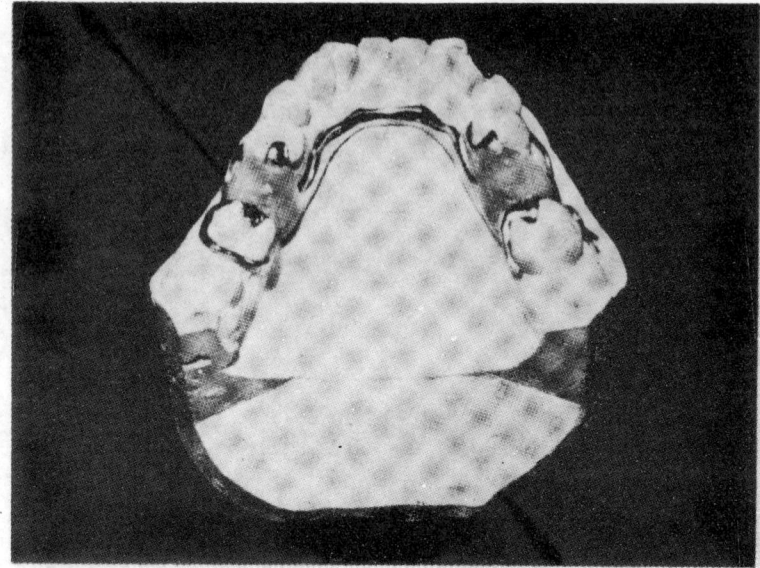

FIG. 355. – A lingual bar.

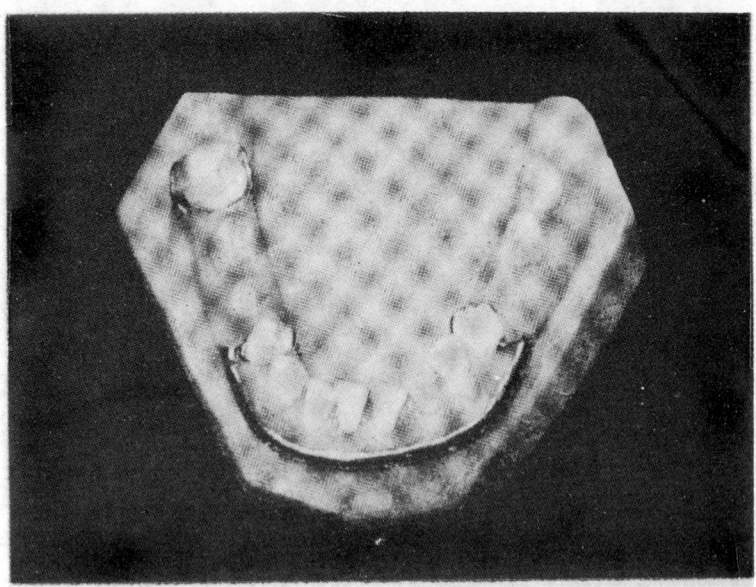

FIG. 356. – A labial bar.

Palatal Plates. – These should be kept as thin as possible consistent with the required strength and they should be dammed along free anterior and posterior borders in order that:

(i) The tongue may pass from mucous membrane to denture and vice versa, without encountering an edge.

(ii) Food particles may not so readily collect under the denture.

This damming must not be in any way excessive because in many parts of the hard palate the mucous membrane covering the bone is rather thin.

The advantages of palatal plates as opposed to palatal bars are:

(i) They are wider and therefore can be thinner in section than bars.

(ii) They can pass some of the loadings to the palate.

(iii) They can be constructed in non-metallic denture base materials when economy is a factor of construction.

(iv) They do not worry the tongue as much as the thicker palatal bar.

The disadvantage of the palatal plate is that it covers more tissue than a bar.

Palatal Bars. – These are always made of metal and should be as thin as possible commensurate with strength. They must fit accurately the palatal tissue, otherwise the wearer is conscious of a space existing between the bar and tissue and of food packing in this space. To ensure this close fit, when using alginate as the impression material, it is usually necessary to gently scrape the plaster model over the whole area covered by the bar (*see* fig. 357). If the denture is to be tooth-borne a compression impression will aid in establishing this close fit of bar to tissue. A combined composition and alginate impression as illustrated in fig. 358 will produce a close fit of the bar to the tissues. The composition and alginate are both loaded soft in the tray together. In tissue-borne dentures it may be necessary to form a relief on the model where the bar crosses a bony prominence covered by a thin mucosa.

The position of a palatal bar will vary according to the positions of the saddle areas to be connected and will be either in the region of the posterior third of the palate, or the middle

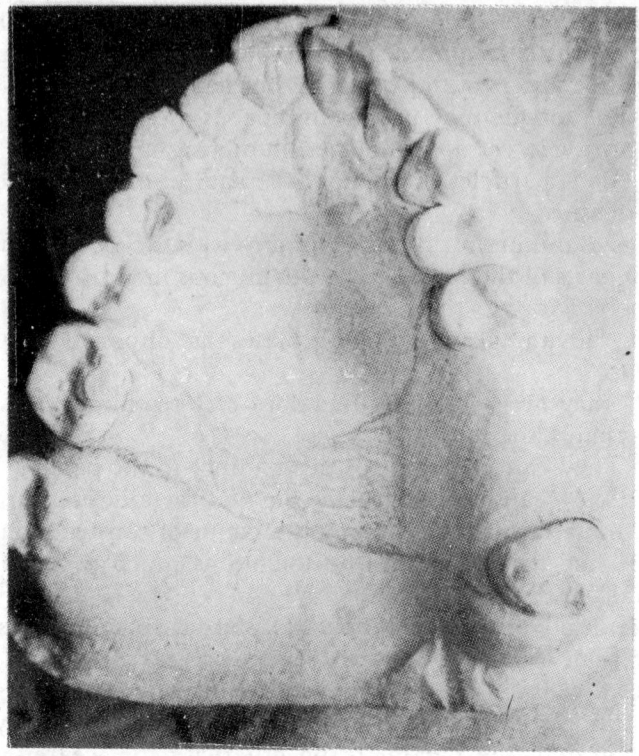

Fig. 357. – Model should be scraped slightly in area indicated by pencil shading to ensure close fit of palatal bar.

third, or the anterior third. The posterior palatal bar is the most suitable since it:

(i) Is less conspicuous to the tongue than the middle or anterior bars.

(ii) Often fulfils the function of an indirect retainer (page 525).

(iii) Is in an area less frequently associated with bony prominences or with thin mucosa.

The middle palatal bar is usually a source of annoyance to the patient, as it is positioned in an area where the tongue makes frequent contact with the palate during swallowing and speech.   It can seldom act as an indirect retainer.

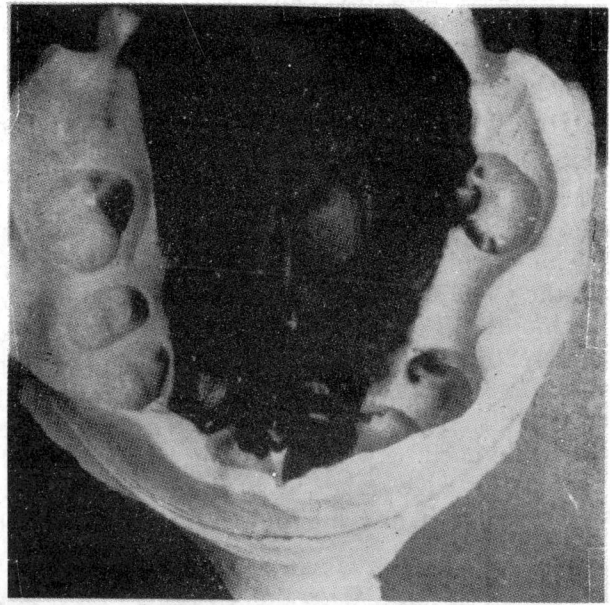

Fig. 358

The anterior palatal bar can be used in conjunction with the posterior bar to increase the rigidity and strength of the denture. It can also act as ·

(i) An indirect retainer
(ii) A link to an anterior saddle from posterior saddles.

When narrow, and therefore thick in cross section, they are not well tolerated by the tongue especially during speech. If a link between bilateral saddles is necessary in the anterior region then the broad bar or plate of thin section is tolerated better, particularly if the free edges are situated in the troughs between the rugae.

Lingual Plates. – These may be made of acrylic resin or metal. Acrylic is rather bulky and constricts the tongue in many instances, and should be avoided whenever possible. After construction, the gingival margins should be relieved by stoning away and polishing the projecting ridge of acrylic which is the counterpart of the gingival trough. Metal plates, provided adequate gingival relief is given are eminently satisfactory. They may be kept pleasantly thin and are delightfully smooth to the tongue. They must fit accurately around the cingulae of the teeth, and between the embrasures, or food will pack down on to the gingival margins and cause damage.

Lingual Bars. – These are usually made of metal and are used to connect two lower side saddles, or occasionally one lower side saddle with a clasp or stabilizer on the opposite side (*see* fig. 359). They should be placed midway between the gingival margins of the teeth and the highest functional position of the floor or the mouth. The cast lingual bar is the most satisfactory type to employ, but if a wrought bar is used then the long axis of the oval cross-section of the bar should be parallel with the underlying soft tissue; if it stands away on its superior edge food will more readily pack between it and the mucous membrane whilst if its inferior edge stands away the tip of the tongue is more likely to catch it and lift the denture. Tissue relief is

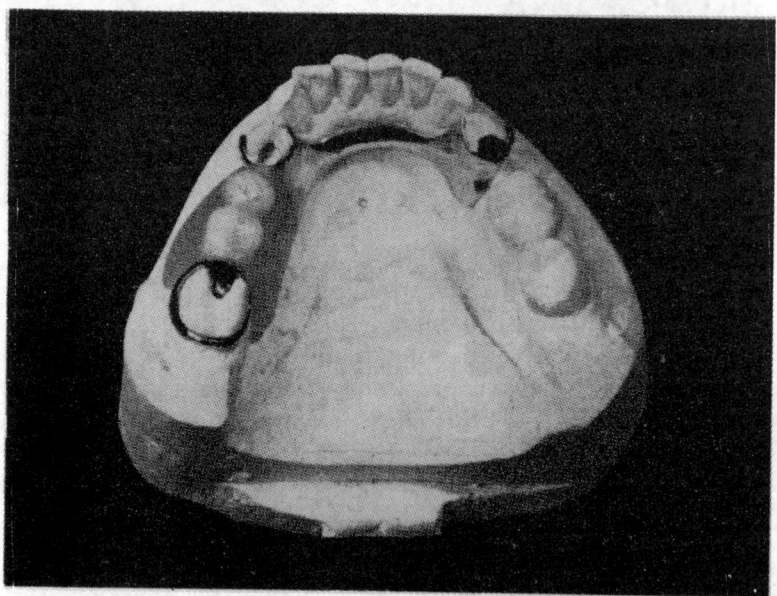

Fig. 359. – A lingual bar connecting one side saddle to a clasp on the opposite side.

provided during construction of the bar by swaging one thickness of gauge 4 tin foil over the surface of the model.

Contra-indications
   (i) Lack of space between functional position of the floor of mouth and gingival margins.
  (ii) Undercut lingual alveolar process.
 (iii) Lingually inclined teeth.

A second connecting bar, termed continuous clasp, positioned on the cingulae of the incisor teeth is sometimes incorporated with a lingual bar to act as an indirect retainer or rest, in tooth-borne dentures. It has the advantage over plates of keeping gingival margins free but it is not well tolerated by the tongue.

Labial and Buccal Bars and Plates. – These are always made of metal but are not used very extensively as they tend to worry the patient's lips. They may be used when lingual connectors are impracticable, due to lingual inclination of the standing teeth, or the presence of excessive lingual undercuts. They should be made as broad and as thin as the sulcus depth and strength of the metal will allow and relief must be provided during their construction, to allow for movement during mastication, similar to that for lingual bars. As they are longer relatively, than lingual bars, they must be greater in cross sectional area.

3. DIRECT RETAINERS

Unlike full dentures that rely on peripheral seal to establish retention by atmospheric pressure, adhesion and cohesion, partial dentures obtain their retention mainly from clasps attached to the denture which embrace natural teeth and thereby hold the denture in place (*see* figs. 360 and 361). Atmospheric pressure, adhesion and cohesion, however, do aid slightly in the retention of extensive partial dentures of the Kennedy Class I type, particularly in the case of the upper as the remaining natural teeth may stabilize the denture against excessive lateral movement enabling the limited peripheral seal obtained to be more effective in action. The tongue is a potent factor in the retention of a partial denture which has a broad palate (*see* fig. 362). The natural teeth also aid retention by presenting surfaces in contact with the denture which offer areas for frictional resistance to movement but, next in order of importance to clasps as a retaining factor is the use of under-

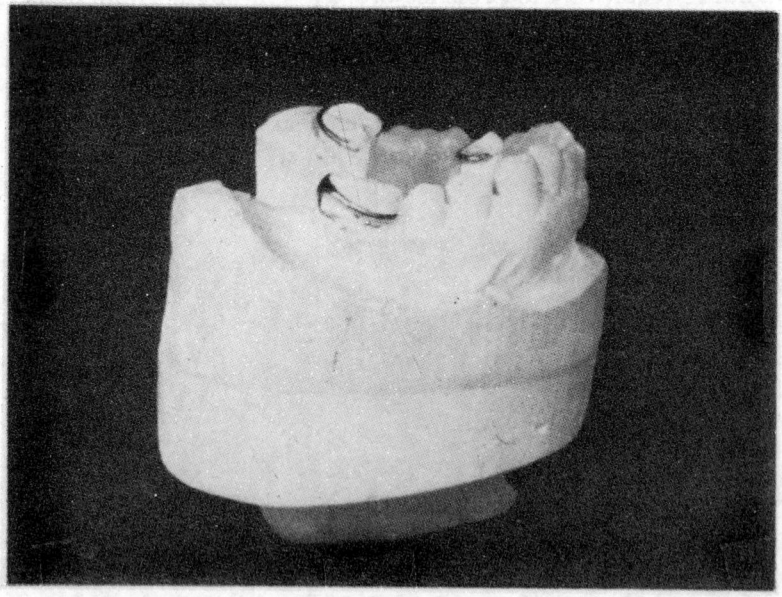

FIG. 360. – Clasps.

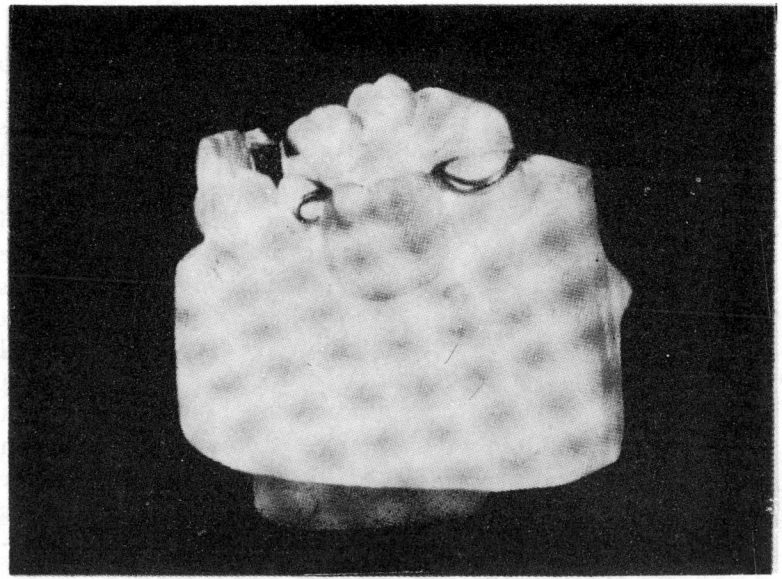

FIG. 361. – Various types of clasp.

cut areas both of the teeth and the soft tissue. In order to use these undercut areas it is necessary to know their precise limits; this requires the use of a surveyor.

REASONS FOR SURVEYING

A partially edentulous mouth has many undercut areas which result from:

(a) The naturally bulbous shape of the crowns of the teeth (fig. 363).

(b) The fact that the long axes of the teeth are frequently inclined at an angle to a vertical taken from the occlusal plane (fig. 364).

(c) The soft tissue and underlying bone being inclined at an angle to a vertical taken from the occlusal plane (fig. 365).

Rigid denture bases and the rigid parts of clasps will not pass

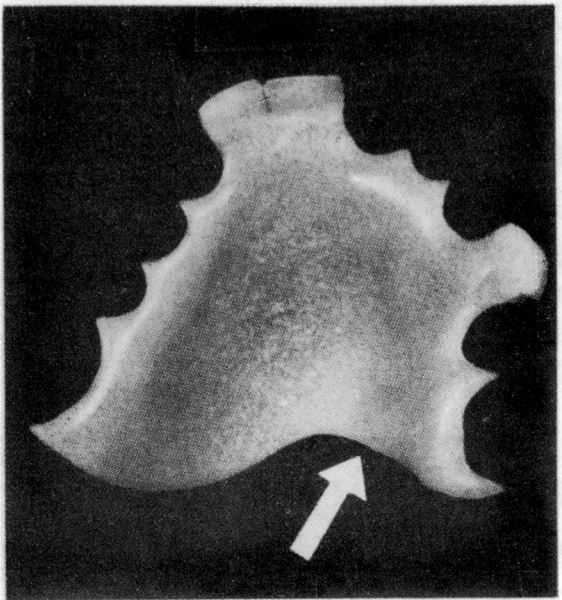

Fig. 362. Note tartar deposited on this denture and the area on the left completely free (arrowed). This is due to the constant pressure of the tongue in that area to counteract the tilting loads applied to the incisor teeth.

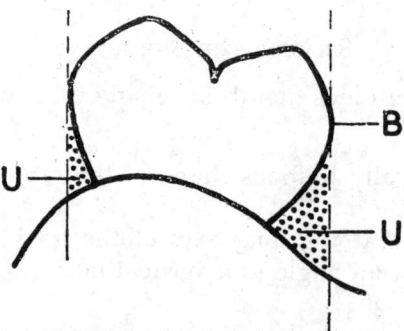

Fig 363. – Illustrating how the naturally bulbous shape of a tooth produces undercut areas.
B = the most bulbous part of the tooth.
U = the undercut areas.

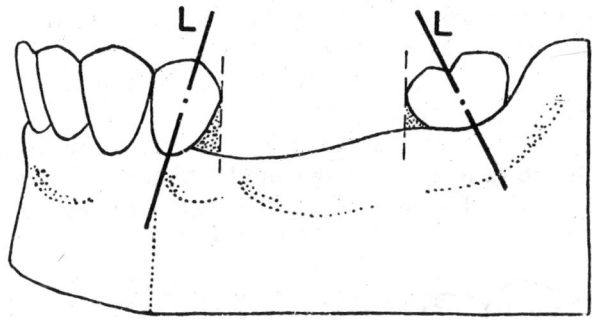

FIG. 364. – Illustrating how a slope of the long axis (L) of a tooth produces an undercut area.

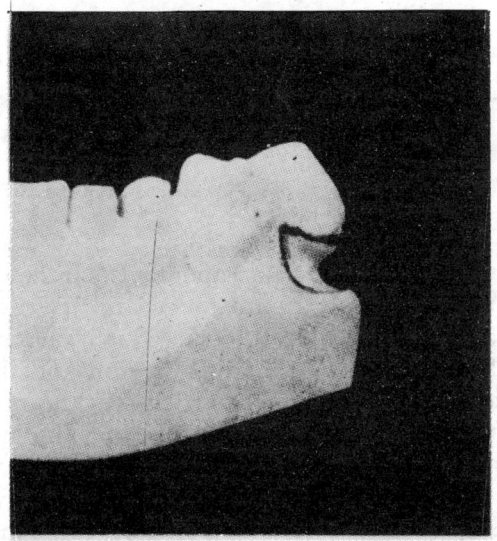

FIG. 365. – Undercuts in tuberosity region surveyed for blocking out.

into undercuts. (An undercut may be defined as an area which is out of contact with any vertical dropped from a given horizontal.) Therefore it is essential for the designer of a partial denture to be able to determine these areas on the model. The technique of this is termed surveying.

Surveying is accomplished by holding a vertical marking device such as a graphite lead, in contact with the crown of the tooth and moving either the model or the lead so that the side of the lead draws a line around the circumference of the crown and its point draws a line, which is the projection of that on the crown, on to the model of the soft tissues (*see* fig. 366 *a* and *b*). The area enclosed between these two lines is

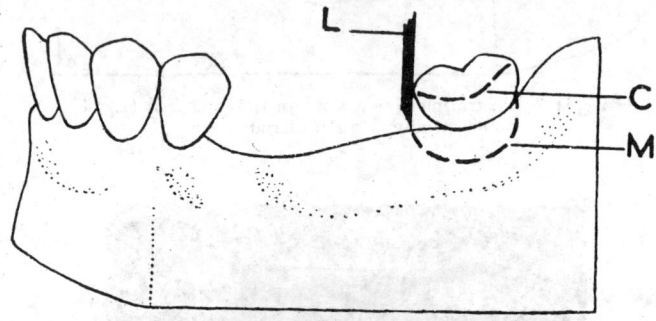

Fig. 366(*a*). – The basis of surveying.
L = vertical graphite lead.
C = the line drawn by the lead on the crown of the tooth.
M = the line drawn on the model.

undercut. Similarly the soft tissue undercuts can be delineated by a line marking the maximum bulge and its vertical projection on to the adjacent soft tissue. Such undercut areas are frequently found in the tuberosity region and the lingual alveolar region of the mandible, particularly the molar area. If these soft tissue undercut areas are not indicated and eliminated the rigid denture base will not pass over the maximum bulge and enter the undercut, except in cases where the undercut is slight and the mucosa covering the bone is thick and compressible.

SURVEYORS

Many different instruments are available for surveying but they all work on the principle of the vertical lead. They consist of a firm horizontal base, a mechanism which supports the marking device and enables it to be raised and lowered, and a table to which the model may be attached, and which may be tilted so as to alter the horizontal axis of the model. The

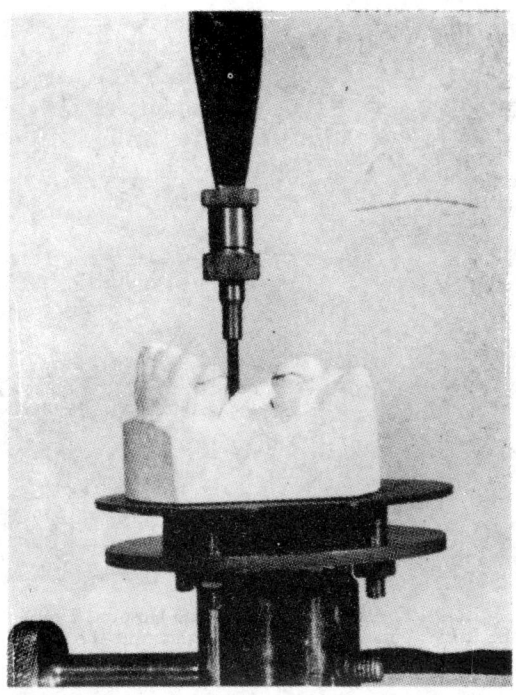

FIG. 366 (*b*). – Lead of surveyor marking the most bulbous
part of the tooth and its projection on the model.

reason for tilting will become apparent in due course. Such an
instrument is shown in fig. 367.

THE VALUE OF SURVEYING A MODEL

Surveying serves six purposes:

(1) It enables undercuts to be accurately blocked out on the
model prior to the processing or casting of the denture, so that
the material of the base does not enter the undercuts and
prevent the denture from being inserted (*see* figs. 368 and 369).
Two methods are commonly employed for blocking out the
undercuts on the model.

(*a*) The area between the survey line on the tooth and that
on the mucous membrane may be filled in with plaster of

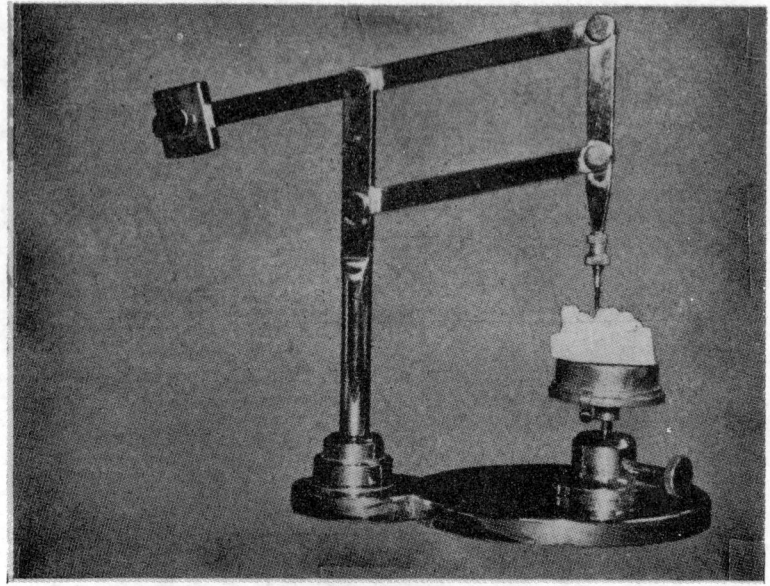

Fig. 367. – A Surveyor (King's College Hospital Type). The tilting table contains a powerful magnet and the model has an iron ring cast into its base; this obviates the necessity for any fixing agent such as plasticine.

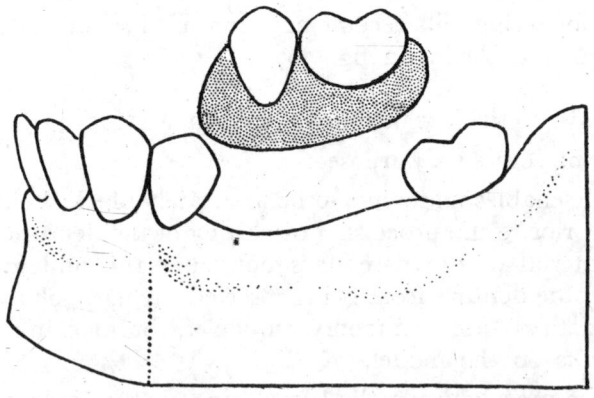

Fig. 368. – A denture which has been processed on a model, the undercuts of which were not blocked out. The denture will not go into place.

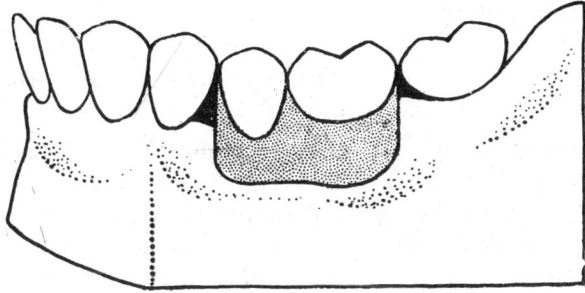

FIG. 369. – Undercuts correctly blocked out, the denture goes into place.

Paris, dental cement, wax, or composition, using the lines drawn by the lead as guides.

(b) The area may be overfilled with hard wax and this may then be trimmed, using a vertical cutting knife on the surveyor instead of a graphite lead (*see* fig. 370).

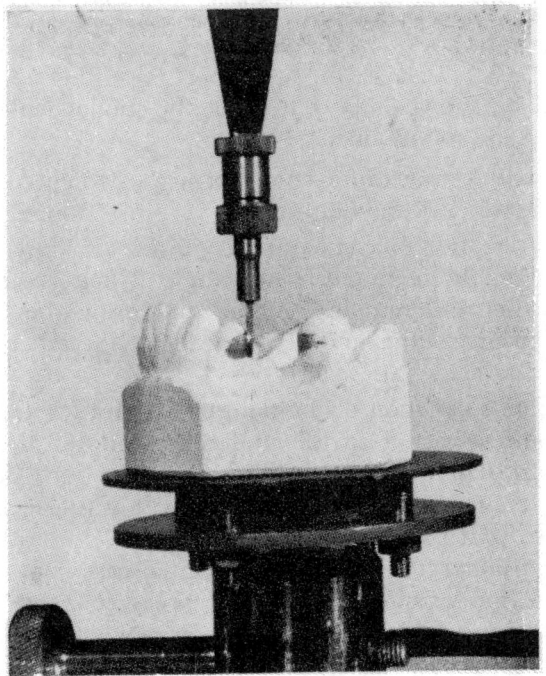

FIG. 370. – Undercuts blocked out and being trimmed with knife on surveyor.

This method, which is the more accurate, is useful when a duplicate model is to be used for casting or processing or when a wax pattern for a metal casting is removed from the model.

(2) It marks the most bulbous part of a tooth which is to carry a clasp. This enables the technician to place the rigid part of the clasp, above the undercut area, and the flexible arm, which does the work of retaining the denture, into the undercut (*see* fig. 371).

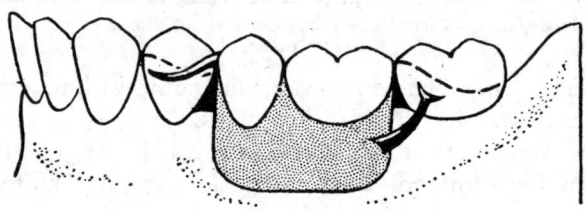

FIG. 371. – Survey lines (broken lines) enabling the prosthetist to select the correct type of clasp and place it accurately.

As will be shown later, tilting of the model will affect the position of the survey line.

(3) It will demonstrate undercut areas which can be used for the retention of the denture.

Such utilization of undercuts requires the horizontal axis of the model to be tilted at an angle which is sufficient to eliminate the undercut in question and bring the side of the tooth adjacent to the undercut parallel with the lead of the surveyor (*see* fig. 372).

The line of insertion of the denture is parallel with the side of the tooth adjacent to the undercut, and the denture will only go into place if inserted in this direction, because all other undercuts, which develop as a result of tilting the model, are blocked out parallel with this line.

Fig. 373 illustrates a more complicated case in which tilting the model has enabled 3 undercut areas (one mesial to the 1st molar, one mesial to the 1st premolar, and the labial undercut of the ridge) to be used for retaining the denture against vertical withdrawal.

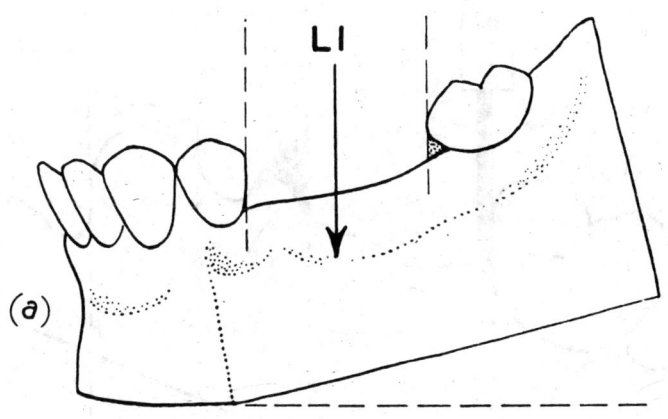

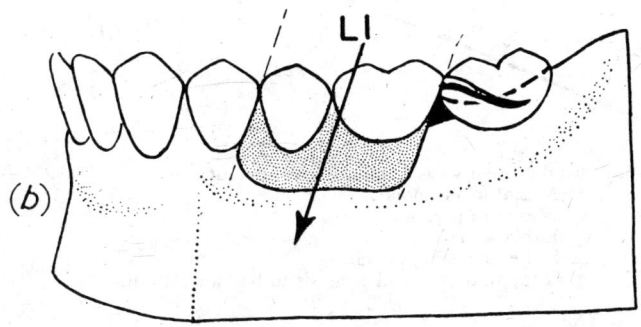

FIG. 372

(a) The model has been tilted sufficiently to bring the lead
of the surveyor parallel to the distal surface of $\overline{4}$, thus
eliminating completely the undercut behind this tooth
but accentuating somewhat the undercut mesial to $\overline{7}$.
LI = the line of insertion of the denture. This is parallel
with the lead of the surveyor.

(b) The denture inserted along the direction of LI. It fits
into the undercut distal to $\overline{4}$ and will thus resist a
vertical withdrawal force. A clasp is necessary, however,
on $\overline{7}$.

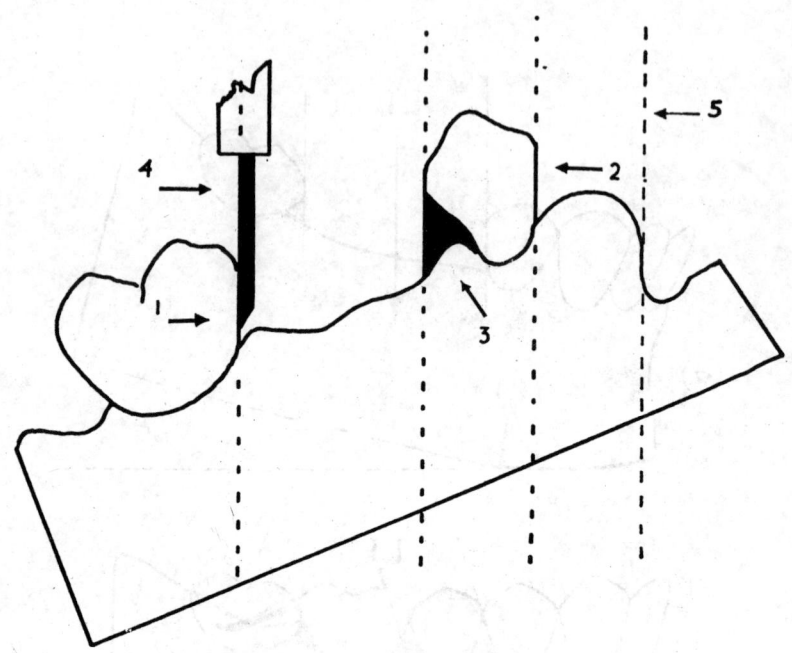

FIG. 373.
(a) Model tilted so as to eliminate undercuts.
    1. Mesial to 1st molar.
    2. Mesial to premolar.
    5. Labial to ridge.
    4. is the surveying pencil.
    3. is the undercut which needs to be blocked out.

(4) It enables those parts of the denture base which fit against the crowns of the teeth, to be placed above the survey line, and therefore against the teeth. This ensures that the denture fits snugly against the tooth and does not leave a gap into which food debris may pack, a fault which is commonly seen in dentures which have been relieved empirically (*see* fig. 374).

(5) It permits the operator to select, and design, a denture about one path of insertion so that all saddles and clasps are designed about this predetermined path and not as individual units.

Frequently a path of insertion is determined by the under-

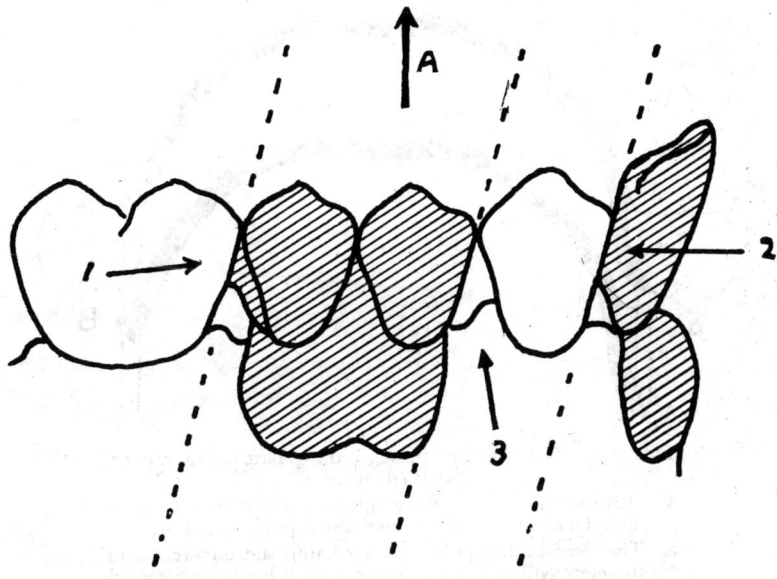

FIG. 373.
(b) Denture fitted to this model along path of insertion
shown by dotted lines will be retained against withdrawal along line of arrow by undercuts detailed above.

cuts revealed during a preliminary survey of the abutment
teeth of an anterior saddle. The tilting table often has to be
adjusted to obtain the minimal undercut area in order to avoid
unsightly spaces showing when the denture is in the mouth.

(6) It enables the operator to measure, with undercut
gauges, the depth, horizontally, of an undercut below the
survey line marked on a tooth and thereby determine the type
of clasp to be used and the material of which it is constructed.

Undercut gauges are usually of 3 sizes having heads with
lips of 10- 20- and 30-thousandths of an inch (fig. 375).
They are interchangeable with the vertical surveying lead
and when in use the shank touches the tooth at the survey line
and the rim of the head touches the tooth in the undercut.
By using the various size heads the horizontal depth of the
undercut can be measured anywhere between the survey line
and the gingival margin and the clasp arm can be then placed

Fig. 374. – Cross-section through the palate of an upper partial denture.

A. Denture finished correctly just above the survey line – note the close fit and the relief of the gingival margin.

B. The denture has been processed into the undercut and therefore will not go into place until it has been trimmed away by the amount indicated by the parallel lines, and when in place a gap is left, indicated by arrow, into which food will pack (*see also* fig. 337*d*).

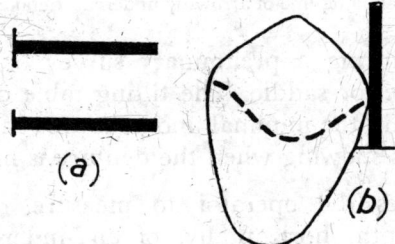

Fig. 375.–Undercut Guager

(*a*) Two sizes of head.

(*b*) Illustrating the method used to determine the degree of undercut.

in a position appropriate to the material and type of clasp. A rigid type of clasp would not need the same depth of undercut that would be required by a more flexible type of clasp.

THE TECHNIQUE OF SURVEYING

These six functions of surveying have been described

separately, for convenience, but in practice all six merge and are closely interrelated. Therefore, to show clearly how surveying is carried out, an actual survey will be illustrated on an upper model with the following teeth standing, 76 321|123 67.

The model is fixed to the table of the surveyor with the occlusal plane horizontal and the lead passed round 6 3 | 3 6. The lines resulting from this survey are shown in figs. 376, 377, 378.

The conclusions drawn from this survey are as follows:

(a) Undercuts are present mesial to 6|6, and the extent of these is shown.

(b) The survey lines are very high on the crowns of all the teeth, especially on the proximal surfaces, and therefore no room exists for the rigid bodies of encircling clasps and projection clasps must be used.

(c) If projection clasps are used on 3|3 and correctly placed just below the survey lines, they will be visible when the patient talks and smiles.

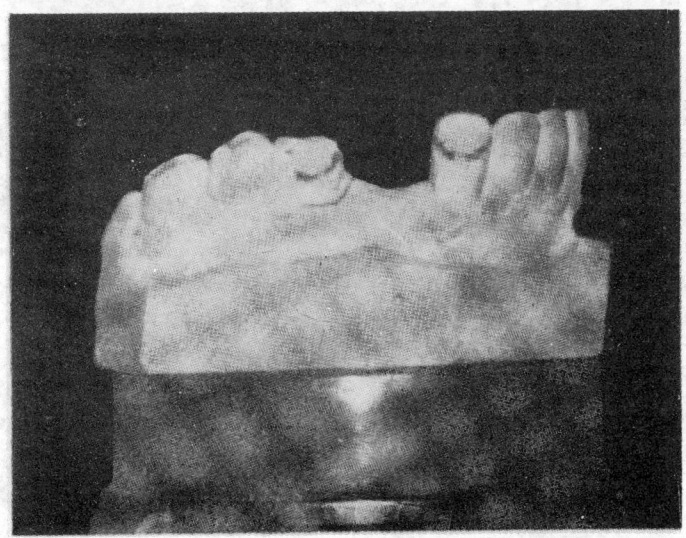

Fig. 376. – Survey with model horizontal. Left side,

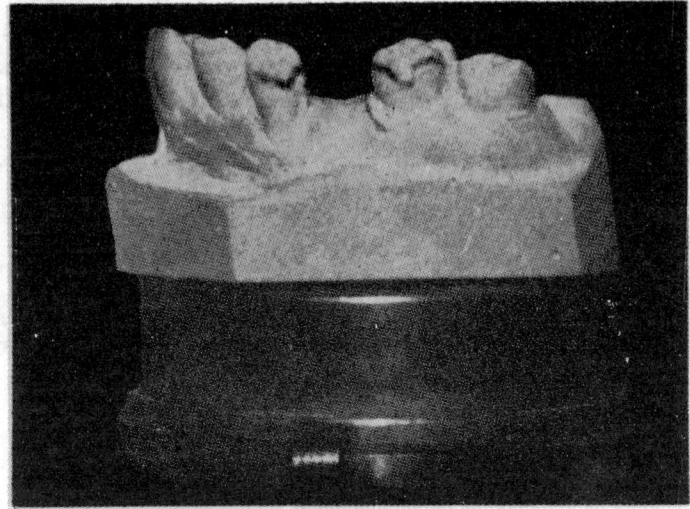

Fig. 377. – Survey with model horizontal. Right side.

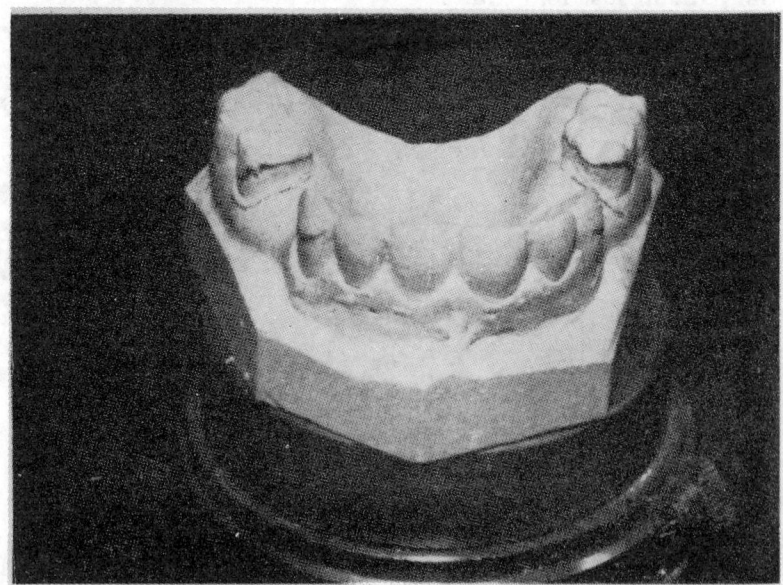

Fig. 378. – Survey with model horizontal. From in front.

(*d*) No use can be made for purposes of retention of the undercuts mesial to 6|6.

Summing Up. – A denture could be designed on this model surveyed horizontally if the undercuts mesial to 6|6 are blocked out and all clasps are of the projection variety. Even so it would be difficult to fit a reciprocal on the palatal aspect of 6|, because the survey line is so high on the mesio-palatal corner that this part of the reciprocal would have to cross the occlusal surface of the tooth if it is to remain above the survey ine at its attachment to the denture.

If having surveyed the model horizontally and considered the implications of the lines drawn, they do not appear as satisfactory as could be desired the next thing to do is to survey the model tilted at various angles, in an effort to develop survey lines which are more suitable for the design of clasps, or which will eliminate undercuts and thus enable them to assist in retention, or both.

In the case illustrated it was considered that a backward tilt of the model, so that the pencil of the surveyor was parallel to the mesial surfaces of 6|6, would eliminate these undercuts and enable them to assist in the retention of the denture. The model was also tilted slightly downwards on the right-hand side to produce more favourable survey lines on 3|3. The straight lines drawn on the base of the model indicate the tilt as these are parallel to the pencil of the surveyor.

The lines developed when the model was surveyed in the position described are illustrated in figs. 379, 380, 381.

The conclusions drawn from this survey are as follows:

(*a*) The undercuts mesial to 6|6 have been eliminated.

(*b*) Slight undercuts have developed distal to 3|3.

(*c*) The position of all the survey lines has been markedly altered and they are now favourable for the use of encircling clasps with the exception of that on |3.

(*d*) The survey line on 3| has been lowered on the tooth, and an encircling clasp used on this tooth would be almost invisible.

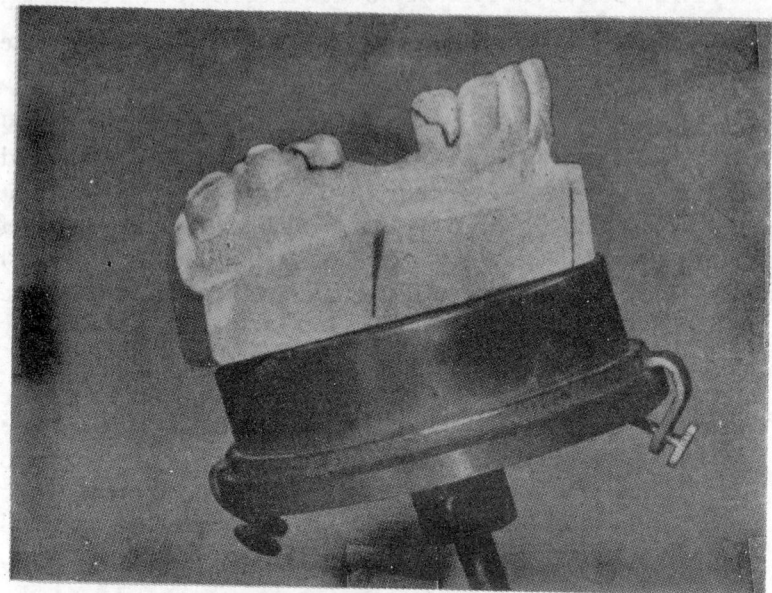

FIG. 379. – Survey with model tilted. Left side.

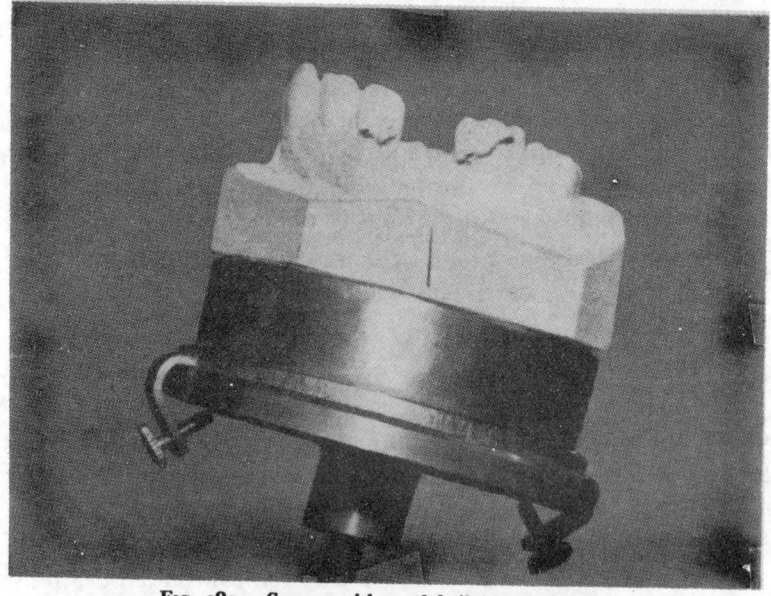

FIG. 380. – Survey with model tilted. Right side.

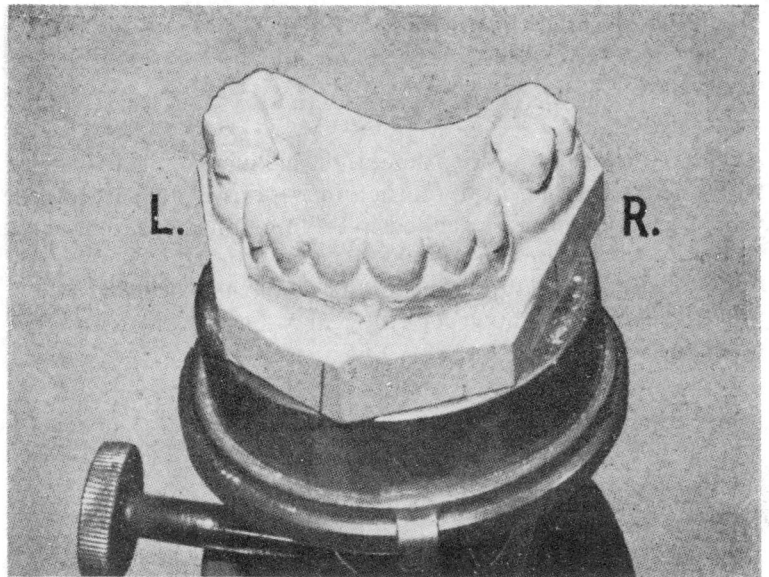

FIG. 381. – Survey with model tilted. From in front.

(*e*) The survey line at the mesio-labial aspect of |3 is also low on the tooth, and a projection clasp correctly positioned here would also be almost invisible.

(*f*) No difficulty now exists in positioning the reciprocals on the molar teeth.

Summing Up. – A denture designed on this model surveyed with a backward tilt would be superior to that designed on it when surveyed horizontally for the following reasons:

The main retention would be by encircling clasps which collect far less food debris and possess superior bracing properties.

The undercuts mesial to 6|6 will also assist in the retention of the denture, and if desired clasps need not be fitted at all on 6|6.

The appearance of the patient will not be marred by conspicuous clasps on 3|3.

The case illustrated is an extremely simple one, but the principles of surveying described hold good for the most complex type of case, and in these both patience and experience are needed before the most favourable tilt of the model is discovered.

CLASPS

A clasp consists of a resilient metal projection from the denture, which grips the natural tooth, and retains that part of the denture, to which it is attached, in its functional position.

The types and designs of clasps are numbered in scores, and many of them are known by the name of their originator. For practical purposes, however, they may be classified into two main types:

1. Encircling Clasps.
2. Projection or Gingivally Approaching Clasps.

1. *Encircling Clasps*

These consist of two arms which encircle the tooth on opposite sides, and are in contact with it along their whole length, gripping it at their extremities (*see* fig. 382). Generally one of

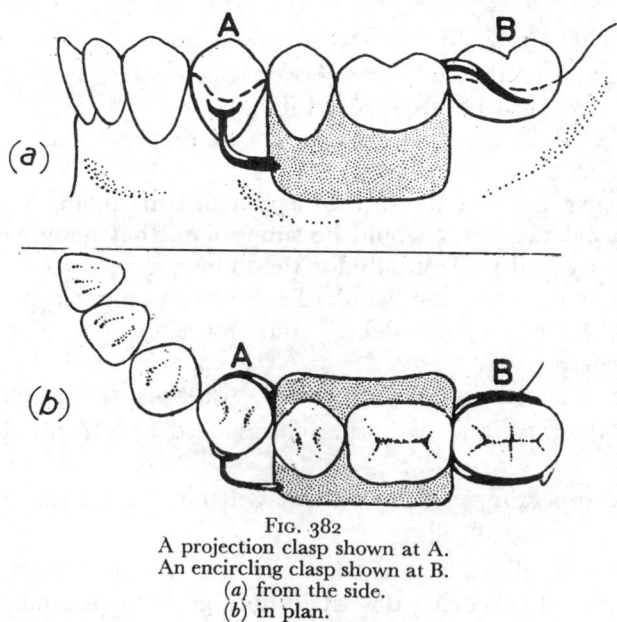

FIG. 382
A projection clasp shown at A.
An encircling clasp shown at B.
(*a*) from the side.
(*b*) in plan.

the arms is rigid, merely acting as a reciprocal to the force of the other functional arm and so preventing movement of the tooth. If pressure is applied to one side of a tooth only, that tooth will eventually move, irrespective of the patient's age; therefore a clasp should always be envisaged as grasping a tooth, never merely pressing against it. Not infrequently this reciprocal is formed by an extension of the denture on to the appropriate surface of the tooth. If both arms of the clasp are flexible, each acting as a reciprocal to the other, very careful adjustment of each arm is required because if one presses more strongly on the tooth than the other the tooth will be moved.

Projection or Gingivally Approaching Clasps

These differ from the encircling type by not being in contact with the tooth along their whole length and by approaching the undercut area from the gingival aspect.

How a Clasp Functions

Basically, any type of clasp consists of a flexible metal arm which is attached to the denture. If the arm is flexed, and then prevented from returning to its position of rest, it will possess energy in the form of spring pressure. Thus, if the extremities of a clasp press on an inclined plane, the clasp will endeavour to travel down the plane, in an effort to release its potential energy.

The basis of correct clasp design, therefore, resolves itself into placing the flexible part of the clasp arm on an inclined plane, which is sloping in the right direction. Thus the clasp will retain the denture in place and any force which attempts to withdraw the denture will draw the tip of the clasp up the inclined plane, thus flexing the arm more and increasing its energy to resist the withdrawing force. If on the other hand the flexible part of the clasp is placed on an inclined plane which is sloping in the wrong direction, the pressure of the clasp will force the denture out of place.

The following diagrams should clarify this (*see* fig. 383):

If a force F which represents the spring pressure of a clasp is applied to an inclined plane AB, it is resolved into two forces, one XY at right angles to the plane and one XZ along the

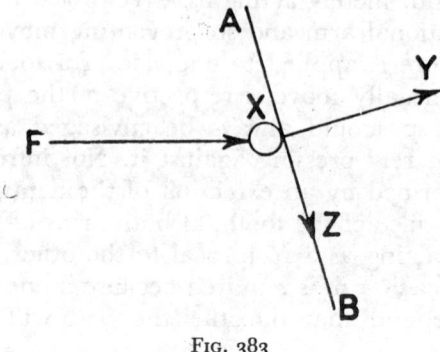

FIG. 383

plane. It is the force XZ which retains the denture in place if the plane slopes in the right direction, or expels it if not.

The surfaces of the natural teeth are planes inclined at various angles. This will be clear from fig. 384 which shows an average tooth in cross-section and in plan.

If the flexible part of the clasp arm is placed on the inclined planes DE and BC, excellent retention will result. If, however, it is placed on AB or EF, expulsion will ensue. In

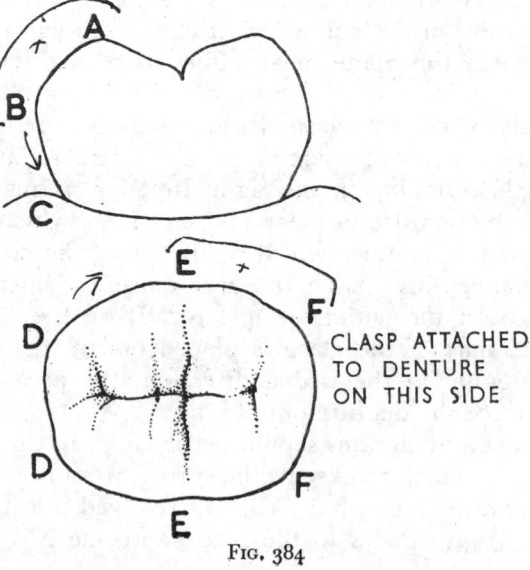

CLASP ATTACHED TO DENTURE ON THIS SIDE

FIG. 384

other words the flexible part must be placed in an undercut area and the clasp must encircle more than half the circumference of the tooth.

The phrase 'the flexible part of the clasp' has been used deliberately because its flexibility is not uniform throughout its length, for two reasons:

(1) Attachment to the denture makes it rigid at one end.
(2) Tapering towards its free extremity increases its flexibility out of proportion to its length. A clasp is like a fishing rod, the handle being rigid and unyielding and the tip the most flexible part.

It will also be obvious from fig. 384 that the point B represents the most bulbous part of the tooth and that only the flexible part of the clasp will pass over it into the undercut area beneath. Therefore, before the correct type of clasp to be employed on any tooth can be decided upon, the positions of the favourable and unfavourable inclined planes of the tooth must be known. The simplest way of discovering this is to delineate the most bulbous circumference of the tooth, and it then follows that any part of the tooth on the gingival side of this line must slope in a favourable direction for clasp retention, whilst for any area to the occlusal side of it, the converse must hold.

This contour line is drawn by means of a surveyor, and a description of this and the technique of its use is dealt with on page 489 *et seq.*

Survey lines on teeth vary widely, and whilst every effort should be made when surveying to develop lines which will enable an encircling type of clasp to be used, this is not always possible, and it is for these cases that projection clasps are particularly useful.

The reasons why the encircling clasp is superior to the projection type are that: (1) The rigid part of the clasp which is in contact with the tooth provides valuable bracing for the denture against lateral movement. (2) It holds the minimum of food debris in contact with the teeth, provided it is highly polished on the fitting surface. This is because it is in close contact with the tooth along its whole length, whilst the arms of projection clasps are separated from the teeth and soft tissues by $\frac{1}{2}$ mm. to 2 mm. and consequently food tends to pack into this space.

The value of projection clasps is great, however, because:
  (1) They can be used in situations unfavourable to the use of encircling clasps.
  (2) Any degree of flexibility can be obtained by lengthening the arm which passes over soft tissue.
  (3) They are less conspicuous.
  (4) They can be placed in the area of the greatest undercut.
  (5) They can be used as stress breakers.

Factors Affecting the Selection of a Clasp

It will be realized from the foregoing that the main factor which guides the operator in his selection of a clasp form, for any particular situation, is the type of survey line. Other factors do, however, affect this selection, and these are:

1. *The Situation of the Tooth which is to be Clasped*

For example the tooth may be adjacent to the edentulous space, or it may be separated from it by other teeth or the width of the mouth. The tooth may be isolated or have another tooth in contact with it. Clasps will vary in relation to these factors.

2. *The Occlusion of the Teeth*

In some clasps it is necessary to carry an arm across the contact point between two natural teeth. If the occlusion will not allow room for this to be done another clasp may have to be selected, or a space made for the arm by grinding the teeth and this is not always desirable.

3. *The Appearance*

In the front of the mouth clasps may require to be subservient to the appearance. Retention, however, may often be obtained by adjusting the tilt of the surveying table in such a manner that an undercut adjacent to the anterior abutment tooth can be entered by the denture.

Types of Clasp

It is intended, therefore, to illustrate the various types of clasp primarily in relation to the types of survey line, and the other factors will be mentioned when they have a bearing. Eleven types of clasp will be described which experience has shown to be most commonly useful. These eleven forms are far from being exhaustive of the clasps available, but they point to the basic principles of clasp design, and if these are grasped the usefulness of other forms may be assessed.

A. *Encircling Clasps*

1. *The Two Arm Encircling Clasp*

   (a) *Normal Arm Form* (*see* fig. 385). – This is a very useful

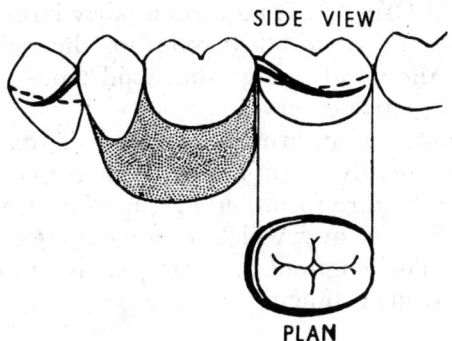

SIDE VIEW

PLAN

FIG. 385

clasp which can be employed whenever the tooth to be clasped is adjacent to an edentulous space, and the survey line on that part of the tooth nearest to the space allows room for the rigid part of the clasp. The design of the arms should be such that the flexible terminals of the clasp travel for as long a distance as possible in the undercut area (*see* fig. 386).

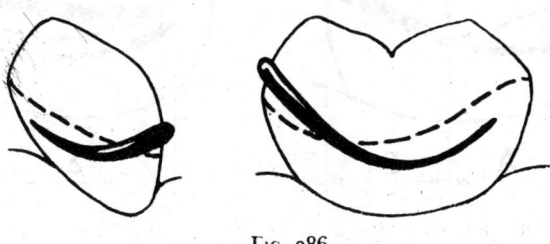

FIG. 386

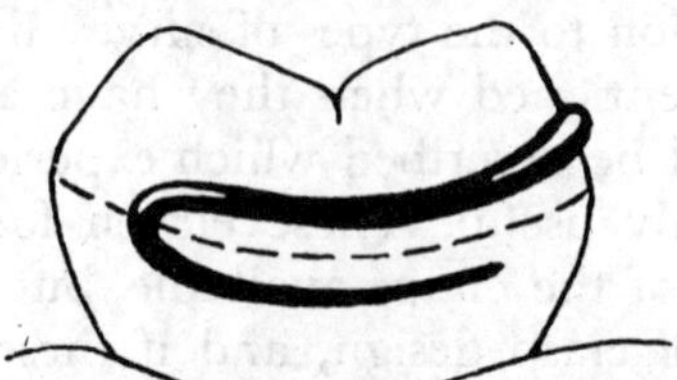

FIG. 387

(*b*) *The Recurved Arm Form.* – In this clasp the length of the arm is increased by curving it on itself as shown in fig. 387.

It can be employed in situations similar to those suitable for the normal form (*a*). It requires a fairly large area of tooth above the survey line to allow room for the rigid part of the clasp. It has the disadvantage that food tends to pack in the space where the arm recurves.

The advantage of an arm of this shape is that it allows the length of the retentive terminal to be increased and brings it nearer to the denture so providing superior retention. This is because the distance over which leverage is effective is reduced (*see* fig. 388). The length of the rigid part is also increased and so provides excellent bracing.

2. *The One Arm Form*

This type of clasp is similar in every way to the two arm variety, except that only one arm is flexible, the other arm, or

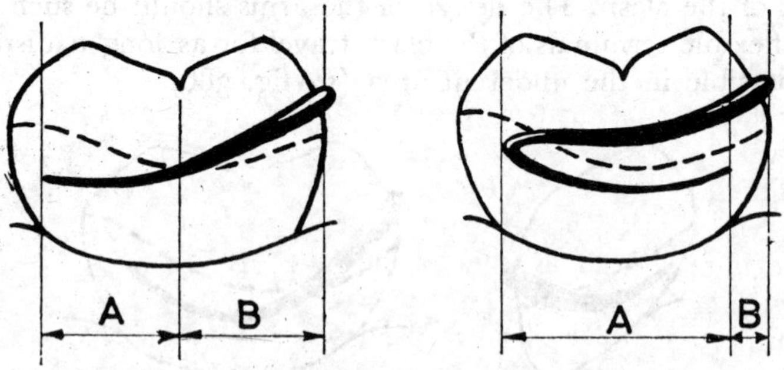

FIG. 388. – A = length of retentive terminal. B = distance from the denture to any part of the retentive terminal.

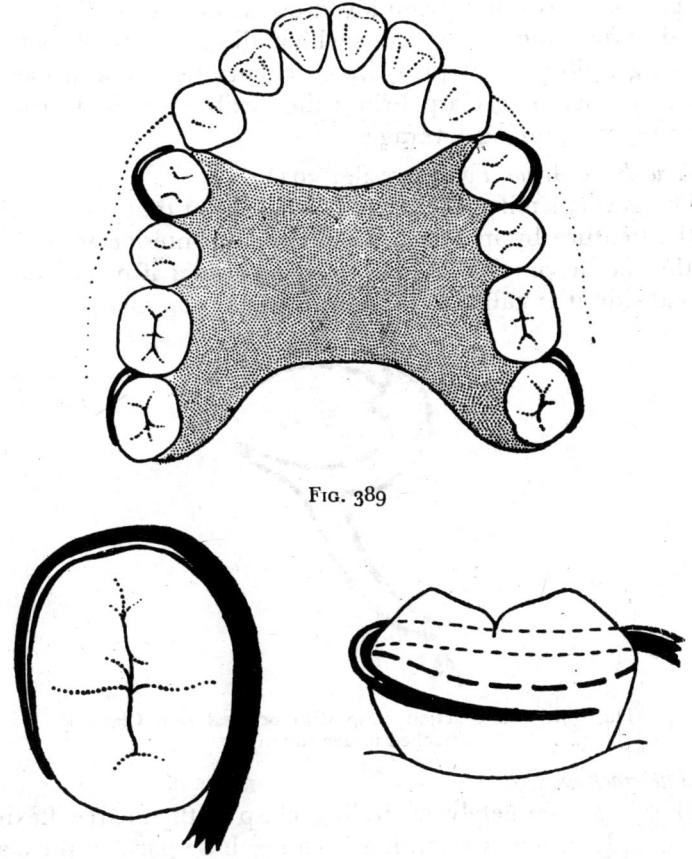

Fig. 389

Fig. 390

reciprocal, being formed by an extension of the denture (*see* fig. 389). The form of the single arm may be normal or re-curved.

This type of clasp does not provide such good retention as the two-armed clasp, because there is only one flexible terminal. The lateral bracing is good, however, being provided by the unyielding reciprocal. This type of clasp is easy to make and is commonly employed with plastic-based dentures.

3. *The Circumferential Form (Ring Clasp)* (*see* fig. 390)

In this type of clasp the flexible arm is an extension of the reciprocal. It is usually employed on isolated teeth, e.g. lower molars exhibiting a survey line which allows plenty of room for the long rigid part. It provides excellent bracing, and like the recurved encircling clasp brings the flexible terminal near the denture, so reducing leverage.

4. *The Back Action Form* (*see* fig. 391)

This is very similar to the ring clasp except that it is attached to the denture by means of a strut placed anterior or posterior to the saddle on the lingual or palatal side; if placed on the buccal side it is called a Reverse Back Action Clasp.

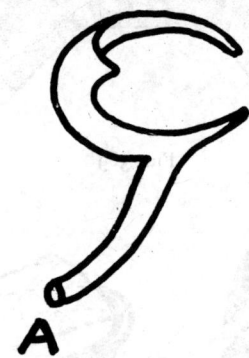

A

FIG. 391. – Back action clasp with occlusal rest. Clasp is attached to denture at A.

5. *The Jackson Crib*

This is a completely encircling clasp with no free flexible terminal. It provides retention because those parts of the clasp which are situated on the proximal embrasures of the tooth are springy and grip the undercuts which exist in these areas (*see* fig. 392). This clasp is valuable when no edentulous space exists on either side of the tooth to be clasped. Room must exist, or be made by grinding, for those parts of the clasp crossing the occlusal surface.

B. *Projection or Gingivally Approaching Clasps* (*Roach Type*)

1. *The T-shaped* (*see* fig. 393)

This is a useful clasp form to employ when the survey line indicates that no room exists for the rigid part of an encircling clasp and yet there is a large undercut area.

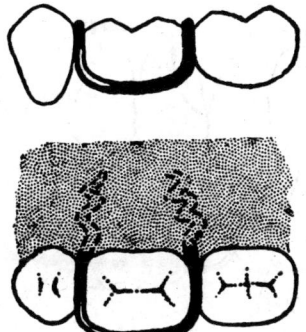

FIG. 392

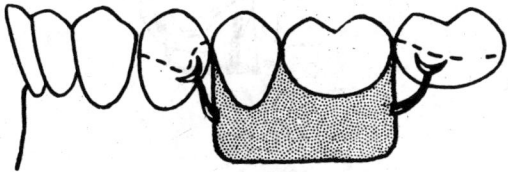

FIG. 393

The length of both the arm and the part which makes contact with the tooth, may be varied to suit the requirements of retention and flexibility. This clasp may be made with two flexible arms or the reciprocal may be rigid, if the survey line on the lingual or palatal aspect of the tooth allows.

This clasp is valuable for use on canine and incisor teeth with the added advantage that it is the least conspicuous type because it approaches from the back, and not the occlusal surface (*see* fig. 394).

2. *The U-shaped* (*see* fig. 395)
This clasp is useful when the survey line dips to the gingival margin, on the buccal aspect of the tooth.

3. *The L-shaped* (*see* fig. 396)
This type of clasp is usually employed on premolar or canine teeth when the area under the survey line is extremely small and where no other type of clasp can be used.

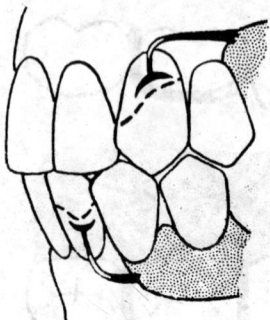

FIG. 394

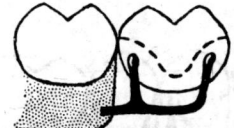

FIG. 395

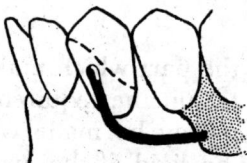

FIG. 396

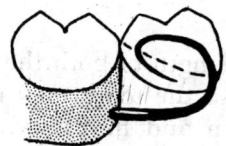

FIG. 397

4. *The C-shaped* (*see* fig. 397)

This type of clasp is almost exclusively reserved for use when a tooth exhibits only a small undercut area mesially or distally. The long curved arm increases the flexibility and thus enables the terminal portion to be placed in the undercut area. It also provides lateral bracing.

5. *The Ball and Socket* (*see* fig. 398)

This type of clasp is invaluable when the slope of the tooth surface is such that no undercut area exists. A round platinized gold wire, which has been melted to form a ball at one end,

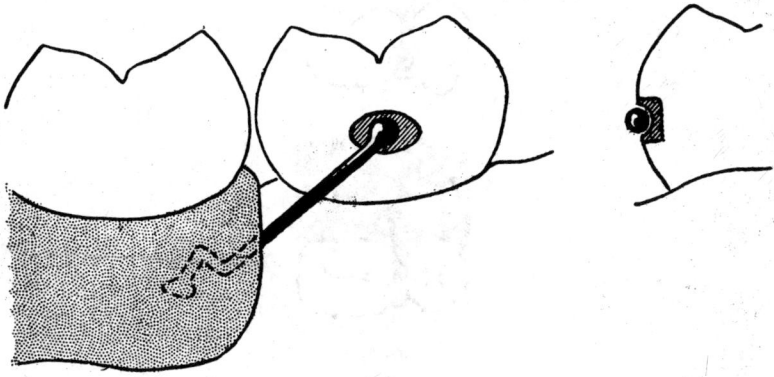

FIG. 398

is constructed to terminate on the buccal surface of the tooth, and a gold inlay is let into the tooth at this point. When the denture is fitted a thin piece of articulating paper is inserted between the ball and the inlay, and the ball given a smart tap. When the denture and articulating paper are removed a small blue spot will be found on the surface of the inlay which coincides with the ball when in position. At this point a cup-shaped hollow is drilled in the inlay with a rose-head bur, and the clasp arm bent slightly inwards so that when the denture is inserted the ball of the clasp clicks into the hollow. This clasp gives a very positive retention and need not be restricted to teeth which exhibit no survey line.

6. *The Interdental* (*see* figs. 399 and 400)

This clasp has two forms. The first consists of a round wire which has been fused at the end, to form a ball. The wire is carried across the occlusal surface at the contact point of the teeth, and the ball fits into the undercut area between the embrasures.

The second, which is usually cast, substitutes a small triangular wedge or two clasp arms in place of the ball.

Interdental clasps are employed when no edentulous gap exists between the teeth. Room must exist or be made for the arm which crosses the occlusal surface.

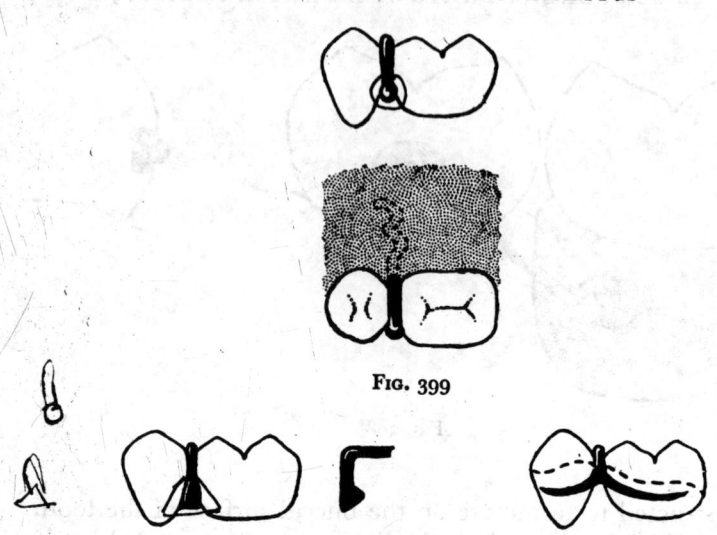

FIG. 399

FIG. 400

LOCATION OF CLASPS

A clasp will retain only that part of the denture to which it is attached. Clasps should thus be located as regularly as the case requires round the periphery of the denture, so that the resultant of their several forces falls as near the centre o gravity of the denture as possible (*see* fig. 401).

In such a case as that depicted in fig. 402 indirect retention is required to retain the back of the denture. This is dealt with later in the Chapter.

Whilst it is quite impossible to lay down hard and fast rules with regard to the number of clasps required, the following precepts are broadly applicable to most cases:

(1) Tooth-borne dentures, particularly if of skeleton design, require more clasps than other types.

(2) When only two clasps are used, a straight line joining them should bisect the denture as nearly as possible.

(3) If a denture would tend to rock about a line joining two clasps, then a third clasp should be added and the farther it is away from the other two the better.

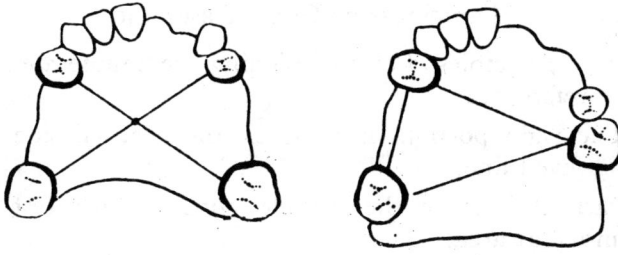

Fig. 401

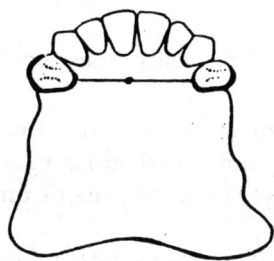

Fig. 402

Which Teeth to Clasp

The following list gives the teeth in order of suitability for clasping from the point of view of shape, strength and size, assuming normal, healthy teeth in normal relation to each other in every case:

(1) Molars.

(2) Premolars.

(3) Canines.

(4) Upper central incisors.

(5) Upper lateral and all lower incisors are almost useless.

When the location and type of the clasps to be used on any case have been decided, there still remains the question of the type of material to be employed in their construction. In order to be able to select intelligently a material for making a clasp, a knowledge of the important mechanical properties required should be possessed.

Principles of Clasp Designing

The main principles of clasp designing are enumerated below for easy reference:

(1) The rigid portion must be on the occlusal side of the surveyed line.

(2) Part at least of the flexible portion must rest in an undercut area.

(3) The flexible portion must not fit more deeply into an undercut area than its elastic or proportional limit will permit.

(4) The terminal of the clasp must remain in contact with the tooth.

(5) Any pressure must be opposed by equal and opposite pressure or by some unyielding part of the denture, i.e. a clasp must never press on one side only of an unsupported tooth.

(6) The clasp, together with its rigid opponent or reciprocal, if it is of the single arm type, must embrace more than half the circumference of the tooth.

(7) Unless fitted with an occlusal rest the clasp must not rest too near to the gingival margin.

Mechanical Properties of Clasp Alloys

Clasps require to be strong enough to resist permanent distortion in the mouth, elastic enough to regain their original shape when flexed, flexible enough to spring over the bulbous parts of the teeth, and springy enough to apply the force required to hold the denture in place. Such terms as these, however, are loose and as expressed lack definite meaning and cannot be accurately assessed. If, however, they are defined and the implications of the definitions grasped, the correct selection of a material for any given clasp is simplified.

Specifications issued by manufacturers of alloys suitable for clasps and denture bases usually quote figures for the following mechanical properties:

1. *The Proportional Limit*

This may be defined as the greatest stress to which a material may be subjected without becoming permanently deformed. Sometimes the figures for Elastic Limit or Yield Point are given instead of the Proportional Limit, and for practical purposes all three may be taken to correspond. Proportional Limit is the criterion of useful strength of the material, and in a clasp this property requires to be high otherwise the clasp may bend during use and no longer function as a clasp. The Proportional Limit varies in heat-treatable materials, being higher in the hardened than the softened state. A figure of 60,000 lb. per square inch in the hardened condition is the minimum acceptable figure for proportional limit, and figures of 100,000 lb. per square inch and over are desirable.

2. *The Modulus of Elasticity*

This is computed from the formula $\dfrac{stress}{strain}$ therefore the greater the stress and the smaller the strain up to the proportional limit the larger will be the figure for the modulus and vice versa. It may be taken therefore as the criterion of stiffness. A material with a high figure for the modulus of elasticity will be stiff, and one with a low modulus, flexible. Figures for the modulus of elasticity vary from about 15×10^6 lb. per square inch in some of the gold alloys, to 32×10^6 lb. per square inch in the cobalt chrome alloys and some of the stainless steels.

The arm of a clasp acting as a reciprocal, or brace, or an indirect retainer, requires to be stiff and unyielding, and therefore should be made of a material with a high modulus of elasticity. The functional arm of a clasp, on the other hand, requires to be flexible and ideally should be made of a material with a low modulus of elasticity.

3. *The Percentage Elongation*

During fabrication and during the final fitting and adjustment of a denture, clasps require to be bent or plastically deformed. If the material from which they are constructed is highly ductile they will withstand considerable adjustment without developing weakness or breaking. If, however, they are not ductile, a slight adjustment may fracture them. Percentage elongation is a measure of the ductility of a material or the degree of adjustment to which it may be subjected. It varies in heat-treatable alloys, being much greater in the softened than the hardened state.

A figure of 10 per cent or above in the softened state is desirable, and this should not fall to less than 2 per cent in the hardened state.

Resistance to fatigue and creep are properties which should be highly developed in materials for clasp construction. Unfortunately little information is available on these properties in relation to clasp alloys. The only guide is the higher the proportional limit, the higher the resistance to fatigue is likely to be.

Before these facts can be applied to clasp design the relationship of them to the dimensions and form of the material must be known. These are as follows:

Resistance to Permanent or Plastic Deformation

This varies directly with the cross-sectional area of the material.

If cast clasps are to be used the dimensions should be related to both the proportional limit and the stress to which the clasp is likely to be subjected. Unfortunately no reliable data are available to guide the novice on this matter, except clinical experience. It is probably true, however, that clasps are more frequently deformed out of the mouth than in.

Stiffness and Flexibility

These vary with the square of the cross-sectional area. This means that if the cross-sectional area of a clasp is doubled the stiffness will be increased four times and the flexibility reduced four times. The practical application of these facts may be summarized as follows:

(1) A highly platinized wrought gold alloy is the best material available for constructing a clasp, because it develops to the highest degree the desirable mechanical properties. It is essential that it is correctly heat treated to develop these properties to the full.

(2) If a high degree of flexibility is required in the terminals, whilst preserving rigidity in the body of the clasp, the arms should taper towards their tips (*see* fig. 403).

(3) If it is desired to carry the terminal of a clasp deeply into an undercut to provide superior retention, a material with a high proportional limit and a low modulus of elasticity must be chosen or the distance which the clasp arm is required to travel may cause its plastic deformation (*see* fig. 404).

(4) If great stiffness is required in the reciprocal or bracing part of a clasp, and yet it is required to keep the dimensions small, a material with a high modulus of elasticity must be chosen.

(5) If the clasp arm has to be long the modulus of elasticity should be high or the tip of the clasp may be too flexible.

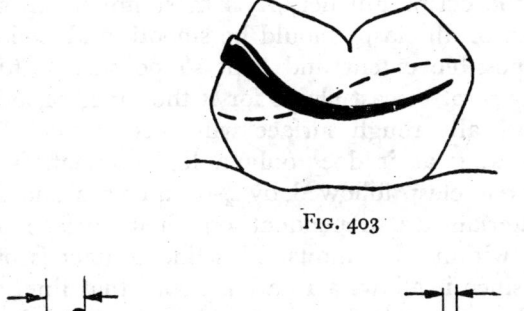

FIG. 403

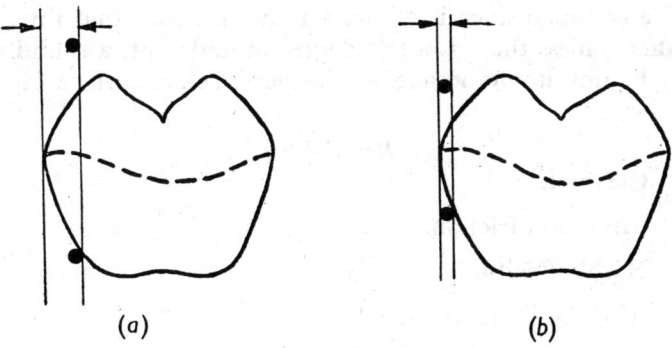

(*a*)   (*b*)

FIG. 404. – Illustrating the amount which a clasp must deform as the denture is inserted, if placed –
(*a*) a long way below the survey line,
(*b*) only just below the survey line.

Finally, clasps may be constructed of wrought wire, wrought plate or cast metal, and the following information is given regarding the advantages and disadvantages of each of these forms:

THE PHYSICAL FORM OF CLASPS

It is generally accepted that the retention of minute particles of foodstuff in contact with the enamel of the teeth is at least a predisposing cause of dental caries, and so it must be accepted as a fact that any form of clasp is potentially dangerous to the well-being of the tooth clasped. It follows, therefore, that any form of clasp should aim at creating the minimum amount of food stagnation, but as it is impossible for any clasp to fit so closely to the tooth as to prevent saliva laden with minute particles of food from lodging between it and the surface of the tooth, it also follows that the smaller the surface area the less dangerous the clasp. Further, it is most important that the inner surface of all clasps should be smooth and polished to the highest possible extent and kept so polished. This is particularly important in cast clasps for if the inner surface is neglected its naturally rough surface will become very foul. Round wire, making as it does only a line contact, is the cleanest form for a clasp followed by $\frac{1}{2}$-round wire and then plate. Cast materials are dependent on their surface area which can vary within wide limits. This line contact is often a disadvantage since it allows a rotation about that line, and further, unless there is a fair degree of undercut, a round wire may be unsuitable because of this very lack of surface friction.

Round Wire

(1) Cleanest.

(2) Minimum friction.

(3) Highly flexible.

(4) Most easily constructed.

(5) Probably most suitable for cases requiring several clasps.

(6) Does not transmit every movement of the denture to the tooth, i.e. it possesses stress-breaking properties.

Half-round Wire

(1) Physical characteristics between those of round wire and those of plate.

(2) Used under the same conditions as round wire but the improved frictional grip does not necessitate so much undercut.

Plate

The use of clasps made of this material is not advised and the following is only included for comparison:

(1) Definitely the worst fitting form and so, coupled with its area, the most liable to cause damage.

(2) Flexibility reduced by its dimensions and the fact that it should be doubly concave, i.e. mesio-distally and occluso-gingivally.

(3) Gives a very firm retention but special care must be taken that it does not impose a tilting strain on the clasped tooth.

(4) Can be used as an indirect retainer, but as this will be bound to put a tilting strain on the tooth it should only be so used in cases where there is no possible alternative.

(5) The most difficult type to construct.

Cast

(1) Accurately fitting.

(2) Easily varied in thickness, form and taper.

(3) Easily thickened to act as an inelastic brace.

(4) Can easily include an occlusal rest.

(5) Can be cast as an integral part of a gold denture or cobalt chrome base.

(4) INDIRECT RETAINERS

An indirect retainer is so called because it retains in position some part of a denture remote from itself. It works on the principle of the counter balance (fig. 405). In the illustration AB represents a bar suspended off centre at C. Point B will drop and A will rise until equilibrium is attained. If, however, point A is prevented from rising by placing an immovable block, D, above it, then point B cannot drop. This principle

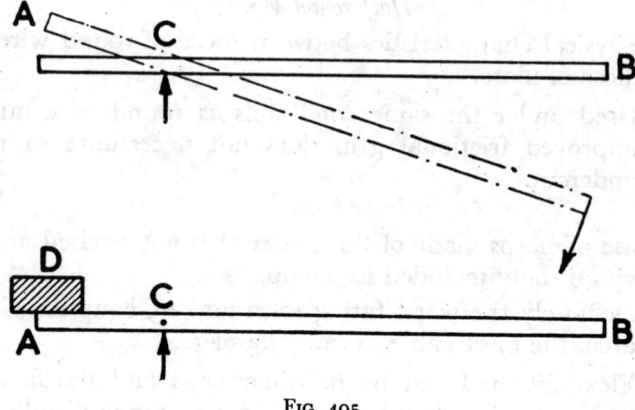

FIG. 405

can be employed in partial dentures whenever a free-end saddle is so long that it cannot be retained adequately by the clasp fitted to the abutment tooth. A typical example is shown in fig. 406. The denture is retained directly by clasps C, C, the free-end saddles being long tend to fall away from the tuberosities. In addition they exert excessive leverage on the pre-

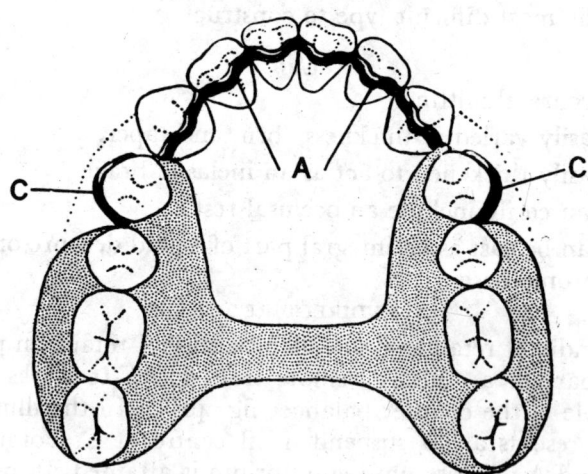

FIG. 406. – Denture retained by clasps C,C. Extension A rests on the lingual surfaces of the upper front teeth and therefore prevents the free-end saddles dropping.

molar teeth carrying the clasps. If an extension, A, of the saddles of the denture is made on the opposite side of the line joining the clasps, and this extension rests on the palatal surfaces of the canines and incisors, then provided that the retention supplied by the clasps is adequate to retain the dentures against normal dislodging forces, the saddles cannot drop unless the indirect retainer for A forces the incisor and canine teeth out of position; provided these teeth are firmly rooted this will not happen.

Indirect retainers are best made of metal, preferably cast so that they fit the teeth accurately. They should be placed as shown in fig. 407. In this position they are low enough on the

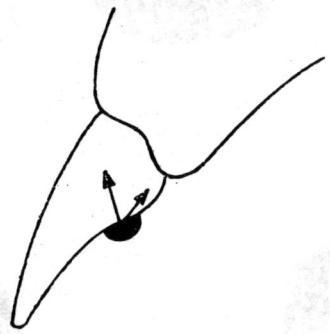

FIG. 407

tooth to prevent excessive leverage developing, and any tendency for the retainer to slide down the tooth is resisted by its cingulum. Indirect retainers may be made of plastic material as part of a tissue-borne denture, as illustrated in fig. 408.

An occlusal or incisal rest, a connector or a saddle may act as an indirect retainer provided its position is such that it is on the opposite side of the line or lines joining the direct retainers or clasps to that part which requires to be retained. Fig. 408 illustrates how various parts of a denture may act as an indirect retainer.

The more remote the position of the indirect retainer from the line joining the points of direct retention the more efficient becomes the indirect retainer. That shown in fig. 408(b) is more

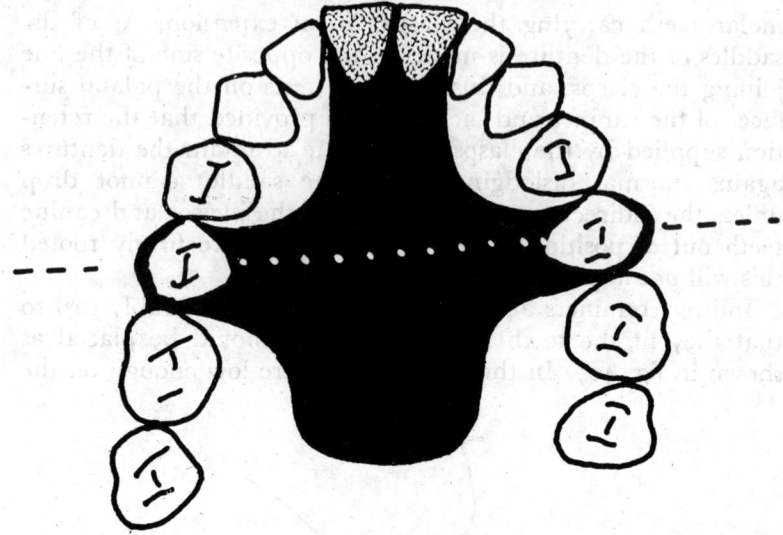

FIG. 408(a)

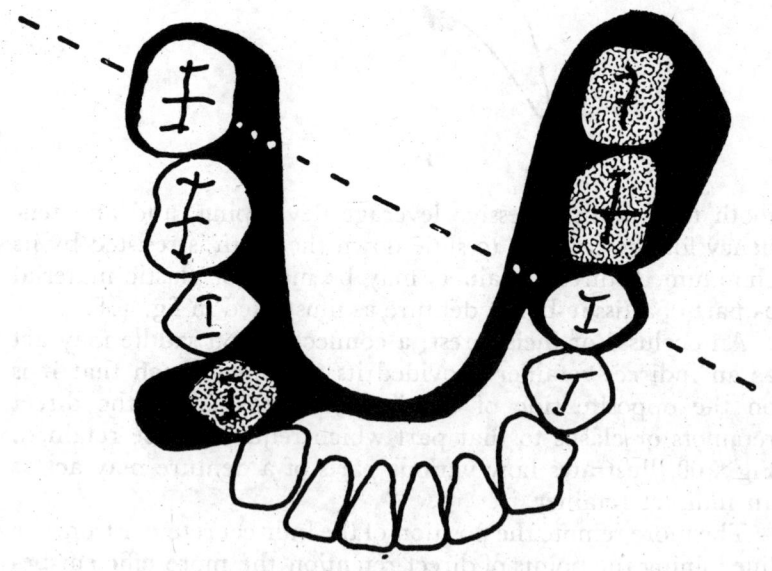

FIG. 408(b)

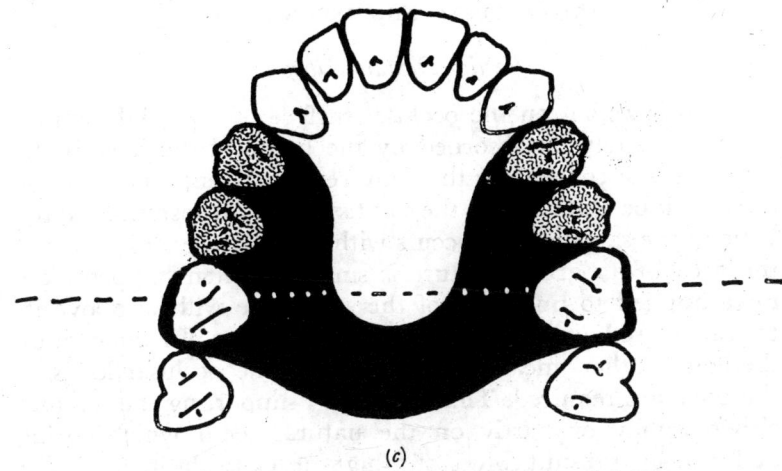

(c)

FIG. 408. – Three examples of the principles of indirect retention. The dotted lines indicate the fulcrum of clasp retention in each case and that part of the denture on one side of the line indirectly retains that part on the opposite side and vice versa.

If as illustrated only two clasps are employed there is inevitably a tendency for the denture to rock about the fulcrum of retention and in case (b) this could be prevented by clasping $\overline{5/}$ as well as $\overline{7/5}$ also if no saddle existed in $\overline{4/}$ region then an occlusal rest placed on $\overline{4/}$ would act as an indirect retainer.

efficient in action than that shown in fig. 408(c) since the parts being retained are approximately equidistant from the line of direct retention, whereas in C the palatal bar is closer to the line of direct retention than the points to be retained.

The points to bear in mind regarding indirect retainers are these:

(a) They can be used only on firmly rooted teeth.

(b) They should be borne by as many teeth as possible, to reduce the possibility of moving teeth by the application of excessive force.

(c) They can only function in conjunction with a direct retainer, i.e. a clasp or clasps.

(5) OCCLUSAL AND INCISAL RESTS

Partial Denture Support

The forces acting on the occlusal surface of a partial denture must ultimately be absorbed by the bones of the jaw. If the area of tissue covered by the denture is sufficiently large, these forces will be absorbed by the soft tissues and transmitted to the bone in the same way as occurs with full dentures. However, if the area of a partial denture is small, as often happens, the force applied to unit area of the soft tissue will be above its tolerance, and pain and ulceration will ensue. In these cases, therefore, other means of transferring the occlusal loads to the bone are required. This is done by supporting the denture either wholly or partly on the natural teeth which, being designed to transmit forces of a high order to the bone, suffer no damage if their supporting tissues are sound and the denture properly designed. The parts of the denture which transmit the loads to the teeth are called rests. The main function of rests is to transfer some, or all, of the masticatory loads to the natural teeth. In addition they may serve two other important functions:

(a) They act as contact points and thus prevent food packing between the denture and the natural tooth.

(b) They retain clasps in their correct position and prevent them sinking and pressing into the gingival tissues.

Rests are of three types: occlusal, cingulum, and incisal.

1. *Occlusal Rests* (*see* figs. 409, 410, 411)

These are made to fit into a mesial or distal fossa on the occlusal surface of a tooth and to be satisfactory they must comply with the following requirements:

(a) They must fit the tooth accurately in order to minimize the collection of food debris beneath them and also to locate them correctly in relation to the tooth.

(b) They must be strong enough to bear all normal masticatory loads without deformation.

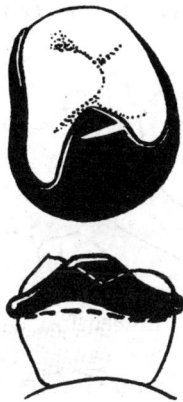

Fig. 409

(c) They must not 'gag' the occlusion. In the majority of cases a certain amount of preparation of the tooth surface is necessary in order that room may be made for the rest and the shape of the occlusal surface may be favourable for it (*see* fig. 413).

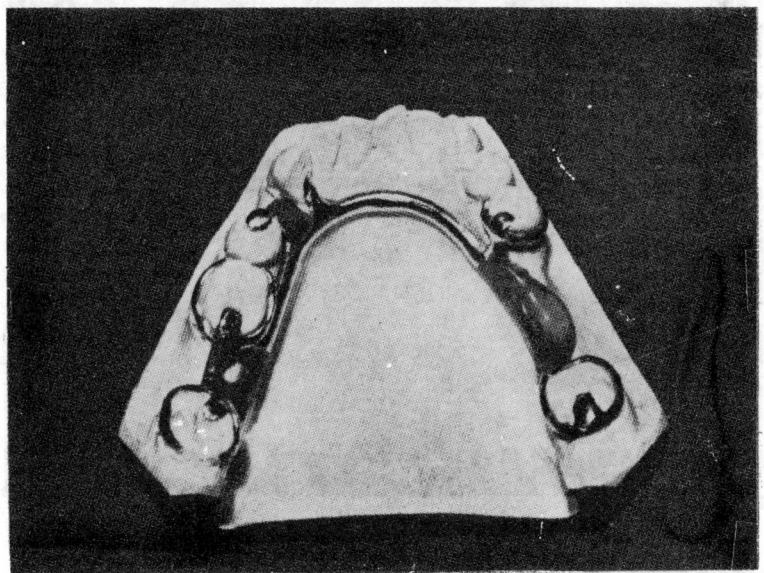

Fig. 410. – A case with sufficient occlusal rests to spread the load.

Fig. 411. – The form of an occlusal rest in section.
(A) incorrect.
(B) correct.

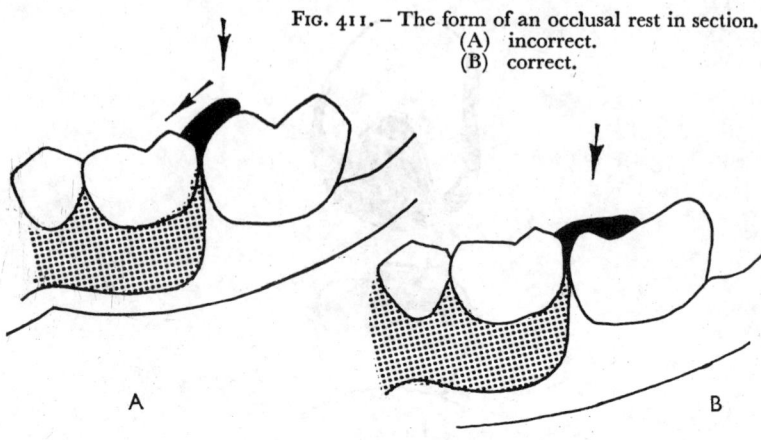

A   B

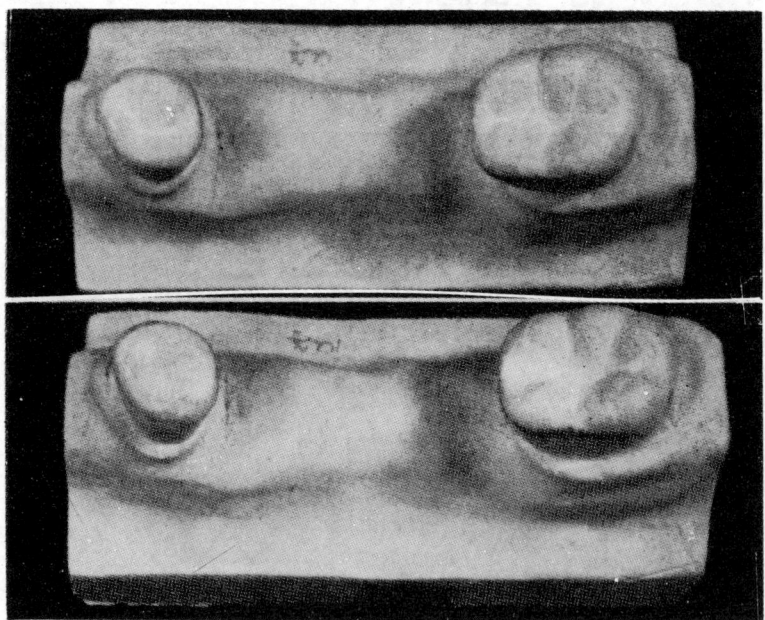

Fig. 412. – Upper illustration shows mesial and distal fossae and fissures in teeth. Lower illustration shows rest seat preparations in mesial and distal fossae. Note how the fissures have been removed and the preparations are smooth and saucer shaped.

This preparation is carried out with carborundum stones or diamond points and does not damage the tooth as it is rarely necessary to penetrate the enamel. If such penetration is necessary an inlay must be fitted to support the rest or caries will occur. If an opposing cusp is ground to make room for a rest the exposure of dentine is unimportant since it is a self-cleansing area and hence unlikely to be attacked by caries (*see* fig. 412).

(*d*) They must transmit the stress down the long axis of the tooth as this is the only direction in which the load can be increased without damage to the periodontal membrane.

(*e*) They must be at right angles or less to the long axis of the tooth otherwise the pressures of mastication will tend to force the denture away from the tooth or vice versa.

An undue load will be placed on the resilient portion of a

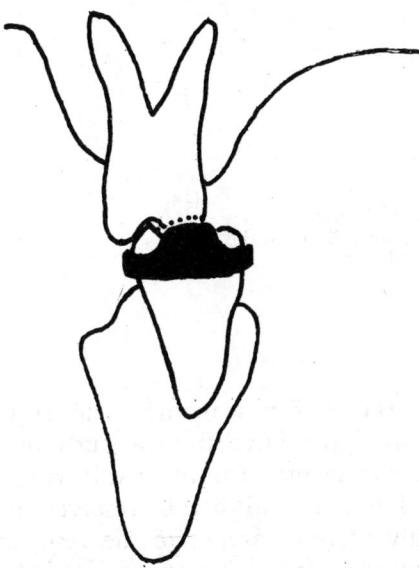

Fig. 413. – A clasp carrying an occlusal rest is fitted to the lower molars. Dotted line indicates the grinding of the palatal cusp of the upper molar necessary to provide room for the rest.

clasp which is made in conjunction with an obtuse angled occlusal rest.

2. *Cingulum Rests* (*see* fig. 414)

These are made to rest on the palatal or lingual surface of <u>front</u> teeth. They are usually unsatisfactory rests because the shape

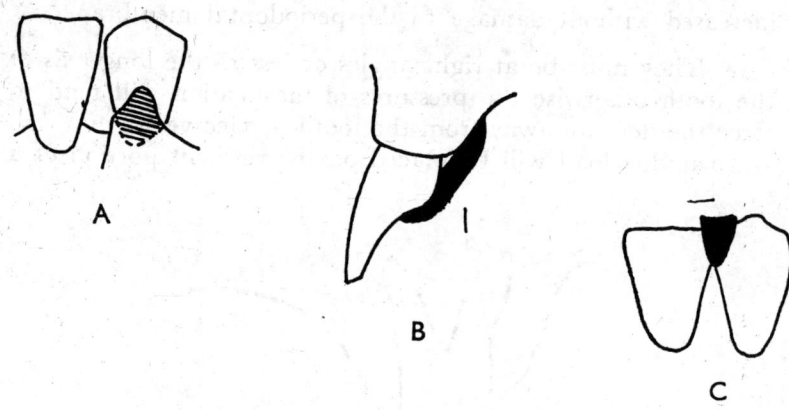

Fig. 414.
(*a*) Cingulum rest.
(*b*) Cingulum rest from the side.
(*c*) Incisal rest.

of the palatal surfaces of most teeth are not suitable to carry a rest. This will be appreciated from a study of fig. 415. If an occlusal load A is transmitted to the rest it will in turn transmit it to the tooth. This load will then be resolved into two loads B, which is broadly at right angles, to the rest, and C which is broadly parallel to it. It will be appreciated that at least half the load, which the rest is supposed to transmit to the tooth is actually devoted to forcing the rest down the tooth, and must be absorbed by the underlying soft tissue.

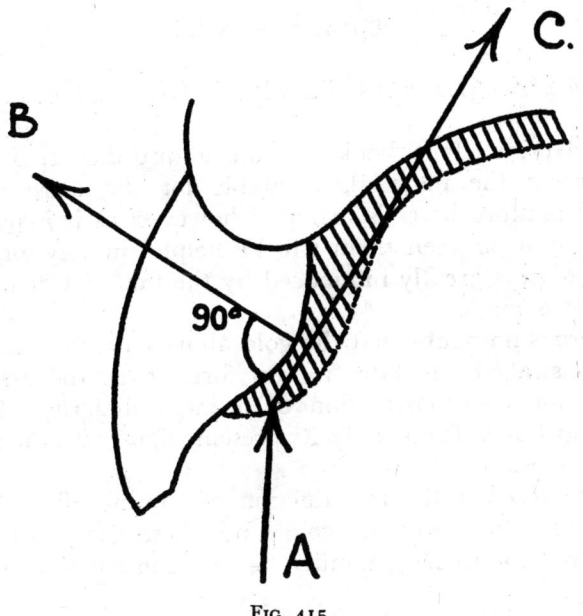

FIG. 415

3. *Incisal Rests* (*see* fig. 414(*c*))

These are mainly used in cases where only six lower front teeth are standing. They tend to be unsightly and are only used when no other rest can be provided.

The use of indirect retainers and occlusal rests is discussed further in the next chapter.

Chapter XXI

MATERIALS FOR PARTIAL DENTURE BASES

This is primarily a book on clinical prosthetics. This short section on the materials available for the construction of partial denture bases is included however, as it is felt that a comparison between them will be helpful in view of the fact that design is greatly influenced by the material of which the denture is made.

There is no doubt that the gold alloys have for a long time, first in swaged and later in cast form, been the material of choice for the construction of a large majority of partial dentures but unfortunately its present high cost now seriously limits its use.

More recently the introduction of chrome alloys has provided an alternative to gold and these materials will be compared for their suitability for the construction of partial dentures.

The bases for partial dentures may be made of either plastic materials or metal alloys.

Plastic Materials

In the past many plastic materials have been used for dentures and most of them have been discarded as their unsuitability for this purpose became apparent, celluloid and phenol-formaldehyde resin for example, to mention only two. Research for the ideal plastic material still continues but at the present moment only vulcanite and polymethyl methacrylate (acrylic resin), are in general use.

For nearly a hundred years vulcanite was the material of choice and it still possesses many excellent properties which render it highly suitable as a base material. Unfortunately its manufacture in this country has now been discontinued though it is still obtainable from foreign sources.

Although the acrylic resins are now virtually the only bases used, a comparison of them with vulcanite is useful.

536

Advantages of Acrylic Resin

(1) It simulates the appearance of natural gum to a greater degree than vulcanite or metal.

(2) The technique is simple and quick and requires little special apparatus.

(3) It can be used for all cases although it is not necessarily the best material for the majority.

(4) It can be used for the whole denture, including the teeth.

(5) It forms a chemical union with acrylic teeth thus giving a very strong attachment.

(6) Repairs and additions can easily be made.

(7) It is light in weight.

(8) It is easy to keep clean.

Disadvantages of Acrylic Resin

(1) The design of dentures is greatly limited by the weakness of the material.

(2) Its resistance to fatigue is low, and it frequently fractures after a few months in the mouth.

(3) It has a tendency to warp during de-flasking, as the stresses induced in the material during processing are released. This may lead to inaccuracy of fit. It also warps when re-cured for repairing.

(4) Its softness leads to rapid wear when used for posterior teeth in contact with natural ones. It is also easily abraded by cleaning with a stiff brush.

Advantages of Vulcanite

(1) It is very accurate and warps to a much lesser degree than acrylic resin.

(2) It is highly elastic, very flexible and possesses a high resistance to fatigue. It is thus capable of passing into and out of small undercuts and rarely fractures in use.

(3) It can be repaired without distortion.

(4) The technique is simple and quick.

Disadvantages of Vulcanite

(1) Its appearance is very unlifelike and this is the main reason why it has been so largely displaced by acrylic resin.

(2) Its surface hardness is very low and in use it soon loses its polish and, in consequence, is difficult to clean.

Vulcanite is unlikely again to be used as a sole base material, but in view of its many superior physical properties it is sometimes very valuable as the main base material if acrylic resin is used in conjunction with it as a facing for those parts of the denture which show.

METAL ALLOYS

Advantages of Metals

(1) Their superior physical properties enable them to be used in thin section and this factor allows great latitude in the design of the denture. It is also appreciated by the patient, as partial metal dentures take up little space in the mouth.

(2) Their resistance to fatigue is great and fracture in the mouth is uncommon.

(3) Their high thermal conductivity enables normal sensations of heat and cold to be appreciated.

Disadvantages of Metals

(1) The techniques of their fabrication are time-consuming, require a high degree of skill and need special apparatus.

(2) Their appearance does not simulate the natural gum.

(3) Additions and repairs cannot be performed easily because these operations entail either soldering or welding and in the majority of cases before either can be performed the teeth need to be removed from the denture.

(4) They may cause electrolytic action if the denture is in contact with a dissimilar metal filling.

INDIVIDUAL METAL ALLOYS

Casting Alloys

(Yellow Gold)

This is an excellent material for use in constructing any type of partial denture.

Its advantages are:

(1) If cast into an investment which gives compensatory thermal expansion for the casting shrinkage, the final denture is accurate.

(2) Due to the fact that all properly constituted gold alloys contain from 12–15 per cent of copper, they are susceptible to heat treatment. The value of this is that the casting may be softened for the final adjustment of clasps, and then given the hardening heat treatment which endows the denture with:

(a) *A high proportional limit;* thus enabling it to resist all normal stresses brought to bear on it, in and out of the mouth.

(b) *A modulus of elasticity* which is sufficiently high to allow the connectors to be made thin, but not so high as to rob the clasps of adequate flexibility.

(3) Any additions, such as wrought clasps or metal backings for porcelain-faced teeth, may easily be soldered on to the main base.

Disadvantages of Gold:

The only true one is its high cost, although some individuals consider its colour to be a disadvantage.

Palladium Silver Alloys (*White Golds*)

Advantages:

(1) They produce accurately fitting dentures.

(2) They are, like yellow gold, susceptible to heat treatment but the final mechanical properties are not so satisfactory as yellow gold.

(3) Attachments can be added easily by soldering.

(4) Are cheaper than yellow gold although the cost is still considerable.

Disadvantages:

(1) Alloys containing a high silver content tend to turn black in use due to the formation of silver sulphide.

(2) The high rate of occlusion of oxygen and hydrogen tends to produce porosity.

(3) Care must be taken, and the manufacturers' instructions rigidly adhered to, when heat treating these alloys or brittleness' will result.

Cobalt Chrome Alloys

Advantages:

(1) They are so far the only completely corrosion-resistant base metal alloys which can be cast.

(2) The denture is an accurate fit, provided a special compensatory investment is used for its casting.

(3) Compared with the precious metal alloys they are extremely cheap.

(4) The majority of them have a satisfactory proportional limit and a high modulus of elasticity.

(5) They can be added to by soldering or welding.

Disadvantages:

(1) They require a considerable amount of special apparatus for their fabrication.

(2) They take longer to trim and polish than other metal alloys.

(3) Their flexibility is low.

(4) They are not susceptible to heat treatment.

(5) They lack the 'kindliness' of gold, and are extremely hard.

Wrought Alloys

Gold or palladium silver alloys and stainless steel can be fashioned into partial dentures by swaging between special dies and counter dies.

Since the mechanical properties of wrought metals are superior to those of cast, due to the difference in grain structure, swaged dentures can be made even thinner than those which are cast.

The main disadvantages of wrought metal denture bases are:

(1) The fit is far less accurate than with castings.

(2) Skeleton dentures are very difficult, if not impossible, to fabricate.

(3) Strengthening of individual areas can only be done by soldering or welding on an extra thickness of metal.

Stainless steel for many years has been the main wrought alloy used in dentistry but its usefulness for partial dentures has been greatly limited by the difficult technique, which requires a special hydraulic press and a welding machine.

The Composition of Cobalt Chrome Alloys

No detailed specifications of the alloys available in this country are published.

As is the case with the gold alloys the individual chrome alloys on the market differ slightly from each other but their general composition is roughly within the range of either

(a)	Chromium	30%	or	(b)	Chromium	30%
	Cobalt	60%			Cobalt	30%
	Molybdenum	5%			Nickel	30%
					Molybdenum	5%

The other 5% is made up by small quantities of Carbon, Iron, Manganese, Silicon, Aluminium, and Beryllium which are added to modify the properties of hardness, stiffness and ductility. It is the large chromium content which produces the corrosion resistance exhibited by these alloys and this is their main claim for use in dentistry.

The Mechanical Properties of Cobalt Chrome Alloys

The mechanical properties of these alloys in the cast condition given as an average are as follows:

Proportional Limit 60,000 lb./in.^{2}

This figure means that the material is strong enough to resist any normal stresses it is likely to encounter in dental use and compares favourably with many casting golds.

Modulus of Elasticity 30×10^6 lb./in.^{2}

This indicates that a large force is required to produce a

small deformation of the material, in other words it is stiff. Such a property is desirable in such parts of a partial denture as connectors, rests and indirect retainers. Taken together with the proportional limit, however, it means that the alloy possesses a low flexibility which is a disadvantage in clasps.

Brinell Hardness 250–320

This means that the material is a little difficult to polish but once a lustre has been obtained it will remain during long use in the mouth. The higher figure of 320 is above the hardness of tooth enamel which is on an average about 250.

Percentage Elongation 3–4 per cent

This figure refers to the ductility of the material and gives an indication of the amount of adjustment to which it may be subjected once cast. 3–4 per cent is not high but some gold alloys in the heat treated condition are lower than this.

Specific Gravity 7·9

For a given volume its mass is less than half that of gold and it may, therefore, be considered a very light material.

The Application of these Properties to Denture Design

(1) The cross-sectional area of connectors such as lingual bars, palatal bars and continuous clasps may be less than that usually employed when using a gold alloy. This is due to the greater stiffness of the material and not to its greater strength.

(2) The dimensions of clasps should be as small as possible, never greater than British Dental wire gauge B and they should taper towards their tip. The reasons for this are:

(*a*) The flexibility of the material is low and its stiffness great. These factors vary with the square of the cross-sectional area and if this is kept as low as possible and further reduced by tapering the tip of the clasp less force is required to insert and remove the denture and the tooth will not be gripped too rigidly.

(*b*) If the clasp arm is placed too deeply into a severe undercut it will have to travel outwards a great distance to pass over the most bulbous part of the tooth and then a corresponding distance inwards to grip the tooth. As the flexibility is so low, the force required to drive the arm outwards this distance may be greater than the proportional limit of the material will withstand and consequently it will bend.

(3) Clasps must be accurately positioned and accurately cast because the percentage elongation is insufficient to allow of much adjustment.

CHAPTER XXII

THE BASIC PRINCIPLES OF PARTIAL DENTURE DESIGN

The requirements of a partial denture may be summarized as follows:

(1) It must spread the forces which will act on it evenly over the supporting tissues to a degree within their physiological limit and be adequately retained in position in the mouth during all normal functional movements.

(2) It must prevent the dental arch from collapsing by preventing the teeth from drifting or tilting into edentulous spaces. It must also cause the minimum amount of damage to either soft or hard tissues.

(3) It must maintain the health of previously unopposed teeth by restoring their function and preventing their over-eruption.

(4) It must restore masticatory efficiency and appearance and be comfortable to wear.

To satisfy all the above requirements it will be apparent that the designer of a partial denture must take into account many things, satisfy many needs and solve many problems. The group of problems which it is intended to deal with here is restricted, for simplicity of explanation, to the method of designing a denture so that it may satisfactorily transmit to the supporting tissues the loads which will be applied to it in function in such a manner that the tissues themselves do not have to bear loads above their tolerance and the denture itself will remain stable under all normal conditions.

In order to produce a design which satisfies the above conditions the simplest manner in which to proceed is to divide the complex loads which are applied to a partial denture into the four basic component loads which are: (1) vertical occlusal, (2) lateral, (3) antero-posterior, (4) vertical dislodging[1]. Then, taking these one by one, ensure that the denture is designed to transmit each to the supporting tissues without

[1]*Partial Dentures*, Osborne, J. and Lammie, G. A., Blackwell Scientific Publications, First and Second editions.

overload and at the same time ensure that it is adequately braced against movement by the load.

The first question the designer asks himself therefore is:

How are the vertical occlusal loads to be transmitted?

When deciding whether a given denture is to be tooth-borne, tissue-borne or tooth and tissue-borne the following points should be kept in mind.

(*a*) A fully tooth-borne denture will resist the greatest loads and provide the most efficient mastication.

(*b*) If the denture is opposed by natural teeth, tooth-borne support is desirable, because, under these circumstances the load applied to the denture will be at the maximum.

(*c*) A denture can only be fully tooth-borne by molar and premolar teeth, with sound or adequately restored crowns, supported by well-formed roots whose long axes are almost vertical and are embedded for an adequate distance in healthy bone (the information to enable one to make a decision on this aspect will be available from the clinical examination).

Canines and incisors cannot alone provide sufficient support for a tooth-borne saddle, due to the inclination of their palatal or lingual surfaces, unless suitable inlays are fitted with occlusal rest seatings prepared in them. Taken together as a group of three or more teeth, however, they may be able to support a denture without the necessity of inlay preparation.

(*d*) If the occlusal rests are to transmit effectively to the teeth the loads imposed on the denture there must be sufficient room for them to be adequately seated. Study models will show if there is sufficient room for the rests with the teeth in occlusion and if there is not room it can frequently be made by grinding the opposing tooth. The seat should always be prepared for the rest in the enamel of the tooth which is going to carry it and obviously any such preparation must be completed prior to the taking of the working impressions.

(*e*) If the saddle areas are extensive, that is where more than two natural teeth are missing from any saddle, it will probably be necessary to design the denture so that the loads applied to it are transmitted via the soft tissues. Under these circumstances as great an area as possible of the ridge must be covered so as to reduce the load applied per unit area.

If the denture-bearing area of the tissue-borne denture is considered inadequate to withstand the anticipated vertical loading, such for example as some instances of the Kennedy Class I lower in which there is a narrow, knife-like ridge with shallow sulci, it will be necessary to reduce the vertical load applied during mastication by:

(1) reducing the bucco-lingual width of the artificial teeth,
(2) leaving off the last tooth from the saddle.

The problem of the tooth-tissue borne method of transferring the load is a vexed one and frequently the subject of misconception and the opinion of the authors on this question has been discussed in Chapter XIX.

A few examples of individual cases will be given to illustrate how a decision is arrived at.with regard to resistance to vertical loading.

Except where the outline is completely black the following diagrams are not intended to show the shape of the finished denture but are purely concerned with illustrating the approximate areas which will receive and resist the loads which are applied to the denture. The direction of the applied load and the area resisting it is delineated thus:

Occlusal loads

Lateral loads

Anteroposterior loads

Tortional loads

Mixed loads

*and the artificial teeth are drawn with a thick line to differentiate them
from the natural teeth.*

Fig. 416 represents a partially edentulous maxilla of the
Kennedy Class III type with 65|56 missing. It is opposed by a
full natural lower dentition. The crowns of 74|47 are sound
(the word 'sound' as used in this book means that the crown or
the tooth is either caries free or has been satisfactorily con-
served) and the roots are supported for more than two-thirds
of their length by bone.

In a case of this type the choice of method for supporting the
vertical loads is by occlusal rests on 74|47. A tooth-borne
denture will enable the patient to chew forcefully, it will not
tend to sink or be driven into the mucous membrane and the
rests themselves will prevent food being forced down between

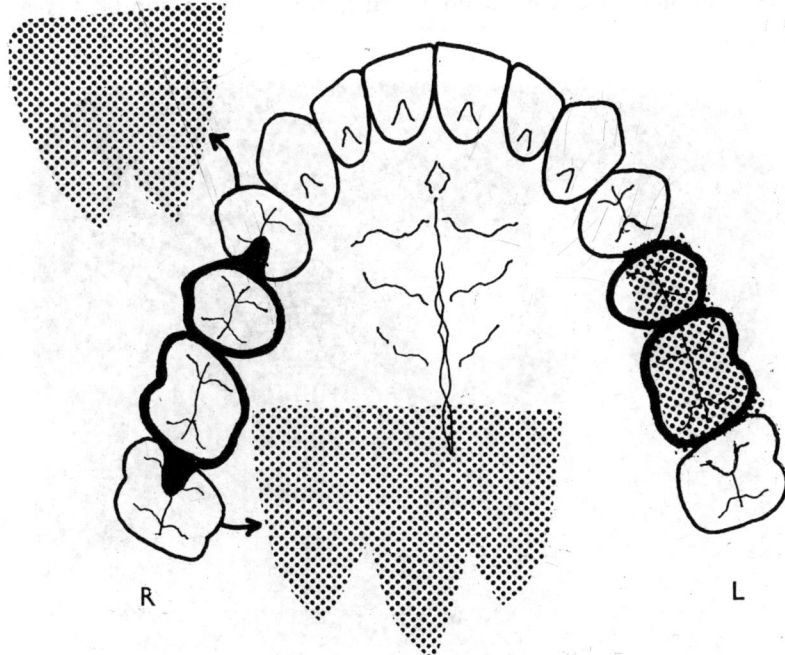

R   L

Fig. 416. – On the right the approximate area of the
periodontal membrane available for supporting the occlusal
loads is illustrated. Compare this with the area available on
the left if tissue support only is enlisted, *see also* fig. 418.

the denture and the abutment teeth on to the gingival margins. Before a final decision can be made that occlusal rests can be used on this case the models must be examined in occlusion to see, either that room exists for the rests or that it can be provided by limited grinding of the opposing teeth. Rest seats must be prepared in the fossae of the teeth carrying the rests.

If the supporting bone in a case of this type is considered on examination of the X-ray negatives to preclude the carrying of the additional load of the denture, that is, if the roots of the abutment teeth, or any one of them, is supported for less than one-half of its length by bone, or if the negatives show that the bone is undergoing rapid absorption (*see* fig. 417) then the saddles will have to be tissue-borne and they should be outlined on the models to cover as large an area of the ridge as possible so that the vertical load applied to the denture is spread as widely as possible. In a case such as this, tissue-borne saddles as a

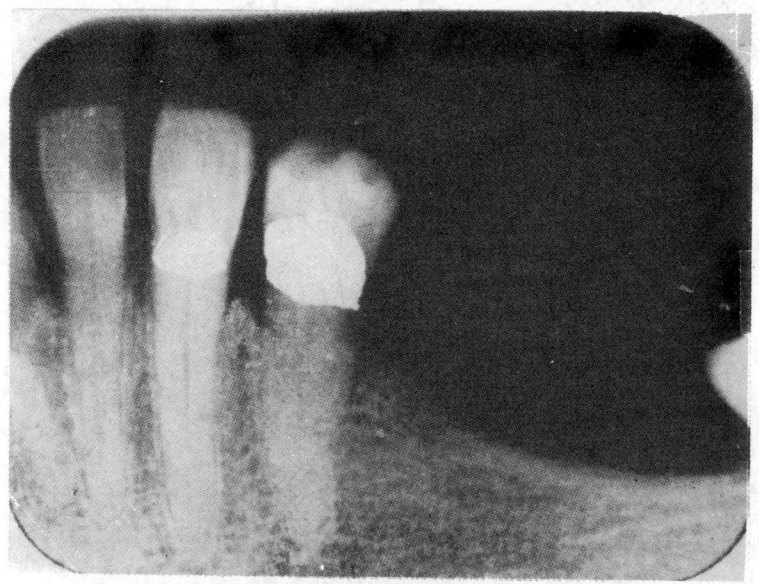

FIG. 417(a). – Illustrates a lower premolar which is quite unsuitable for carrying a rest: the bone is undergoing rapid absorption and a rarefying osteitis is present in the bone supporting the distal surface of the root.

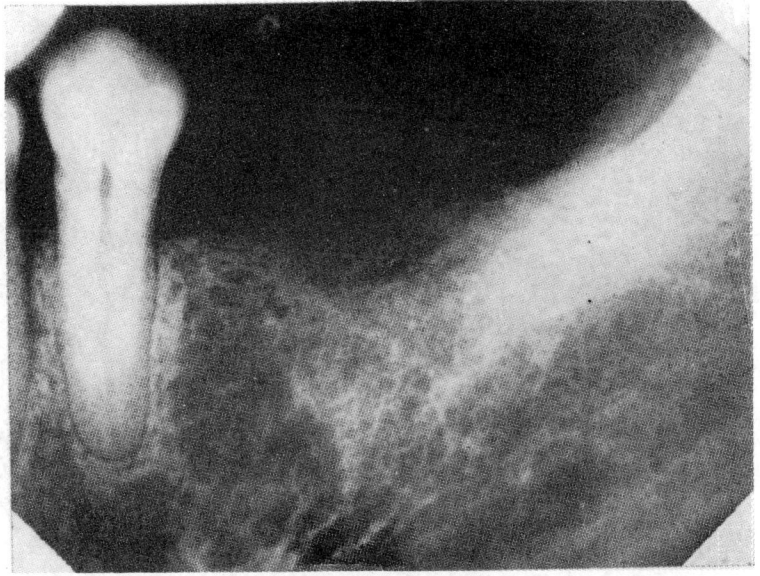

FIG. 417.

(b) Although this premolar is only partly supported by bone that immediately surrounding the root is showing a condensation of bone (condensing osteitis) which results in providing extra support for the tooth, and if this tooth is subjected to extra stress by placing a rest on it the bone will react favourably.

The surface of the edentulous ridge is not very suitable to support a tissue-borne denture because it shows evidence of rarefaction and the surface is rough in spite of the fact that the last tooth was extracted over two years ago.

means of transmitting the vertical load are very definitely inferior to occlusal rests as will be appreciated by studying fig. 418 which shows a comparison between the surface area of the periodontal membranes of the |47 available to support a tooth-borne saddle and the surface area of the mucous membrane which will support a tissue-borne saddle[1]. In addition, the mucous membrane will, in function, distort unevenly and therefore only some of its surface will actually transmit the load and finally absorption of the ridge will further upset the equilibrium.

[1] Watt, D. M., MacGregor, A. R., et al. (1958) Dental Pract. **9** : 2 (see also fig. 418).

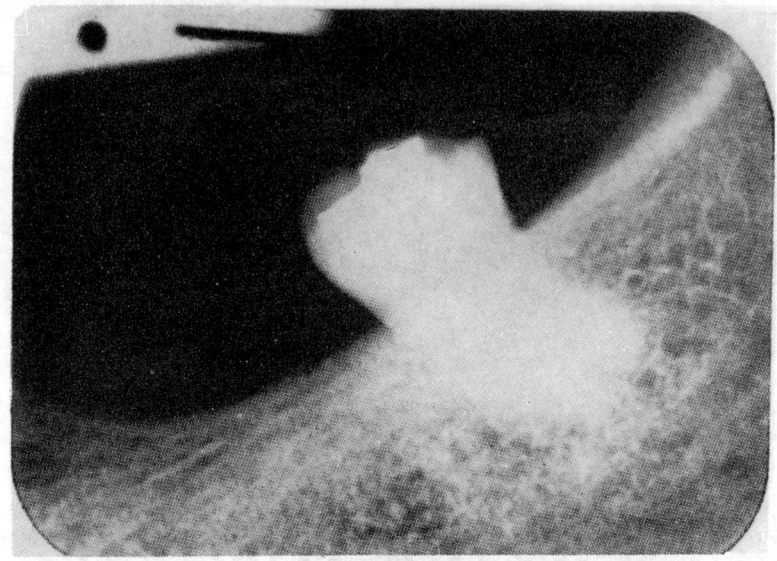

FIG. 417.
(c) Although the lower molar is leaning mesially it is well
supported by bone which shows signs of condensation
anteriorly. It would be wise to place the rest posteriorly
on this tooth so that the tilting movement of the load
would be reduced.

Nevertheless, in many cases of this kind, tissue-borne saddles
do provide a satisfactory foundation for transmitting the
vertical load and such dentures are frequently worn for many
years with satisfactory results.

Fig. 419 illustrates a case similar to fig. 416 with more extensive
lateral saddles, 654|456 being missing. Here the decision
between tooth- and tissue- borne saddles is not quite so simple
to make. The 7|7 can certainly carry rests, but with three
teeth on each saddle instead of two, as in fig. 416, the extra load
which the 7|7 can be called upon to bear will be proportionately
heavier and unless the roots of these teeth are long and very
well supported in dense bone such extra load is likely to cause
loosening and tilting of the teeth. Further, 3|3 by themselves
are not suitable teeth for carrying occlusal rests because the
palatal and cingular slopes of these teeth form an inclined

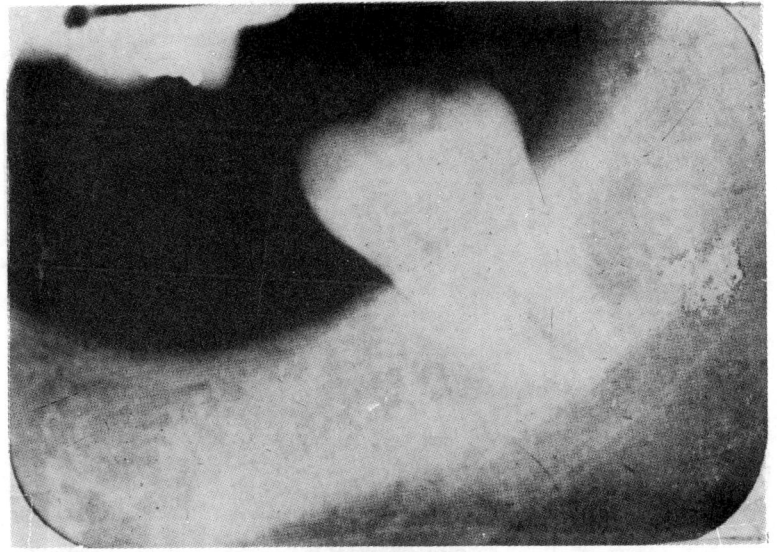

FIG. 417.

(d) The roots of this molar are short but the bone supporting
     it is dense and although it is tilted mesially it should be
     capable of supporting a distally placed rest.
     The surface of the edentulous ridge in both (c) and
     (d) is smooth and covered with a thin layer of cortical
     bone and should support a tissue borne saddle with little
     absorption.

plane and reference to fig. 415 will show that a vertical
occlusal load applied through a rest to such a surface is
resolved into a force along the surface and one at right angles to
it and if the angle of inclination of the palatal surface is steep
then most of the occlusal load is converted into a force tending
to drive the rest off the tooth. If, as in a case like this, the
posterior movement of the saddle which such a force will
engender is resisted by the buttressing effect of the mesial
surfaces of the upper second molars then an additional and
unfavourable backward load is applied to these already over-
loaded teeth. If it is decided that the canines must carry rests
then proper inlay preparations must be made in them with
rest seats designed to transmit the vertical loads straight down
the long axes of the canines. In a saddle of the length of that

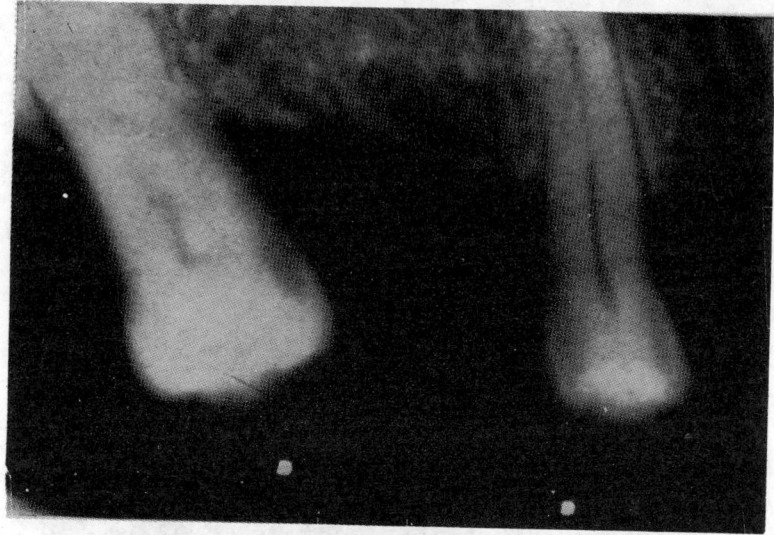

FIG. 417.

(e) The bone supporting both these teeth is rarefying rapidly and there is no evidence of condensation; the surface of the bone in the edentulous area shows no cortical bone and these teeth are quite incapable of supporting occlusal rests. A tissue-borne saddle would not fit for long because rapid absorption of the ridge would probably occur. These teeth are best extracted.

(No illustrations are given of ideal bone support for teeth carrying rests or for ridge surfaces carrying tissue-borne saddles as these are self evident. The above figures show X-rays of cases in which doubt may exist.)

shown in fig. 419, however, it is considered that this method of using the rest would overload the attachment of the canine and such techniques are best reserved for saddles carrying only two artificial teeth.

If the six front teeth in this case are considered as a group, and the denture carried up on to the cingulae of each tooth as shown in fig. 420 then possibly sufficient resistance to occlusal loading will be provided to make the saddles truly tooth-borne. If the slope of the palatal surfaces of these teeth is steep, however, an even greater backward thrust of the denture is likely to be engendered. In addition, a continuous rest of this type will, of necessity, cover the palatal gingival margins of these teeth which is detrimental to the health of these tissues. The

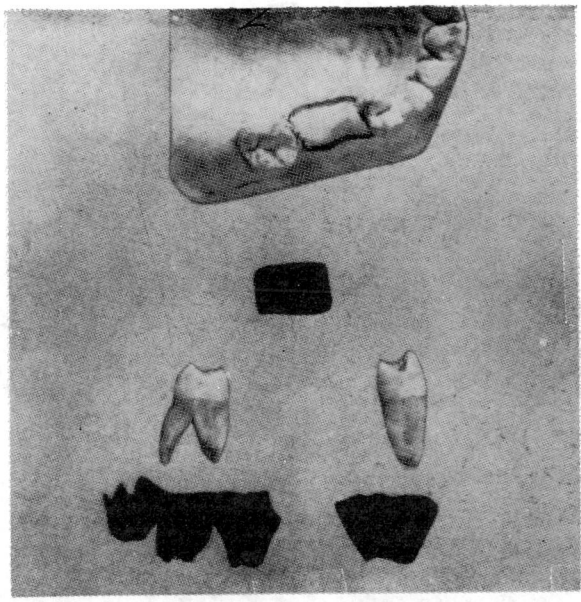

Fig. 418. – The black shape immediately below the model represents the area of mucous membrane available to support the occlusal load of a tissue-borne saddle replacing |56. Compare this with the black shapes below the molar and premolar teeth with represent the areas of the periodontal membranes of the |47 which are available to support the occlusal load of the saddle if it is tooth-borne. (After Watt and MacGregor *et al.*)

Kennedy bar can be used to overcome this difficulty but patients frequently dislike the narrow, raised ridge which such a bar presents to the tongue and finally a large majority of patients will present such a deep overbite that room is rarely available for either a continuation of the plate to provide a continuous rest or a Kennedy bar.

From the foregoing considerations it will be obvious that in the majority of cases a tissue-borne denture, as illustrated in fig. 419, will be the method of choice, the shaded areas in the diagram being the saddle areas which will resist the occlusal loads.

Fig. 421 illustrates, in the lower jaw, a similar case to fig. 419.

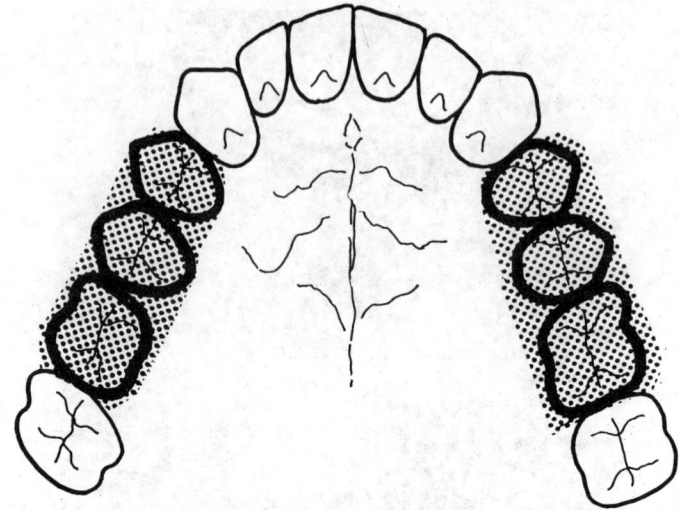

FIG. 419. – The approximate area available for tissue support in this case is shown.

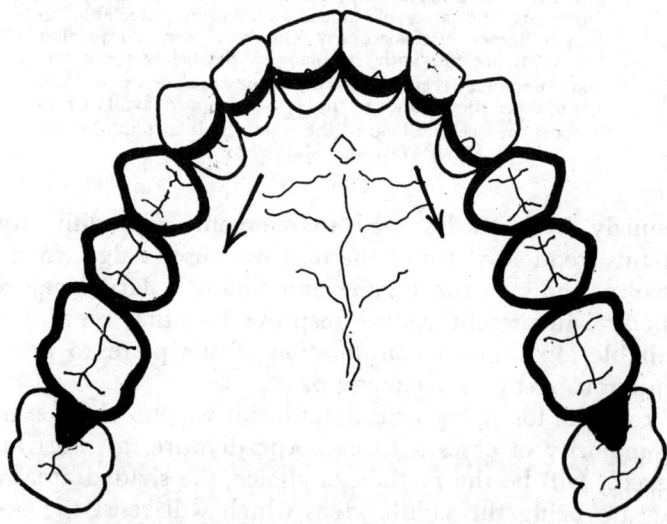

FIG. 420. – If the six anterior teeth are enlisted to provide tooth support for the two saddles then a powerful backward load is applied to 7|7 which may cause these teeth to shift.

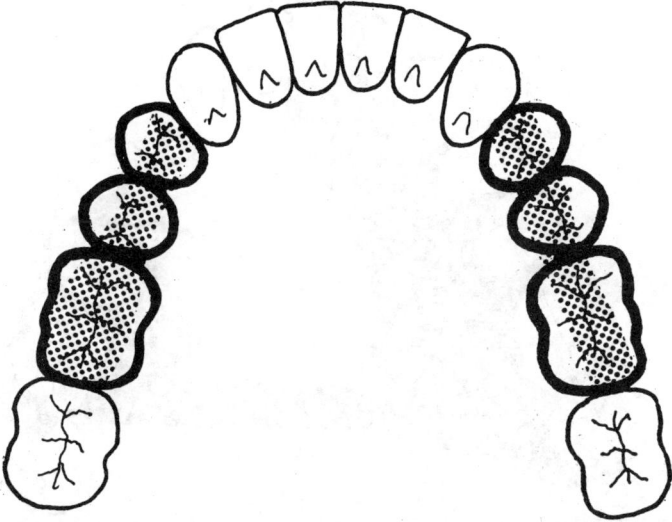

Fig. 421. – The only area available for the support of the saddles in this case is the shaded tissue shown in the diagram, because the acute slope of the lingual surfaces of 321|123 precludes the use of a continuous rest.

Here the remarks regarding the effect of a continuous rest on the inclined lingual surfaces of the lower front teeth apply even more forcefully because the angulation of the inclines of these teeth is steeper as a general rule than those of the upper teeth.

Fig. 422 illustrates a case with three saddles. Here the choice of support of vertical load is complex. Following the above reasoning the right saddle carrying 7654| should be tissue-borne, the front saddle also should be tissue-borne unless properly prepared inlays are to be inserted into the 3|1. The left hand saddle, however, carrying only |56 and having as abutments the |47 which can well support the two artificial teeth, can be tooth-borne. If it is considered desirable to make this saddle tooth-borne, perhaps because it is opposed by natural teeth in the lower jaw, then the connector between this saddle and the other two must be of such dimensions that it allows the slight but definite differential movement between it and the other two tissue-borne saddles.

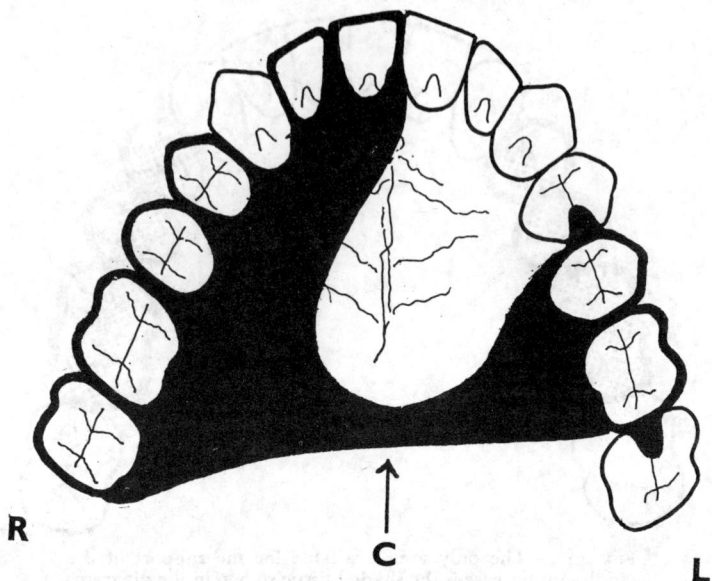

FIG. 422. – 7654 21| are tissue-borne and |56 are tooth-borne. The connector between the tooth and tissue-borne saddles (C) must be·of such dimensions that while being rigid it still allows a slight differential movement between the two classes of saddle otherwise as the tissue-borne one sinks slightly on chewing the tooth-borne saddle will rise.

In such cases as are illustrated in figs. 423 and 424 the problem of choice of the method of transmitting the occlusal load is simplified because these saddles are so extensive that they can only be tissue-borne.

The second question:

How are the lateral loads to be resisted?

These loads are imposed during the lateral movements of the mandible during normal mastication; they can be varied by tooth form, tooth area and the balance of the articulation, but they cannot be eliminated. Even if the teeth are left out of any possible contact a lateral load can still be applied through the medium of intervening foodstuff. The greatest lateral stresses arise where there is cuspal interference and when this is absent the lateral stress is proportional to the occlusal area.

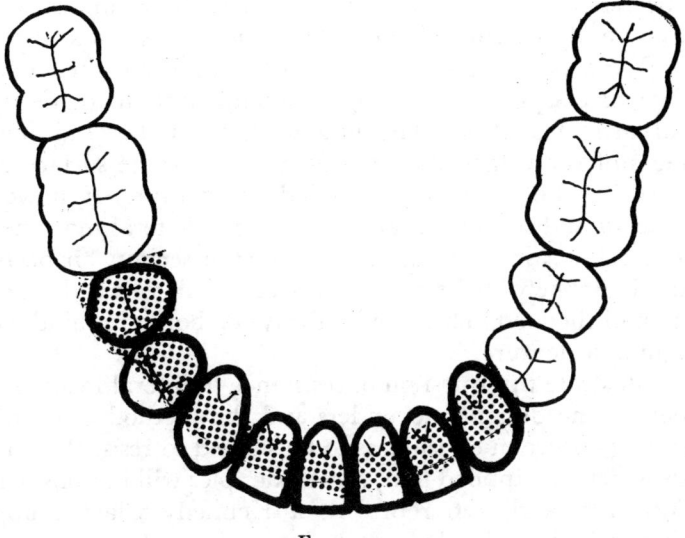

FIG. 423.

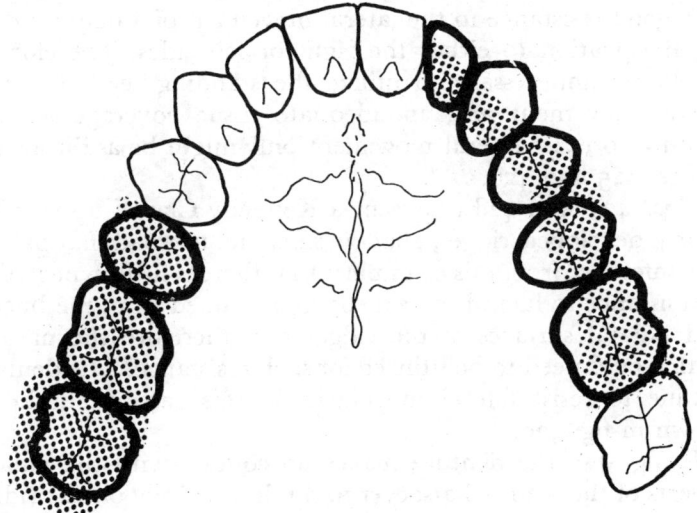

FIG. 424.
The area for supporting the occlusal load is shown dotted.

The tissues which will resist the lateral movements of the denture and transmit them to the underlying bone are the lingual and palatal surfaces of the teeth and also their buccal surfaces if clasps incorporating a bracing section to the functional arm are fitted. The lingual and palatal and buccal surfaces of the ridges also provide a considerable surface area for resisting the lateral loads applied to a denture. If, however, both teeth and soft tissues are used to resist lateral movements, then, for the same reasons as given in the section on occlusal loads, it is likely to be the teeth which will carry the major portion of the load. This should always be borne in mind when designing a denture.

To illustrate this question of resistance to lateral loading and to enable the designer to understand the method of deciding how the denture in question is to be shaped to resist the lateral loads which are applied to it, three examples will be considered.

Figs. 425 and 426 represent a Kennedy Class I upper, having well formed ridges, with deep sulci and a deep, broad palate.

The observations made when studying such a case would be that the well-developed ridges of the saddle areas would provide good resistance to the lateral movement of a denture during mastication to either the right or left sides. Therefore it would be unnecessary to utilize the standing teeth to resist lateral movement and an adequate tissue coverage for the denture to resist lateral movement only might be as illustrated in figs. 425 and 426.

Figs. 427 and 428 represent a Kennedy Class I upper with poorly developed ridges, shallow sulci and a broad, flat palate. The inference from this example is that there is little expectation of resistance to lateral movement to be gained from the buccal and palatal surfaces of the ridges and therefore the natural teeth would need to be utilized for such resistance. The denture outline to resist lateral movement in this case might be as shown in fig. 429.

In fig. 427 the denture makes no contact with the palatal aspects of the teeth whatsoever and relies entirely on the ridges for support against lateral movement, whereas in fig. 429 all the palatal surfaces of the teeth are covered by the denture to brace

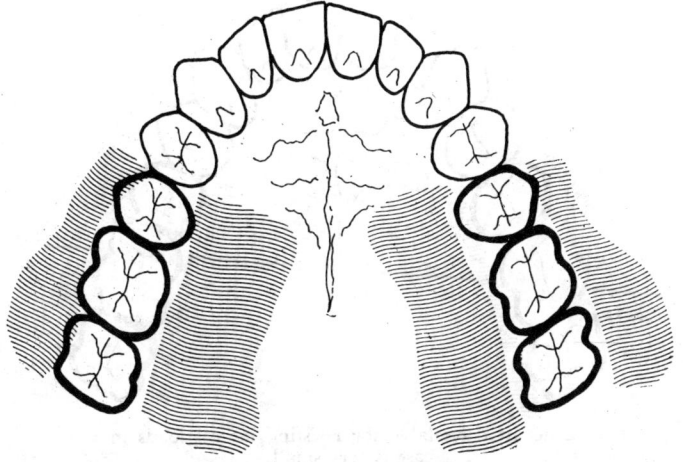

The shaded area is the tissue available for resisting lateral
loads applied to this case.

FIG. 425. – In plan.

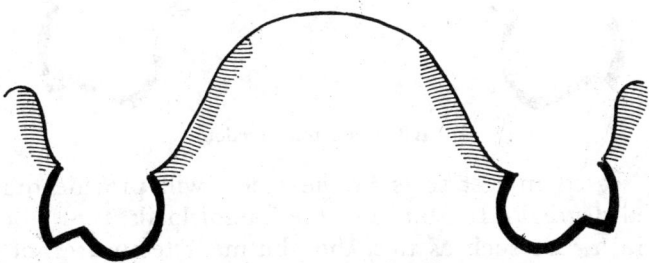

FIG. 426. – In coronal section.

it against lateral movement and additional bracing is also
obtained from the rigid parts of the clasp arms.

Fig. 430 represents a Kennedy Class III Modification I type
of case, either upper or lower with 65|56 missing. The abut-
ment teeth are sound and well supported by dense bone and
under these circumstances, the occlusal load being taken by the
rests, the lateral loads can safely be accepted by these teeth
and resistance to lateral movement can be gained by carrying
clasps and reciprocals on the buccal and palatal aspects of
these teeth. In addition, of course, the occlusal rests themselves

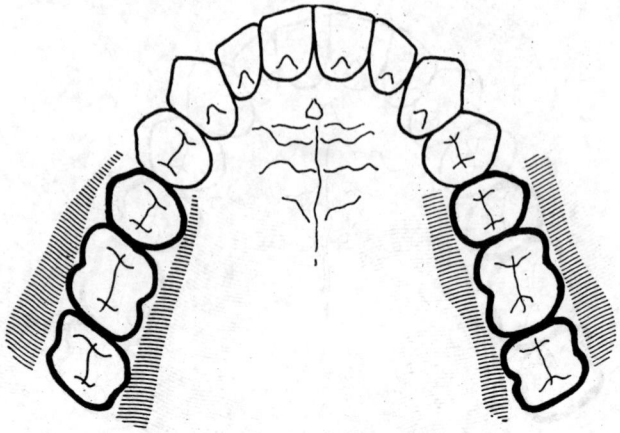

The tissue area available for resisting lateral loads in this case is very small:

FIG. 427. – In plan.

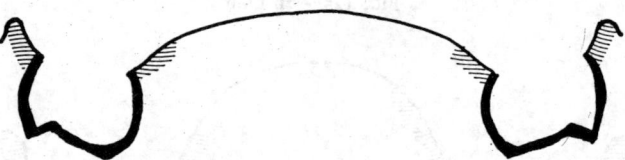

FIG. 428. – In coronal section.

being seated in rest seats in the teeth, will provide quite a marked degree of resistance to the lateral loads.

If, in a case such as this, the abutment teeth are not well supported by bone, it may be necessary to transmit the lateral load entirely by means of the palatal and buccal slopes of the ridges and in this case a decision will have to be made as to whether the resistance afforded by these surfaces is adequate to provide sufficient resistance to lateral movement on the same lines as the decision was made in the cases illustrated in 425 and 427. If the lateral slopes of the ridges are capable of resisting the load then a possible outline might be similar to that illustrated in fig. 426. This shows how the broad coverage of the lateral slopes of the ridges will enable adequate resistance to lateral movement to be provided. If the lateral and palatal slopes of the ridges are considered inadequate to provide

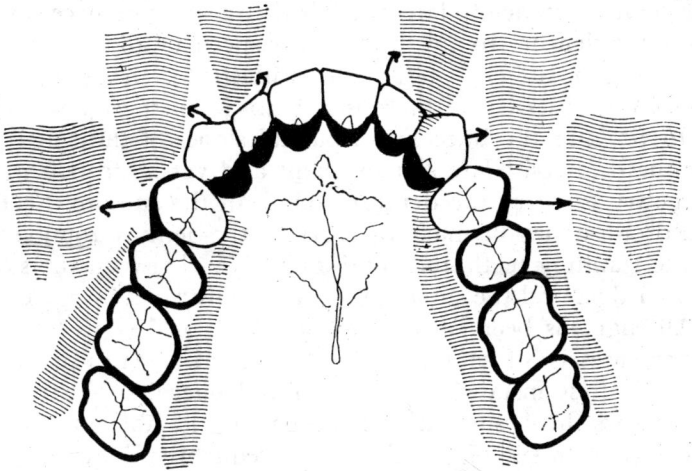

FIG. 429. – By carrying the denture round the natural teeth (shown in black) a much greater area is made available to resist the lateral loads: compare with fig. 427.

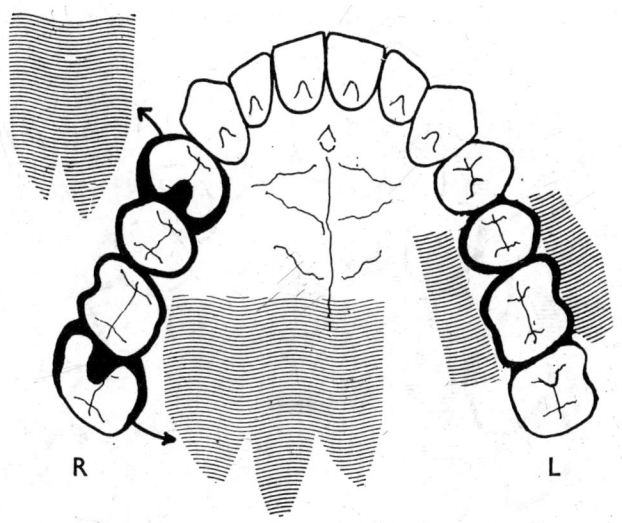

R   L

FIG. 430. – The right side illustrates the approximate area available if the saddle carrying the second premolar and first molar rely on the teeth to resist lateral loads. The left side illustrates the approximate area available if the soft tissues are employed.

sufficient resistance to lateral loads then it may be necessary to carry the denture round the palatal aspects of all the standing teeth to gain sufficient resistance as illustrated in fig. 429.

In some cases where there is a doubt in the designer's mind as to whether the buccal and palatal slopes of the ridges are adequate to resist lateral movement and yet he feels it is unnecessary to carry the denture round all the standing teeth a compromise may be made by carrying the denture round some of the standing teeth and sharing the load between the slopes of the ridges and the standing teeth, as illustrated in fig. 431.

All that has been said about the types of designs for these upper cases is, of course, applicable to lower cases of similar type, in these instances the lingual and buccal surfaces of the ridges are the tissue surfaces which are capable of resisting lateral movement of the denture. Frequently, however, it is found in lower cases, that the ridges are less well developed than the uppers and often, therefore, greater support must be enlisted from the standing teeth.

When designing a denture to resist lateral movement, care must be taken that no individual tooth is subjected to too

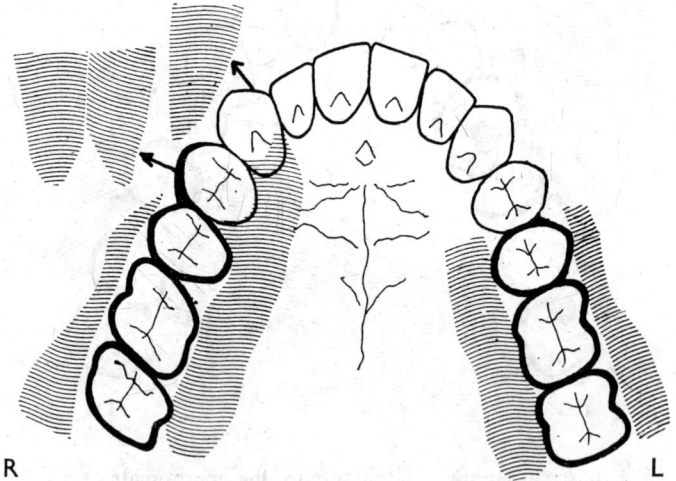

R   L

FIG. 431. – The left side illustrates the area available if the soft tissues only are used to resist lateral loads and the right side shows the additional area available if the denture is carried round 43|.

severe a load neither in a direct lateral direction nor in the form of a rotary one.

The case illustrated in fig. 432 is an example of how this possibility may develop. The case illustrated is a Kennedy Class I lower Modification I, the left saddle being completely edentulous and the right side being edentulous except for the isolated lower second premolar. The ridges are absorbed and the sulci are shallow and if the denture is designed with a lingual bar as illustrated then the tendency of the denture to move sideways is resisted almost entirely by its contact with the isolated standing premolar. In addition there is a tendency for the saddle on the left hand side to move backwards during mastication and to inflict a torsional strain on this isolated tooth. In such a case the resistance to lateral movement must be increased by carrying the denture around the lingual aspects of all the lower standing front teeth, as illustrated in fig. 433 and also by placing a bracing type of clasp on the lower canines.

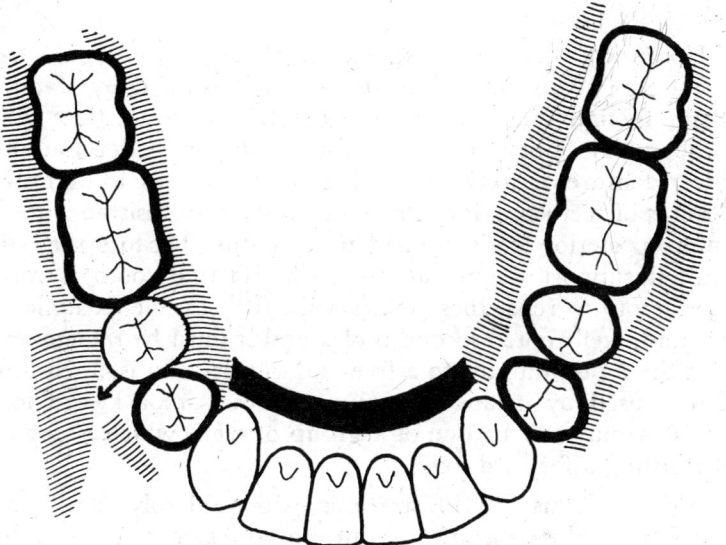

Fig. 432. – Note the small area of the soft tissues available to resist the lateral loads applied by this denture if a lingual bar is used as a connector and how the major resistance must come from the 5|.

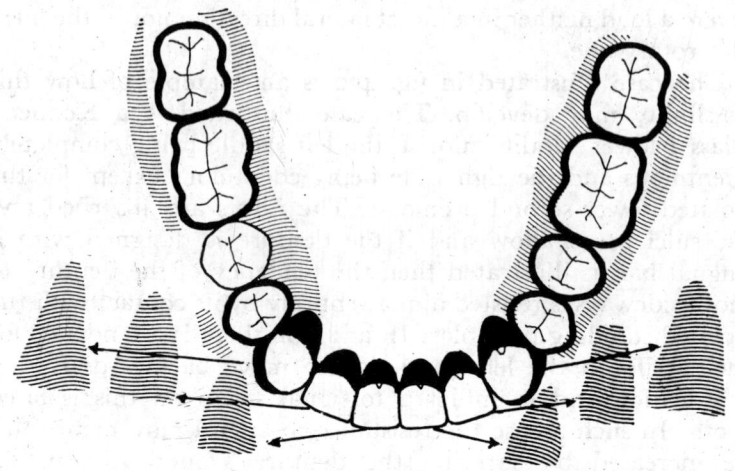

FIG. 433. – If 3|3 are clasped and the denture is carried round the lower front teeth the area available for resisting the lateral load is greatly increased.

The Third Question

How are the antero-posterior loads to be resisted?

These, like the lateral loads, are best resisted by standing teeth, though they may be resisted by the soft tissues via a large labial flange or, less satisfactorily, an extension of a lower denture on to the anterior slope of the ascending ramus. Groups of teeth provide the most satisfactory resistance to the antero-posterior loads applied to a denture because they give mutual support to one another. An isolated tooth is rarely satisfactory to resist these loads, with the possible exception of a sound, well-rooted second molar and it must be remembered that the tooth anterior to a free-end saddle is an isolated tooth if it is used by means of a clasp to resist a backward load, whilst it may still be one of a group of teeth which is capable of resisting a forward load.

Again the use of illustrations will probably clarify this question of the resistance to antero-posterior loads. Fig. 434 represents a Kennedy Class III Modification I case in which there are two bounded saddles. The resistance to the anterior movement of this denture is provided by the distal surfaces of

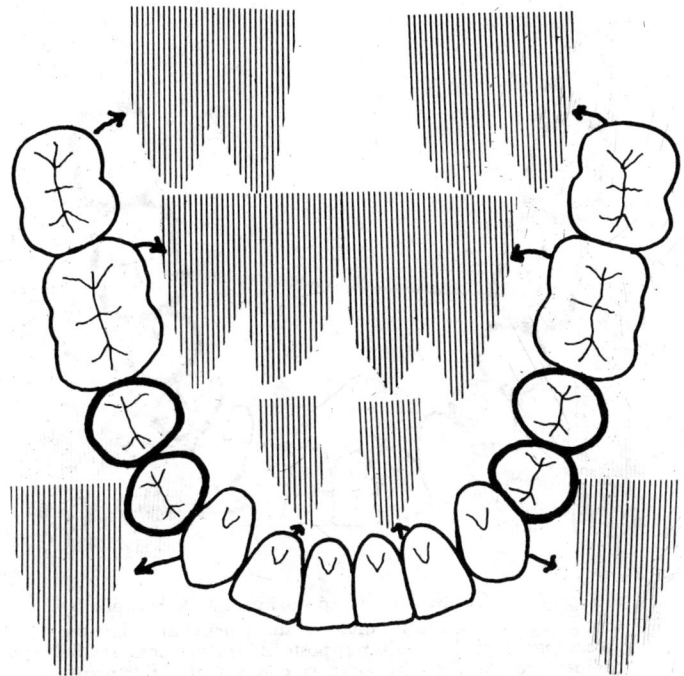

Fig. 434. – The large area available for resisting antero-posterior loads in a case carrying a bounded saddle is shaded.

the canines which themselves are supported by the four incisors and provided these teeth are adequately supported by bone they are quite capable of resisting all the anterior loads which are likely to be applied to this denture during function. The posterior loads are similarly satisfactorily resisted by the mesial surfaces of the first molars, which themselves are buttressed again by the second molars. In this type of case no real problem arises with regard to the antero-posterior type of movement. The main problems of designing a denture to resist antero-posterior movement are concerned mainly with the Kennedy Class I free-end saddle type of dentures and the Kennedy Class IV anterior saddle dentures. Fig. 435(a) illustrates a Kennedy Class I lower. The resistance to anterior movement of this saddle is adequately provided by the distal surfaces of the canines which, as in the previous illustration, are

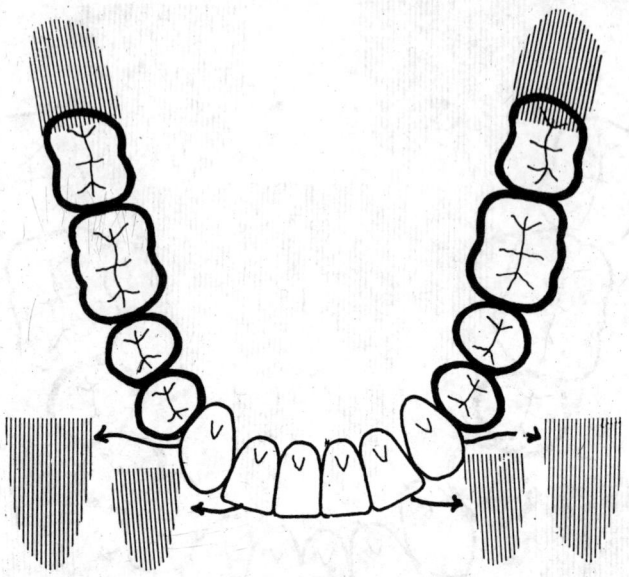

FIG. 435(*a*). - Illustrating the approximate area provided by the 32|23 for resisting anterior movement and by the ascending rami for resisting posterior movement. If the canines are clasped with bracing clasps some of the area provided by the teeth will resist posterior movement also.

well buttressed by the other standing teeth. The resistance to posterior movement, however, can only be achieved by carrying the distal extension of the base of the denture as high up the ascending ramus as the case will allow. Fig. 435(*c*) shows how

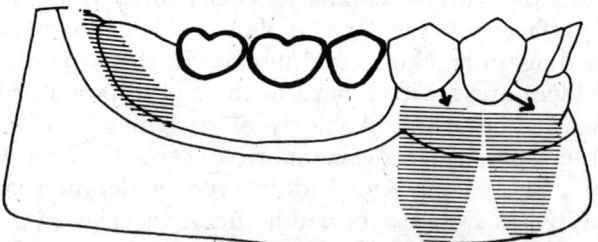

FIG. 435(*b*). - Plenty of area to resist anterior loads but little to resist posterior movement. If 4| is clasped some of the area available for resisting anterior movement can be utilised to resist posterior loads.

finishing the saddle short distally provides no resistance to posterior movement, whereas fig. 435(*b*) shows how the extension of the base of the saddle up on to the ascending ramus will provide a resistance to posterior movement. If, in addition, clasps are fitted to the lower canines with satisfactory bracing action, these also will provide additional resistance to posterior movement. Care must be taken, however, that these clasps are not so rigid that they tend to place abnormally high loads on these teeth.

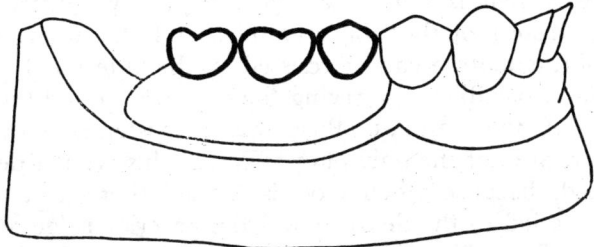

Fig. 435(*c*). – No resistance to posterior movement at all because the heels of the denture are finished short of the ascending ramii and there is no clasp round the $\overline{4|}$.

In Kennedy Class I uppers there is no anterior slope of the ascending ramus such as exists in the lower to buttress the denture against posterior movement. Fortunately, however, most of the loads applied to an upper denture during mastication are in a forward direction due to the upward and forward movement of the lower jaw and the inclines of the cusps and in these cases the distal surfaces of the canine teeth and the anterior slope of the palate provide adequate resistance to anterior movement.

The Kennedy Class II type of case sometimes presents considerable problems in relation to resistance to posterior movement and here it is sometimes necessary to provide really rigid bracing by carrying a rigid connector round to the other side of the mouth and firmly clasping the standing natural teeth on that side. Although this is likely to produce a torsional movement of these teeth, provided they are well rooted and two or sometimes three of them are clasped, they are usually capable of standing up to the torsional load thus applied to them. If, in addition, the lower canine on the side of the saddle is also clasped and the denture carried round it and up on its lingual surface, and in addition the posterior aspect of the saddle is carried on to the ascending ramus, adequate resistance to posterior movement can be provided. The carrying of the bracing connector round to the opposite side of the mouth also provides considerable resistance to lateral movements applied to this denture. The area resisting labial loads is illustrated in fig. 436.

Kennedy Class IV cases present one or two special problems. In the case illustrated in fig. 437 the posterior movement of the denture, which is slight, can be adequately resisted by the mesial surfaces of the upper canines and the anterior movement of the denture can be resisted by the anterior slope of the palate and possibly by carrying the denture around the palatal aspects of the canines. Pure antero-posterior movements, however, are not the only ones to which this type of denture is subjected, because when food is incised there is a torsional strain applied to the denture and the anterior ridge and some of the surface of the palate acts as a fulcrum. This action is

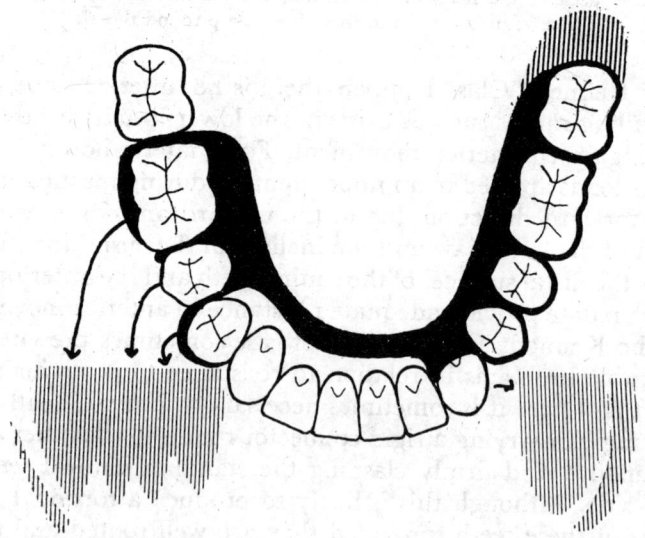

FIG. 436. – Areas available for resisting antero-posterior loads in Kennedy Class II type of case. A lingual plate carried round the lower anterior teeth would be even better.

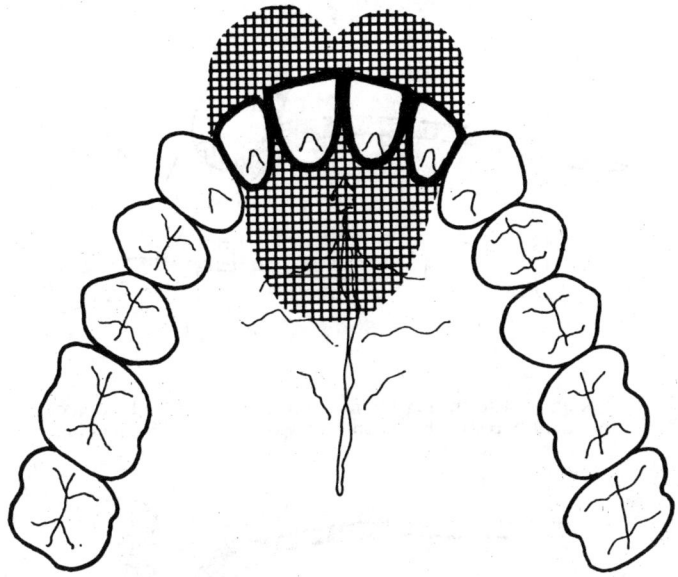

FIG. 437. – Area available to resist torsional loads applied during incision in the case of an upper Kennedy Class IV.

illustrated in fig. 438. This torsional action frequently produces considerable damage to the ridge and anterior surface of the palate, producing quite rapidly, a flabby and inflamed mucous membrane with loss of supporting alveolar bone. It is, therefore, particularly important in this type of case that some means of spreading this torsional strain is incorporated in the design of the denture. The fitting of a labial flange will do much to reduce torsional stress by providing a broad bearing surface anteriorly and thus helping to resist the tilting load applied to the denture, as illustrated in fig. 439. Further resistance to the torsional stress may be gained by clasping the last molar teeth and this will provide a very definite resistance to the torsional movement of the denture because the anterior ridge is acting as a fulcrum and the application of the load is not very far from the fulcrum, whereas the application of the resistance by a clasp placed on the last molar is a long way from the fulcrum and therefore its mechanical advantage is great

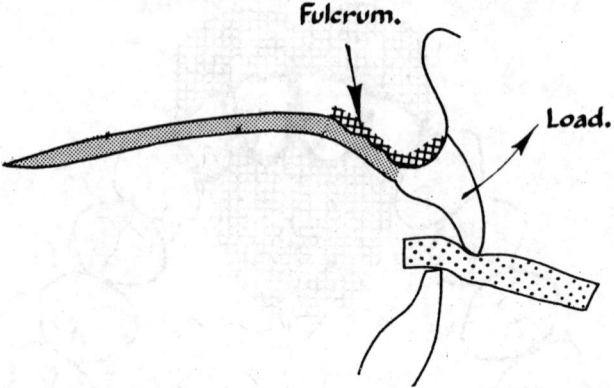

FIG. 438. – Illustrating the fulcrum which is the only area of this mouth resisting torsional loads applied when incising.

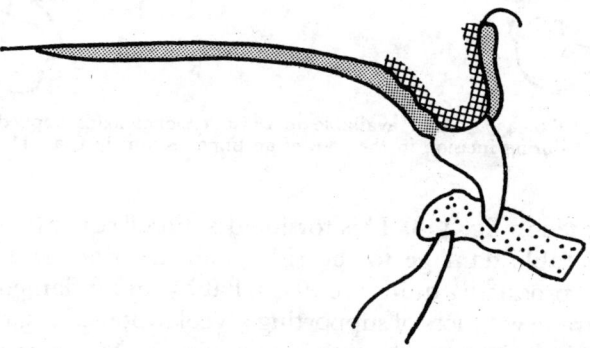

FIG. 439. – Illustrating how the fitting of a labial flange to a Kennedy Class IV denture produces a larger area for resisting the torsional loads applied during incising.

see fig. 440). In some cases it is impossible to put a labial flange on this type of case because the patient's appearance would be spoiled by its presence. When it is necessary to 'gum-fit' the anterior teeth a clasp or clasps must be fitted as far posteriorly as is practicable in order to resist torsional movement.

The Fourth Question

How are the vertical dislodging forces to be resisted?

Forces which tend to dislodge a denture are:

(*a*) Gravity. Upper denture only.

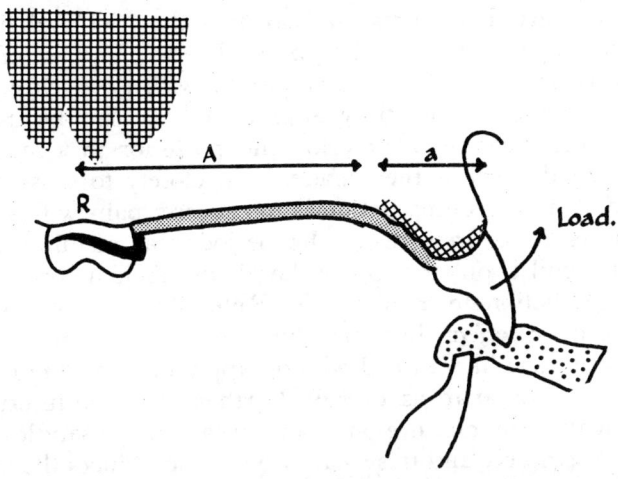

FIG. 440. – If a posterior tooth on either side of the mouth is clasped the area available for resisting the incising load is greatly increased and the further back in the mouth the teeth are the greater the mechanical advantage because the fulcrum is in the area of the anterior ridge and palate and the distance 'A' is much longer than 'a'.

(b) Sticky foods. Both upper and lower dentures.

(c) The tongue. More applicable to the lower denture but may apply to either if the patient has formed a habit of playing with the denture.

(d) Part of the lateral and antero-posterior loads will be resolved into torsional stresses.

Peripheral seal plays little or no part in retaining partial dentures because even if the periphery is located for a considerable part of its length in the sulcus, its seal is broken wherever it makes contact with a natural tooth. Adhesion will play a small part, being proportional to the area of the tissue covered by the denture, but this will only be effective if a large area of the palate is covered and therefore adhesion plays in most cases practically no part at all in the retention of lower dentures. Muscular control will play a part in the same way as it does with full dentures and is proportional to the size of the denture: the larger the dentures the more effective will muscular control become. The use of undercuts, as described in the chapter on surveying, plays an important part in the retention of partial dentures, and so does the frictional fit of the denture against the standing natural teeth. The use of friction to assist retention must be employed with great care and the limitations of its use fully appreciated. It can be used only when there are teeth anterior and posterior to a saddle area and the denture is then made to fit closely to these adjacent teeth. If the wedging action is too severe, pain will be caused as a result of pressure on the periodontal membrane of the tooth whilst on the other hand insufficient pressure will reduce friction to a minimum. Retention by friction is soon reduced in effect because the constant pressure from the dentures acts like an orthodontic appliance and the teeth will move slightly apart as a result. Further, repeated insertion and removal of the denture will cause wear on the saddle where it fits most closely and this wear also in time reduces the frictional effect.

The main method, therefore, of retaining a partial denture against withdrawal forces is the use of clasps and the selection and design of these is fully discussed in Chapter XX.

Thus, when the retention of a partial denture is under consideration, careful thought must be given to the following:

(a) The use of clasps (Chapter XX).

(b) The material from which these clasps are to be made and the dimensions of them in relation to the physical properties which each material can be expected to produce in function.

(c) The use of undercuts (see Chapter XX).

(d) The frictional grip which is likely to be obtained by the contact between the denture and the teeth.

(e) Adhesion, the larger the area covered in tissue-borne dentures the greater will this retentive force be.

(f) Gravity, this need hardly be considered because it only applies to the lower and the mass of a lower denture even if it is made of metal is so small in relation to the power of the dislodging forces that it is of little importance.

(g) Indirect retainers, these are fully discussed in Chapter XX and, at this stage of designing the denture, full consideration must be given as to whether they are needed and if so, how they are to be designed to produce effective indirect retention.

While considering the problem of designing the denture to resist withdrawal, thought should also be given to the occlusion because if the occlusion is likely to be locked in any position, the load which may be applied to the denture will probably be greater than the method of retaining it will withstand. Every effort should be made when setting the teeth for a partial denture that at least half a cusp's movement laterally is allowed before the cusps lock.

Preservation of the Health of the Tissues (*see also* pages 462 *et seq*).

The health of the tissues covered by the denture will not maintain the same level that would have been expected if no dentures were fitted.

This is because: (i) the denture holds food debris in contact with the tissues which is irritant and also tends to ferment; (ii) by covering the tissues the frictional stimulation and cleansing from the rough surface of the tongue and fibrous foods, which maintain a healthy keratinization, is prevented from occurring; (iii) the movement of the denture, which although slight is definite, tends to cause a low grade trauma.

With these facts in mind the design of the denture should be such that only those areas of the mouth are covered which are required to fulfil the attainment of the aforementioned basic principles.

A denture may cause damage to the following tissues:

(1) The mucous membrane generally.
(2) The gingival margins specifically, leading in time to severe damage to the supporting structures of the teeth.
(3) The bone of the edentulous alveolar ridge.
(4) The teeth.

Figs. 338 and 339 illustrate these types of damage.

All tissue-borne dentures transmit the load to the bone via the mucous membrane during mastication and damage can be inflicted to this tissue:

(1) By failing to cover a sufficiently large area of the supporting tissues and thus overloading the area which is covered.
(2) By fitting a denture which is insufficiently supported,

either by bracing against the natural teeth or the lateral slopes of the ridges, and which therefore moves from ide to side or backwards and forwards and causes trauma o the mucous membrane by friction. This is especially so in a case which presents deep, convoluted surfaces of the palate and the impression for which has been taken in an alginate impression material which faithfully copies those deep convolutions. This results in a denture with a fitting surface which has a roughness comparable to that of coarse glasspaper. Fig. 278(a) illustrates a cross-section of an alginate impression depicting the sharp detail of the palate which it copies. Fig. 278(b) is a silhouette of a cross-section of a denture made from a model cast from such an impression and illustrates the sharpness of the fitting surface of such a denture. Figs. 53 and 277 illustrate the granular type of hyperplasia which such a denture will ultimately cause. Clinically the tissues are red and inflamed and the condition is often diagnosed as sensitivity to acrylic resin.

(3) By fitting a denture which opens the vertical dimension, be it only a small amount resulting in the entire load applied during chewing being taken on the denture and little or none on the natural teeth, with the consequence that a severe overload is placed on the mucous membrane and the underlying edentulous alveolar ridge.

Frequently the damage remains confined for some time to the mucous membrane, showing as a localized or generalized inflammation, but often the consequences of the overload result in absorption of the alveolar ridge leading to an inaccurate fit of the denture base with the consequent worsening of the condition and loss of occlusion.

(4) By gross cuspal interference and locking of the articulation. This results in a drag being applied to the denture which inflicts traumatic damage to the supporting tissues.

Any or all of the above-mentioned conditions may cause damage to the gingival margins, but in addition there are damaging factors which are specific thus:

(1) If a denture is made to fit the gingival margins accurately, its every movement will cause that part of it which fits the

gingival margin to press or drag on the margin with consequent traumatic injury and any settlement of the denture (and a very small initial degree of settlement of a tissue-borne denture is normal) will tend to cause the fitting part of the denture to cut into the margin.

In fig. 333 is illustrated a sharp damaging denture margin, and indicates how it will fit against the gingival tissues in the mouth and literally tear the gingival margin away from the tooth with any movement of the denture. Fig. 336 shows how such sharp margins should be trimmed and polished before the fitting of the denture and fig. 334 shows how a denture margin trimmed and polished will be free of the gingival margin.

(2) Any failure of fit of the denture around a standing natural tooth will leave a space down which food will be driven under full masticatory force directly on to the gingival margin. Such a denture might in fact be thought to have been designed specifically to direct food on to the margin. Fig. 337(d) illustrates this condition and fig. 374 shows in cross-section on the left side how a space between the tooth and the denture, made by incorrect easing when inserting the denture, leaves a gap down which food will be forced under great pressure when the individual is chewing. The right side of fig. 374 illustrates the correct manner in which a denture should fit in close contact with the tooth just on or above its most bulbous part, thus directing the food during chewing from the occlusal surface of the tooth on to the polished surface of the denture and not down between it and the tooth on to the gingival margin.

Caries may be caused by food being held in contact with the teeth due to a poorly fitting denture or to roughness of its surface.

The supporting tissues of the teeth may be damaged by excessive lateral or antero-posterior load being applied to them by the dentures or by using the teeth for lateral or antero-posterior bracing where attachment is insufficiently robust to withstand the load applied to it.

Although emphasis has been placed on the damage which may result from partial dentures, careful design of them can generally reduce this damage to a minimum and the advantages of fitting good partial dentures generally outweigh the disadvantages. In many cases the partial denture prolongs the life of the remaining natural teeth by supporting them and reducing the masticatory loading placed on them and it also prevents drift and over-eruption of natural teeth.

The basic principles of partial denture design have now been considered individually, but in practice they are obviously inter-related and considered together and in order to illustrate how a partial denture should be designed one or two examples of the method of proceeding will be given.

The Economic Position

It may perhaps be considered out of place in a textbook to consider such a mundane matter as cost, but in practice, in the opinion of the authors, it is a factor of considerable importance and in most cases the designer of a denture is faced with the problem of producing a design and using a material which will confer the maximum benefit on the patient for the minimum cost; or if the case is being treated under the National Health Insurance Scheme of only increasing the cost when clinical necessity demands it. Therefore, in the following examples, the economic position will be considered as an important factor.

When designing dentures it is helpful to use a diagram of the outline of the teeth, both upper and lower, as illustrated in fig. 441. The shape and extent of the various parts of the denture can be outlined on this diagram in coloured pencil. As the design of the denture proceeds its ability to resist each of the component loadings should be given a rating of 'good', 'fair' or 'poor'. This will bring out clearly which loadings the denture is unable to resist satisfactorily and then, either as the design proceeds, or when it is completed the designer can see on which part of the design he must concentrate his attention to perfect it. If no improvement of the design can be effected because of mouth conditions, he will know which loading the denture will be unable to resist and therefore which must be reduced by attention to the occlusion. The following examples should help to make the meaning of this paragraph quite clear.

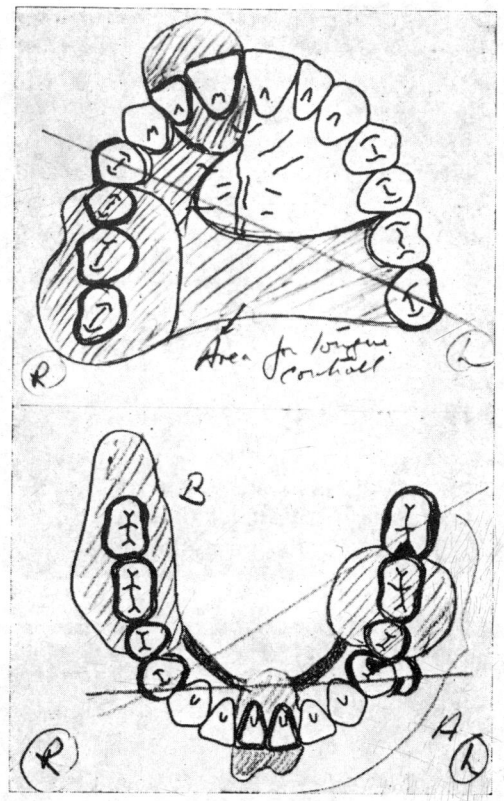

FIG. 441. – Typical outline diagram for use when designing partial dentures with design of dentures partly completed in pencil.

Examples of the Technique of Designing Partial Dentures

Fig. 442 illustrates a partially edentulous case: the upper dentition is a Kennedy Class II Modification II with 8765|12458 missing and is opposed by a lower dentition of Kennedy Class II Modification I with 865|5678 missing.

The technique of designing dentures for this case is as follows:

(1) The clinical examination has produced the following information: $\dfrac{|6}{|4}$ have sound M.O.D. amalgam fillings in them.

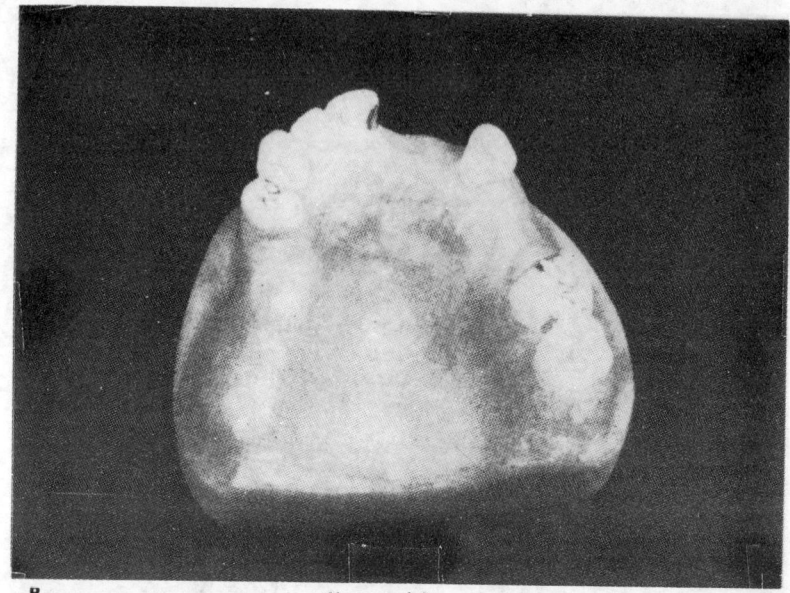

R   FIG. 442(a).   L

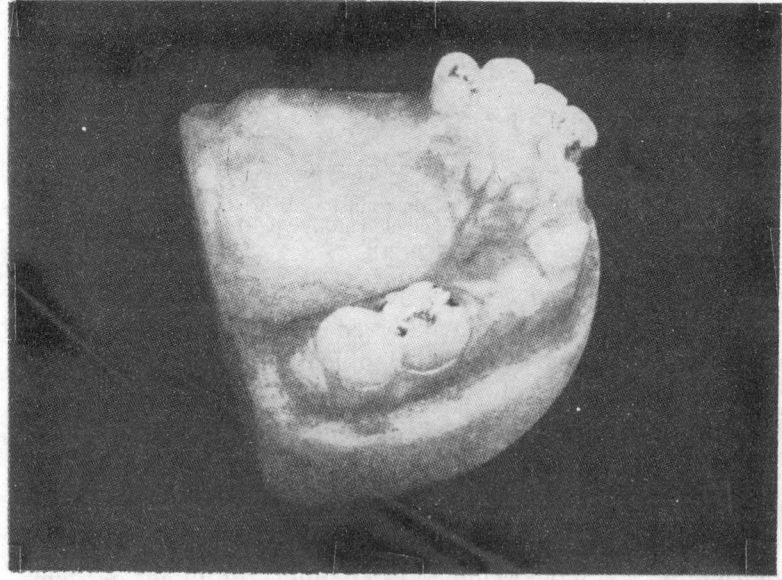

FIG. 442(b).

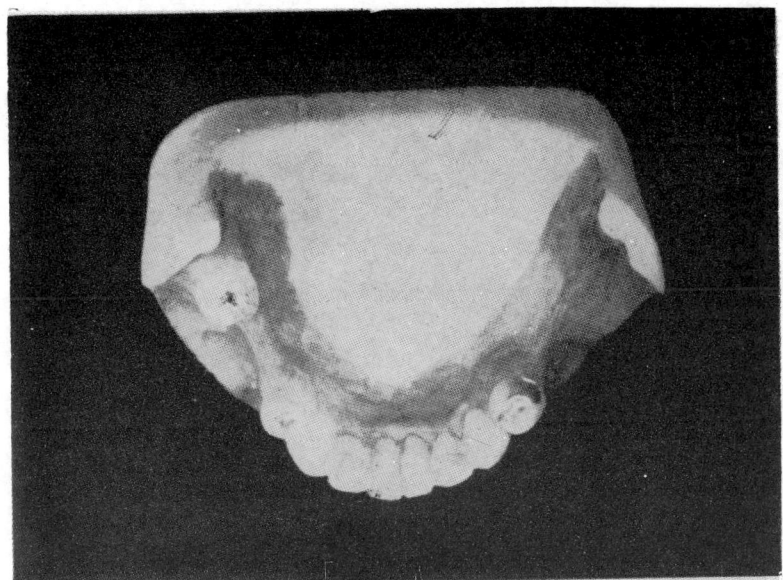

R FIG. 442(c). L

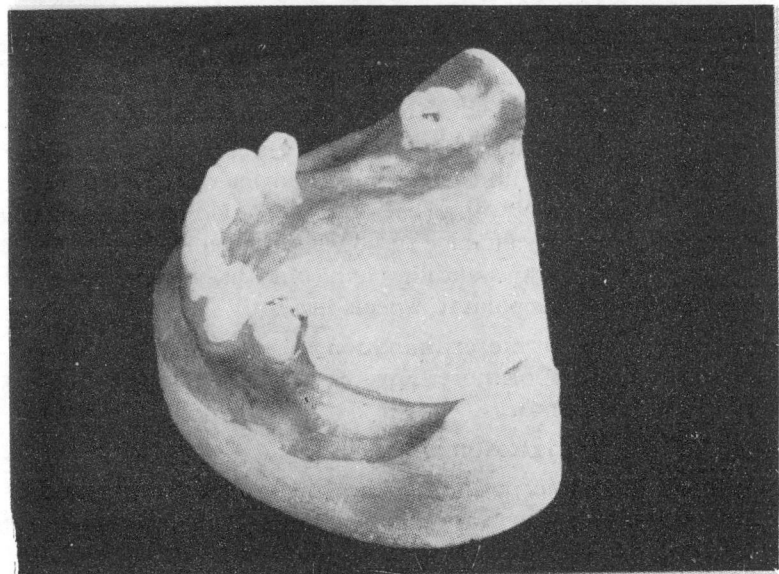

FIG. 442(d).

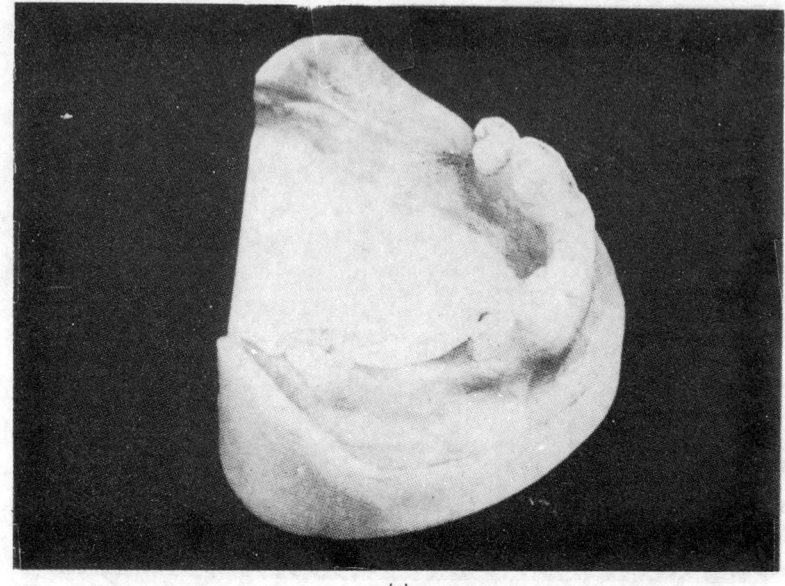

(e)

FIG. 442. – Models of case for partial dentures from various aspects showing the different areas available for support.

1| has a Class IV mesial silicate filling which is functional but not strong; 4| has an M.O. amalgam filling and lower 74| have occlusal amalgams. The mucous membrane of the ridges and palate is healthy and firm, but the lower ridge on the left hand side is extremely absorbed and the mylohyoid ridge is prominent. There is evidence of pocketing around most of the gingival margins of the standing teeth, but it is not severe, with the exception of the palatal aspects 321|.

(2) The radiographic examination shows that all standing teeth are supported for more than two-thirds of their length by normally dense bone.

(3) The patient is a woman, aged 30.

(4) The economic position is that these dentures are to be constructed under the National Health Insurance Scheme.

With the above information in mind, the models before him and outline diagrams at hand, the designer commences his task.

Decision One

The designer's first problem is to decide how the vertical occlusal loads are to be borne in this case.

Holding the models in articulation (*see* fig. 443) he observes that the natural $\overline{7|}$ will occlude with the artificial teeth of the upper denture and that the $|\underline{67}$ will occlude with the artificial teeth of the lower denture. This means that the load applied to these saddles will be greater than if they were opposed by artificial teeth. The question therefore arises: can either of these saddles be made tooth-borne to resist this extra load better than if they were tissue-borne?

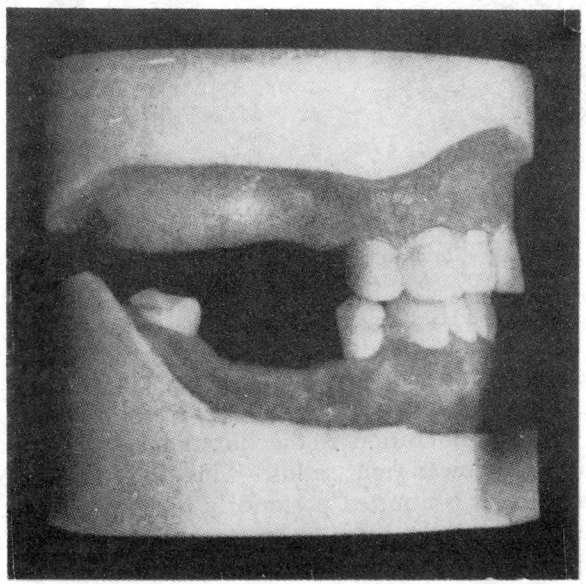

FIG. 443. – Models of partial case articulated.

Both these saddles are free-end with no posterior abutment tooth, so no effective tooth support against the vertical loads can be enlisted. The decision with regard to these saddles, therefore, is that they must be tissue-borne and cover as wide an area of the ridge as possible so as to resist the loads applied by the natural teeth effectively. The first stage of the design, therefore, is to outline the area of these saddles resisting occlusal

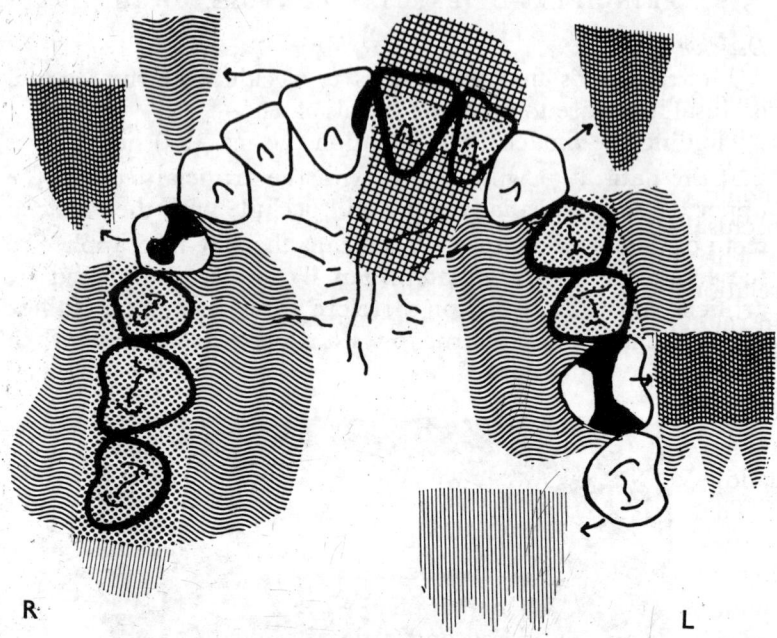

Fig. 444. - Illustrating the areas resisting the loads applied
to the upper denture depicted in fig. 446. Note the centre
of the palate resists no load and merely acts as a connector
and helps the tongue to control the dentures.

loading and this is shown in fig. 444. (*see* page 546 for key to
shading).

The next consideration is the question of vertical load in
relation to the lower right saddle. This saddle could be tooth
borne because it is abutted posteriorly by a well-rooted molar
tooth and anteriorly by a premolar, both of which could
support rests. To make this saddle tooth-borne, however,
would be a bad decision for three reasons:

. (1) If tooth-borne it will be capable of applying greater
vertical loads to its opposing saddle of the upper denture which,
as has already been decided, must be tissue-borne.

(2) If this saddle is made tooth-borne and the free-end
saddle on the opposite side of the lower denture must be tissue-
borne, then a stress-breaking connector will be required to join
the two saddles.

(3) As the load-bearing capacity of the upper tissue-borne saddle is the limiting factor in the power with which the individual will be able to chew on the left side nothing will be gained in this respect from making this saddle tooth-borne.

The decision in relation to this saddle, therefore, is that it should be tissue-borne and the area of the ridge resisting the occlusal loading is shown in fig. 444.

The next consideration is the question of the vertical load in relation to the upper left saddle. Here the same remarks apply in relation to making the saddle tooth-borne as applied to the lower right saddle, with the addition of the fact that the anterior abutment tooth, being a canine, is unsuitable for supporting a rest unless a special inlay is inserted into it and that is certainly not called for in this case. The outline for this saddle is therefore as shown in fig. 444.

The final saddle requiring consideration in relation to the vertical load is the anterior saddle of the upper denture, carrying the $\lfloor$12. This also must be a tissue-borne saddle. Here the question of the tilting load applied when the patient incises also requires to be considered and a decision must be made as to whether a labial flange is to be fitted to assist in resisting this tilt or whether the $\underline{4}\lfloor 7$ are to be clasped to provide a resistance against the tilting force if $\lfloor$12 are gum fitted. If the patient's upper lip does not rise above the gingival margins of the upper front teeth when smiling the labial flange can be fitted without fear of spoiling the appearance and if sufficient alveolar absorption has occurred to produce a hollow in the labial surface of the ridge in this region then a flange will also enhance the appearance by supporting the lip. If, on the other hand, the patient does show a lot of gum when smiling a labial flange will be unsightly and the $\lfloor$12 should be gum fitted and $\underline{4}\lfloor 7$ should be clasped.

In the case under consideration the patient does not show any gum when smiling and therefore a labial flange will be fitted. The areas of the anterior saddle are shown in fig. 444.

Decision Two

The designer now turns his attention to providing adequate resistance to the lateral movement of the dentures. Considering the lower denture first; from the clinical examination it is evident that the resistance to be gained from the buccal and lingual slopes of the ridges is poor and because of the prominent mylohyoid ridge on the left side no use whatever can be made of the lingual surface of the ridge in this area. In addition, as the left saddle of the lower denture occludes with the natural |67, the lateral loads applied to this saddle are likely to be great. The flanges of these saddles will need to be carried as deeply into the sulci as muscular function will allow, but no coverage of the mylohyoid ridge should be attempted. The area of the saddles for ridge resistance to lateral movement is shown in fig. 445 and it is rated 'poor', therefore in this case it is necessary to ensure that adequate resistance to lateral movement is gained from the standing teeth. What possibilities do these offer?

The denture can be carried round the lingual surfaces of the 74|4 and this will provide excellent resistance to movement towards the right, but resistance to movement towards the left will fall entirely on the |4 which would overload this tooth. Carrying the denture round the lingual surfaces of the 321|123 would produce some extra stability against movement towards the right and left by the impingement of the denture against the lingual surfaces and embrasures of these teeth, but the additional resistance to lateral movement to the left would be outweighed by covering the gingival margins of these teeth. A better method would be to use highly bracing clasps on the buccal surfaces of 74| if the survey lines on these teeth allow such clasps to be designed. If these teeth show an unsuitable survey line, however, the only course will be to carry the plate round the lingual surfaces of 321|123.

In the case under discussion, bracing clasps can be used on these teeth and are shown in black in fig. 445.

Resistance to lateral movement of the upper denture must now be considered. Here the problem is not so difficult as in the lower because this case has a deep palate and well formed ridges and soft tissue resistance to lateral movement is good. The area in this case for tissue-borne resistance to lateral movement is shown in fig. 444. As the upper right saddle is

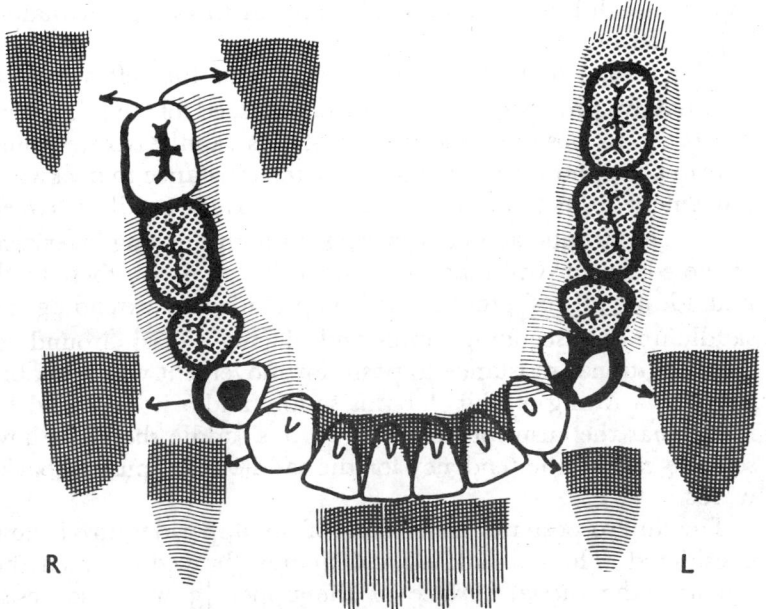

FIG. 445. – Illustrating the areas resisting the loads applied
to the lower denture depicted in fig. 446
(*see* page 546 for key to shading).

opposed by a natural lower $\overline{7|}$ and therefore greater lateral
loads will be applied by this tooth than if the saddle were
opposed by artificial teeth only, it will be wise to gain extra
resistance to lateral movement by carrying the denture round
the palatal surfaces of $4|6$. Resistance to lateral loads will be
gained automatically by the fitment of the denture against the
mesial surfaces of $1|3$. The rating given to resistance to the
lateral movement of this denture in general is 'good'.

Decision Three

Resistance to antéro-posterior loads now need to be considered.

In the lower denture the right saddle presents no problem
because it is buttressed against forward movement by the distal
surface of the $\overline{4|}$ which is itself supported by $\overline{32|}$, and against
backward movement by the mesial surface of $\overline{7|}$. This is a

solitary tooth but is double rooted and in this case adequately supported by bone.

The resistance to forward movement of the left saddle is adequately provided by the distal surface of the $\overline{4}$. The resistance to posterior movement of this saddle is rated only 'fair to poor', however. It will gain some resistance to backward movement from the keying effect of the right saddle between $\overline{74}$ but the torque action occurring through the long lever arm of the connector will place a considerable strain on these teeth and additional resistance should be provided by extending the saddle up the ascending ramus and placing a clasp around $\overline{4}$. This additional resistance to posterior movement will probably prôduce a rating of 'fair' for this saddle and a note should be made that the cusps of the teeth on this saddle should be low so as to reduce the tendency for the saddle to be pushed backwards.

The antero-posterior movement of the upper denture is now considered. The left saddle is adequately braced between the $\underline{|36}$ and the mesial surface of the upper $\underline{|3}$ will also resist posterior movement to some extent. The distal surface of $4|$ will resist forward movement of the saddle on that side and it is well supported by $\underline{321|}$. The anterior slope of the palate will also resist forward movement.

In this case the resistance to backward movement of the right saddle is questionable and should be rated only 'fair'. But there is a keying effect against backward movement of this saddle provided by both the anterior and the left saddles and taking into account the fact that the tendency of an upper denture to move backwards is less than a lower such keying effect is considered safe in this case. It is still advisable, however, to make a note that the cusps of the teeth of this saddle should be low in order not to provide inclined surfaces for the development of posterior forces.

Decision Four

The question of resistance to withdrawal forces now needs to be considered.

In the lower denture clasps have been placed on $\overline{74|4}$ for the virtue of their bracing action against lateral movement. These clasps will also provide retention of the denture. The centre of their retentive action will fall much nearer the right saddle than the left, however (*see* page 518) and the resistance to withdrawal of the distal end of the left saddle, which is a long one, will be rated 'poor'. It must therefore be considered whether it is necessary to place a continuous rest or carry the base of the denture on to the lingual surfaces of the lower front teeth to act as an indirect retainer to resist this movement and in this case, as the left saddle is very long, it would be considered necessary to do this.

The resistance to withdrawal of the upper denture is simpler. There is considerable frictional retention gained by the close fit of the denture against mesial surfaces of $1|3$ and $|36$ and in addition a large area of the palate is being covered by the base of the denture to resist lateral and antero-posterior movement and therefore adhesion and tongue control will markedly assist retention. It is not therefore considered necessary to put clasps on this denture and its resistance to withdrawal forces is rated 'fair'.

Decision Five

The final decision of the designer is to produce the complete outline of the denture, make up his mind in relation to the types of connectors and come to a decision with regard to the coverage or freeing of the gingival margins. In the lower denture the question devolves itself into deciding whether the connector between the two saddles shall be a cast lingual bar with a cast indirect retainer that leaves the gingival margins uncovered or whether the acrylic plate shall be carried round and up the palatal aspects of the lower front teeth and in the upper denture whether to carry the acrylic of the palate round all the standing teeth or leave the $321|7$ free. The need to secure firm resistance to lateral movement and adequate indirect retention of the left saddle dictates the use of a lingual plate as the lower connector. The question of cost decides that it shall be made of acrylic.

The $321|7$ are relieved from coverage by the denture because they show evidence of gingival damage (*see* fig. 446).

The following pages carry illustrations of a variety of denture designs based on the principles discussed in this chapter.

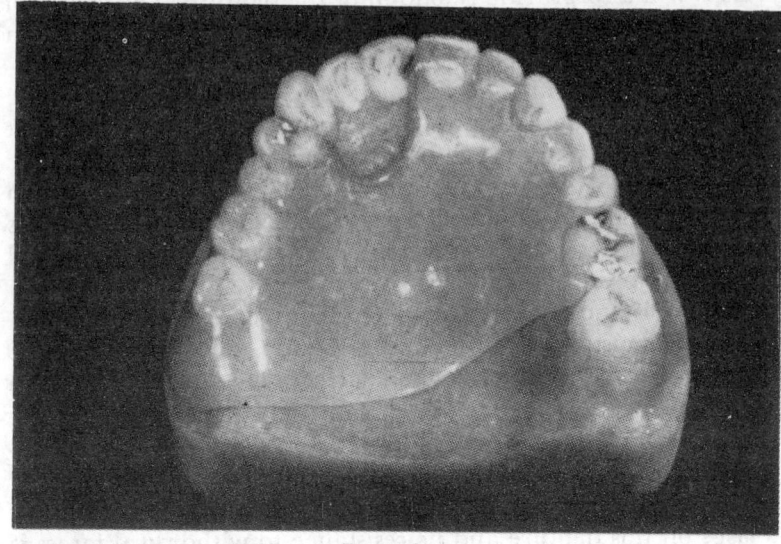

FIG. 446(a).

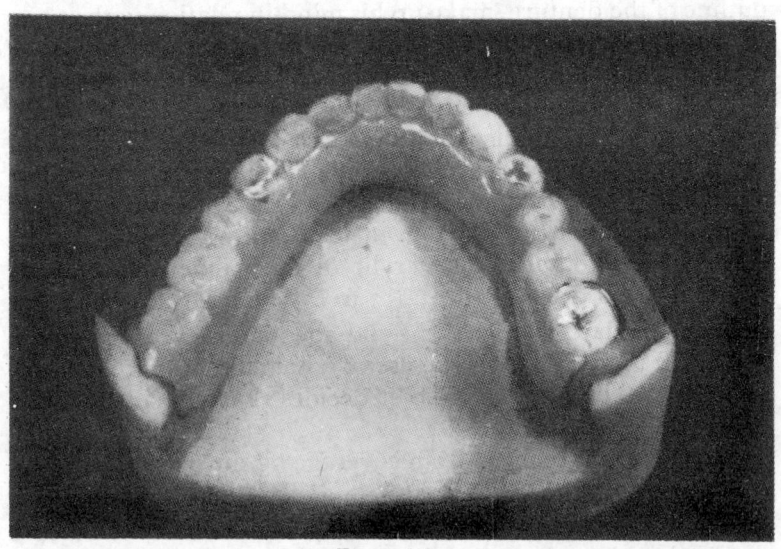

FIG. 446(b).

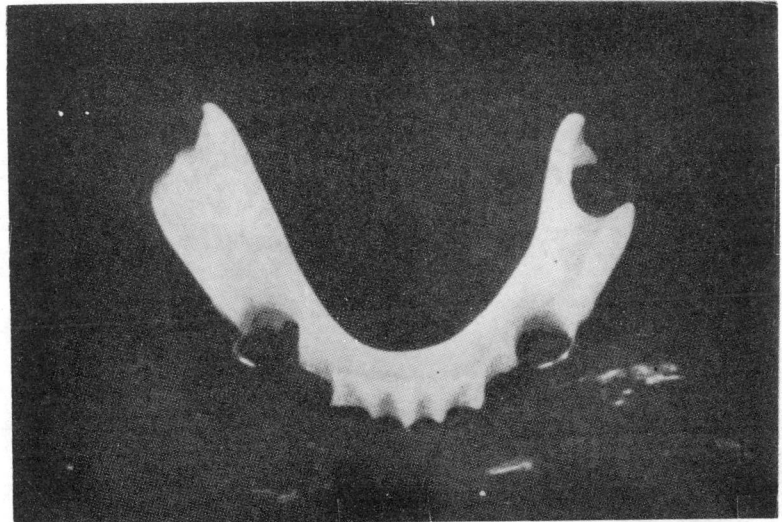

FIG. 446(c).

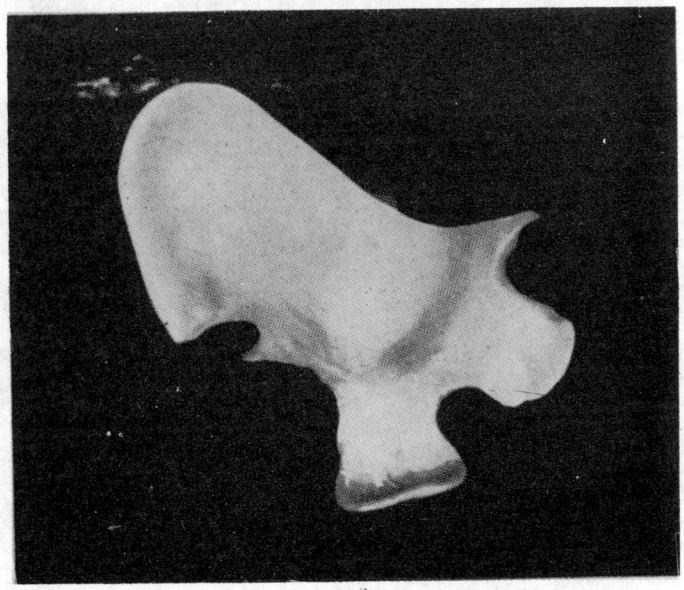

(a)

FIG. 446. – Finished acrylic dentures on and off the models of case illustrated in 442 and 441.

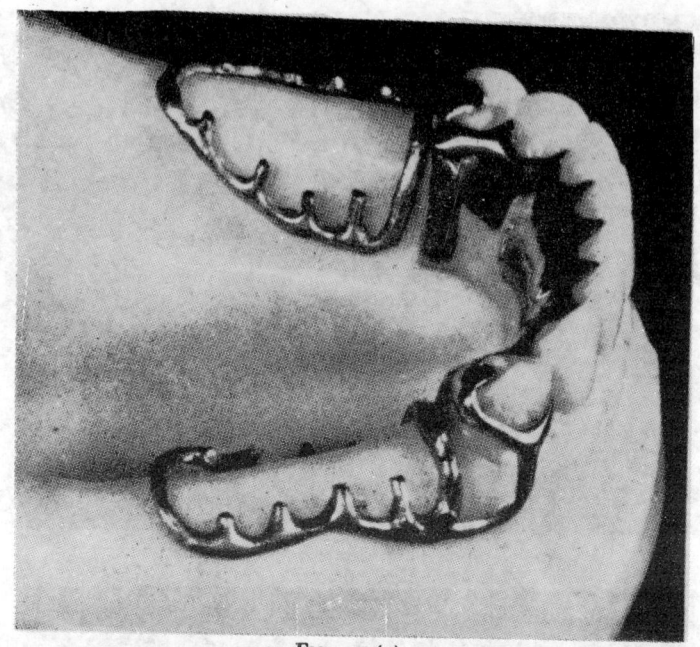

FIG. 447(a).

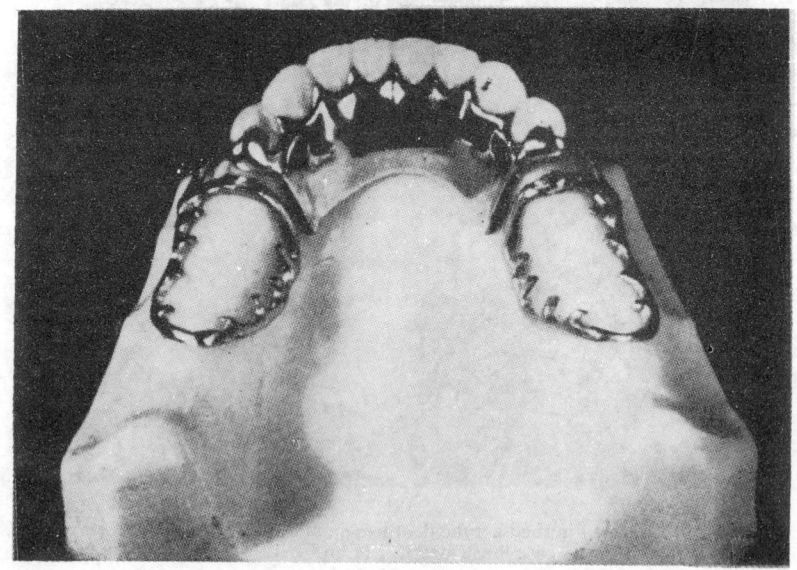

FIG. 447(b).

Figs. 447(*a* and *b*). – Metal Lingual Plate. Class I.
Modification O.

Occlusal loading. Partly tooth-borne on the premolars and
anterior teeth, partly tissue-borne in the saddle regions.
The lingual plate is prevented from sinking into the gingival
margins by being tooth-borne on $\overline{4|4}$ (*b*). The saddles are
attached to the plate by stress-breaking clasps (*a*), thus
reducing the tilt action which otherwise would be applied
to the $\overline{4|4}$ by saddles rigidly connected to the lingual plate
and carrying occlusal rests and clasps.

Lateral loading. Resistance is shared by the alveolar ridges,
anterior teeth and clasped premolars. Advantageous in
cases with shallow ridges.

Antero-posterior loading. Movement is resisted by the clasps and
collets of the lingual plate. The finished denture would be
extended to give maximum buttress against the retromolar
pad region.

Vertical displacement. Movement is resisted by direct clasping
of the $\overline{4|4}$ and by indirect retention from the lingual plate
resisting the upward movement of the distal aspect of the
saddles through the line of direct retention across the
premolars.

By using a stress-breaking design it is possible to have the
denture partly tooth-borne which is contra-indicated in
designs of rigid unit construction as a tilt action is introduced
across the occlusal rests and the lingual plate lifts out of
contact with the anterior teeth.

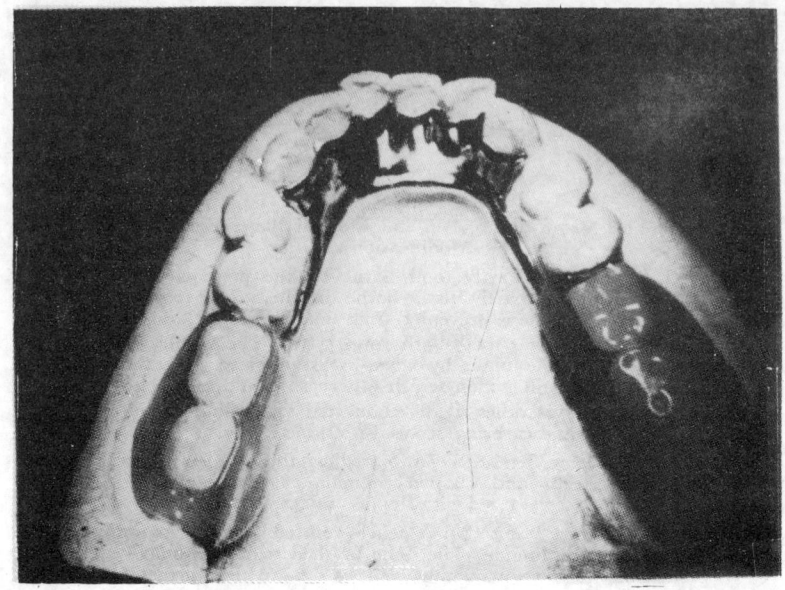

FIG. 448(a).

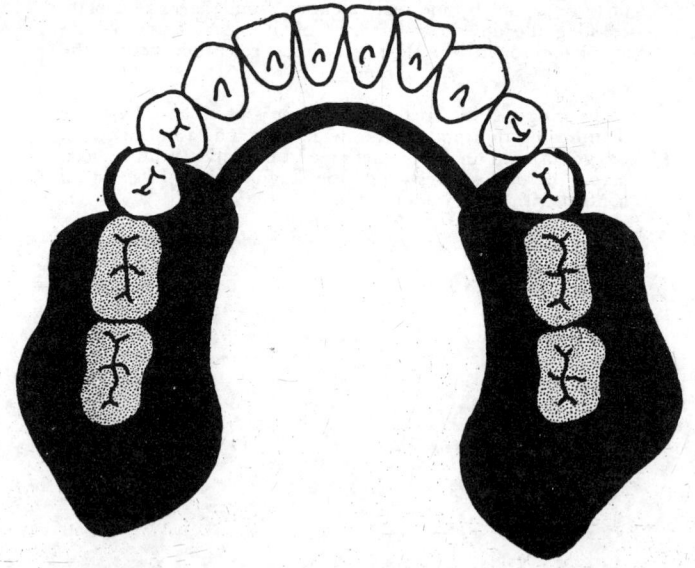

FIG. 448(b).

Fig. 448(*a*). – Metal Lingual Plate and Bar. Class I. Modification O.

Occlusal loading. Tissue-borne saddles (free-end).

Lateral loading. The well developed ridges are considered adequate support as the saddle areas are of short span.

Antero-posterior loading. The distal aspect of the collets of the $\overline{3|3}$ rest against the mesial surface of the $\overline{4|4}$ resisting distal movement and are assisted in this by correct coverage of the retromolar pads.

Vertical displacement. By surveying the model with an anterior downward tilt the undercut zones of the distal surfaces of the $\overline{5|5}$ may be used combined with the frictional grip of the lingual plate against the mesial surface of the $\overline{3|3}$.

Lingual bars pass the $\overline{54|45}$ to clear their gingival margins and to overcome the lingual inclination of the second premolars. An anterior plate is used instead of a bar to give greater stability.

Fig. 448(*b*). – A line diagram of an acrylic design incorporating a wrought lingual bar. The $\overline{5|5}$ are clasped to provide direct retention and to aid resistance to posterior movement. A less expensive denture.

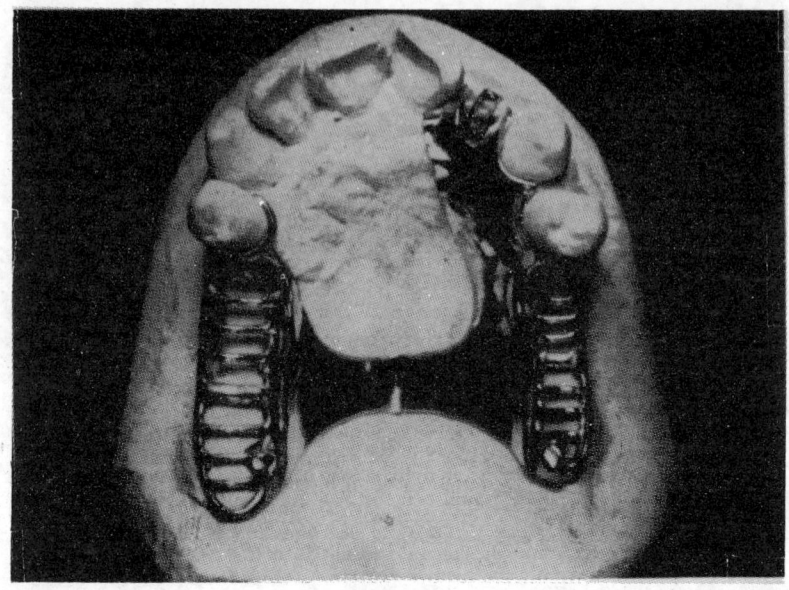

FIG. 449(a).

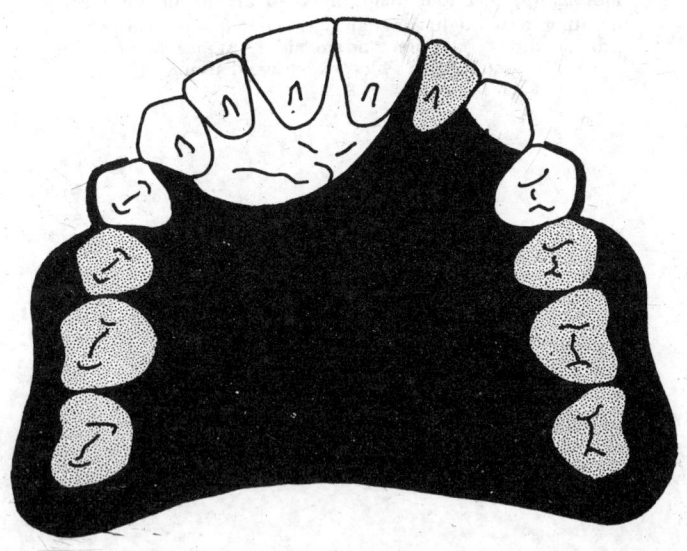

FIG. 449(b).

Fig. 449(*a*). – Metal Partial Upper Denture with a Posterior Palatal Bar. Class I. Modification I.

Occlusal loading. Tissue borne saddles (free-end).

Lateral loading. Movement laterally is resisted by 4|34, the saddle of |2 and clasping of the 4|4. Provided that the 4| is firmly supported by sound alveolar bone this tooth should support the lateral load adequately. The ridges are of average size and will aid in the resistance to movement.

Antero-posterior loading. Movement will be resisted on the left side by the |2 saddle and |4 clasp. The right side relies mainly on the clasping of the 4| but receives support from |2 saddle and clasped |4.

Vertical displacement. Direct retention from the clasped 4|4 and indirect retention of the posterior saddles by the anterior saddle and vice versa.

This design minimizes the coverage of gingival and palatal mucosa. The posterior bar is kept reasonably wide in order that it may be suitably thin thus avoiding the thicker narrow bar which sometimes cannot be tolerated by the patient.

Fig. 449(*b*). – A line diagram of an alternative design using acrylic. The main difference is in the coverage of palatal mucosa which patients often state causes loss of taste and temperature sensations.

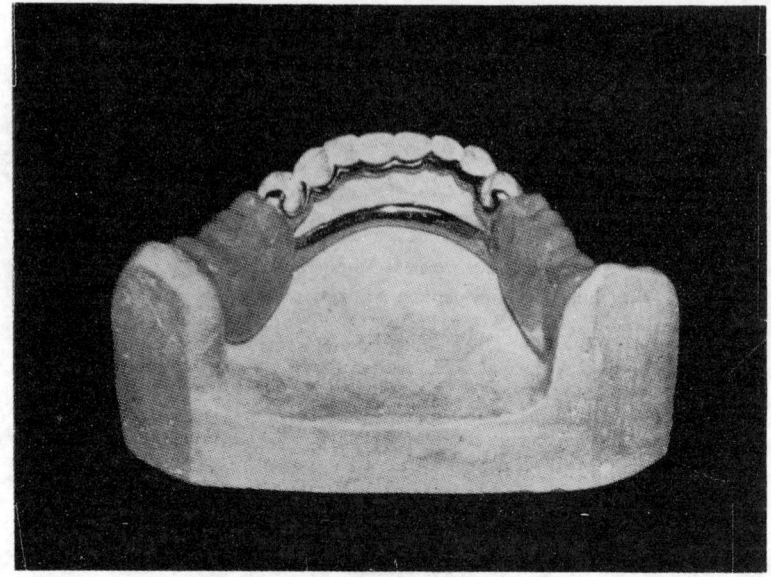

FIG. 450(*a*).

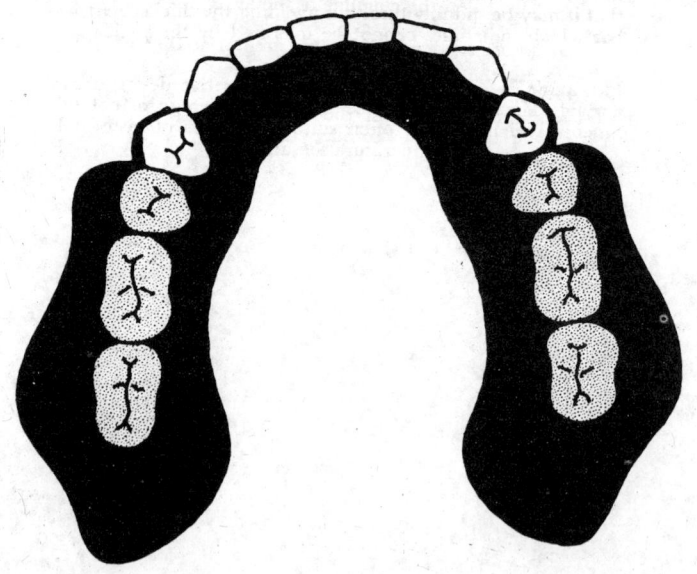

FIG. 450(*b*).

Fig. 450(*a*). – Metal Lower Lingual Bar and Continuous Clasp (Kennedy Bar). Class I. Modification None.

Occlusal loading. Partly tooth-borne on the premolar and anterior teeth and partly tissue-borne on the saddle areas. This design cannot be solely tooth-borne as occlusal loading must compress the mucosa of the saddle areas thereby causing the denture to tilt across a line joining the occlusal rests. Such movement, when the $\overline{4|4}$ are clasped in addition, will have an adverse effect on these teeth as they will be moved with the denture movement, and will soon be lost.

Lateral loading. Well supported against lateral movement by the clasping of $\overline{4|4}$ and the continuous clasp in addition to ridge support.

Antero-posterior loading. Movement resisted by the clasps, continuous clasp and the correct coverage of the retromolar pads.

Vertical displacement. Direct retention by clasping $\overline{4|4}$. Indirect retention of the saddles by the continuous clasp placed on the cingulae of the anterior teeth.

This design is not advised as too great a stress is applied to $\overline{4|4}$ due to the tilting movement of the denture across the occlusal rests and encircling clasps. Also many patients complain of annoyance from the lingual bar and continuous clasp, which also may collect food debris.

Fig. 450(*b*). – A line diagram of an alternative design using acrylic.

This illustrates the all-acrylic lingual plate denture. It is tissue-borne as opposed to being partly tooth-borne but is otherwise similar in its resistance to the displacing forces. Direct retention is obtained by clasping $\overline{4|4}$, and indirect retention by the lingual plate. This should be relieved along the gingival trough line by carefully trimming and polishing the finished denture in that area.

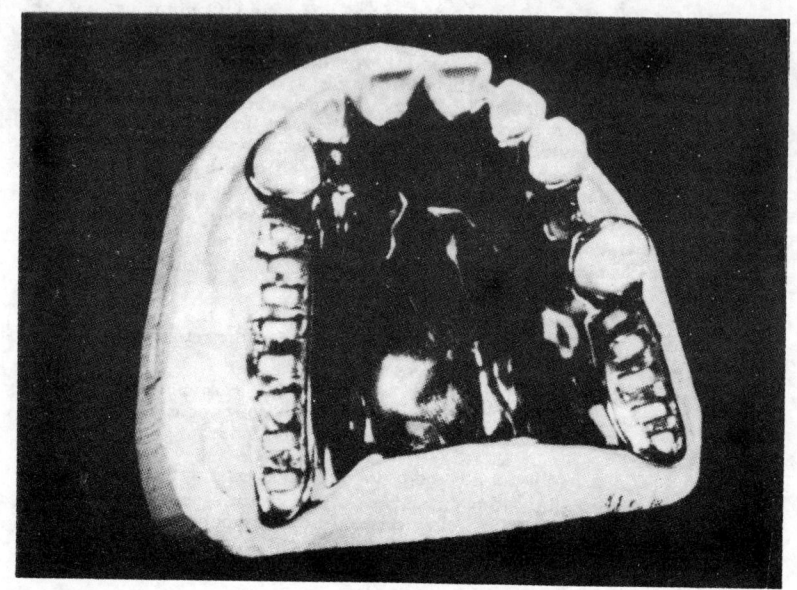

FIG. 451.

Fig. 451. – Metal Partial Upper Denture. Class I. Modification I.

Occlusal loading. Tissue-borne.

Lateral loading. Shallow ridges and a rather shallow palate call for maximum support from the standing teeth hence the complete coverage of all the standing teeth.

Antero-posterior loading. Resistance to movement on the right side is obtained from clasping the 3| with additional support from the saddle of |4. There is no problem on the left side as the saddle of |4 prevents movement.

Vertical displacement. The |5 can be clasped adequately but there is only slight retention from 3|, therefore use is made of the distal undercut of the 3| by suitably tilting the surveying table. Some degree of indirect retention is obtained by fixing the plate on to the anterior teeth, and the maximum use is made of the factors of adhesion and cohesion by covering the maximum denture bearing area. Retention of the denture was considered to be the main problem.

An identical design could be carried out in acrylic denture base material but metal was used in this instance because of a history of continual fracture of a previous acrylic denture.

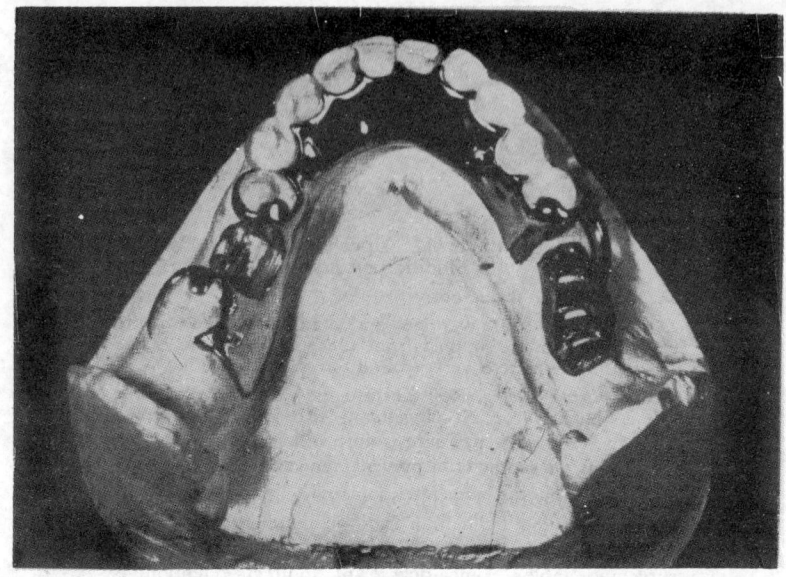

FIG. 452(a).

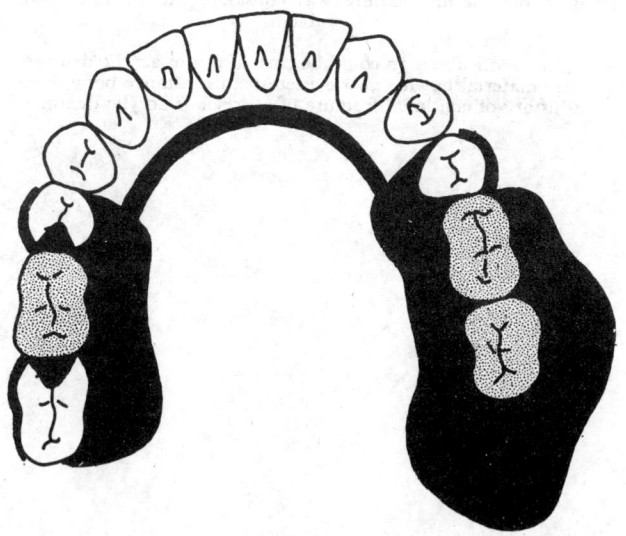

FIG. 452(b).

Fig. 452(*a*). – Metal Lingual Plate Tooth-borne Lower Denture. Class II. Modification I.

Occlusal loading. The left saddle is tooth-borne with occlusal rests placed on $\overline{|57}$, the right saddle is partly tooth-borne by the occlusal rest on the $\overline{5|}$ and partly tissue-borne by the saddle having a stress breaking connector.

Lateral loading. Movement resisted by the clasps $\overline{5|57}$ and the lingual plate collets around the anterior teeth.

Antero-posterior loading. The bounded saddles of the left side present no problem, the right saddle being prevented from moving by the collets around $\overline{54|}$ and the clasped $\overline{5|}$.

Vertical displacement. Direct retention from clasps and indirect retention from the lingual plate.

The greater part of the denture can be tooth-borne thereby preserving the health of the gingival tissues. The lingual plate is considered advisable as little room exists between the gingival margins and lingual sulcus for a lingual bar, and also the plate aids retention.

Fig. 452(*b*). – A line diagram illustrating an alternative and less expensive design incorporating a wrought lingual bar, a tooth-borne left saddle and a tissue right saddle. This combination is possible since the long lingual bar accommodates the movement of the right saddle during tissue compression under occlusal loading. The $\overline{5|57}$ are clasped for direct retention but this design loses the indirect retention of the lingual plate denture. The lateral and antero-posterior loading are resisted in a manner similar to that in design (*a*).

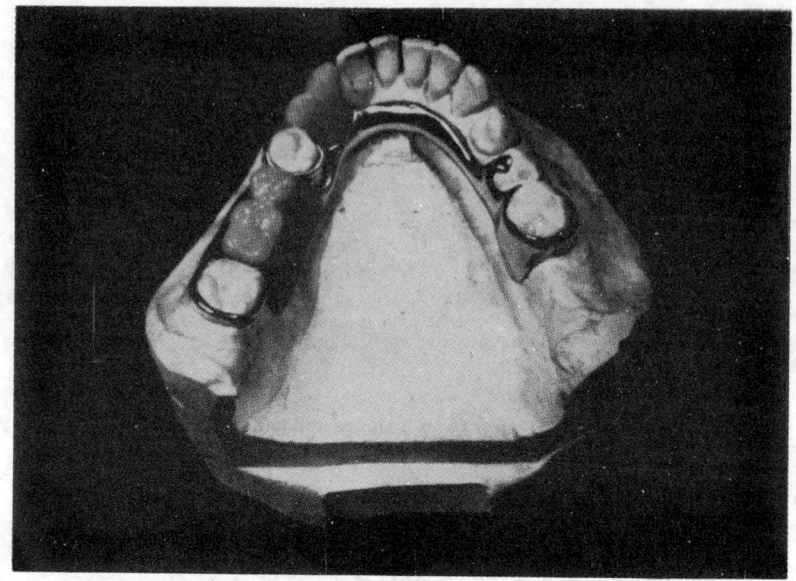

FIG. 453(a).

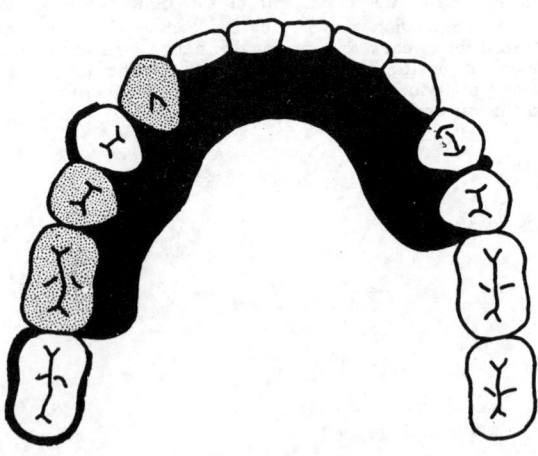

FIG. 453(b).

Fig. 453(*a*). – A Lingual Bar Tissue-borne Partial Denture. Class II arch. Modification II.

No tooth opposed the right free end saddle and for this reason this denture saddle is omitted from the design.

Occlusal loading. The two saddles on the left side are tissue-borne because no additional loading could be placed on the anterior teeth due to their slight 'looseness' and considerable alveolar absorption around $\overline{2}|$. The $|\overline{58}$ are considered inadequate for the support of the occlusal loading which would be placed upon the four artificial teeth of the left saddles. An occlusal rest has been placed on $\overline{5}|$ to prevent the plate around the $\overline{65}|$ from sinking into the gingival margins.

Lateral loading. Movement resisted by the well formed ridges of the left saddles and by the clasps around $\overline{6}|\overline{58}$.

Antero-posterior loading. No problem of movement since the saddles have abutment teeth either end.

Vertical displacement. Direct retention by clasps around $\overline{6}|\overline{58}$. Since the $|\overline{5}$ is clasped the saddles on the left side act as indirect retainers to each other.

A bar is used to join the two left saddles in preference to a plate since the lingually inclined $|\overline{5}$ presents a marked undercut zone.

Fig. 453(*b*). – A design of an acrylic denture for a similar case in which the $|\overline{356}$ are missing.

Being tissue-borne gingival damage may be expected as alveolar absorption occurs in the saddle regions. For this reason frequent inspection of the mouth should be carried out and tissue changes noted and dealt with followed by relining, or making a new denture.

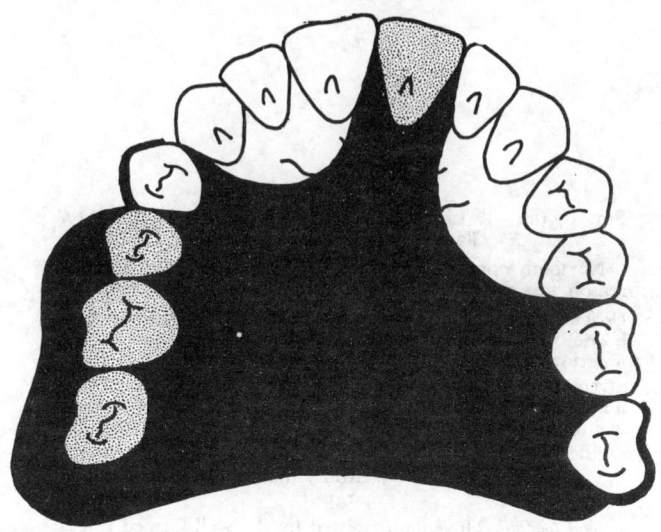

Fig. 454(a).

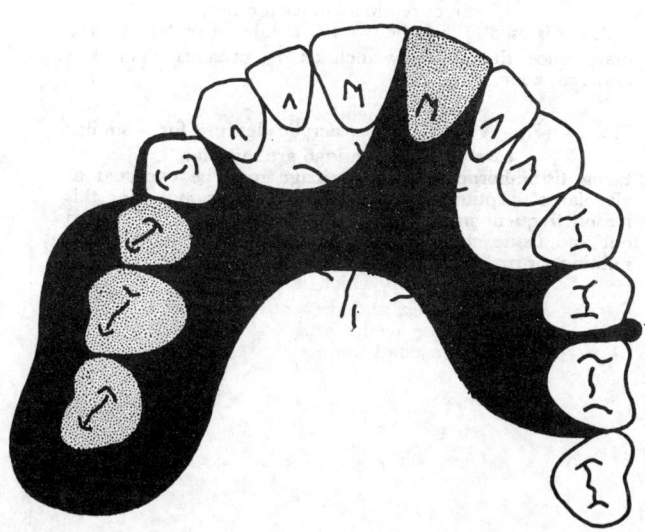

Fig. 454(b).

Fig. 454(a). – Acrylic Partial Upper Denture (line diagram).
Class II. Modification I.

Occlusal loading. Tissue-borne.

Lateral loading. Movement is resisted by clasping 4|7 and by
the anterior saddle of |1 and the collet around the 4|.

Antero-posterior loading. Movement is resisted by the collet
and clasp around the 4|, a small flange on the anterior
saddle and the collets and clasp of |67.

Vertical displacement. Direct retention from the clasps around
the 4|7 and indirect retention of the posterior saddle by the
anterior saddle and vice versa, since each falls well outside
the line of direct retention between the clasped 4|7. Adhesion
and cohesion become a factor in retention due to the large
area covered by the denture.

In surveying a model for such a design it may be possible
to tilt the surveying platform in a manner which enables
the palatal undercuts of the |67 to be used for retention
purposes. This is an asset when the buccal survey lines of
|67 are unfavourable for placing clasp arms. As many gingival
margins as possible have been left uncovered to minimize
tissue damage by the denture.

Fig. 454(b). – A line diagram illustrating a design which
could be used when a metal denture is contemplated. It
cannot be fully tooth-borne since there exists a free-end
saddle.

A thin metal plate is preferred to the thicker cross-section
required for narrow palatal bars. The loading forces are
resisted in a similar manner to those described in (a),
as also are the displacing forces, except for loss of adhesion
and cohesion due to limited coverage of the palate.

The interdental clasp which is placed between the |56
acts as an occlusal rest and prevents the plate sinking into
the gingivae of those teeth. This design minimizes palatal
coverage which is a point frequently welcomed by patients.

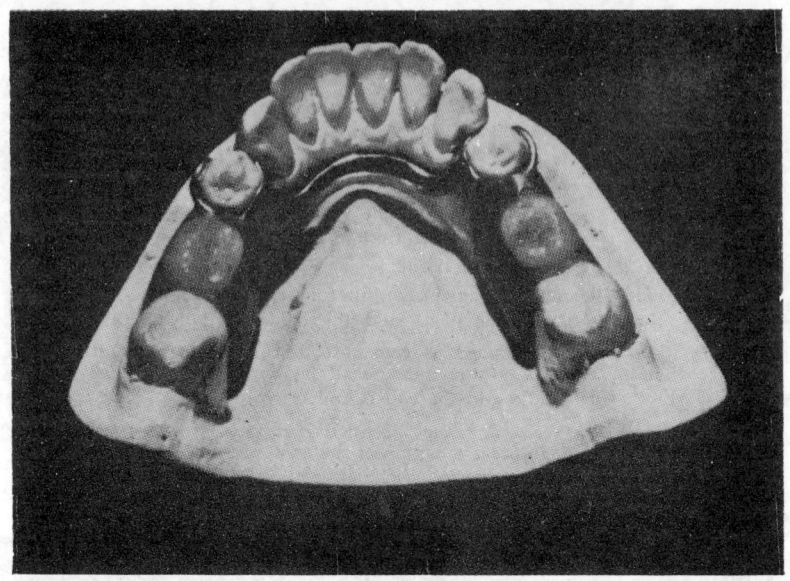

FIG. 455(a).

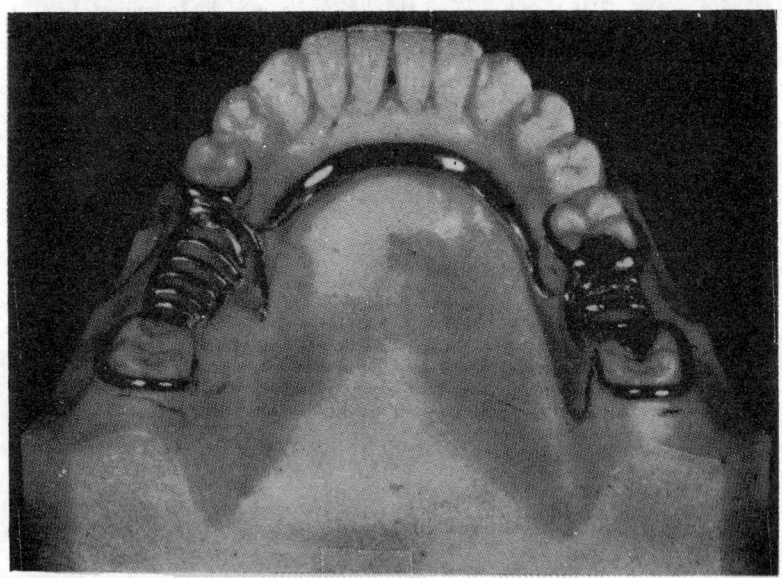

FIG. 455(b).

Fig. 455(a). – Cast Lingual Bar Partial Lower Denture.
Class III. Modification I.

Occlusal loading. Tissue-borne. This is necessary since both
$\overline{7|7}$ are somewhat loose and show bone degeneration on
X-ray examination, otherwise it is an ideal case for a fully
tooth-borne denture.

Lateral loading Movement is resisted by adequate ridge form
and by the collets and clasps around the $\overline{4|4}$.

Anterio-posterior loading. No problem presents since there are
abutmet teeth either end of the saddles.

Vertical displacement. Movement is resisted by the clasps
around the $\overline{4|4}$ and by the use of the mesial undercuts of
the $\overline{7|7}$ obtained by a suitable inclination of the surveying
platform.

A similar denture can be constructed with a wrought
lingual bar and all acrylic saddles and collets.

Fig. 455(b). – Cast Lingual Bar Partial Lower Denture.
Class III. Modification I.

Occlusal loading. The right saddle is tooth-borne and the
left saddle is tissue-borne. This saddle is not made tooth
borne since it is considered inadvisable to place the occlusal
loading of the two artificial molars upon the one natural
molar and one premolar.

Lateral loading. Movement is resisted by the alveolar ridge
and the clasps around $\overline{86|58}$.

Antero-posterior loading. No problem exists as the saddles are
bounded either end.

Vertical displacement. Direct retention is obtained by placing
clasps in a quadrilateral form making indirect retention
unnecessary so that a lingual bar can be used as a connector,
which, being long, accommodates for the movement between
the tissue-borne saddle under occlusal load and the stable
tooth-borne saddle.

This design permits the maximum clearance of gingival
margins. A completely tissue-borne denture with acrylic
saddles and a wrought lingual bar could be an alternative
and a less expensive denture, the saddle outlines remaining
the same.

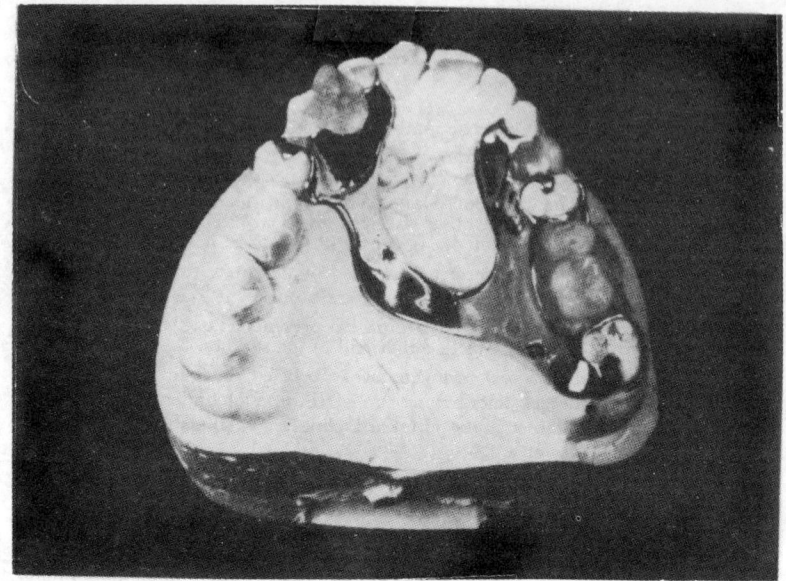

FIG. 456(a).

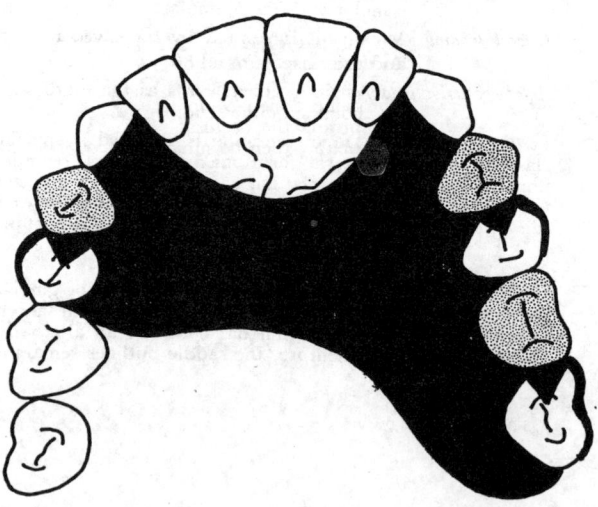

FIG. 456(b)

FIG. 456(a). – Metal Palatal Bar. Partial Upper Denture. Class III. Modification II.

Occlusal loading. Tooth-borne upon 532|358.

Lateral loading. No problem exists as clasp placing necessitates sufficient reciprocals to resist lateral movement adequately.

Antero-posterior loading. The bounded saddles prevent movement.

Vertical displacement. Direct retention by placing clasps in a triangular pattern using 4|58

The palatal bar is made wide and therefore it can be thinner in cross-section than the narrow type of bar. There is no anterior connecting bar since this may interfere with speech.

FIG. 456(b). – A line diagram illustrating a similar case where the denture is constructed in acrylic with cast occlusal rests on the 5|57. The occlusal rests and clasp arms may be unit construction in chrome cobalt. Resistance to the various loadings is similar to that described in (a). Retention is also based on the triangular placing of the clasps. Palatal coverage needs to be greater because of the weaker denture base material. The same design could be used as a tissue-borne denture by omitting the occlusal rests. The gingival margins would probably then be subjected to trauma.

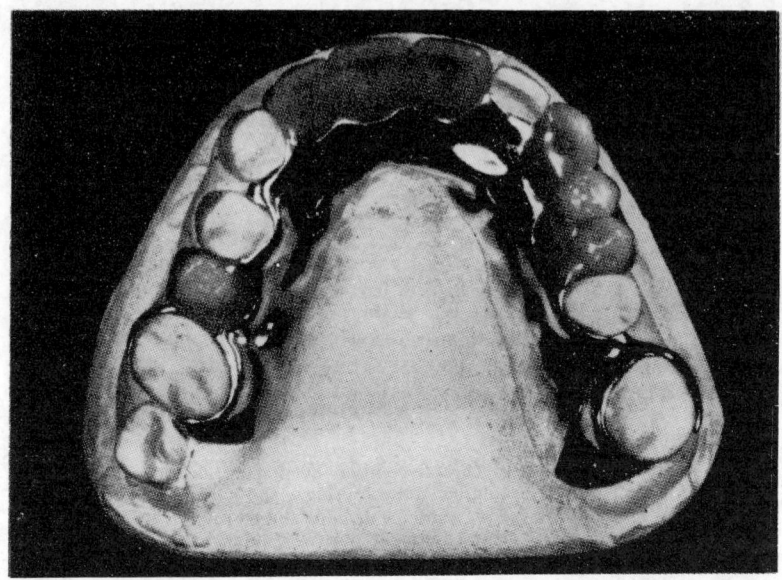

Fig 457(a).

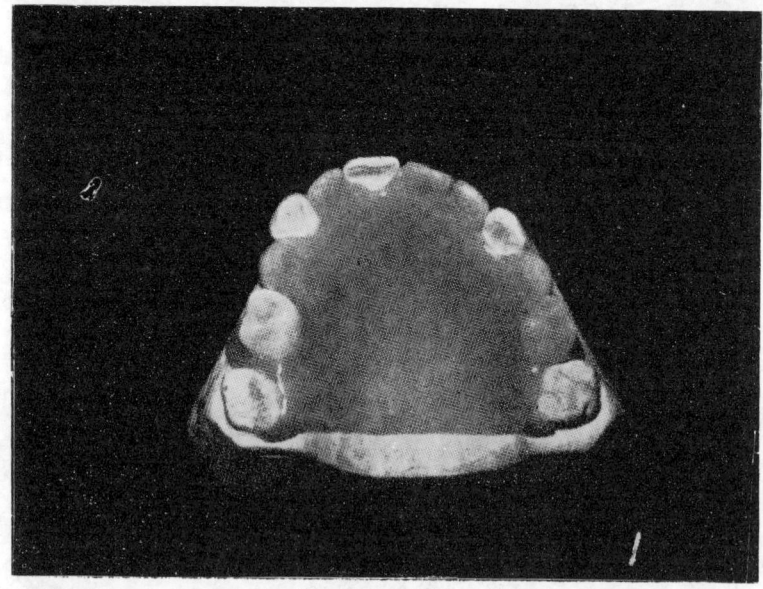

Fig. 457(b).

Fig. 457(a). – Metal Partial Upper Denture. Class III
Modification II.

Occlusal loading. Tissue-borne. This cannot be tooth-borne
since the quadrilateral placing of occlusal rests necessary
in such a case cannot be achieved as there is only a lateral
incisor at the left corner of the arch, and a tooth-borne
denture would subject this tooth to too great an individual
load.

Lateral loading. Movement resisted by the anterior bounded
saddle and the posterior collets of the denture.

Antero-posterior loading. As with a Class III case no problem
exists as the saddles are bounded mesially and distally.

Vertical displacement. A suitable tilt of the surveying platform
makes use of the mesial undercuts of the 4|2 for anterior
retention whilst the 7|7 are clasped to retain the posterior
part of the denture.

Fig. 457(b). – A similar type of case in which the denture
is all acrylic using no clasps. Retention is by adhesion and
cohesion and frictional grip between the many saddles and
the standing teeth.

Careful surveying is necessary in this instance together with
extremely accurate blocking out of the undercut areas as
denture trimming at the chairside results in spaces between
the collets and the teeth leading to food packing, caries and
gingivitis.

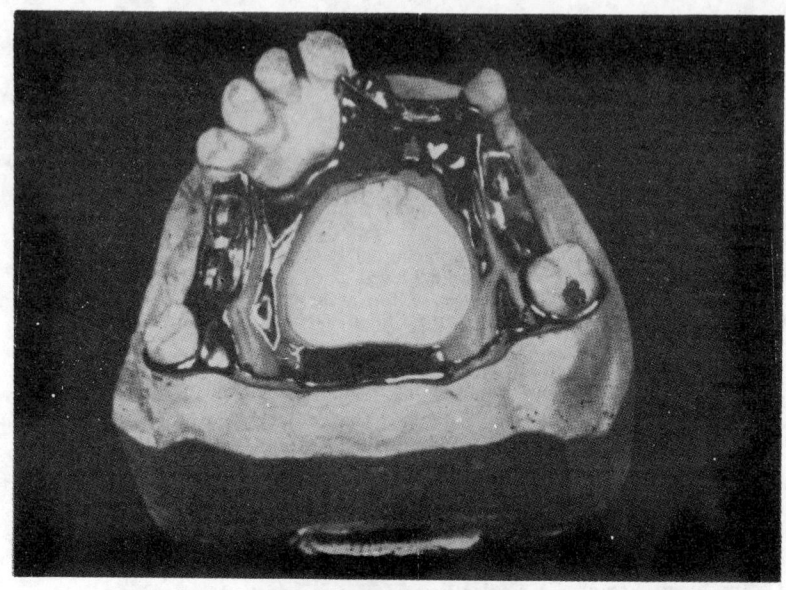

Fig. 458(a). – Metal Partial Upper Denture. Class III.
Modification II.

Occlusal loading. Tissue-borne. The saddles are too extensive
for this denture to be tooth-borne.

Lateral loading. The anterior saddle plus the collets and
clasps of 8|7 provide sufficient resistance to lateral movement.

Antero-posterior loading. No problem exists as the posterior
saddles have abutment teeth either end.

Vertical displacement. The surveying table is inclined to allow
the mesial undercuts of 1|3 to be used for retention, the 8|7
being clasped to retain the posterior part of the denture.

The connecting bars have been made wide so that they
may be suitably thin. This type of design is sometimes
called a skeleton denture. The outline for an acrylic denture
would be similar but the palate would be covered.

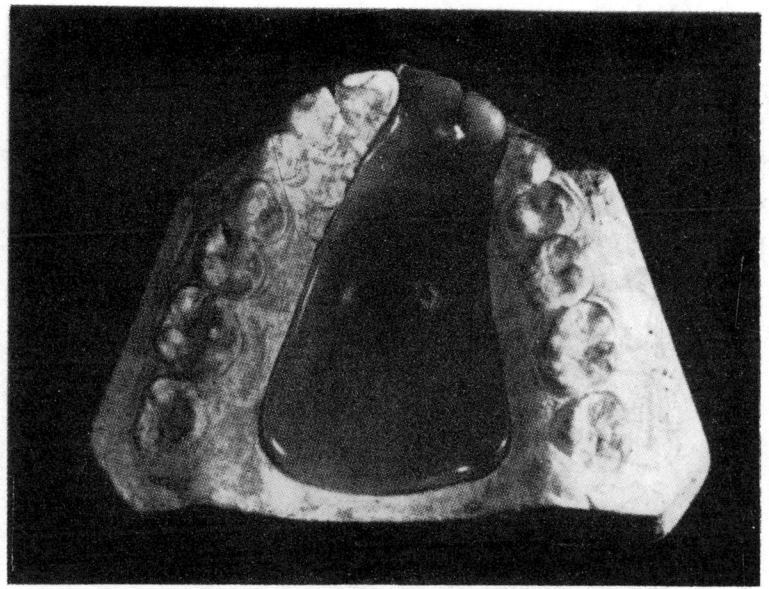

Fig. 458(*b*). – Acrylic Partial Upper Denture. Class IV.

Occlusal loading. Tissue-borne. Maximum palatal coverage without encroaching upon the gingival margins.

Lateral loading. Bounded anterior saddle prevents movement laterally.

Antero-posterior loading. Anterior movement prevented by the slope of the anterior part of the palate and by the contact with the palatal aspect of 1|3. Posterior movement is prevented by incorporating a labial flange in the |12 saddle area.

Vertical displacement. Retention is by frictional grip against the abutment teeth of the saddle, by adhesion and cohesion, but mainly by the patient developing tongue control of the denture during the incising action. The labial flange assists in this by counteracting the forward tilt during this incising action.

This design is referred to as a spoon denture and is ideal from the point of view of maintaining normal conditions for the gingival tissues but lacks firm retention. For this latter reason it is not advocated for young children and teenagers, in most cases, since it may be dislodged easily during robust activities. The T-shaped denture with interdental clasps is preferred for such patients (*see* fig. 458(*c*)).

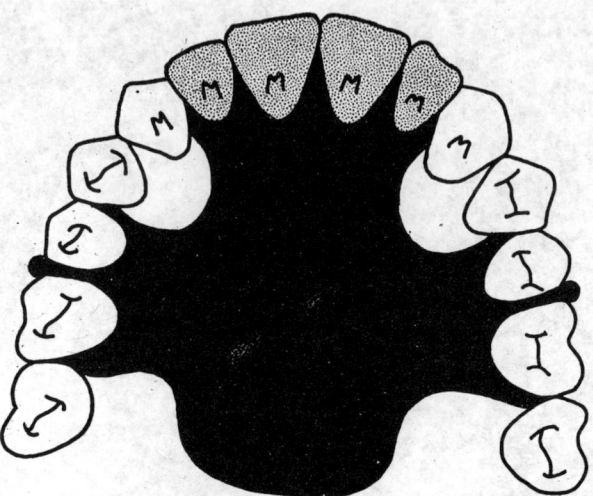

FIG. 458(c). – Line Diagram Illustrating the T-shaped
Partial Denture. Class IV.

Occlusal loading. Tissue-borne, except for the areas associated
with the interdental clasps which become tooth-borne
where the clasps cross the occlusal surface between 65|56.

Antero-posterior loading. Movement is prevented by the collets
and clasps of 65|56. A labial flange is not so important in this
design as it is in the case of a spoon denture.

Vertical displacement. Direct retention from the interdental
clasps and indirect retention of the anterior saddle by
extension of the palate of the denture posteriorly, thereby
also providing a more accessible area for tongue control.

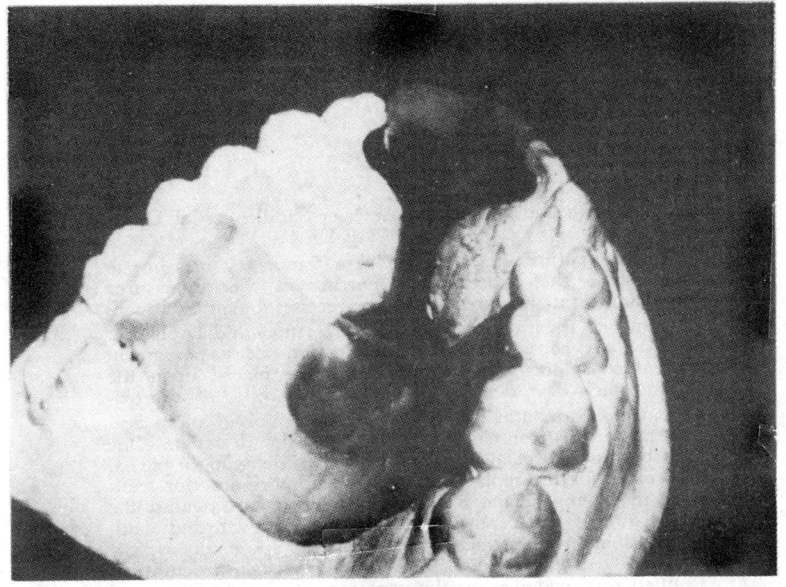

FIG. 459(a).

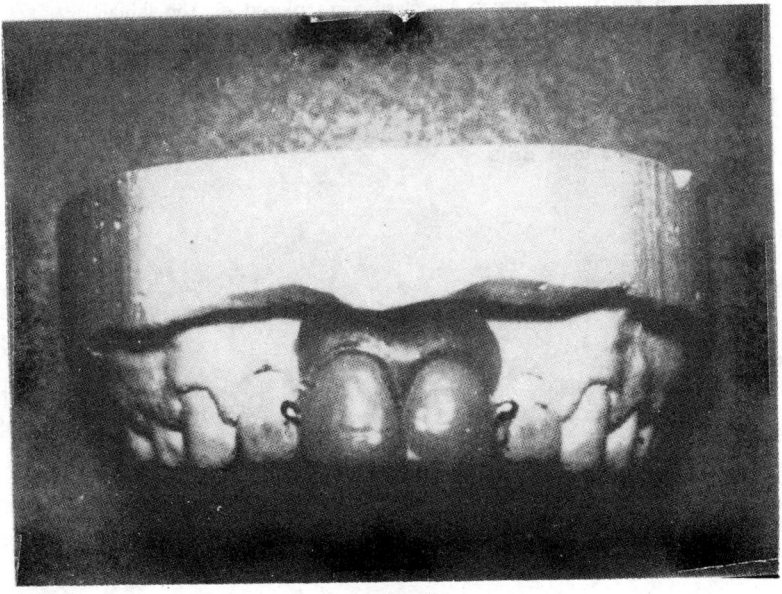

FIG. 459(b).

FIG. 459 (*a* and *b*). – Metal Anterior Saddle Partial Upper Denture Class IV.

This denture was designed as a temporary measure to overcome the hyperplasia occurring in the rugae area palatal to the 32|23 resulting from recesses for spring attachments in the fitting surface of an orthodontic appliance. It is not considered a suitable design for a permanent denture as too great a load would be placed upon the 2|2 which bear cingulum rests. After a period of approximately two months the hyperplasia had resolved and a new denture was constructed of a conventional design. One important aspect to be considered when designing a partial denture for the replacement of one or more anterior teeth in the young person is stability of the denture against the pressure of tooth movement during jaw growth and tooth eruption. In the young person an anterior space may rapidly close when a natural tooth is lost. Even when a denture is fitted this tendency for the gap to close may continue and displace the denture palatally unless the denture is held firmly in the saddle region by clasp arms placed on the labial surface of the abutment teeth and the denture base carried onto the cingulum of these teeth so that the anterior saddle is virtually wedged between the abutment teeth (fig. *a* and *b*). A labial flange is also considered to be of assistance in such cases.

A spoon denture is contra-indicated when any possibility exists of tooth drift.

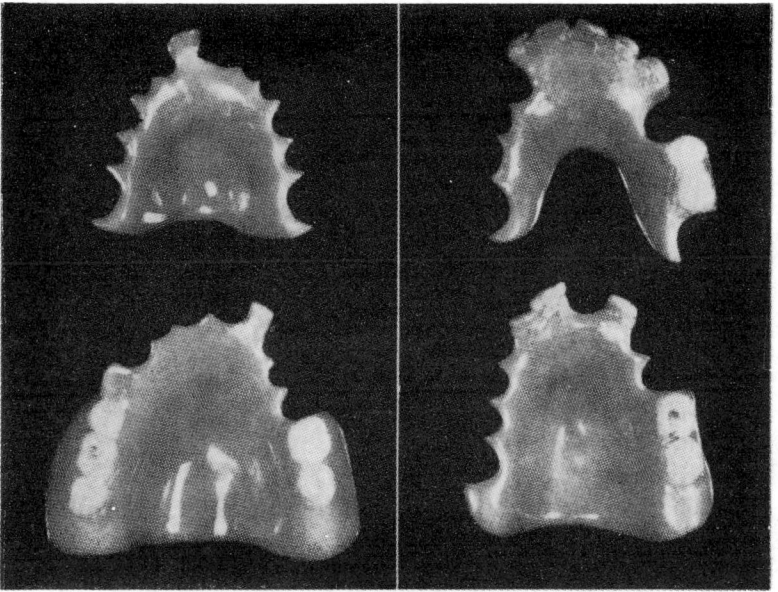

Fig. 459(c). – This figure shows four acrylic partial dentures which could be improved, either slightly or considerably, in design from the consideration of maintaining normal gingival conditions for the standing teeth.

Bottom left: Kennedy Class I. A denture could be designed to clear the gingival margins of the 21|134 provided that adequate support against lateral loading could be obtained from the saddles.

Bottom right: Kennedy Class II. This design could be changed to allow clearance of the gingival margins of the 543|. The 6|4 could be clasped to form a line of direct retention so that 21| and |67 act as reciprocating indirect retainers.

Top right: Kennedy Class III. The gingival margins of the 54|7 could be left uncovered and the palate extended posteriorly to provide for tongue control. If the 7|4 are clasped there would be direct and indirect retention.

Top left: Kennedy Class IV. All gingival margins could be freed by a spoon denture in the adult person, or a large proportion of the gingival margins freed by the use of the T-shaped denture when greater retention is required.

Chapter XXIII

THE POSITION OF PARTIAL DENTURES IN RELATION TO THE TREATMENT OF THE MOUTH AS A WHOLE

Treatment Planning

In order to co-ordinate the treatment of a patient requiring a partial denture it is advisable to formulate a plan which may be used as a routine at the initial examination. Such a plan could be:

1. *History*
   (a) Previous partial denture experience, recorded as:
      (i) Satisfactory
      (ii) Unsatisfactory
      (iii) None
   (b) What are the patient's reasons for requesting a denture?
      (i) For restoration of appearance
      (ii) For improvement in mastication
      (iii) Old denture now ill-fitting or broken.

2. *Clinical Examination*
   (a) Condition of remaining natural teeth:
      (i) Carious
      (ii) Periodontally involved
   (b) Condition of mucosa
   (c) Type of ridge in the edentulous areas
   (d) Occlusion of the natural teeth
   (e) Articulation of the natural teeth
   (f) Condition likely to cause instability

3. *X-ray Examination*
   (a) For caries undiscovered at the clinical examination
   (b) For evidence of the condition of the bone surrounding the natural teeth and that of the saddle areas.

4. *Study Models*

(1) *History.* This information is extremely useful. A patient not wearing a denture, who really needs one, may have had

one previously but discarded it because it was painful, moved
during mastication or was a general source of annoyance. An
examination of such a denture, if available, may lead to the
discovery of a basic error of design or, by questioning the
patient further, the discovery of some aspect of the design
which the patient found irritating, thereby providing the
operator with valuable information for consideration when
designing the new denture. For example on the basis of this
information the retention of the new denture may be increased
to overcome movement during mastication and speech, or
the position or shape of connectors may be changed to overcome irritation to the tongue. (Figs. 460 and 461 show a
case in which alteration of design led to improvement.)

The reasons why a patient requests a denture may be due
to his inability to chew food adequately or to the fact that lost
anterior teeth have spoilt his appearance and speech.
Information on these points provides the operator with knowledge of the aspect of the denture with which the patient is most

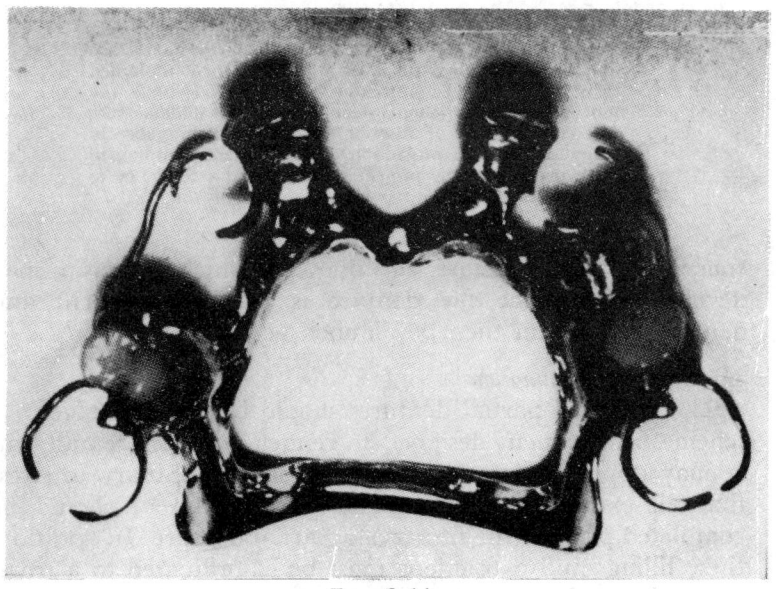

FIG. 460(a).

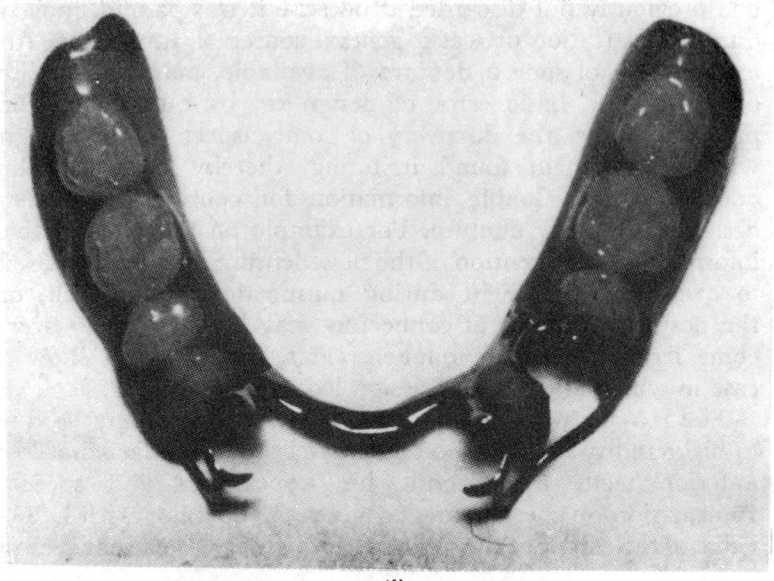

(b)

FIG. 460

(a) Upper skeleton design with encircling clasps and projection clasps – note the long arm projection clasp on the left side of the illustration. Patient complained of irritation from (1) numerous 'wires,' (2) food under the posterior palatal bar, (3) thick posterior palatal bar, (4) consciousness of anterior palatal bar during speech.

(b) Lingual bar and projection clasps. Patient complained of 'worry' from the projection clasps and a tendency to play with the lingual bar with the tip of his tongue.

concerned and therefore the lines on which criticism may develop when once the denture is fitted. Treatment and denture design can then be planned accordingly.

(2) *Clinical Examination*

The fitting of partial dentures should be the last stage in a scheme of treatment designed to render a person dentally fit. It may appear axiomatic and therefore unnecessary to stress that all extractions, fillings and gum treatment should be completed prior to the fitting of a partial denture. In addition, these fillings and extractions must be co-ordinated to a treatment plan and not performed as isolated operations. The con-

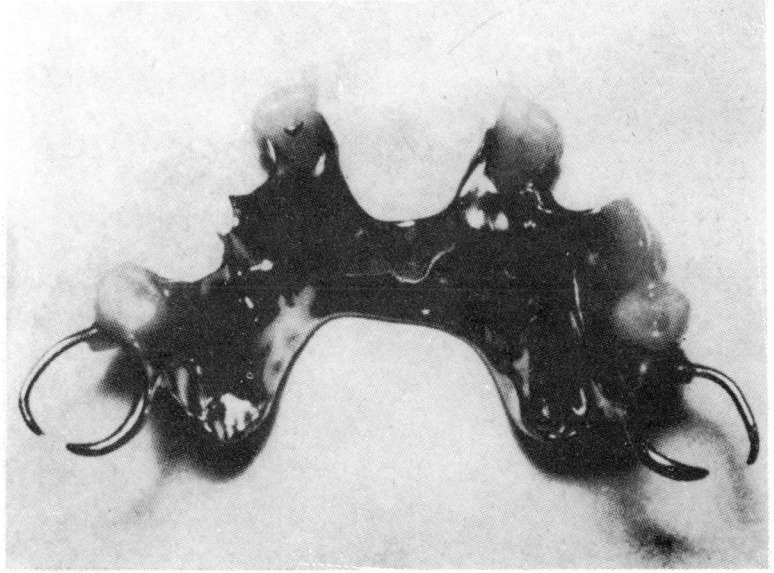

FIG. 461 (a).

sideration of the necessity for a denture, therefore, *should not be left to the end of the treatment but should be planned at the patient's first visit* so that the mouth may be prepared suitably for the contemplated prosthesis.

The initial examination must be a careful appraisal of all the remaining teeth. Carious teeth are noted and a decision made regarding their conservation or extraction. It is most irritating having planned treatment, designed a partial denture, and discussed their case with the patient, to be faced with the extraction of a tooth at a later date and the possible need to re-design the denture. Those teeth which require conservation may require a special type of restoration to fit in with the denture design, e.g. a gold inlay or a gold crown, and for this reason the conservation treatment and denture design must be co-ordinated.

Details of the gingival condition are recorded so that this information is at hand during the study of the X-ray negatives.

The mucosa is examined and any areas of inflammation

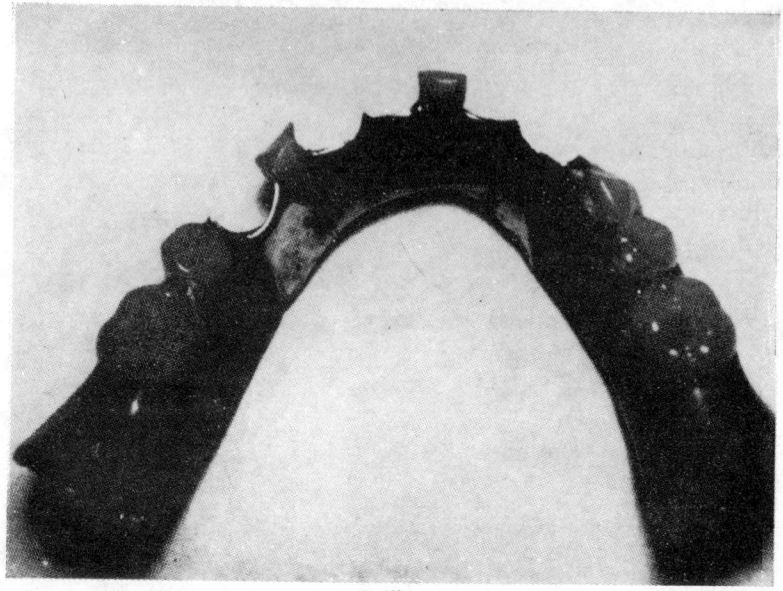

(b)

Fig. 461

(a) Upper metal plate with minimum clasp attachments.
(b) Lower metal lingual plate – no clasps.
  Patient reported complete toleration of new dentures
and had no complaint relating to inadequate retention or
stability as a result of the reduction in number of teeth
clasped.

noted. Assessment of the health or otherwise of the mucous membrane is based largely on its colour and texture, and its attachment to the remaining natural teeth. It should be a uniform reddish-pink colour, a colour which, though difficult to describe is easily recognised after one or two healthy mouths have been examined. Redness is a sign of reaction to irritation which may be either mechanical, chemical, bacterial or any combination of these, but whatever the cause it should receive attention before the tissue is covered by a denture. Although redness is the commonest change in colour to be noted, whitish patches or spots are frequently seen, and the cause of any variation from the normal colour must be diagnosed and, if necessary, treated.

The texture is assessed by palpation and the ideal is an even thickness of firm mucosa neither very thin nor pendulous and flabby.

The form of the edentulous ridge should be noted as hard and well shaped, knife edged or flat (*see* Chapter II). This information when considered in conjunction with X-ray photographs will enable an assessment to be made of the load which the saddle areas may be expected to withstand and the denture design related to it.

The depth of the sulci should also be noted. A clinical estimation of their depth is important since study models (*see* page 628) cast from impressions taken in stock trays may produce an inaccurate picture of the true depth of the sulci due to over or under extension of the stock tray. This may result in an inaccurate design of the dentures on the study models the error only being discovered when the working models, cast from functionally trimmed impressions, are to hand.

The natural dentition with the teeth in occlusion should also be observed as part of the examination and any teeth which are considerably over-erupted noted for possible extraction. In cases with close bites where the upper incisors have been lost the lower teeth may be in, or almost in contact with the palatal mucosa (fig. 462). Such cases may require periodic grinding of the lower incisors during visits for conservation treatment to reduce the tooth height gradually so that a partial denture may be fitted later.

This may consist of a very thin stainless steel or chrome cobalt plate to attach the anterior teeth to the denture if the lower incisors are not quite in contact with the mucosa of the palate. If they are in contact then the attachment of the teeth to the denture may have to be by a buccal bar approaching from the buccal side and not from the palate. In very severe cases the vertical dimensions may have to be increased by an overlay denture in order that a partial denture may be fitted at all (*see* fig. 463).

The teeth should also be examined when articulating from centric to lateral occlusion. If good balance and tooth contact is maintained during these excursions the dentures should be set up to follow this pattern. This will require the use of an

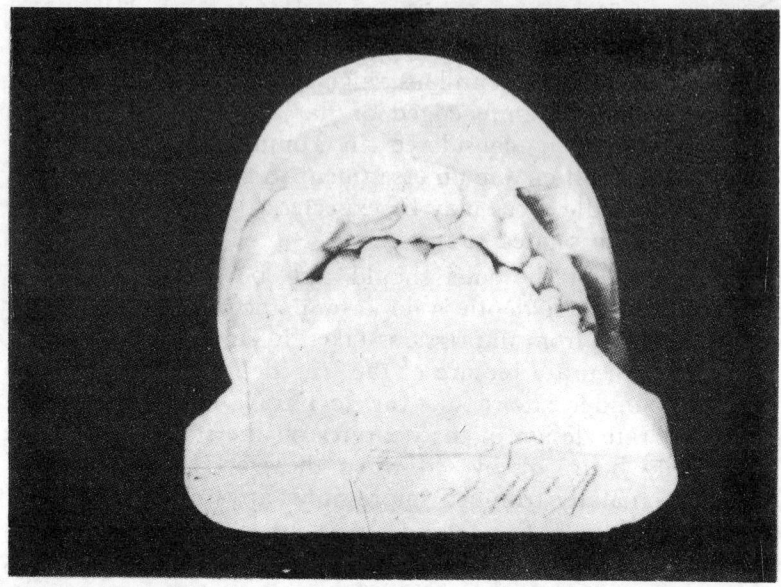

FIG. 462. – Patient with a very close bite anteriorly who has to have 1|1 extracted.

adjustable articulator and a face-bow recording so that the artificial teeth may be set in balance with the natural teeth.

In many instances however only a limited articulation occurs in lateral movements before posterior tooth contact is lost owing to the depth of the anterior over-bite which may cover half, or more, of the labial surface of the lower incisors: in such cases when the anterior teeth are brought into edge to edge contact the posterior teeth are completely out of occlusion. Dentures in these cases are unlikely to result in cuspal interference posteriorly and can therefore be set-up using a plane-line articulator, any slight cuspal interference being reduced by the careful use of articulating paper and carborundum stones. Obviously such deep overbites cannot be eliminated by grinding the natural anterior teeth to bring the posterior teeth into contact without drastic loss of tooth substance, which in the authors' opinion is not justified.

Factors likely to unstabilize a partial denture are noted so that the denture design may be developed to overcome them.

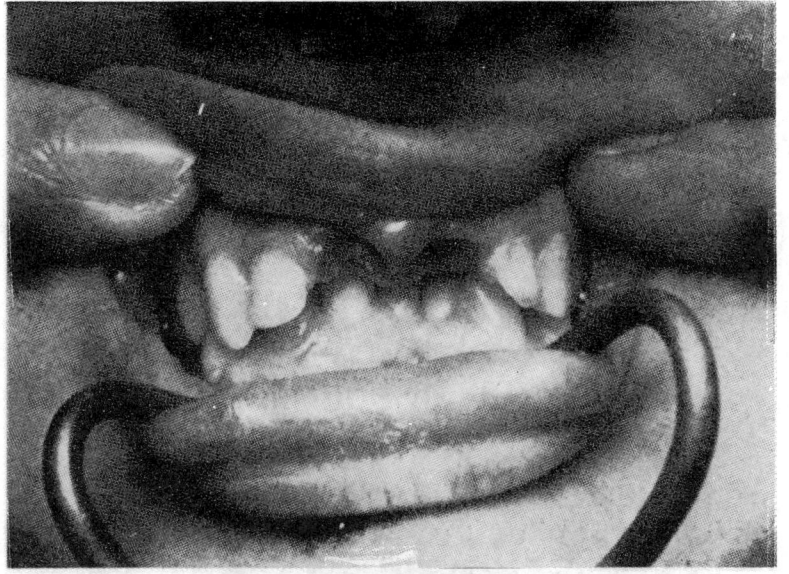

FIG. 463

(a) Same patient as 462 after extractions. Note how ‾2‾1‾|‾1‾2‾ sink right into palatal mucosa making it quite impossible to fit a denture approaching from the palatal side.

Such factors may be jaw relationship, variation in the relative size of the maxilla to the mandible and tongue size: fraenal attachments which are likely seriously to interfere with the peripheral outline may very occasionally require surgical treatment.

(3) X-ray Examination

Bite-wing films are desirable for the diagnosis of caries either interstitially or under existing fillings and full mouth X-rays may be required in order to estimate the extent of alveolar absorption associated with any existing periodontal lesions. The condition, and extent, of the bone surrounding the natural teeth will give an indication of the probable load to which a given tooth may be subjected without rapid deterioration of its supporting structures. In a similar way the radiographic appearance of the bone structure in the saddle areas will indicate the likelihood of changes occurring in the bone

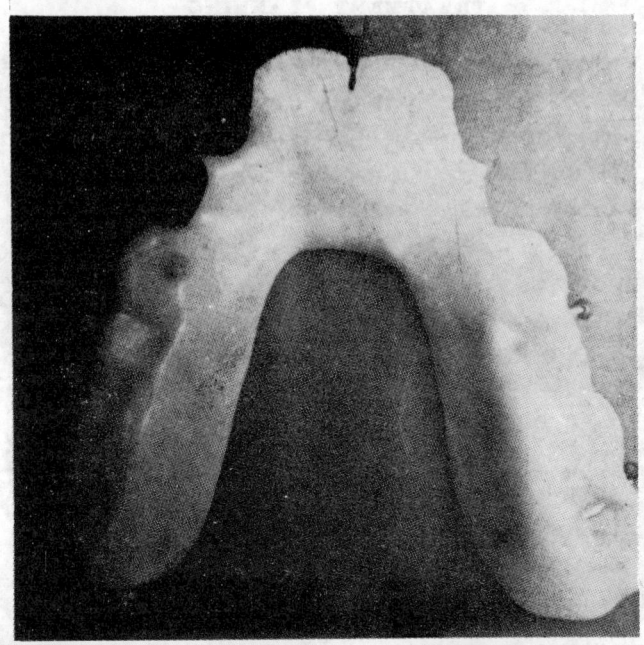

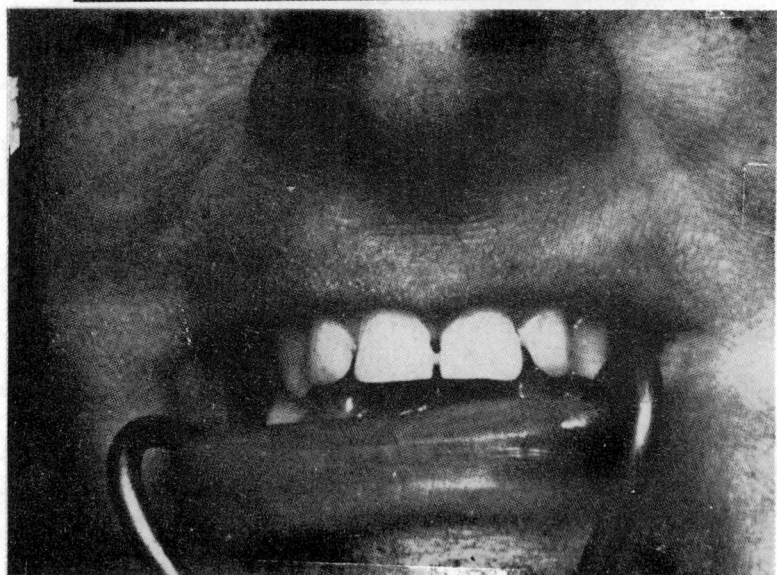

FIG. 463 (b) and (c). Onlay carrying $\underline{1|1}$ fitted as immediate temporary measure. This opens occlusion slightly and allows plate to approach from palatal side.

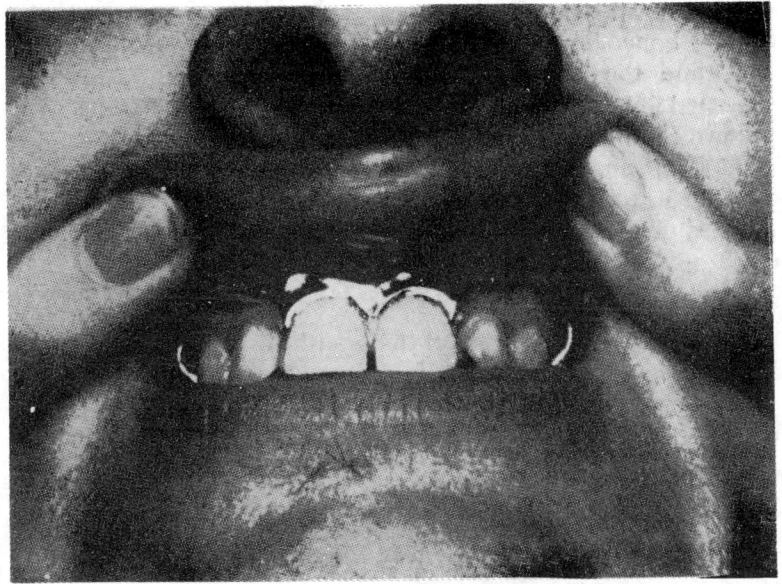

FIG. 463(d).

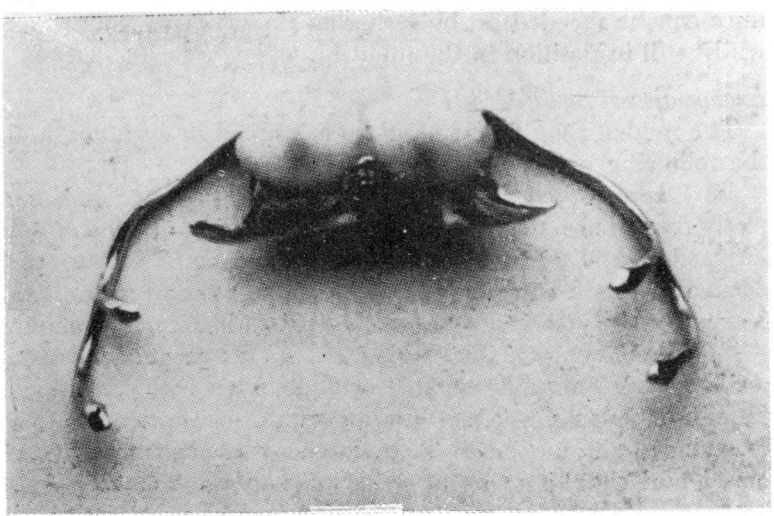

FIG. 463 (d) and (e). Permanent dentures fitted with buccal
bars to avoid palatal approach.

when a masticatory load is applied through a denture, poorly formed bone showing signs of degeneration will obviously not withstand the same loading by a denture which would be tolerated by dense, well formed bone with a good trabecular pattern (*see* fig. 417).

This information, coupled with that of the case history and clinical examination and used in conjunction with study models, gives the operator a sound basis on which to plan the denture design.

(4) Study Models

These are plaster models of the mouth cast from hydrocolloid impressions and set in an articulator either by using the inter-digitation of the teeth as a guide to centric occlusion, or by utilizing a wax template record taken at the same time as the impressions. A wax template record is taken by placing a soften-ed roll of pink wax about as thick as a finger on the edentulous ridges and occlusal surfaces of the standing teeth of the mandible and requesting the patient to close the teeth firmly through the wax, care being taken to see that the teeth are in centric occlusion (fig. 464). It is left in this position for two or three minutes to harden and then removed and chilled. The proce-dure can be speeded up by syringing the wax with cold water whilst still in position in the mouth.

Examination of Study Models

The models should first of all be examined in occlusion and the following points observed.

(a) Over-erupted teeth (fig. 327). The presence of such teeth may make the fitting of a partial denture difficult or impossible and consideration must be given either to the extraction of the offending tooth or teeth if the over-eruption is gross, or the grinding of the occlusal surface if it is only slight.

(b) The closeness of the bite (fig. 463(a)). In the incisor region the lower teeth not infrequently occlude either with the palatal mucosa or so close to it that not more than 1 mm. space exists. In such cases it must be decided whether the vertical height has closed and should be restored as part of the treatment (*see* Chapter XXVI) or whether a thin metal base or other technique should be used in the denture design.

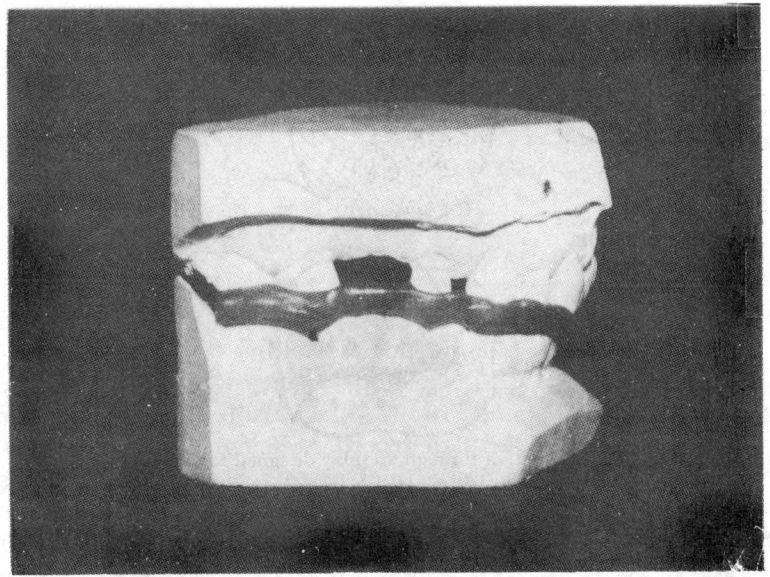

FIG. 464.

(c) The closeness of the interdigitation of the teeth.

If partial dentures are to be tooth-borne (see page 470) rests will have to be fitted upon certain of the natural teeth. Such rests take up space and those teeth which are to carry them frequently require either grinding or the fitting of inlays prepared in such a manner as to provide this space (see figs. 465 and 466). In addition part of the tooth which opposes the occlusal rest may have to be ground. The study models will

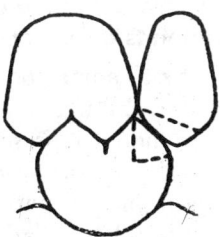

FIG. 465. – The dotted lines illustrate the type of grinding frequently required before an occlusal rest can be employed.

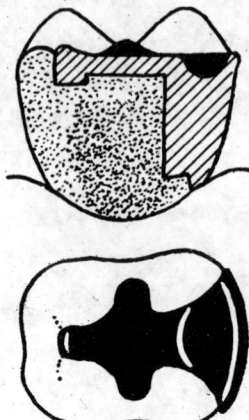

FIG. 466. – A section through an inlay designed to carry a rest.

show if space for rests exists or where tooth grinding will be required.

The study models should then be examined separately and the dentures tentatively designed in pencil. As this is done the value of any isolated tooth may be assessed and a decision reached whether such a tooth will assist in the retention of the denture or make its construction less satisfactory and thus might be better extracted. Teeth which show exaggerated inclinations and which would make the insertion of a denture difficult, should at the same time also be noted and an estimation made regarding the value to be gained by retaining such a tooth. If there is no advantage in retaining the tooth then it should be extracted.

The following case illustrates how study models are used (*see* figs. 467 and 468). The points to be noted are:

(*a*) The upper right first molar tooth considered by itself requires a simple occlusal filling, but when considered in occlusion with the lower model it is seen to be grossly over-erupted and will make the construction of a lower partial denture difficult. In addition the patient requires an upper denture because the upper left quadrant of the mouth is edentulous and to fit a partial denture to such a unilateral

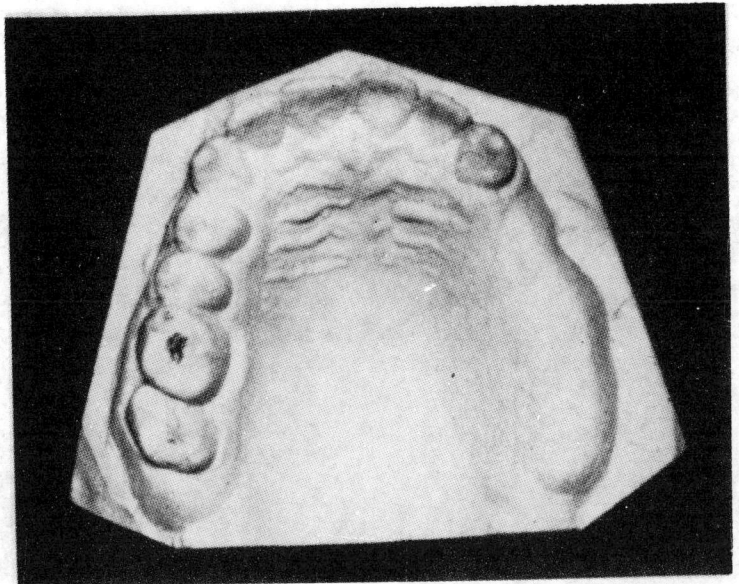

FIG. 467 (a). Specimen study model. Upper.

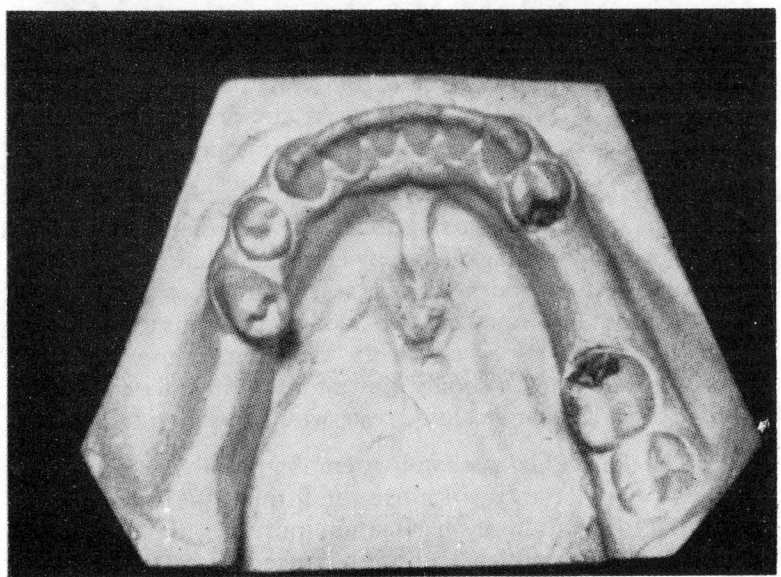

FIG. 467 (b). Lower model.

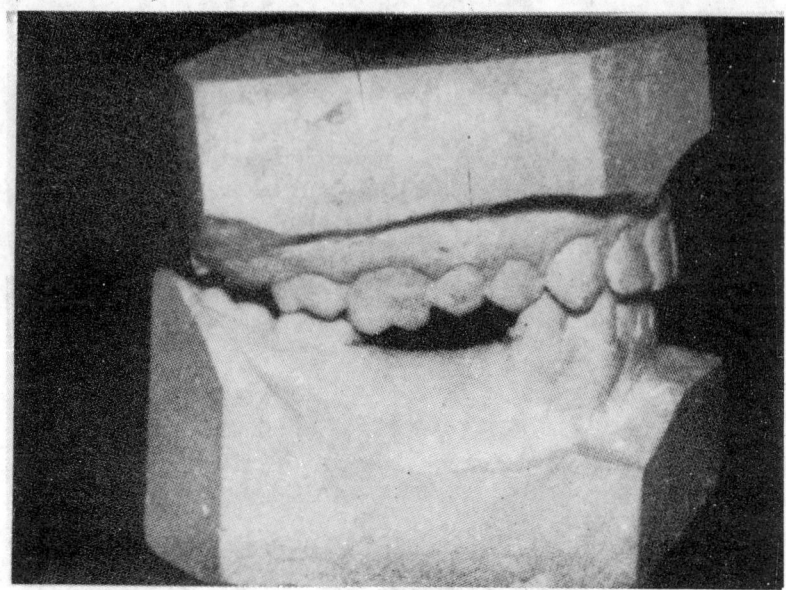

FIG. 468. – Specimen study models seen from right side.

case presents difficulties of retention which the provision of an edentulous space in the upper right quadrant will simplify. Therefore, for two reasons it is better not to restore the upper right first molar but to extract it.

(*b*) The lower right first premolar and second molar teeth require proximal fillings. The lower partial denture, however, requires to be tooth-borne on this side with occlusal rests seated on these teeth. On viewing the models in occlusion no room exists for such rests as the teeth are closely interdigitating. Therefore, these teeth should be restored with inlays in which suitable seats for the occlusal rests would be prepared.

(*c*) The lower left second premolar tooth is excessively inclined lingually and will make the fitting of a lower denture somewhat difficult. For mastication purposes the tooth is of little value to the patient and on balance it is better to extract than retain this tooth.

Had study models not been taken, and had the case not been considered as a whole with the final fitting of partial dentures in mind, the upper right first molar might have been filled, the lower right first premolar and second molar filled to occlude with the upper teeth and the lower left second premolar left in place, and not until impressions had been taken and model provided for the construction of the dentures would the points which have just been discussed become painfully apparent.

Chapter XXIV

TAKING IMPRESSIONS OF THE PARTIALLY EDENTULOUS MOUTH

All the materials commonly used for impression taking and their methods of preparation have been fully described in the section on full dentures. It is only intended therefore to describe here the essential points in their application to the taking of partial impressions.

Trays for Partial Impressions

The type of tray required for an impression will vary in relation to the number of natural teeth standing. If the majority of natural teeth are standing a stock box tray may be used (*see* figs. 469 and 470) and in some cases no second impression in a special tray will be required. If extensive edentulous spaces exist, a preliminary impression in a stock tray will be required

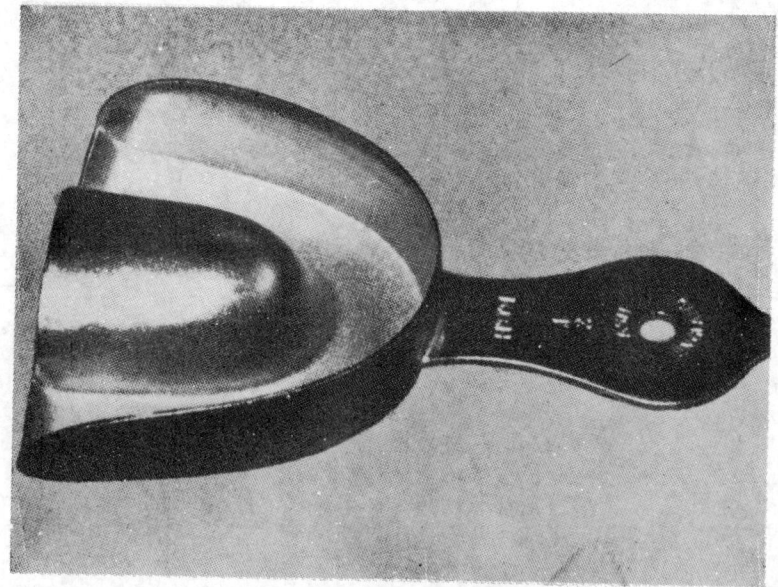

FIG. 469. – An upper box tray.

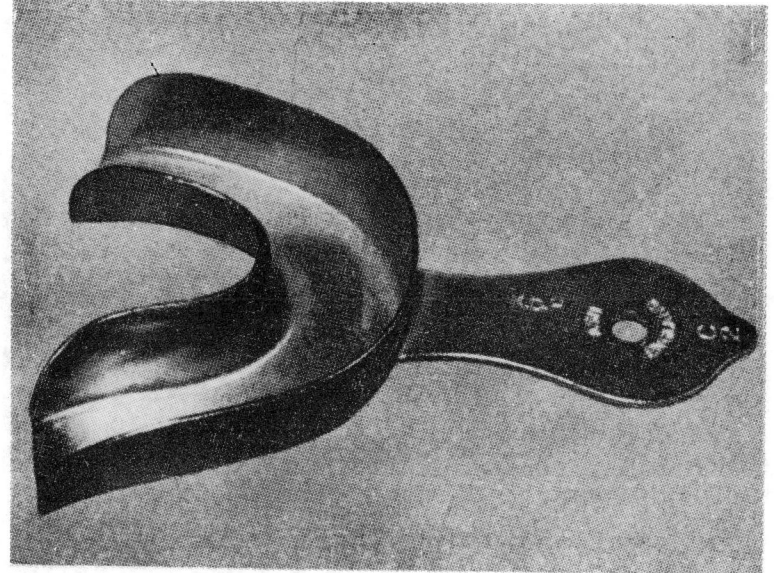

FIG. 470. – A lower box tray.

to produce a model on which a special tray may be made for taking the final working impression. The reason for this difference is that dentures replacing a few isolated teeth will not be carried deeply into the sulci and therefore an accurate impression of the functional depth of this region is unimportant. Where large edentulous spaces exist, however, the denture will be carried into the sulci and the only means of obtaining an accurate impression of them in their functional position is by using a special tray (*see* fig. 471).

Method of Adapting a Box Tray for Taking an Impression when Extensive Edentulous Areas Exist

Mouths are frequently encountered containing both extensive edentulous areas and a group of natural teeth. In such cases a box tray may sometimes be successfully adapted to fit the mouth and thus allow an accurate impression of the functional

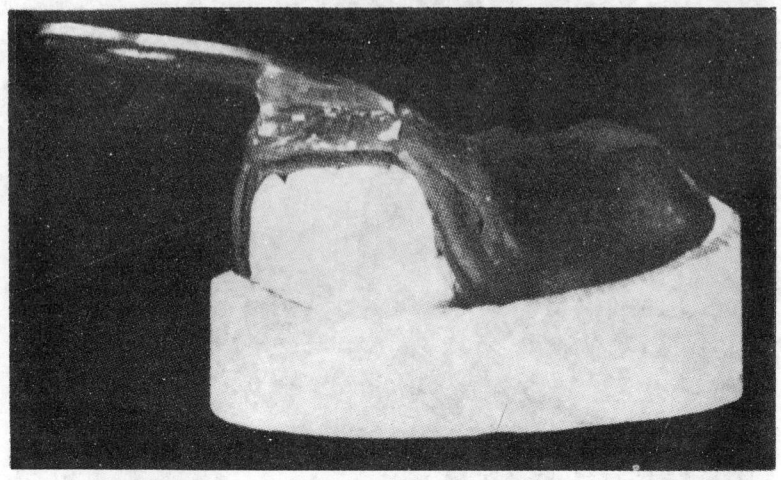

FIG. 471. – Special tray for partially edentulous mouth cut away so as not to include unnecessary labial undercuts.

sulci bounding the edentulous area to be taken. The tray is adapted by filling that part of it which will cover the edentulous area with softened composition and then inserting the tray; when the tray is in place the cheek is manipulated so as to trim the composition in the sulcus. The tray is then removed and the composition impression of the edentulous ridge widened and deepened slightly with the finger to allow room for the material to be used for the final impression (*see* fig. 472).

The problem of producing an accurate model of a partially edentulous mouth is considerably greater than that of the wholly edentulous mouth, due to the fact that natural teeth are normally undercut and are composed of unyielding tissue. Many techniques have been evolved, employing many different materials, in attempts to gain accuracy but the present-day alginates have generally superseded such techniques as the plaster of Paris impression, sectional composition impression and the agar-agar hydrocolloid impression since the alginate impression is both accurate and easy to obtain, provided that the manufacturers' instructions are followed strictly.

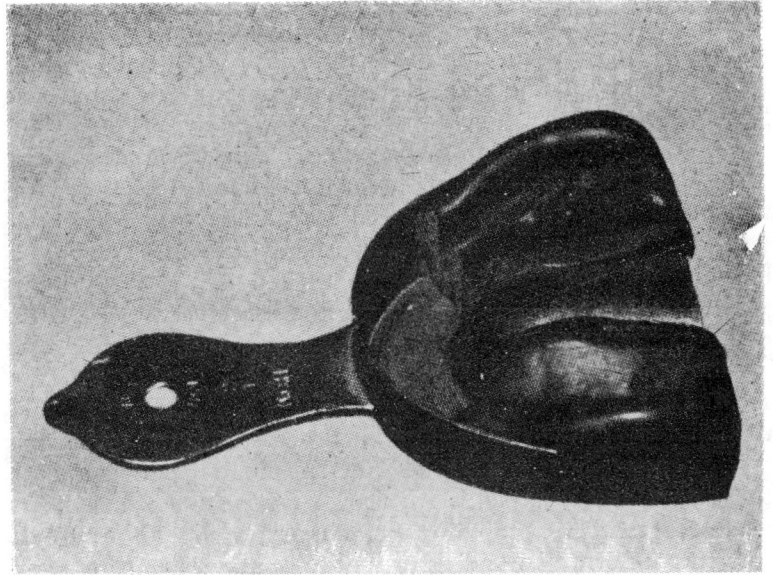

FIG. 472. – A method of adapting a box tray with composition.

IMPRESSION MATERIALS

The Alginates

To produce an accurate impression of the hard and soft tissues of the mouth it is necessary that this material be used in a rigid type of tray which will not be distorted during the working period, particularly the moment of withdrawal from the mouth when considerable force is often employed. This is extremely important when a model is required for the construction of a metal casting in which the slightest distortion in an impression becomes irritatingly obvious when the casting is tried-in in the mouth. For such an impression a rigid tray is essential, it may be either a special tray made of 'cold cure' acrylic or cast in tray alloy or a stock box tray adapted with composition. In the latter case it is desirable when taking an upper impression to post-dam the tray with soft wax and insert the tray so that this soft wax is first seated in close contact with the tissues; this will prevent the impression material escaping posteriorly, which is desirable both from the point of view of the comfort of the patient and also because a mass of alginate unsupported by the tray will tend to pull away from the palate and also distort the impression material farther forward.

The ordinary compound special tray may be used satisfactorily where extensive saddle areas are present, which require the denture periphery to be placed accurately at the functional level of the various sulci, since extensive saddles indicate only a few natural teeth standing which do not usually restrict the easy removal of such an impression and therefore there is little chance of distorting the impression tray.

Alginate material should be placed in those areas of the mouth where it is anticipated that air may be trapped prior to the insertion of the filled tray. Such areas are the palate, the sulci lateral to the tuberosities, the sub-lingual pouch and in the case where a model is required for a casting which bears occlusal rests then a little impression material should be rubbed into the occlusal pits and fissures of the natural teeth to avoid the small bubbles which may otherwise occur in the impression and make the fit of the rest inaccurate.

Only those areas of the mouth required for the construction of the denture should be included in the impression because alginate material distorts easily, and to take an impression of the entire jaw when only the replacement of a few teeth is intended is both undesirable and unnecessary.

Synthetic Rubber Base Impression Materials

Two varieties of synthetic rubber base impression materials have become available in recent years: the Thiocol 'rubbers' and the Silicone 'rubbers'.

Thiocol is the patent name of a polysulphide polymer which when mixed with lead peroxide polymerizes further into a semi-rigid 'rubber'.

The Silicone rubbers are derived from the Siloxane chain (basic unit Sio_2) to which are attached methyl or phenyl groups. This material can be polymerized to form a rubber by the addition of certain organic salts of heavy metals, e.g. dibutyl tin dilaurate together with tetraethyl polysilicate[1].

[1] McLean, J. W. (1958) *Dent. Pract.*

For the purposes of making dental impression materials the polymerizable materials are mixed with such fillers as zinc oxide, chalk or starch to produce a thickish paste. In the case of the thiocol rubbers, the accelerator is similarly mixed into a paste but with the silicones the accelerator is in the form of a liquid.

Both materials when set form soft but adequately rigid rubbers which produce faithful impressions exhibiting excellent surface detail. The polymerization contraction for the thiocols as given by Jørgensen[1] vary from 0·13 per cent to 0·39 per cent; for the Silicones as given by Tomlin and Osborne[2] 0·63 per cent to 080 per cent after twenty-four hours.

For a detailed explanation of the chemistry and properties of these materials the reader is referred to the appropriate texts.

Impression Taking with these Materials

To take an impression of the partially edentulous mouth with either of these materials a close fitting special tray of either acrylic or base-plate material is required. Although when mixed both these materials are sticky they do tend to pull away from the tray when removing the impression from the mouth unless its fitting surface has been well roughened or some fibres of cotton-wool have been fixed to it with sticky wax. Some operators prefer to use perforated trays when employing the Silicone materials.

Mixing the Materials

A suitable length of the impression material is squeezed from the tube on to a glass or porcelain slab and in the case of the Thiocol material an equal length of the accelerator is squeezed beside it: with Silicone materials the accelerator is added drop by drop according to the manufacturer's instructions.

The impression material and its accelerator are then thoroughly mixed with a broad spatula, loaded into the tray which is inserted into the mouth in the usual manner.

The setting time of these impression materials varies from

[1] Jørgensen, K. D. (1956) *Acta Odontologica Scandinavica*, **14**, 313.
[2] Tomlin, H. R. and Osborne, J. (1958) *B.D.J.*, **105**, 407·

4 to 8 minutes or more and depends on the make of the material and the amount of accelerator incorporated. All require to be held steady in the mouth for what appears to the operator and certainly to the patient to be an indefinitely long time.

Removal of the impression from the mouth after the peripheral seal has been broken is simple – the completed impression exhibits a smooth, detailed surface (*see* fig. 473).

In spite of claims by manufacturers that impression taken with either of these materials exhibit little or no dimensional change they should be cast soon after removal from the mouth if the highest degree of accuracy is required.

The Use of these Materials

They can be used for any impression but have little advantage over the alginates save in bulk, so for patients who exhibit a marked tendency to retching they can be employed although in these cases extra acceleration is necessary to shorten to a

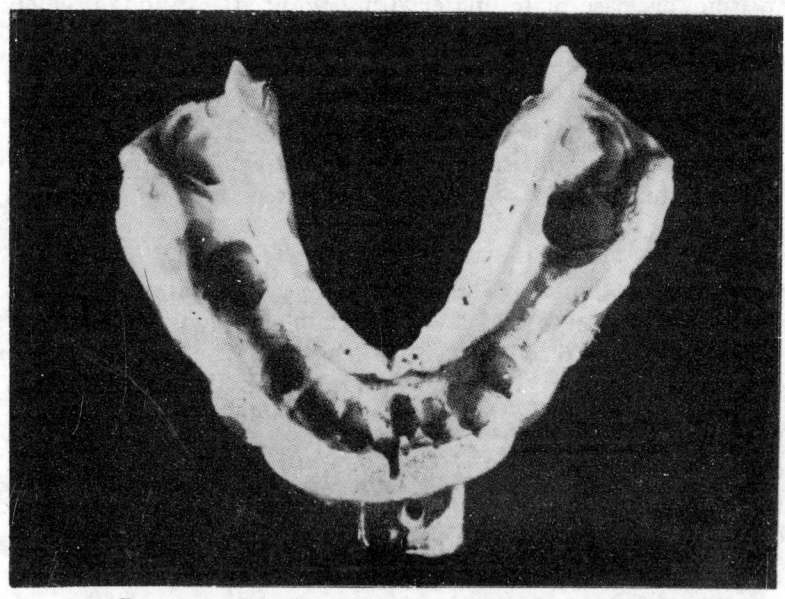

FIG. 473. – Completed impression taken in a synthetic rubber material.

minimum the time required for the impression to be held in the mouth.

The type of case in which their value is greatest is with those patients who are unable to open the mouth fully and yet require a partial denture. In such cases alginate material will tear on the standing natural teeth when the impression is removed from the mouth whereas synthetic rubber will not.

Composition and Alginate

This technique is most commonly employed for obtaining study models. It can be used as a method for obtaining a final working impression, but it must be remembered that it usually produces an impression which is over-extended in the region of the sulci and therefore the peripheries of the denture must be designed accordingly. As large a tray as is convenient, without causing distortion, is filled with softened composition and an impression taken, but before the composition has time to harden, the tray is moved about from side to side and backwards and forwards, thus the impression is finally only an approximate fit. On removal more distortion can be caused with a finger in any area where there is a severe undercut or around isolated teeth; the composition must then be thoroughly chilled in cold water and trimmed if necessary. This distorted impression is now used as a special tray and the impression taken with a wash of alginate: if the composition is dried and quickly flamed immediately before putting in the alginate there is no need to use sticky wax to keep the material in the tray.

Composition

Composition is, for all practical purposes, non-elastic, except for a short time during its cooling period, and it therefore distorts during removal from the mouth and will not accurately reproduce an undercut unless a special sectional technique is employed. It is a valuable material, however, because it is the only material which will compress the soft tissues.

Sectional Impressions. – If it is desired to use composition for taking a detailed impression of a partially edentulous mouth the impression must be taken in sections, each one being removed in a direction which eliminates the undercut area. For example an accurate composition impression can be taken of a single tooth if the labial surface together with part of the mesial and distal surfaces is taken and removed at right angles to the long axis of the tooth, thus: fig. 474.

This first section is chilled, reinserted and the palatal or lingual portion taken in the same way but removed in the opposite direction, thus: fig. 475.

Finally both these sections are replaced and the third impression taken of the occlusal surface thus: fig. 476.

Grooves should be cut in each section so that succeeding sections will key into place and the final collection can be sealed together with a hot knife before the model is poured.

The same principles are used when taking an impression of many teeth for the construction of a partial denture and the number of sections which will be required and the direction of removal of each can be determined by the examination of a

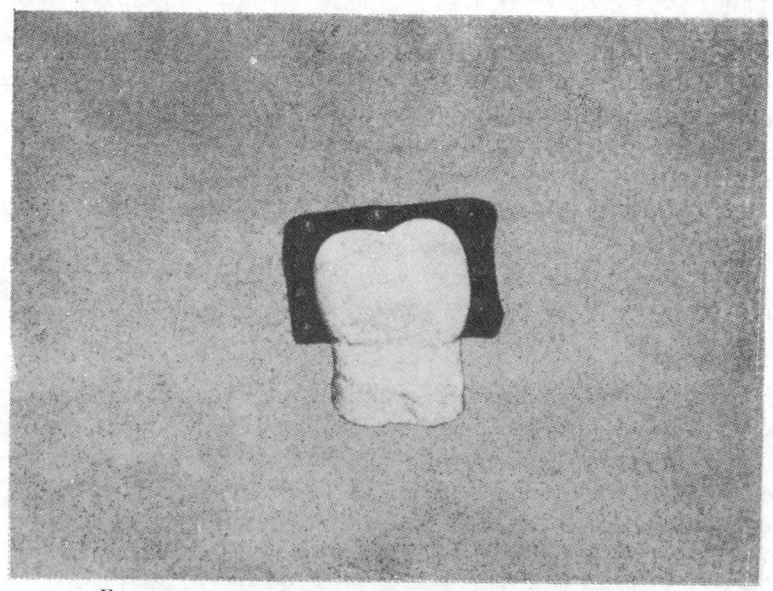

FIG. 474. – Impression of the buccal surface with part of the mesial and distal undercuts. The composition has been trimmed and pits cut for keying with the subsequent sections. Impression withdrawn buccally.

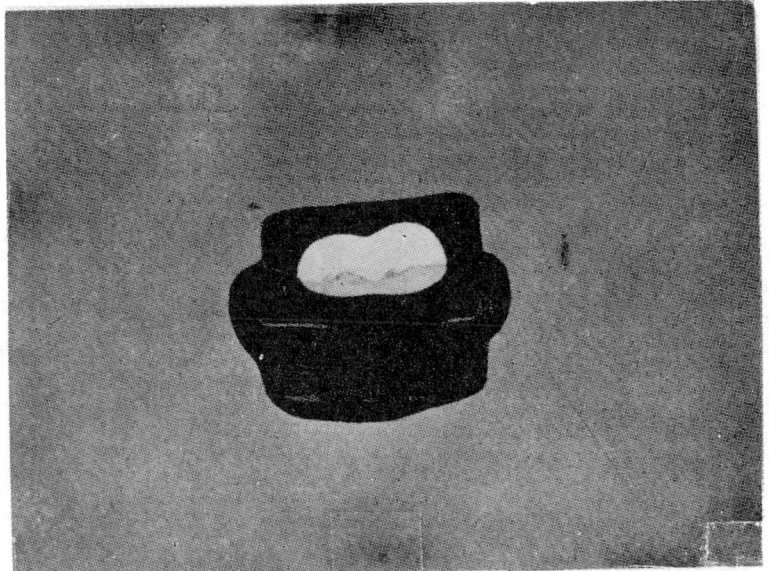

FIG. 475. – The lingual section in position. Impression withdrawn lingually.

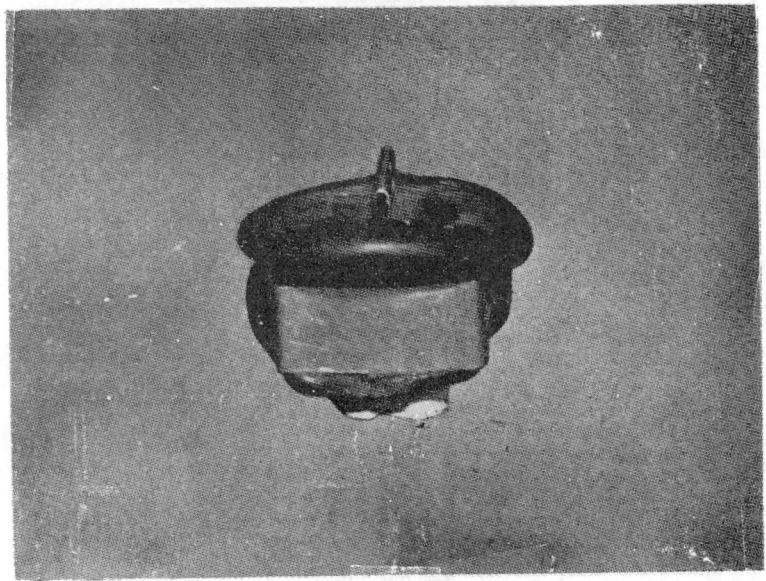

FIG. 476. – The occlusal surface impression taken with the buccal and lingual sections in position. Note the metal supports for all sections.

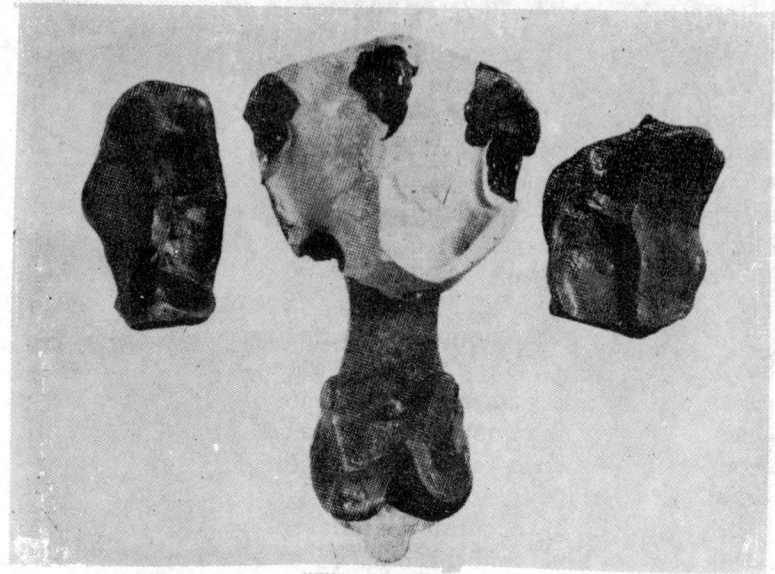

(a) In pieces.

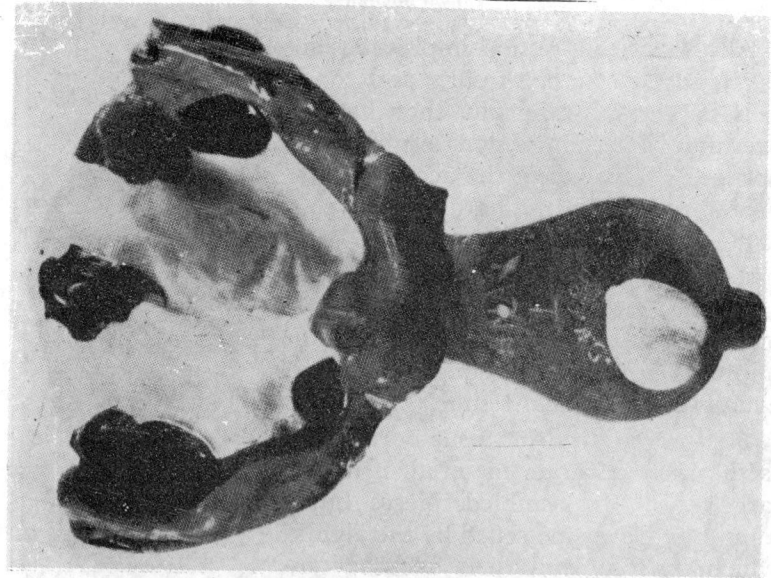

(b) Assembled in tray.

The main impression was taken in white composition; small additions were made with green stick, and the buccal and labial sections completed in brown composition.

FIG. 477. – A completed sectional composition impression.

study model. Each section should have a stiff backing cut from
sheet metal to support the softened material and to allow some
pressure to be applied in pressing it against the teeth or soft
tissues. The composition should be handled in the same way
as has been described for edentulous impressions, i.e. soften,
insert, remove, chill, dry, flame, temper, reinsert with pressure,
remove and chill. A completed impression is shown in fig. 477.

Plaster of Paris

This material is rarely used today for taking impressions of
the partially edentulous mouth because of the difficulty of
technique. It is inserted soft into the mouth in a box tray and
when set the tray is removed and the set plaster fractured into
pieces which are then reassembled in the tray (see fig. 478 a
and b).

Although a highly accurate material small pieces tend to get
lost or badly rubbed and this often invalidates the impression.

Choice of Impression Material

Although compression impressions should theoretically give
the most satisfactory results and so should always be used,
it is found that clinically they have little if any advanatge
over mucostatic impressions even in the case of tooth and tissue-
borne dentures where the accurate distribution of masticatory
pressures between the hard and the soft tissues is desirable.

By mucostatic impression is meant one in which the soft
tissues are in no way compressed or distorted and therefore the
impression material must flow readily and impose no pressure
on the mucosa. Plaster of Paris is the only true mucostatic
impression material though the hydrocolloids often give
equally good clinical results.

For tooth-borne or tissue-borne dentures, plaster of Paris
is the most accurate material, if it can be removed in a few
large, easily reassembled, pieces but nowadays it has been
almost entirely superseded by the alginate impression materials
which have proved their accuracy over many years if the
correct technique of their use is strictly adhered to. The great
advantages of the alginate materials over plaster are that they
are better liked and tolerated by the patient and as they do not

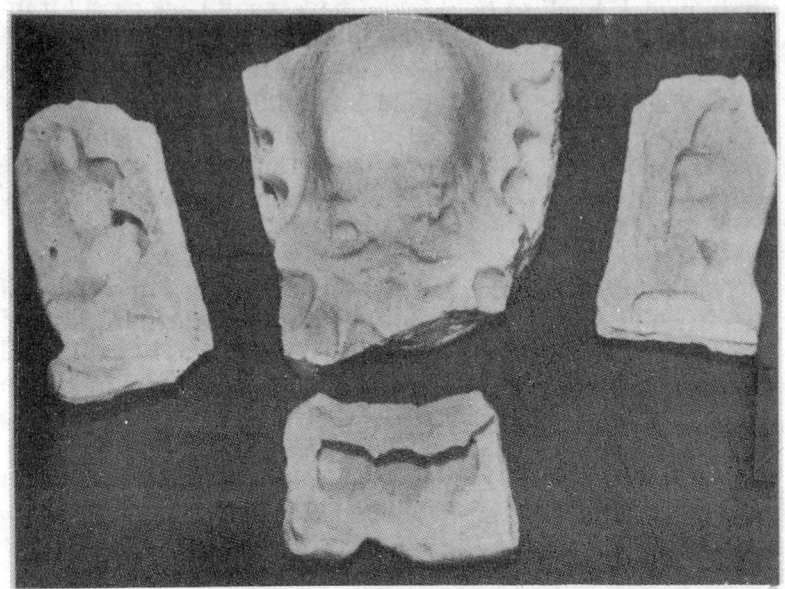

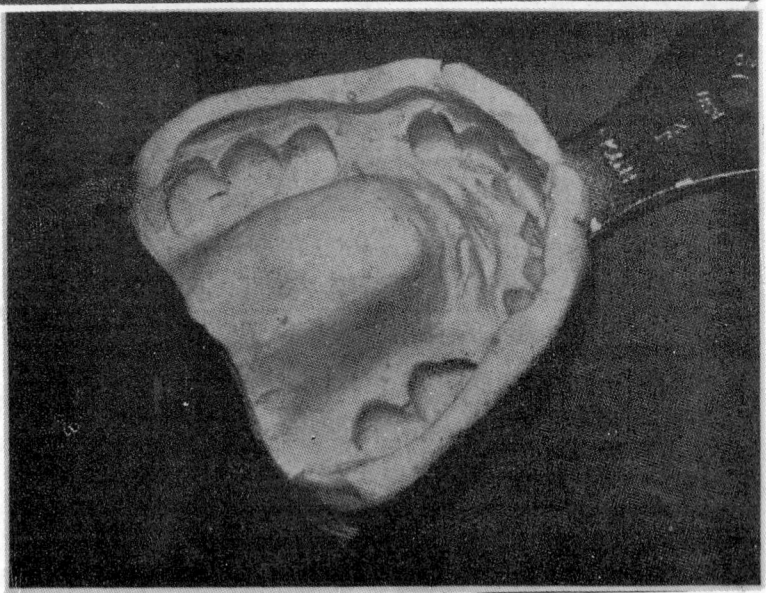

(b) The pieces united in the tray.

FIG. 478. – Plaster impression.

fracture on removal, small pieces are not likely to be lost and invalidate the impression as may be the case with plaster. Where isolated teeth are missing, or where the natural teeth are spaced, an accurate plaster impression may be impossible, and a hydrocolloidal material will then be the material of choice.

For tooth and tissue-borne dentures a sectional, composition impression with some degree of compression must be used if an attempt is being made to distribute the masticatory stresses between teeth and mucous membrane.

MODELS

Although satisfactory models for the construction of full dentures may be made from a mixture of plaster of Paris and artificial stone in equal parts, which has the advantage of being more easily cut and removed from acrylic dentures, only a hard non-expanding plaster or stone should be used for partial denture work, for two reasons:

(1) All partial dentures have some contact with the natural teeth, as distinct from full dentures which are only in contact with soft mucous membrane, and as the teeth are rigid, or at least must be treated as such, the greatest possible accuracy is required.

(2) A considerable amount of constructional work may have to be carried out on the model, such as the designing and fitting of clasps, and unless the model is hard, the resultant wear will naturally spoil the fit of the denture made on it.

CHAPTER XXV

RECORDING THE POSITION OF OCCLUSION IN PARTIALLY EDENTULOUS CASES

In Cases with Many Natural Teeth Standing

Frequently, sufficient natural teeth remain in both jaws to enable the position of centric occlusion to be accurately determined by their interdigitation when the models are occluded.

If any doubt exists, however, as to the exact jaw relationship a squash record, as described for the study models, should be taken and the models articulated with its aid (*see* fig. 464).

In Cases with Large Edentulous Spaces

In cases presenting extensive edentulous areas the models cannot be accurately articulated by the interdigitation of the natural teeth and it is necessary to record centric occlusion. Record blocks for partial cases are made in a manner identical with that employed for edentulous cases, the only difference being that the rims are not continuous but merely fill the edentulous spaces (*see* fig. 479). Sometimes it is only necessary to make a record block for one jaw if sufficient natural teeth exist in the opposing jaw. The relationship and interdigitation, if any, of the mandibular and maxillary teeth should be examined and noted before the record blocks are inserted in the mouth. In the majority of partial cases both the vertical and anteroposterior dimensions are indicated by the interdigitation of the remaining natural teeth. All that the operator is required to do, therefore, is to trim the occlusal surfaces of the rims until they just fail to occlude when the natural teeth are fully in occlusion.

Localization grooves and pits are then cut in the rims as described in Chapter VI and a thin template of softened wax placed on the surface of the lower rim. The record blocks are inserted in the mouth and the patient requested to close the teeth together. The operator should watch carefully and

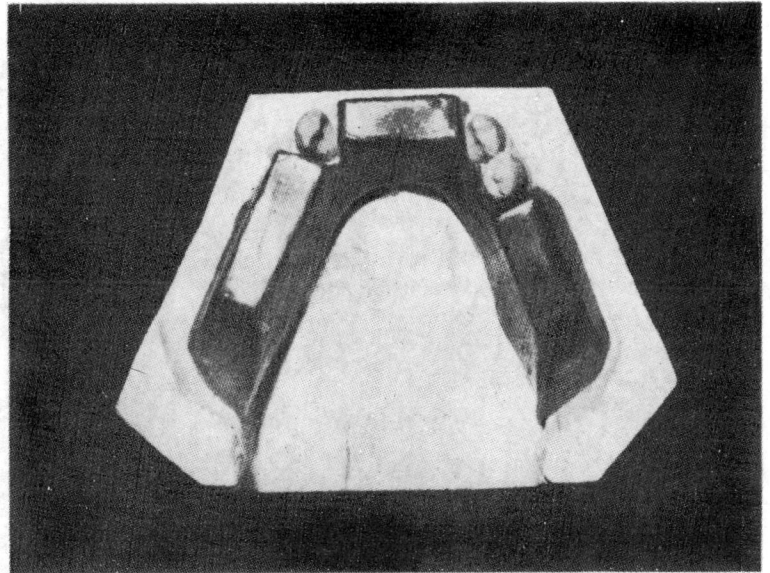

FIG. 479. – An example of a partial bite block.

ensure that *the natural teeth are fully in occlusion and interdigitating correctly*. The blocks are then removed from the
mouth, the plaster models placed in them and the occlusion
and interdigitation of the natural plaster teeth checked.

The firm occlusion and interdigitation of the natural teeth
is emphasized because a very common source of trouble with
partial dentures is that when they are finally fitted they are
found to hold the occlusion open off the natural teeth by
anything from 1 mm. to 4 mm. necessitating extensive grinding
and mutilation of the occlusal surfaces of the artificial teeth (*see
fig. 480).

A contributory cause of this trouble is undoubtedly failure
on the part of some technicians to pay sufficient attention
to the elementary rules of flasking and packing thereby
increasing the height of the denture in processing. The main
cause of the trouble is usually traceable, however, to the fact
that the plaster models were articulated with the natural
teeth slightly out of occlusion.

It sometimes happens that when the record blocks are in the

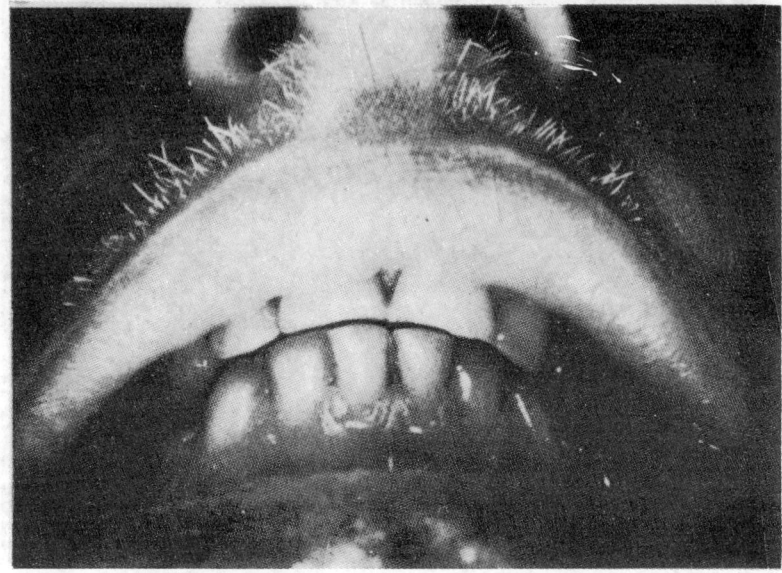

Fig. 480. – Natural teeth out of occlusion when partial
dentures are in place, a bad but common fault.

mouth with the jaws closed the natural teeth are observed to
be fully in occlusion and yet when the blocks are removed
from the mouth and the plaster models inserted in them the
teeth are slightly separated. The cause of this trouble can be
traced to the fact that the rims of the blocks were not trimmed
so as to allow a small space to exist between the occlusal
surfaces when the natural teeth were fully in occlusion and
this has resulted in compression of the soft tissues by the
record blocks and compression of the resilient wax rims of
the blocks allowing the natural teeth to come into occlusion.
When the record blocks are placed on the models, however, the
plaster representing the soft tissues will not compress and
consequently the natural teeth are held out of occlusion.
Theoretically if partial dentures are set up and finished to a
record obtained under such circumstances the dentures should
compress the soft tissues when the jaws are closed and allow
the natural teeth to occlude; in practice, however, this is not
borne out and if this error of recording is made, considerable

grinding of the occlusal surfaces of the artificial teeth is always required; which points to the resilient nature of some dental waxes (*see also* page 653 *et seg*).

Tooth-borne Dentures

Where a metal casting has been constructed for a tooth-borne partial denture it is advisable to record centric occlusion with wax rims attached to the metal casting so that it is recorded under conditions similar to that occurring at the fitting stage of the denture. A word of warning is necessary however as it is easy to overlook incomplete occlusion of the natural teeth due to premature contact against an occlusal rest.

In Cases Where the Natural Teeth Remaining in Both Jaws do not Occlude

In these cases the vertical and anteroposterior occlusal relationships are assessed in the same way as described in Chapter VI. Such cases should be looked upon as edentulous with a few natural teeth standing and edentulous methods of record taking applied to them.

Recording the Occlusal Relationship when Employing an Anatomical Articulator

The stages are identical with those described for the edentulous case. If most of the natural teeth are standing the lateral records are taken by means of wax squash records otherwise blocks are used as described above.

The essential difference between partial and edentulous cases is in the adjustment of the incisal guide table of the articulator. In partial cases the natural teeth provide the guidance and the table should be set so as to allow these teeth to remain in occlusion when lateral movements are made.

Trial Dentures (try-in)

The main considerations at this stage are the verification of centric occlusion, the testing of the stability and retention of the denture and the approval of the appearance, by the patient, of any artificial teeth which are situated in the anterior part of the mouth.

The occlusion of the artificial and natural teeth is checked with celluloid strips for evenness of pressure, it being most important that the pressure is not heavier on the artificial teeth than it is on the natural teeth, the ideal being equal pressure on both. Clasps are assessed for their position and their relationship to the soft tissues – the gingival margins in the case of encircling clasps of tissue-borne dentures, and the sulcus and gum tissue in the case of projection clasps.

The artificial teeth are observed for correctness of match of mould and shade, and any minor alterations of position and angulation of such teeth carried out at the chairside to produce maximum harmony with the natural teeth. Artificial anterior teeth of a tissue-borne trial denture should be left very slightly longer than the neighbouring natural anterior teeth in order to allow for the slight settling which occurs during the first few days after fitting of the finished denture and for any incisal grinding which is contemplated to produce a more natural appearance of the anterior teeth.

Fitting Partial Dentures

If the model has been accurately surveyed and the denture and clasps properly designed (*see* Chapter XX) the denture should fit the mouth easily and accurately. It is frequently discovered, however, especially when acrylic resin is the base material, that the denture binds slightly on the natural teeth and will not go fully into place. If the surveying and blocking out of undercuts has been done carefully, the commonest cause of this trouble is that the plaster teeth on the model have been rubbed or chipped during the fabrication of the denture. In order to fit such a denture the acrylin resin round the teeth must be eased slightly and to do this accurately careful observation is necessary. The denture should be inserted in the mouth and very gently coaxed into place as far as it will go easily. Using a mouth mirror the whole area of the denture in contact with the natural teeth should be inspected and any point where the contact is hard noted. The denture is then removed from the mouth and a little of the acrylic resin in this area stoned away and the denture tried again and further careful observations made. This process must be repeated until the denture slips into place. Under no circumstances should the denture be forced home because if this is done it will be found extremely difficult to remove.

If the exact area of hard contact cannot be discovered by observation a little black carding wax may be run on to the surface of the denture fitting against the suspect tooth and the denture inserted as far as it will go. On removal the black carding wax will be found to have been completely squeezed out of the area of hard contact which may then be eased accurately.

It is emphasized that easing a partial denture into place requires care and patience because if material is removed from the wrong area, or an excessive amount of material removed, the fit of the denture may be ruined. *Such easing is unnecessary and is best avoided by a careful and exact technique both at the chairside and in the laboratory.*

Adjusting the Occlusion

This is carried out with articulating paper and wax templates as described for full dentures (*see* Chapter XII). Care should always be taken to ensure that the occlusion is not heavy on occlusal rests.

The Increased Vertical Dimension

The development of an increased vertical dimension is an ever present problem in partial denture prosthetics. The causes of this may be of clinical or technical origin and all too frequently the technician is blamed for such an occurrance resulting from failure of the dental surgeon to obtain the correct occlusion in the first place.

Clinical Cause

In all partial cases where natural teeth occlude this normal occlusal position of the teeth may be assumed to be correct unless the vertical dimension is to be intentionally increased within the bounds of the free-way space. In cases where the edentulous areas are limited and many natural teeth are present all that is required usually is to occlude the models in the manner indicated by the occlusion of the natural teeth and secure them to the articulator. It is important, however, to check the occlusion of the models against the patient's natural occlusion and to ensure that their relations are identical because it is possible to occlude the models in a slightly incorrect position with disastrous results.

Those cases requiring wax record blocks to register the position of occlusion are the ones in which clinical errors cause opening and what happens is this:

The record blocks are trimmed down until the upper and lower blocks just occlude when the natural teeth are in occlusion; soft wax is then interposed between the blocks and the patient is instructed to close. What occurs then is one of two things. Either the dental surgeon fails to check accurately that the natural teeth are in full occlusion – often the anterior teeth are 1 – 2 mm. out of occlusion and this frequently escapes notice being masked by a deep overbite when viewed from the front (*see* fig. 480) – or otherwise the wax blocks compress under the force of occlusion and then elastically recoil when the teeth are parted. In either case when the plaster models are fitted into the record

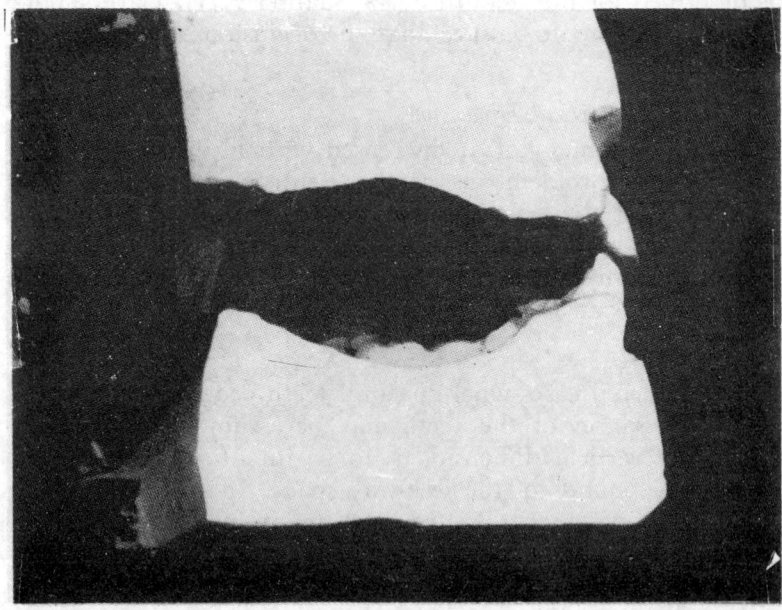

FIG. 481(*a*).

blocks prior to articulating them the plaster replicas of the natural teeth will be slightly out of occlusion and unless very careful comparison is made with the position of occlusion of the natural teeth the error will pass unnoticed (*see* figs. 480 and 481). Frequently this cause will escape notice at the try-in stage because again the wax of the set-up teeth will compress on occlusion. When the unyielding acrylic dentures are fitted, however, the error will become obvious and a lot of time-consuming grinding will be resorted to or otherwise the patient will be instructed to wear the dentures for a few days in the hope that they will settle. If they do settle it will be at the expense of the gingival margins, and soft tissues. Actually the degree of so-called settlement of a properly constructed and designed partial denture is very small.

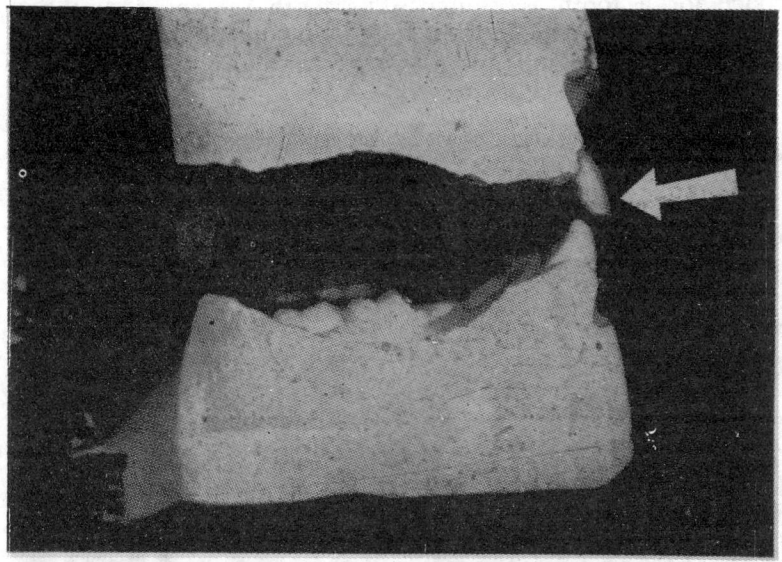

Fig. 481. – A sagittal section through the plaster models of a partially edentulous case with record blocks in place:
(a) Close contact of the upper and lower front teeth which copies accurately the occlusion of these teeth in the mouth.
(b) Lack of occlusion of the front teeth due to recoil of the wax blocks, contact with the baseplate or careless articulation.
Inaccurate occlusion such as this frequently escapes notice if viewed casually from the front in the direction of the arrow (compare with fig. 480).

Technical Causes

The first of these is a continuation of the fault already mentioned, i.e. failure to occlude the plaster models so that the plaster teeth truly represent the occlusal relationship of the natural ones. If the fixing together of the models is left to the technician such things as wax recoil, excess of wax, warping of wax and rubbing of plaster teeth may all contribute to this error, and it is strongly advocated that the union of models by means of wire strips or sticks should be made at the chairside after the comparison with the natural occlusion has been made (*see* fig. 482).

The second and very common technical fault is the gradual opening of the vertical dimension as the artificial teeth are set up. Frequently in partial cases the vertical or inter-alveolar space for a tooth is limited. The tooth is ground, but not sufficiently, the articulator is closed forcefully and the opponent plaster tooth rubbed and the vertical dimension thus opened

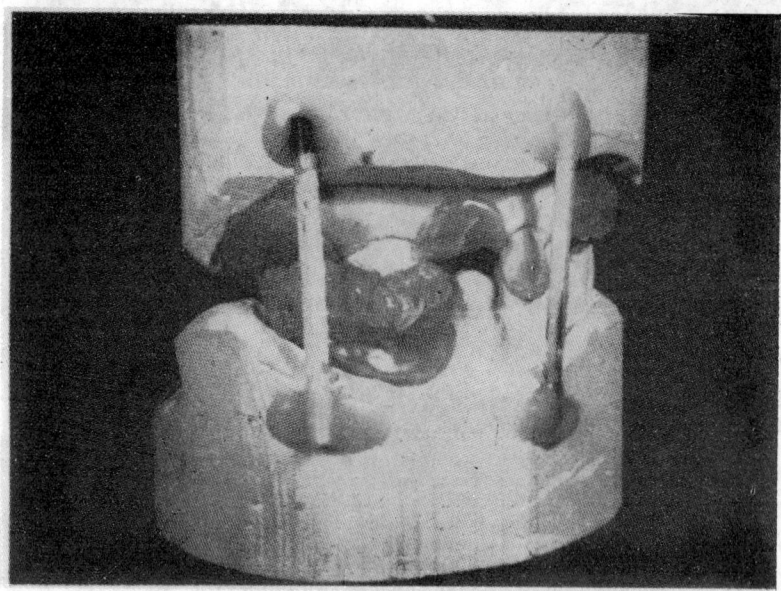

FIG. 482. – Method of uniting models with matchsticks (or wire) and sticky wax, so as to ensure that they are correctly articulated by the technician.

slightly. The posterior teeth are usually the chief offenders in this matter and if such a case is observed critically it will be seen that the anterior teeth are often 1/16 in. out of occlusion, but that this is frequently masked by the overbite on the model if viewed casually from the front. When such a set-up is tried-in, the elasticity of the wax and the normally slack fit of the trial bases often allow these errors to pass unnoticed and they only become apparent when the unyielding finished denture is fitted.

The swaging of thin tin foil over plaster natural teeth will prevent the rubbing of the surface when much fitting of an opposing artificial tooth has to be carried out and the meticulous observance of the position of occlusion of the natural teeth all through the setting-up will prevent this occurrence.

Processing[1]

Finally the cause which is frequently the only one understood and blamed for an increase of vertical dimension in partial cases, i.e. that occurring during processing.

The causes of this are twofold:

(*a*) Failure of the two halves of the flask to meet due to the extrusion of acrylic flash and thus an increase in the vertical dimension by the amount of this failure.

(*b*) The artificial teeth are driven into the plaster containing them either as a result of excessive pressure applied through the acrylic resin or due to softness of the plaster or due to weakness of lack of support of the plaster.

Two methods of flasking are possible for partial dentures. In the first method the model and artificial teeth are invested in one half of the flask and plaster caps built over the occlusal surfaces of the teeth to support and position them during the boiling-out of the wax and the packing and curing of the acrylic. The plaster in the second half of the flask merely acts as a ram to force the soft acrylic into the space which was occupied by the wax. This method will be referred to as packing through.

In the second method the case is flasked so that after boiling out the wax and separating the two halves of the flask the model is in one half and the teeth in the other. This method will be referred to as reverse packing.

[1]The substance of this first appeared in an article by one of us in the *B.D.J.* (1956) **101,** 411.

A cinematograph study through a Perspex window let into the side of a flask has given much information on this irritating phenomenon of the alteration of tooth position during packing in both these methods of flasking.

Fig. 483 illustrates the flask with the Perspex window. The investing plaster, the model, a tooth and the supporting wax can be seen in cross section. In these studies a saddle consisting of four molar teeth set up in the normal manner has been used, the first tooth abutting against the window. The thickness of the plaster caps and the distance between the teeth and the model and the time and rate of closure of the flask being varied with each experiment.

Fig. 484 shows frame enlargements from a Kodachrome cine film showing how the alteration in tooth position occurs in a case packed by the method of packing through. In the first frame the supporting plaster cap (A, fig. 484c) is seen intact supporting the tooth. In the second and subsequent frames as the acrylic (B) flows between the model (C) and the tooth (D)

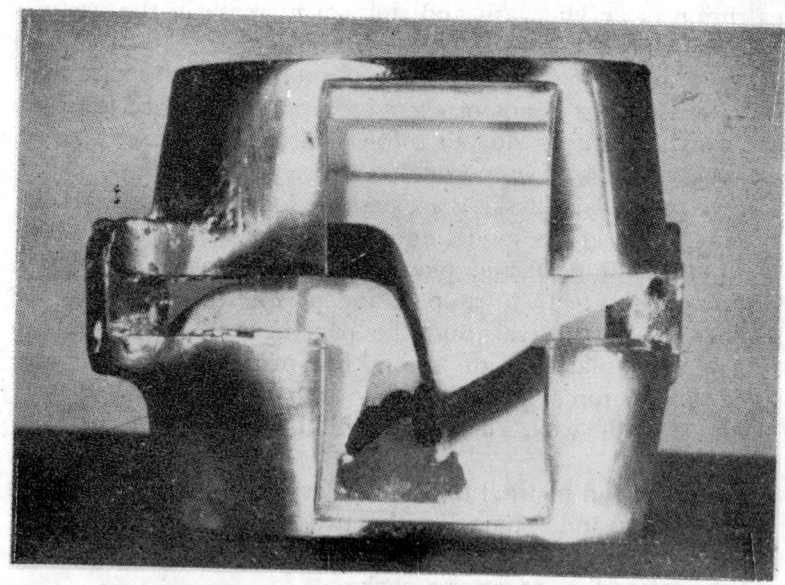

FIG. 483. – Flask with Perspex window; model and wax supporting teeth are coloured to aid photography.

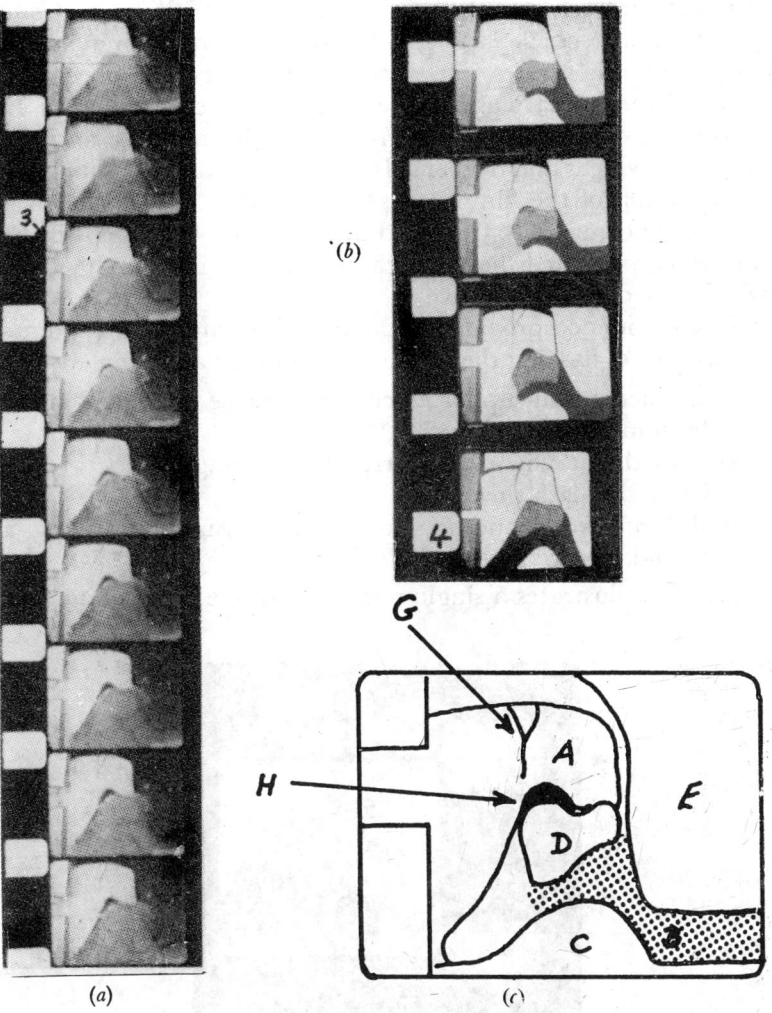

FIG. 484.

(a) Frame enlargements from a Kodachrome cine film
   illustrating the fracture of a plaster cap.
   Note how the first sign of a crack appears in frame 3(a) and
then the cap rises in successive frames producing a space
above the buccal cusp of the tooth.

(b) The first 3 frames are retouched ones from (a) showing
   what happens in greater detail. The 4th frame is from
   further on in the film showing that the buccal cusp of
   the tooth has risen into the space.

(c) Key to frames: *see* text.

under the influence of the plaster wedge (E) of the second half of the flask a crack (G) is just discernible occurring in the middle of the plaster cap, and a space (H) has developed between the buccal cusp of the tooth and the plaster cap. In succeeding frames the space (H) gradually increases and the crack (G) widens and deepens. In fig. 484(*b*), frame 4, which is a continuation of the film some seconds later, the plaster cap is seen to be completely fractured and malpositioned and in the film when projected the tooth can be seen to rise into the space which has developed above it.

From evidence provided by many cinematographic studies of this type of flasking the way to prevent such an occurrence is:

(1) Use deep, well-supported caps, and place the model at the bottom of the flask.
(2) Pack the acrylic at the correct dough stage.
(3) Close the flask slowly.
(4) Refrain from adding extra acrylic and performing a second closure.

Fig. 485 illustrates a single retouched frame from a cine film

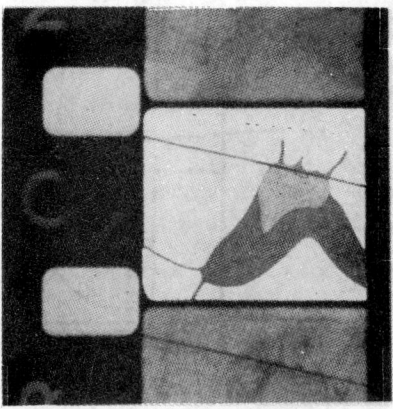

FIG. 485. – The black line on the plane of which the cusps of the tooth were situated before the wax was boiled out runs slantingly across the top third of each frame.
Note the cracks in the plaster radiating up from the cusps and the fact that the latter are above the black line now that the acrylic has been packed (the middle frame has been retouched to illustrate the details more clearly).

taken through the Perspex window of a flask prepared for examining what occurs when the reverse method of packing is employed. A thin black line is scribed across the Perspex window so that it lies on the plane of the extreme tips of the cusps before opening the flask after investment. The wax is then boiled out and the acrylic dough packed and closure of the flask carried out. At first the dough flows easily but when the flask is almost closed and the flash thin the pressure inside the flask obviously increases; suddenly cracks develop in the plaster supporting the tooth and the tooth is driven slightly into the plaster. Fig. 485 shows the cracks in the supporting plaster of the reverse half of the flask and the fact that the cusps now lie above the black line indicate that the vertical dimension has been increased.

Several trials were filmed using the method of reverse packing in which a space is made for the inevitable flash by painting the plaster surface of the first half of the flasked case with a thin film of wax before pouring the reverse half, thus providing a space for the flash. In each case the flow of acrylic continued until complete closure of the flask was obtained and no pressure built up inside and no cracking of the plaster was visible. The cusps of the teeth returned at full closure of the flask to their correct relationship with the black line.

This method in practice gives consistently good results in partial cases with little or no increase in the vertical dimension of the denture due to processing faults and this technique is strongly advocated as a means of prevention of bite opening during processing.

Chapter XXVI

IMMEDIATE DENTURES

The term immediate denture is used to describe a denture which is entirely constructed before the extraction of the teeth which it replaces and is inserted immediately after the extraction of the teeth. This term is used in preference to that of temporary denture which, though often employed, is an unfortunate title for two reasons:

(1) It is used not only for dentures which are made before extractions, but also for dentures made at any time during the two or three months immediately following.

(2) The idea is conveyed to the patient that the denture is temporary, when what is meant is that its usefulness is temporary, owing to the rapid change in shape of the alveolar ridges, during the first few months following extraction.

Many techniques have been described for constructing immediate dentures, most of them differing only slightly in detail, and in general they can be divided into two groups:

(1) Without alveolectomy.

(2) With alveolectomy.

Immediate Dentures Without Alveolectomy
(see figs. 486–492)

This method is most suitable for replacing the single-rooted teeth and is chiefly used for incisors and canines. If some posterior teeth have also to be extracted they should, if possible, be removed three or four months before making the immediate denture. The first step is to examine the patient, paying particular attention to the occlusal relationship of the upper and lower front teeth. If the occlusion of these teeth is such that they give an accurate guide to the jaw relationship only they

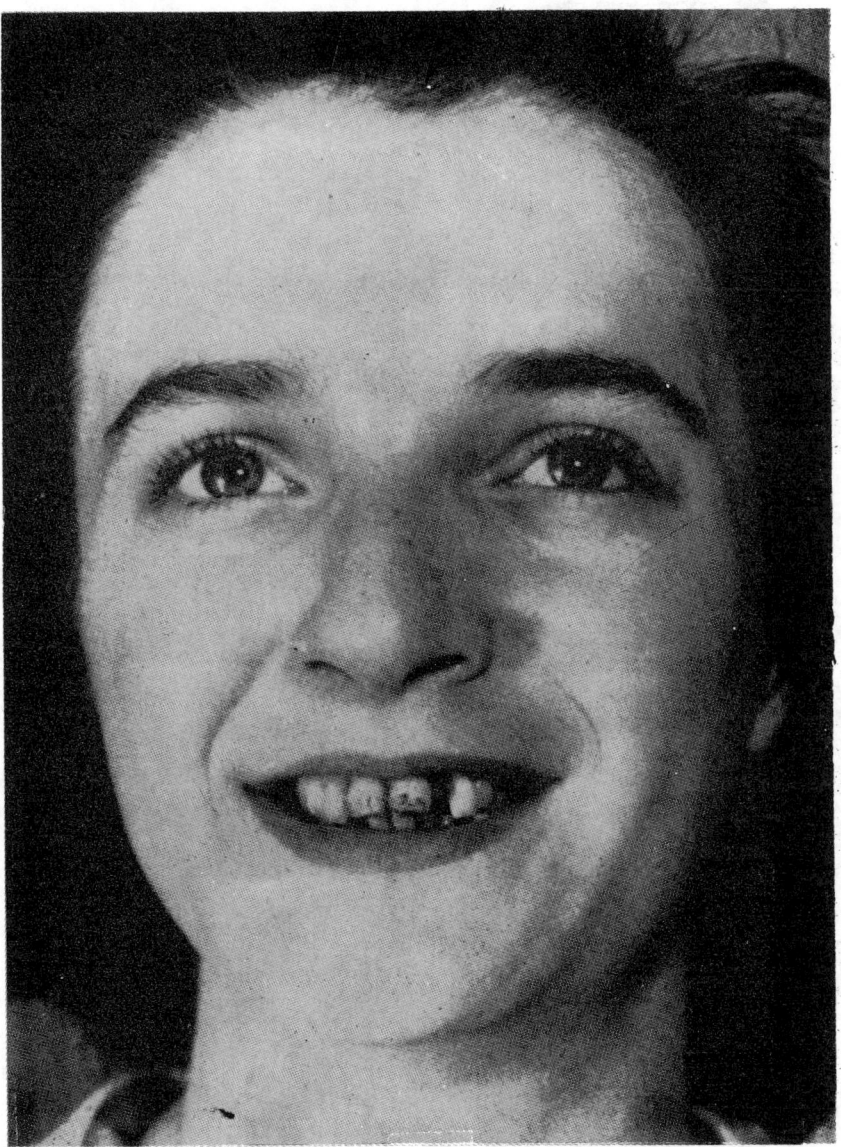

FIG. 486. – The posterior teeth have been extracted and the sockets have healed.

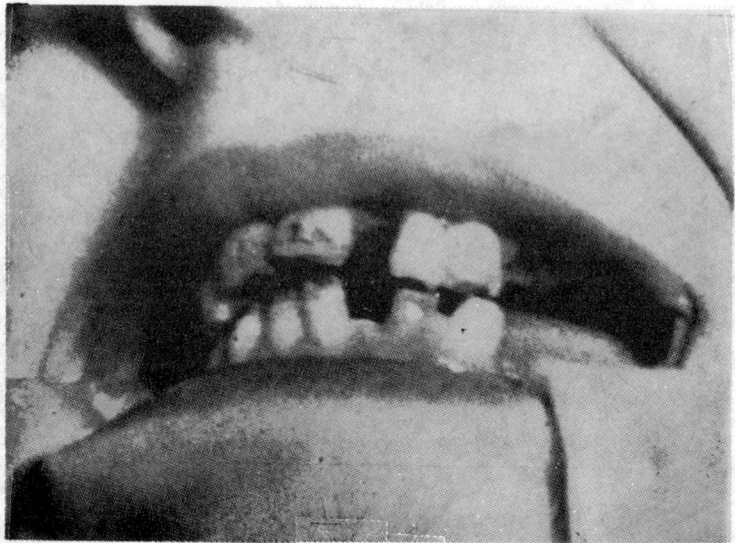

FIG. 487. – Illustrating how the occlusal relationship of the jaws is indicated by the occlusion of $\overline{32|3}$.

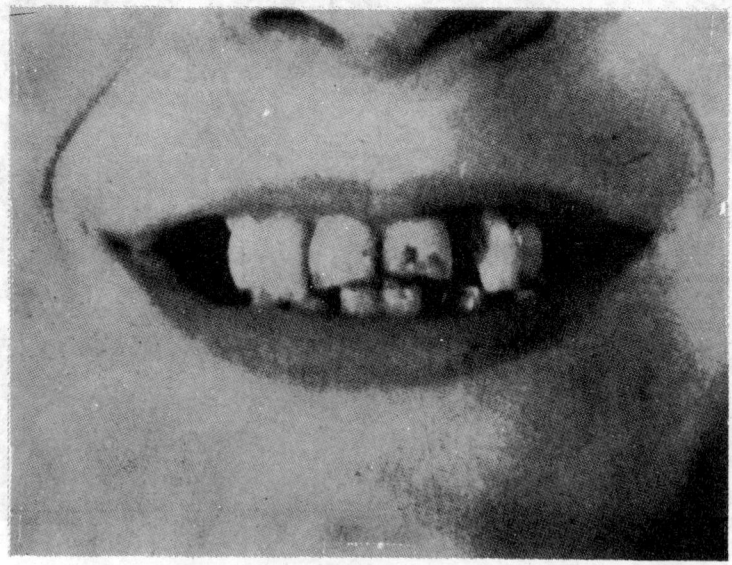

FIG. 488. – Upper and lower partial dentures have been fitted.

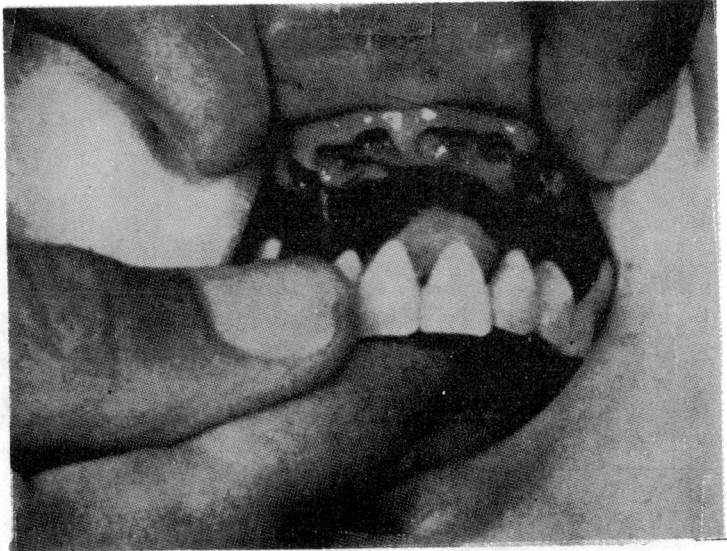

FIG. 489. – The natural upper front teeth have been extracted and the upper denture to which the artificial front teeth have been added is being inserted.

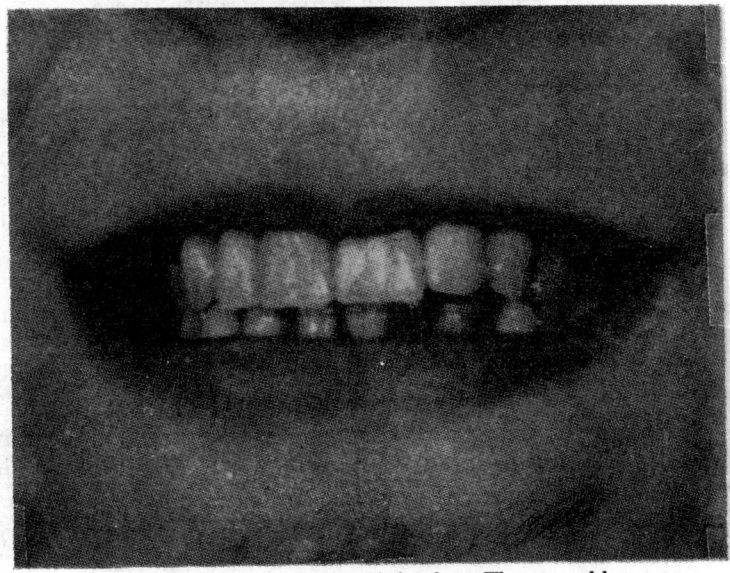

FIG. 490. – The upper denture is in place. The natural lower front teeth are still standing.

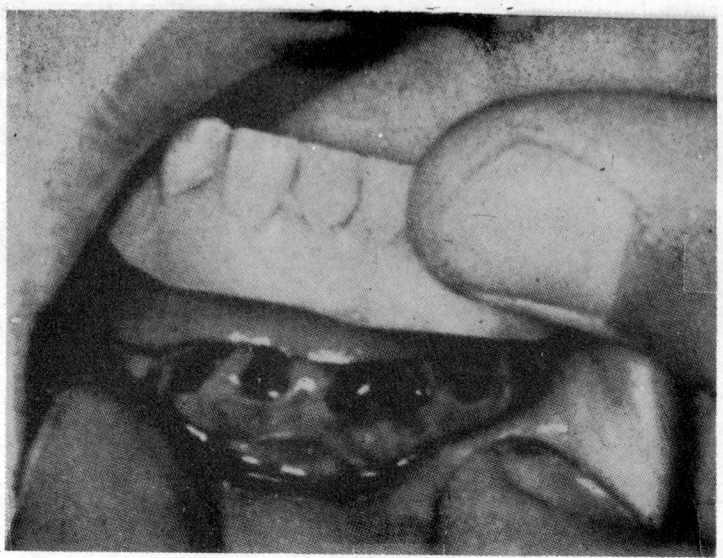

Fig. 491. – The natural lower front teeth have been extracted and the lower denture to which the artificial front teeth have been added is being inserted. Note labial flange.

need be retained for immediate replacement. If, however, as frequently occurs in cases presenting a large overjet, the front teeth do not make contact in the centric occlusion, then the upper and lower first premolars on either side must be retained for immediate replacement.

Once it has been decided which teeth are to be retained, the posterior teeth are extracted. This is conveniently done by removing at one visit the upper and lower back teeth on the side which is not habitually used for chewing, and then a fortnight later extracting those on the other side. Sharp interdental bone is removed with rongeurs at the time of extraction. After the posterior teeth have been extracted the patient should be dismissed for the period of immediate healing and most rapid alveolar absorption. The longer this waiting period, up to six months, the better, for two reasons:

(1) The more rounded will be the sharp edges of the tooth sockets and consequently the more comfortable will be the dentures, even under the pressure of mastication.

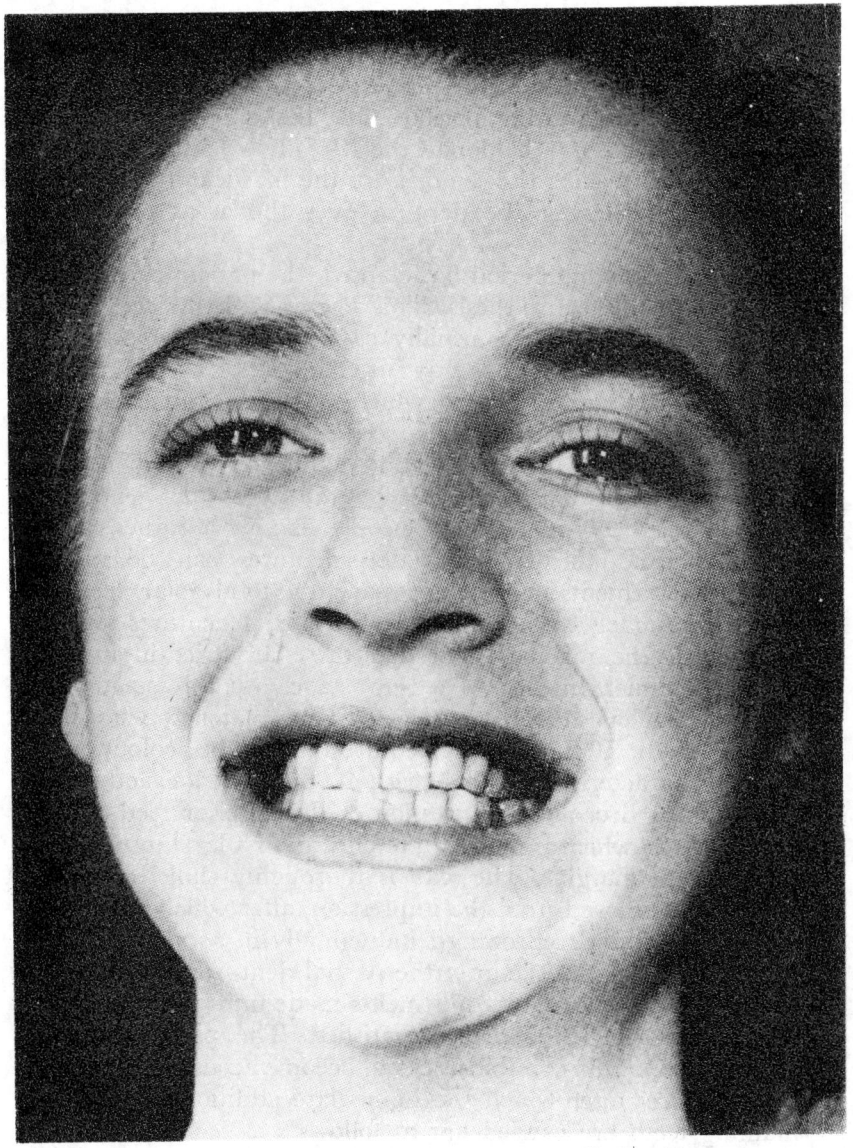

FIG. 492. – The completed case, compare with fig. 486.

(2) The period of rapid absorption will be over and thus the useful life of the dentures will be increased.

In cases where most of the posterior teeth have been lost for some years, the waiting period after the extraction of the remainder need not be long; the already edentulous areas can be made to take the majority of the masticatory pressure by suitably relieving the denture over the areas of recent extraction.

When the healing period has elapsed, the patient is recalled for the immediate prosthesis. This begins with the taking of the primary impressions, usually carried out in composition or a hydrocolloid, in a stock tray (see Chapter XXIV on impressions for partial dentures) from which special trays are constructed and the working impressions secured in a hydrocolloid.

The records are taken in the usual manner for partially edentulous cases. An anatomical setting of the teeth is not generally possible since the majority of people exhibit a rather deep overbite. Anatomically articulated dentures can be made when replacements become necessary due to alveolar absorption. The models are articulated and partial dentures set up to replace the missing teeth and these are tried-in in the normal manner, in the waxed-up stage. At this stage the anterior artificial teeth are selected and matched with the natural teeth. If the patient requires the shape, colour and surface characteristics of his teeth to be copied exactly, an additional hydrocolloid impression of the anterior teeth must be taken into which is poured molten wax to a level just above the gingival margins. The wax is thoroughly chilled in cold water and removed from the impression, after which the teeth are separated and reproduced individually in acrylic resin.

If the try-in is satisfactory, the partial dentures are finished and fitted and necessary adjustments made until the patient is comfortable and the operator satisfied. The patient is dismissed for a period of a few weeks to become accustomed to the new dentures after which the immediate additions of the remaining teeth are carried out as follows.

An impression is taken of the remaining natural teeth and the model cast from it is kept as a record of the position and relationship of these teeth. This model is useful for reference when setting up the artificial teeth even if an exact duplication is not desired. Hydrocolloid impressions are taken with the dentures in position. When the impressions are removed from the mouth the dentures usually come away with them but if this is not the case the dentures must be accurately re-positioned in the impressions before casting. The resulting models are mounted on an articulator by means of a wax wafer or squash record.

The Replacement of the Natural Teeth by Artificial Teeth

The Upper Denture

The plaster teeth are cut from the model and replaced by the artificial teeth. This is best achieved by removing and replacing one tooth at a time so that the form of the arch and the position of each individual tooth can more easily be copied if desired. Root sockets are prepared in the plaster model into which the necks of the artificial teeth are fitted so that when the completed denture is inserted in the mouth after the extraction of the natural teeth, the necks of the artificial teeth just enter the natural sockets (see figs. 493(a) and 494).

The advantages of root socketing are:

(1) It allows for the initial alveolar absorption. No unpleasant gap appears between the neck of the tooth and the alveolar ridge since, as absorption takes place, more and more artificial root becomes exposed and the denture maintains the appearance of fitting to the gum.

(2) It provides an anterior seal. It is equivalent to an exaggerated damming and materially assists in the retention of the denture.

(3) It provides resistance to movement. If during mastication there is a tendency for the denture to be moved on the ridges, root socketing will aid in resisting this movement.

(4) It produces a natural appearance of the teeth growing from the gums.

Three important points should be remembered when preparing the sockets in the model:

(1) The direction of the socket should follow the long axis of the tooth.

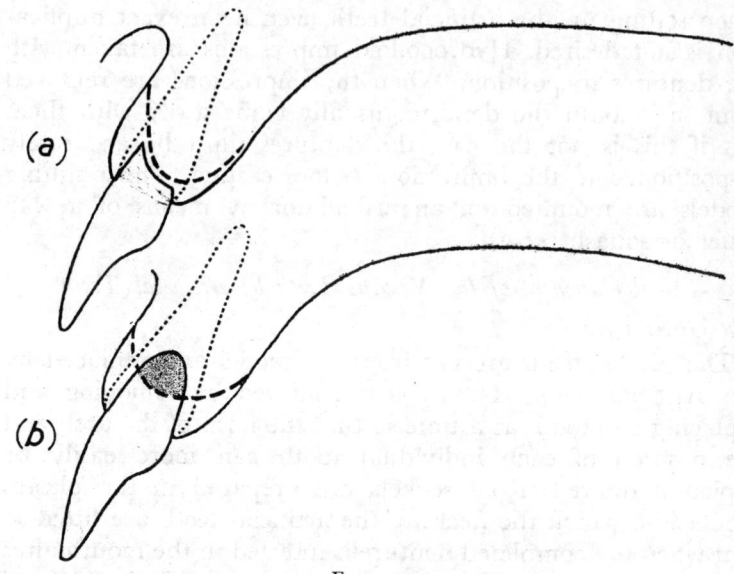

FIG. 493.

(a) Diagram illustrating the correct form of the artificial root of a socketed tooth. This form ensures that no bone destruction occurs and that the artificial tooth will fit the absorbed alveolar ridge reasonably well three months after the extractions.

(b) The type of socketing which leads to bone destruction. Note how the artificial root protrudes above the level of the absorbed alveolar ridge. Compare with fig. 495(a).

(2) Never socket to a greater depth than 5 mm.

(3) Do not carry the socket too far towards the palatal side: the socket should slope from the palatal gingival margin upwards towards the labial aspect.

The reasons for the above statements are:

(1) If the long axis of the root is not followed when preparing the socket in the plaster model the finished artificial root will be out of alignment with the natural socket and the acrylic root will impinge on bone preventing the denture from being seated accurately. Also the pressure exerted on the bone will cause pain and discomfort to the patient.

(2) If the artificial root is carried too far into the natural socket and also allowed to extend too far up its palatal aspect

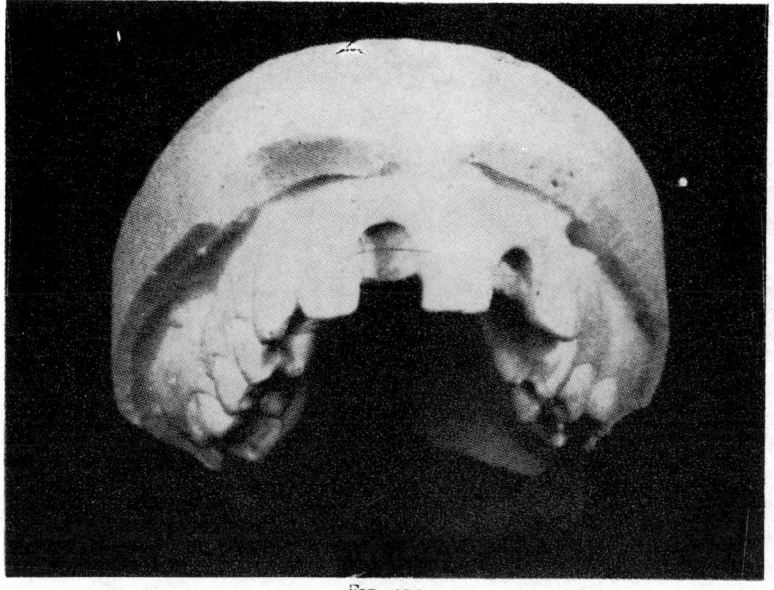

FIG. 494.
(a) 1|2 removed from model and sockets prepared.

the ultimate absorbed ridge will show concavities of varying
extent (*see* figs. 493(*b*) and 495) due to loss of ridge tissue which
might otherwise have been preserved. The reason for this will
become apparent if the following diagrams are studied.
Fig. 496 shows, diagrammatically, a socket directly after the
extraction of a tooth and filled with blood clot. Gradually this
blood clot is replaced by granulation tissue and finally bone.
At the same time absorption of the thin marginal processes
takes place forming the rounded alveolar ridge of the normal
edentulous mouth (*see* fig. 496). It will be seen from the
diagram that in the upper anterior region absorption occurs
in a backwards and slightly upwards direction. When artificial roots are prepared which penetrate too deeply into the
sockets some of the space available for the formation of new
bone is encroached on by the root of the artificial tooth, hence
the development of a depression in the ultimate ridge (*see*
fig. 493(*b*)).

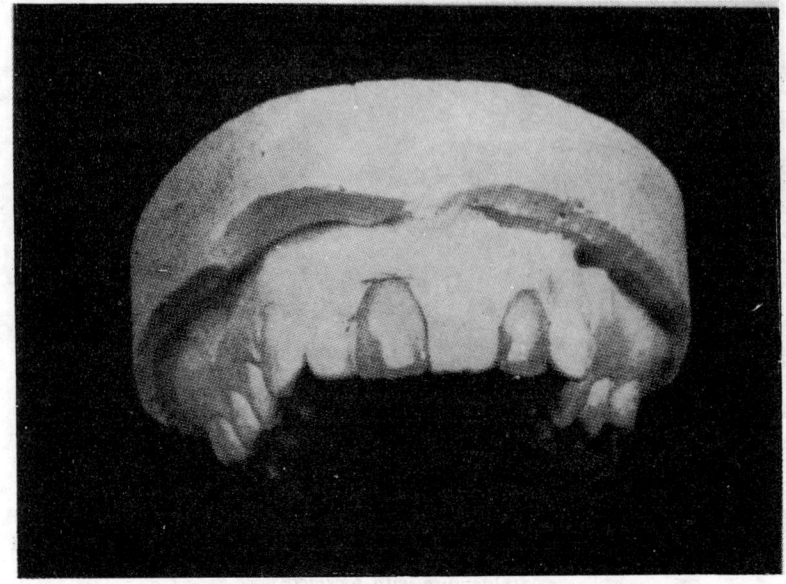

FIG. 494.
(b) Artificial replacements fitted in place, their shape and
position being indicated by the plaster teeth on either
side. The |1̲3̲ are then removed and their artificial
replacements are fitted, their positions being guided
by the artificial 1̲|2̲ and so on.

Careful socketing produces a condition which approximates
to a gum-fit of the teeth when the alveolar absorption has
passed through the initial and fairly rapid stage seen during
the first three months following extraction (*see* fig. 495(*b*)).
In this case there has been no encroachment upon the area of
new bone formation as the artificial root is only resting lightly
against the mucosa covering the ridge.

The Lower Denture

Socketing the anterior teeth is not usually satisfactory in full
lower immediate dentures because the stability of a lower
denture is much less than that of an upper and the movements of the denture during mastication cause pain as the
artificial roots move in the tooth sockets. Greater stability will
be obtained and pain reduced to a minimum if the lower

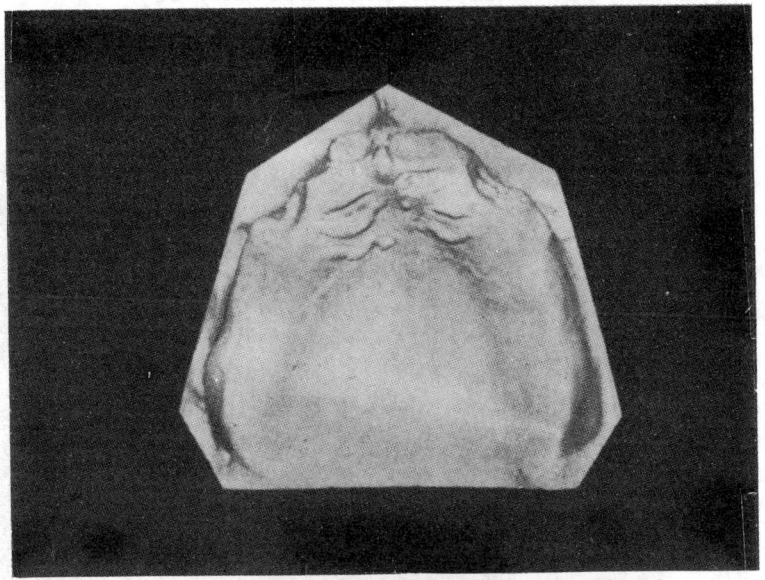

(a) Bone destruction anteriorly resulting from the fitting of an immediate denture with socketed teeth in 321|123, the artificial roots of which were too long and incorrectly shaped (*see* fig. 493(*b*)).

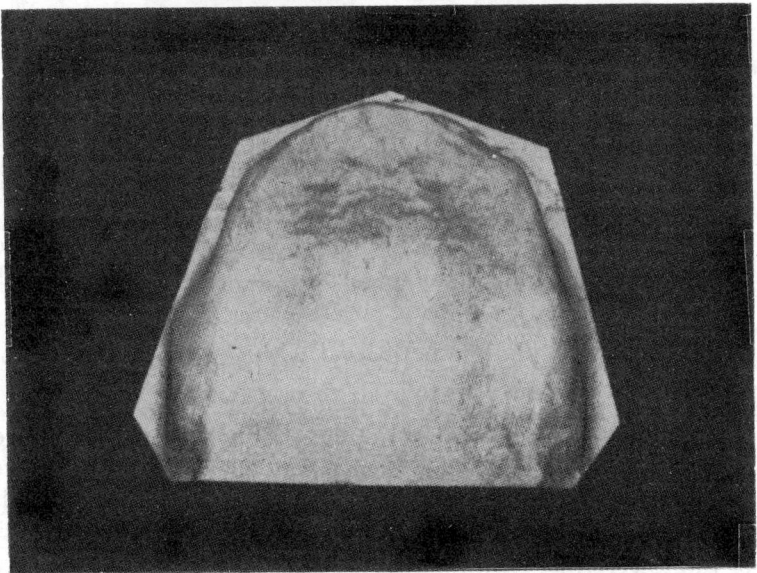

(b) A well-formed ridge resulting from a correctly fitted immediate denture.

FIG. 495. – The effect of socketed teeth on the alveolar ridge after three months.

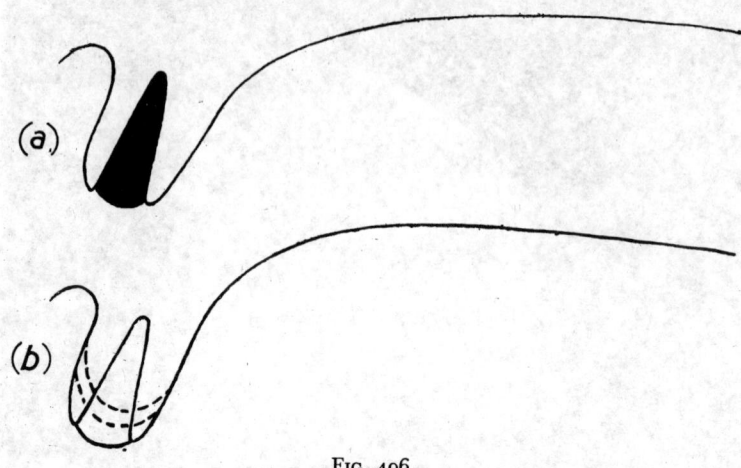

FIG. 496.

(a) Section through a socket immediately after the extraction of an upper central incisor tooth showing socket filled with blood clot.

(b) The dotted lines indicate the direction and give a general idea of the amount of absorption which occurs three months after the extractions.

denture is made with a normal labial flange. In cases, however, where canine or premolar teeth are retained on either side of the mouth to stabilize the denture, the anterior teeth may be socketed with excellent results. When a labial flange is to be fitted, the gingival margins of each tooth are scraped as soon as it is cut off the model. The amount of plaster removed is only sufficient to allow for the collapse of the gingival margins which occurs when the natural teeth are extracted.

The usual method of gingival trimming is as follows (*see* fig. 497):

(1) Cut off the plaster tooth level with the gingival margin.

(2) Hollow out the root to a depth of 2 mm.

(3) Trim and round off the gingival margins to the above level.

The depth to which the upper anterior teeth are carried into the sockets and the amount of plaster trimmed from the model of the lower ridge will depend on the amount of bone lost by

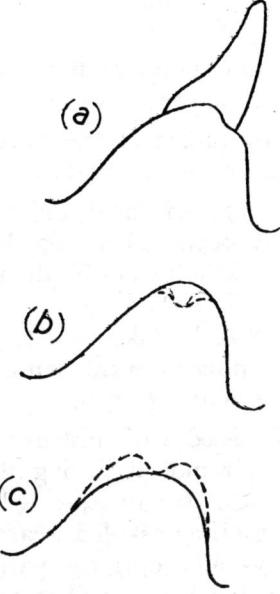

FIG. 497. – Method of cutting the teeth from the model and forming a rounded alveolar ridge. Illustrated in section.

(a) Tooth in position.

(b) Tooth removed and socket hollowed to a depth of 2 mm.

(c) Model rounded to this depth.

periodontal disease prior to the extraction of the teeth. The greater the bone loss the deeper the socketing required and the greater the amount of plaster to be removed from the lower ridge because when the teeth are extracted the greater will be the collapse of the unsupported gingival tissues. X-ray photographs are useful in determining the amount of bone lost.

The Insertion of the Dentures

The artificial anterior teeth are attached with acrylic resin to the original partial dentures, and the completed dentures inserted immediately after the natural teeth are extracted. Some slight adjustments may be necessary, the most usual being:

(1) Slight trimming of the acrylic 'roots' if these impinge on the bone of the sockets.

(2) Removal of the interdental septum if a rocking movement is elicited when fitting the lower denture.

(3) Easing the labial flange of the lower denture if it has been carried too far into an undercut area.

If the extractions are performed under a local anaesthetic, a slight rocking may occur when the dentures are inserted due to the distension of the tissues by the injected anaesthetic: the denture will settle into place after a few hours as the fluid is absorbed. Care should be taken not to confuse this type of rocking with that resulting from the denture impinging on the socket margin or interdental septum.

The patient is dismissed with instructions that a socketed denture must not be removed during the first twenty-four hours since reinsertion of the denture will probably be very painful; particularly by the unskilled wearer of a first denture. At the end of twenty-four hours the patient should be seen again by the dental surgeon who will remove the denture and clean both it and the patient's mouth before reinserting it. Adjustments at this stage are rarely necessary and the patient is given such instructions regarding cleaning and care of dentures as are necessary but in particular he should be told that:

(1) A socketed denture should not be left out of the mouth day or night, for more than a few minutes at a time, during the first few weeks, otherwise the sockets will tend to contract and reinsertion may be difficult and probably painful.

(2) The dentures should be removed and cleaned and the mouth rinsed out after every meal, if possible.

The dentures may require re-lining after three to six months and new dentures, with a balanced occlusion, should usually be constructed after nine to twelve months.

It is often preferable, from the patient's point of view, to carry out the fitting of the immediate dentures in two stages, first the upper denture, followed a week or two later by the lower. The reason for this is that the minimum amount of surgery is performed at each visit, with the result that the minimum amount of post-operative discomfort should be experienced; also the transition from comparatively stable partial dentures to the more unstable full denture condition is brought about in progressive stages.

It is of course possible to proceed directly from the try-in stage to the finished dentures and insert them both together. To do so, however, demands a much greater degree of adaptation on the part of the patient than the technique which has been described.

IMMEDIATE DENTURES FOLLOWING ALVEOLECTOMY

The technique which has just been described will require some modification before it can be used in cases where part of the alveolar ridge requires to be removed. An alveolectomy may be required for one of the following reasons:

(1) A prominent premaxilla.

(2) In order to provide better retention and stability of the dentures.

(3) A very close bite anteriorly.

(4) The preference of the operator.

(1) *A Prominent Premaxilla* (*see* figs. 498–501):

Patients are occasionally seen who have a very prominent upper jaw with the teeth tilted outwards, often spaced and usually resting on the external surface of the lower lip when the mandible is in its rest position. If such a patient requests an immediate denture and, at the same time, wishes for an improvement in appearance, a satisfactory result cannot usually be obtained by the technique previously described, because although some correction of the angulation of the teeth may be achieved (*see* fig. 502) their position is governed by the sockets receiving the artificial roots. Unfortunately this protrusion of the upper teeth is not confined to the incisors but also involves the canines and even if the teeth are brought back to a more acceptable arch the prominent premaxilla and

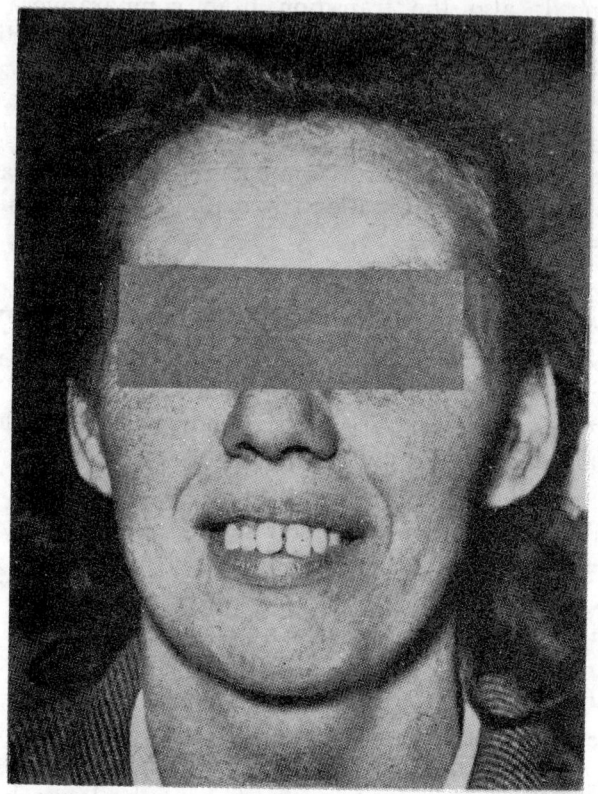

FIG. 498. – A case of superior protrusion. Full face.

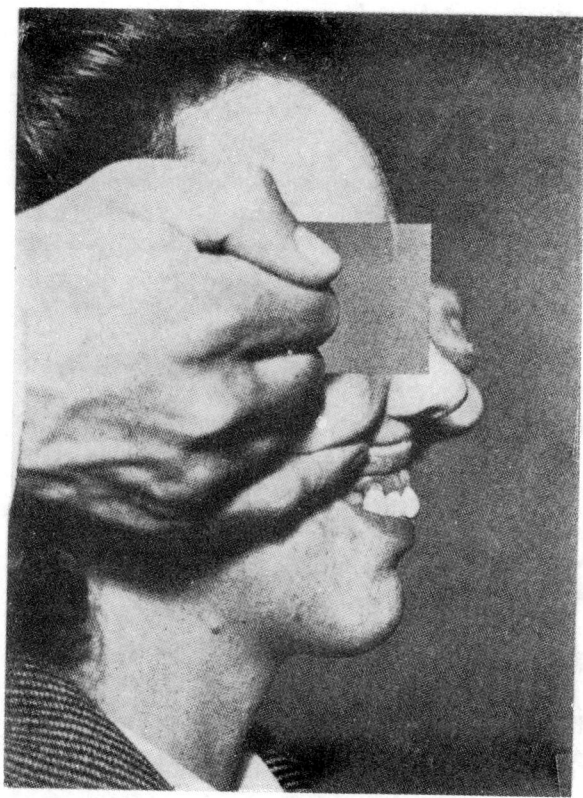

FIG. 499. – A case of superior protrusion. In profile. Note the relation of the upper front teeth to the lower lip.

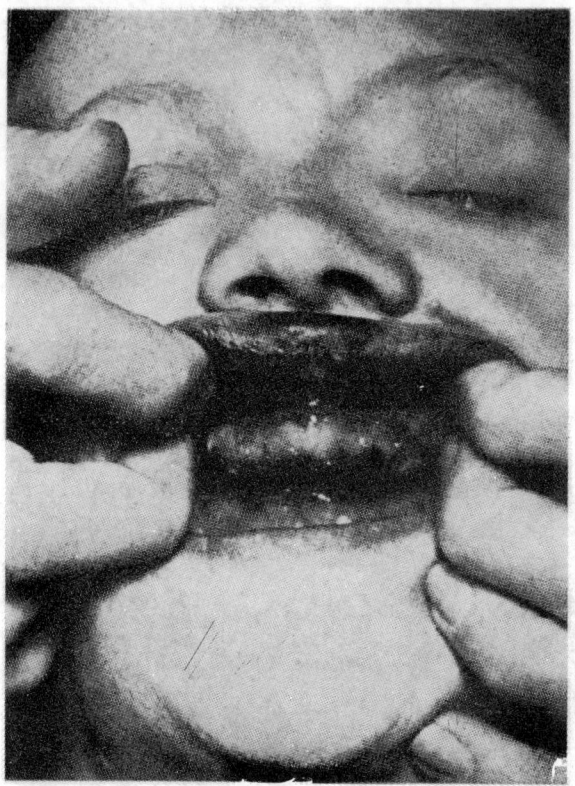

FIG. 500 – A case of superior protrusion. Twenty-four hours after the alveolectomy. The upper denture has been removed to show the alveolar ridge.

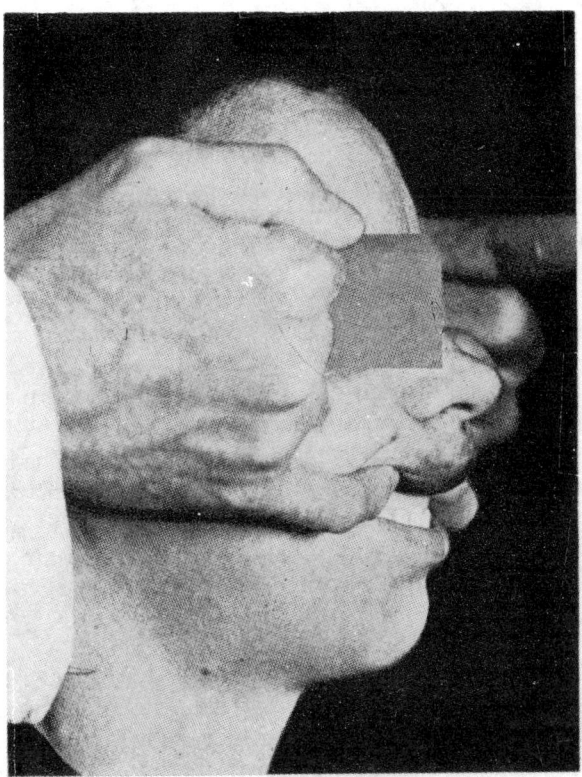

FIG. 501. – A case of superior protrusion. Twenty-four hours after the alveolectomy. Note how the upper front teeth now pass behind the lower lip (compare with fig. 499).

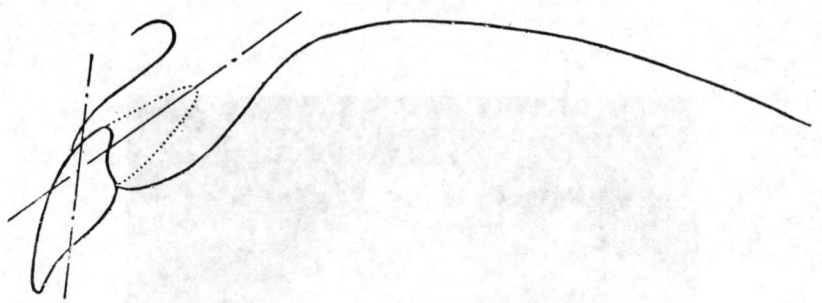

FIG. 502. – Illustrating the method of angulating the artificial root to the crown of the tooth in order to correct, without performing an alveolectomy, the appearance of superior protrusion.

canine eminences still continue to hold the upper lip forward presenting an unpleasant appearance. Such cases call for an alveolectomy at the time of extraction in order to reduce the alveolar process and allow the lip to fall back when the teeth have been set farther palatally. The extractions and alveolectomy can be followed by the insertion of an immediate denture as will be described in due course.

(2) *To Provide Better Retention and Stability:*

In cases where the factors of retention are adverse, such as the V-shaped palate, poor posterior ridge formation, shallow sulci and a narrow upper jaw with a wide lower jaw, it is often advisable to produce an upper immediate denture having a labial flange. This flange increases the peripheral seal and resists lateral and antero-posterior movement of the denture. When a labial flange is added in such cases, it is usual to perform a slight alveolectomy at the time of the extractions in order to form a smooth and rounded denture-bearing surface. Unless this is done there will often be insufficient room for the flange without obviously distorting the lip; also pressure of the flange on the sharp edges of the sockets and the interdental bone will cause considerable discomfort to the patient.

(3) *A Very Close Bite Anteriorly:*

Some patients exhibit a very deep overbite; the incisal

edges of the upper teeth touching the gingival margins of the lowers and the lower teeth occluding with the soft tissues of the palate. Upper and lower alveolectomies are needed in these cases if sufficient interalveolar space is to be obtained to produce satisfactory dentures, although some help may be obtained by slightly increasing the vertical height providing it is within the range of the freeway space. Close bites are not always quite so extreme and often sufficient space can be gained by removing bone from one jaw only.

(4) *The Preference of the Operator:*

It is not intended to enter into the controversy regarding the superiority of the socketed over the flanged type of immediate denture or vice versa; it is sufficient to note that some operators have very strong views on the subject whilst the Authors consider that each technique has its place.

In cases where only a slight alveolectomy is contemplated partial dentures may be constructed and worn by the patient as has already been described. In cases involving an extensive alveolectomy it is preferable to continue the immediate replacements from the try-in stage of the partial dentures since the reduction of the arch anteriorly may require the posterior teeth to be moved farther back and this can easily be done whilst the teeth are still mounted in wax. The trial partial dentures are used in the normal way to check the accuracy of the occlusal registration.

Model Trimming

The incisors and canine teeth on one side are cut from the model and the plaster representing the alveolar ridge is trimmed to the desired shape. This trimming will be from either the labial surface or from the alveolar crest, or both, depending on whether more labial space is required, as in a case with a prominent premaxilla or one presenting severely undercut areas, or whether more interalveolar space is needed, as in close-bite cases. Having completed the trimming of one side of the model the opposite side is treated in the same way and any final adjustments made until the anterior plaster ridge is shaped to correspond as nearly as possible to the condition which will be obtained after the extraction of the teeth and the associated alveolectomy.

A duplicate is now made of this trimmed model and on it a thin template (one thickness of wax) is produced in clear acrylic. This template is for the assistance of the surgeon and should cover as much of the denture-bearing surface as possible, for greater accuracy. The artificial teeth are mounted on the original trimmed model with such variations of the original positions of the natural teeth as may be desired. The set-up is completed with a normal labial gum flange and the denture processed and finished ready for insertion in the mouth.

The surgical operation consists of extracting the teeth and trimming the alveolar ridge to the same extent as the plaster model. In order to ensure this similarity of shape the clear acrylic template is tried in the mouth from time to time during the operation, bone being trimmed away as necessary till it fits snugly without any rocking. In theory it is possible to see through the acrylic template areas where the gum is blanched indicating pressure on high spots: in fact this is often impossible owing to the presence of blood and the surgeon is dependent on his sense of touch.

There are two points which merit emphasis as they are essential to the success of this operation.

(1) Do not encroach on the area covered by the periphery of the denture. This region should not have been touched on the plaster model and accuracy of fit round the periphery is needed for retention.

(2) Remove sufficient bone. If the denture presses on any high spots of trimmed bone it will be too painful to be tolerated and the denture will have to be left out until some absorption has taken place, or a new denture will have to be made. In either case the advantages of an immediate denture are lost. The removal of slightly too much bone, in the upper, is immaterial since the palate and periphery are intact and in any case the exactness of fit over the site of the operation is rapidly lost owing to alveolar absorption.

This technique applies to both the upper and lower immediate dentures and the patient should be instructed to wear them night and day during the first week, only removing them for cleansing after meals. If the dentures are left out of the mouth for long periods during this first week some difficulty may be experienced in replacing them owing to slight swelling of the oral tissues. In time the dentures will become loose and will require re-lining or replacing; this can only be judged by clinical observation but if the peripheries have not been interfered with it is unlikely to occur in under six months.

IMMEDIATE DENTURES WITHOUT PRIOR EXTRACTION OF THE POSTERIOR TEETH

In some cases it is necessary to fit immediate dentures without the prior extraction of the posterior teeth, e.g. when the anterior teeth are causing pain or are excessively loose, or if the patient wishes to shorten the number of visits for extractions. This method is not suitable for general practice and should only be employed if the patient can be treated in a hospital or nursing home.

The technique is briefly as follows:

(1) Impressions are taken in hydrocolloid of both jaws, care being taken to secure a good reproduction of the sulci. Such impressions are best taken in box trays whose peripheries have been built up with composition and functionally adapted.

(2) The models cast from these impressions are mounted on an articulator by means of a wax wafer or squash record.

(3) Duplicates of these models are made for reference when setting the teeth.

(4) The teeth are removed from the model and the ridge trimmed as described for immediate dentures with alveolectomy; duplicates of these models are made and on them clear acrylic templates prepared.

(5) The artificial teeth are set up and the dentures cured and completed with normal flanges.

(6) The patient is admitted to hospital, the teeth removed and the ridges trimmed with the aid of the templates, and the dentures inserted.

This technique gives remarkably successful results, its main drawback being that the rapid absorption renders the dentures an ill fit after a few weeks, and two re-linings are usually necessary within the first three months.

PARTIAL IMMEDIATE DENTURES

The socketing technique can be applied to any of the sixteen anterior teeth which are being replaced by a partial denture, and due to the stability of the partial denture, which has natural teeth to support it, the results are very satisfactory.

COPYING THE APPEARANCE OF IMMEDIATE DENTURES WHEN FITTING THE REPLACEMENT DENTURES

It is quite easy to copy irregularities of an individual's anterior teeth when fitting an immediate denture because the artificial teeth can be placed in exactly the same positions and given the same angulation as the natural teeth.

When the time comes to construct another set of dentures to replace the immediate ones, however, it is sometimes extremely difficult to copy the position and set of the teeth and many a patient who has been delighted with the appearance of the immediate dentures is very disappointed with the final set.

A simple way to ensure an exact copy of the positions of the anterior socketed teeth of an immediate upper denture is to insert the denture and then mould a piece of composition over the labial surfaces of the ridge and the six anterior teeth. The composition is chilled *in situ* and then removed and excess composition trimmed away. It is then slightly softened and replaced in the mouth and given a final moulding followed by a second chilling. This piece of composition will fit the labial surface of the upper model and the artificial anterior teeth of the replacement denture can be placed in the impressions left by the teeth of the immediate denture and then waxed to the base plate (*see* fig. 503). When all the teeth are in position the composition is removed and the labial flange waxed up.

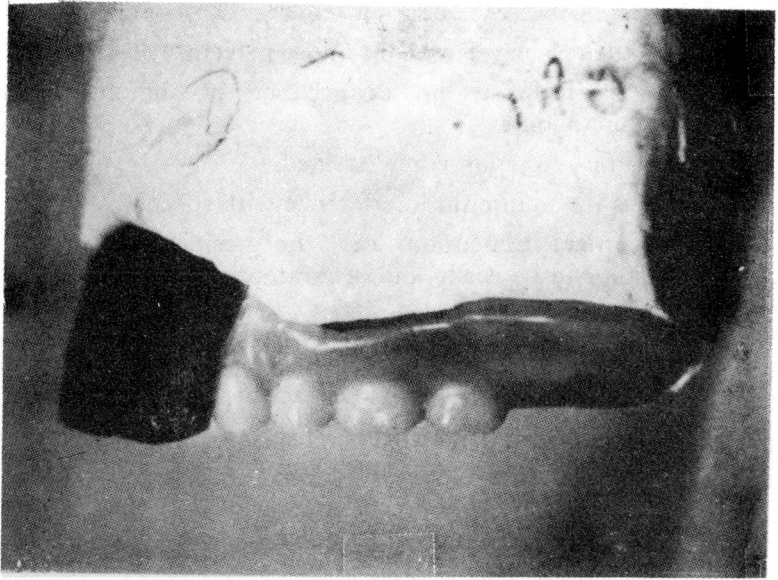

(a) Composition impression in place on model.

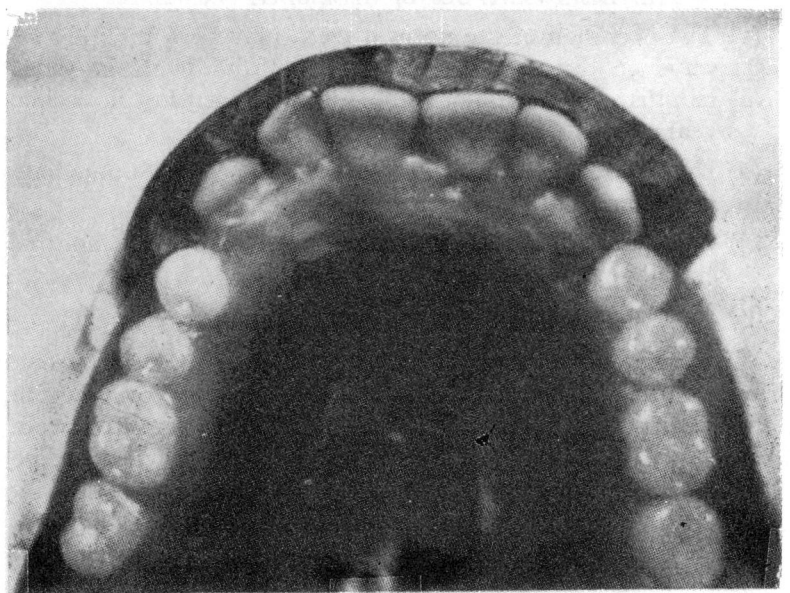

(b) Anterior teeth of replacement denture fitted into impression of the teeth of the immediate denture.

FIG. 503.

The Advantages of Immediate Dentures

(1) The patient is never without anterior teeth.

(2) There is little or no disturbance of the temporo-mandibular joint.

(3) Masticatory function is maintained.

(4) There is the minimum interference with speech.

(5) The vertical dimension and the position of centric occlusion can be easily and accurately reproduced.

(6) The facial contour is maintained.

(7) Changes in the shape of the tongue are prevented.

(8) No unnatural habits of mastication and speech will have been formed.

(9) The position, shape, size and colour of the natural teeth can be reproduced with accuracy.

10) The sockets are protected during the healing period.

The Disadvantages of Immediate Dentures

(1) The occlusion of the natural teeth may be a bite of convenience due to the movement of the teeth in those mouths where some of the teeth have been lost in earlier years.

(2) Naturally deep overbites if reproduced in immediate dentures would produce prosthetic malocclusion.

(3) The patient's general health may not permit multiple extractions.

(4) Additional expense for the patient.

The first two disadvantages mentioned are not direct contra-indications for immediate dentures which could quite satisfactorily be constructed if the necessary alterations were made to the occlusion. They are valid contra-indications to the exact reproduction of the positions of the natural teeth.

Chapter XXVII

OVERLAY OR ONLAY DENTURES

An overlay or onlay denture is one which is designed to alter the shape and height of the occlusal surfaces of the teeth over which it fits.

Overlay dentures may form part of a conventional partial denture, or be fitted in a mouth in which no teeth are missing. They may be constructed of acrylic resin, gold or chrome cobalt (*see* fig. 504(*a*),(*b*),(*c*)).

Conditions Requiring an Overlay Denture

Overlay dentures are fitted to correct faults of occlusion and articulation, and four broad classes of such faults may be identified.

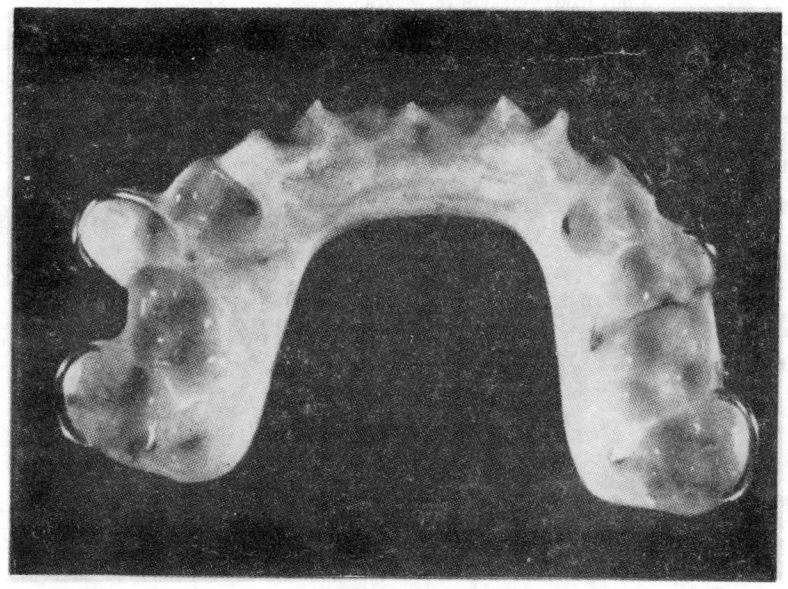

Fig. 504.
(*a*) Acrylic overlay from fitting surface.

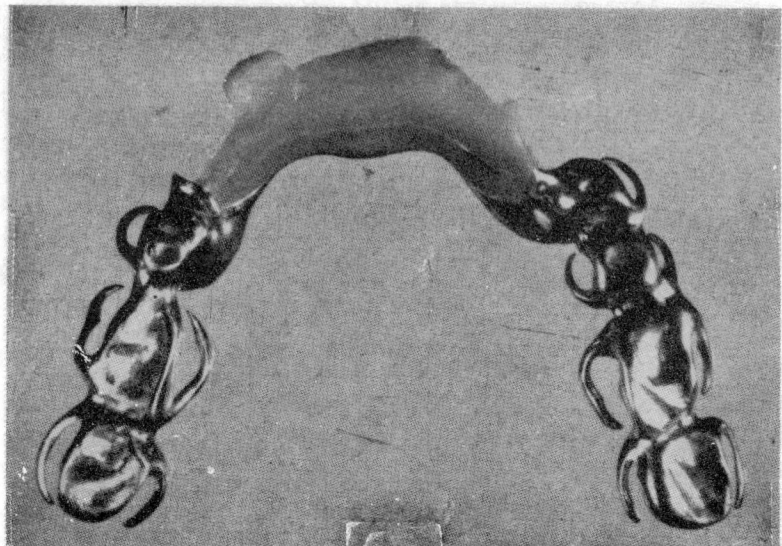

(*b*) Chrome cobalt overlay from occlusal surface; acrylic platform in anterior region is to occlude with lower front teeth and reduce weight.

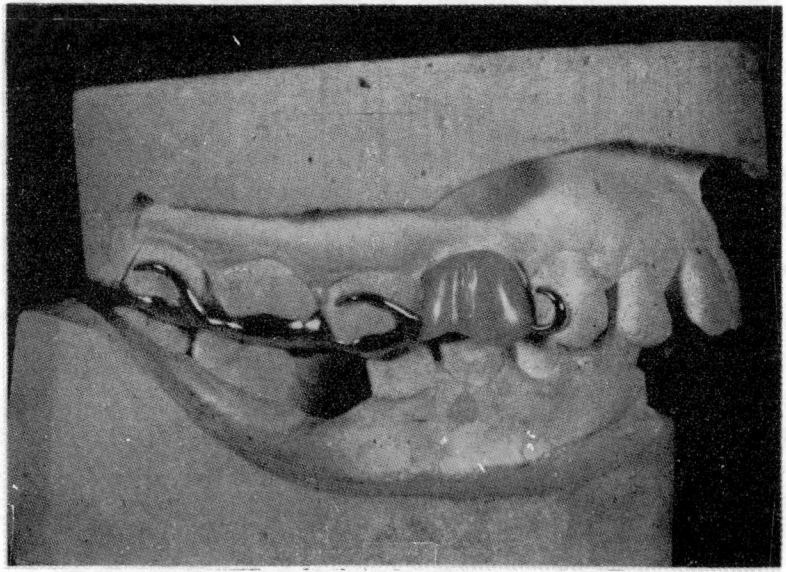

(*c*) Overlay from the side. Note large number of clasps to ensure adequate retention.

FIG. 504.

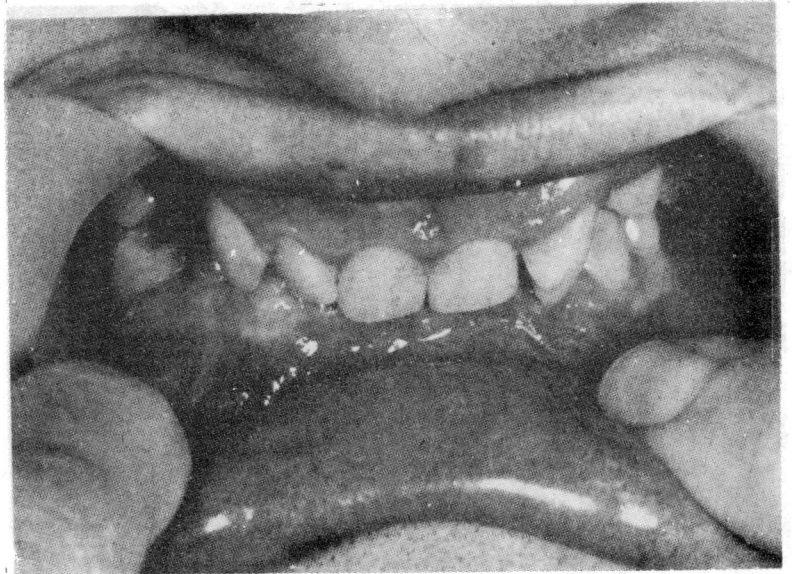

FIG. 505. – A case of abnormal occlusion resulting in trauma
to gingival margins:
(*a*) From the front.
(*b*) From lingual side.
(*c*) From the side.

(*a*) Those causing damage to the tissues. Fig. 505 illustrates
a case in which the occlusion is such that the upper incisors are
biting into the labial gingivae of the lower incisors, and the
lower incisors are traumatizing the palatal mucosa. Fig. 506
illustrates how the fitting of an overlay on the occlusal surfaces
of the upper teeth lifts the incisive edges of these teeth from the
tissues and prevents the damage continuing.

(*b*) Those cases in which the occlusion is such that the lower
teeth occlude palatally to the uppers (*see* fig. 507). Such a
condition makes it difficult or impossible for the individual to
chew. The fitment of an overlay to the upper teeth shaped in
such a manner that it occludes with the lower teeth enables the
individual to masticate.

(*c*) Those cases in which the occlusion is locked in the
position of centric occlusion and attempts to make lateral
chewing movements cause excessive loads to be imposed on the

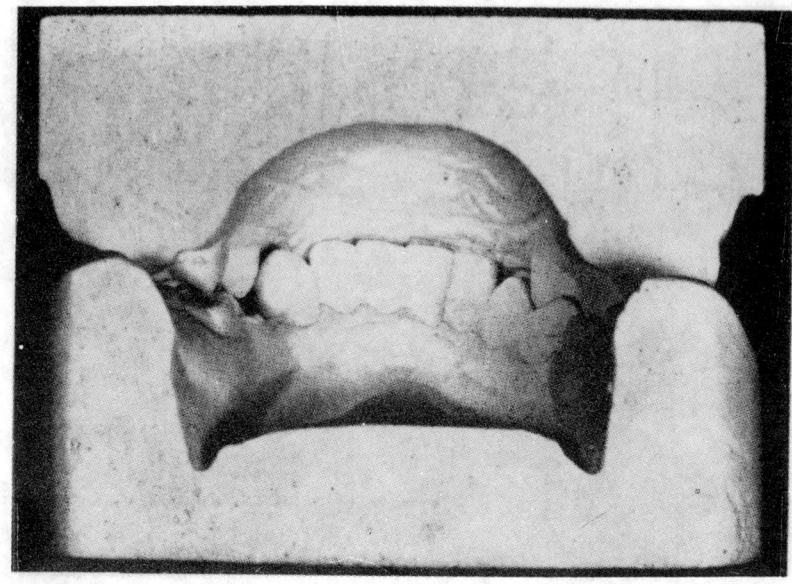

FIG. 505(b).

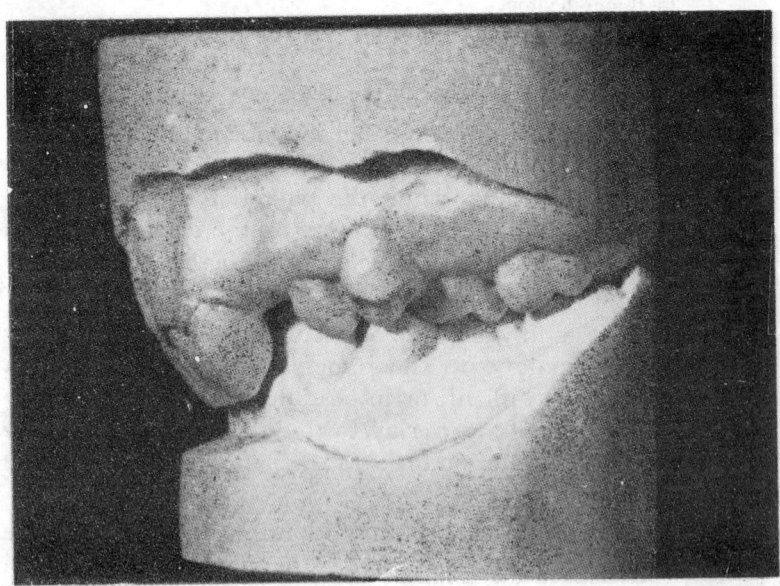

FIG. 505(c).

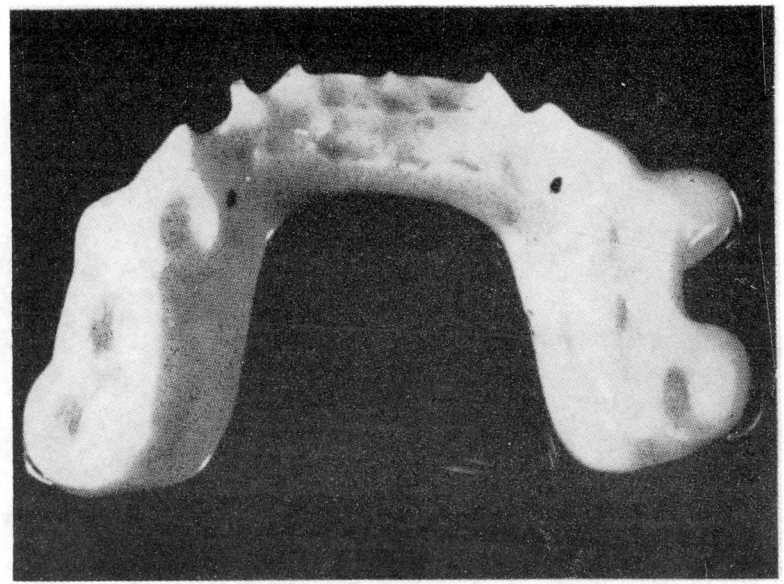

(a)

Fig. 506. – Treatment of case shown in fig. 505 by fitting
overlay.
(a) Note holes worn in it by use.
(b) Fitting over upper teeth.
(c) Compare with 505(a) to see how 21|12 have been raised
from lower gingivae.

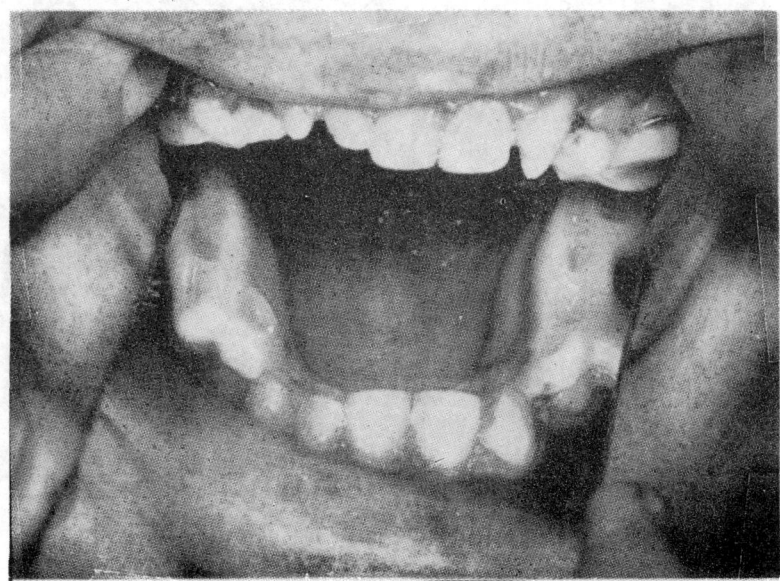

Fig. 506(b).

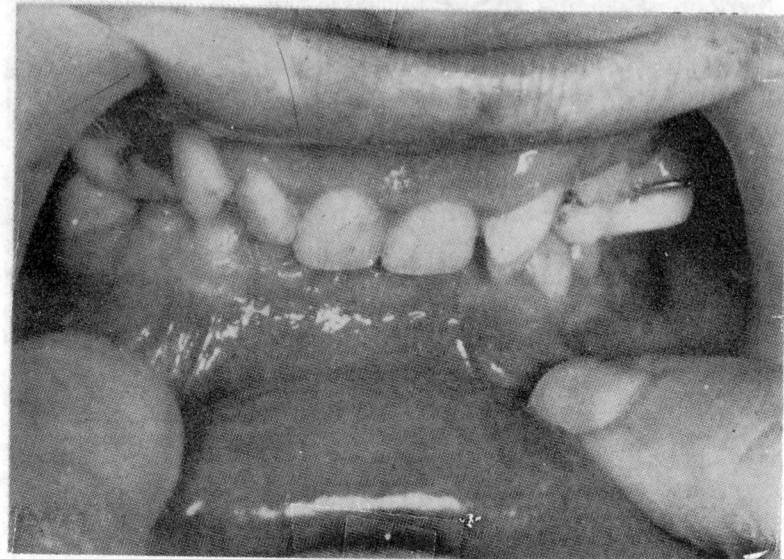

FIG. 506(c).

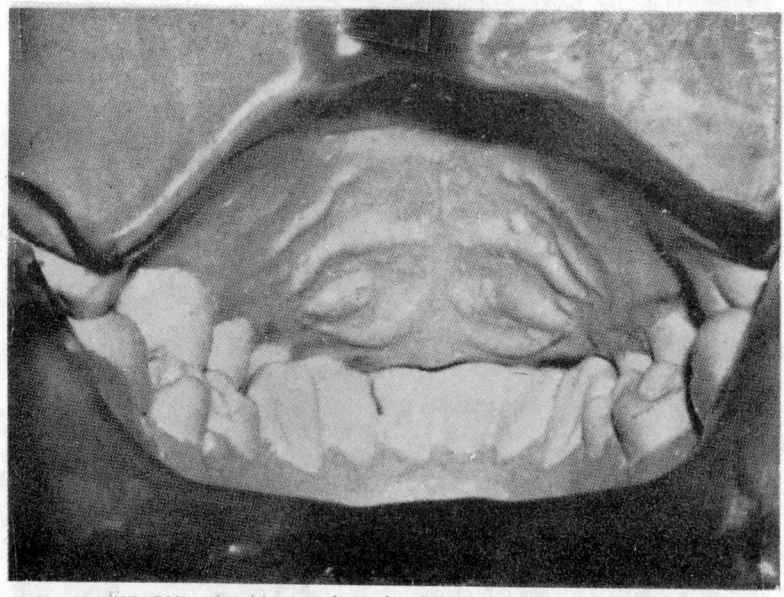

FIG. 507. — Looking at the palatal aspect of a case in which the lower posterior teeth occlude palatally to the uppers.

periodontal membranes of the teeth with consequent damage to these tissues. A traumatic occlusion of this type can frequently be corrected by fitting an overlay to the upper teeth thus providing a change in the cuspal relationships which allows lateral movements to be made (*see* fig. 508).

(*d*) Those cases in which pain or derangement of function of the temporo-mandibular joint results, or is considered to result, from faults of occlusion. This subject of occlusal disharmony and temporo-mandibular arthrosis has become prominent in recent years, and as it is far too extensive to be dealt with in a text on clinical dental prosthetics, the salient points only of the rationale of treatment of this condition by overlays is summarized below. For more extensive information on this subject the student is referred to the appropriate texts.

The present day conception of the articulation of the mandible with the skull is that it is a triple and not a double

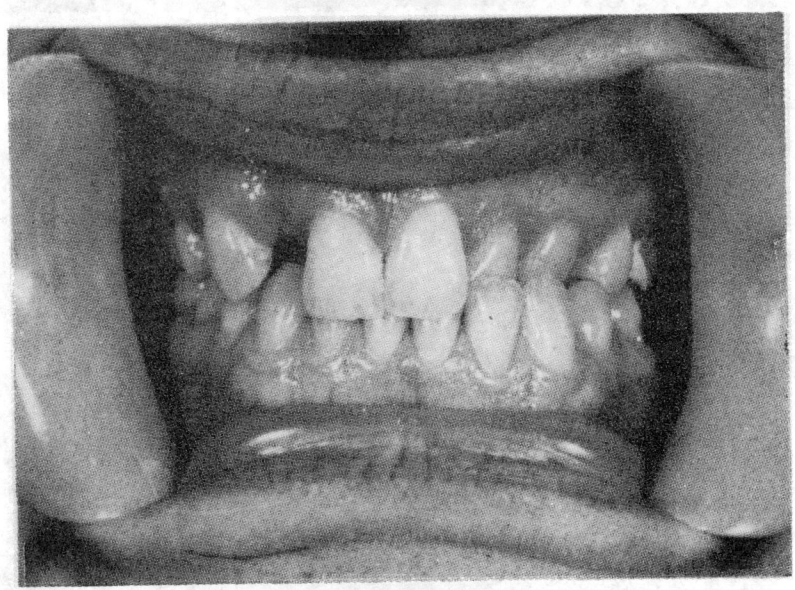

FIG. 508.
(*a*) A locked occlusion.
(*b*) The overlay in place.
(*c*) The occlusion is now freely sliding.

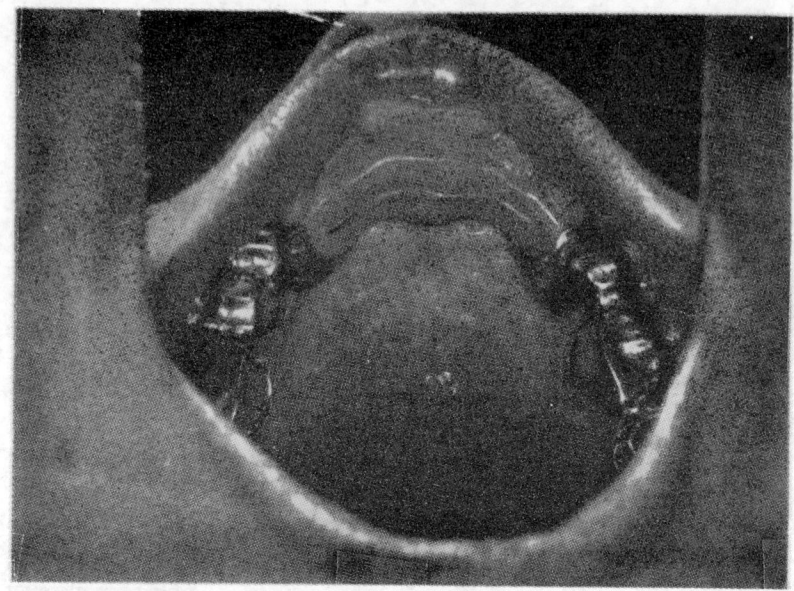

FIG. 508(b).

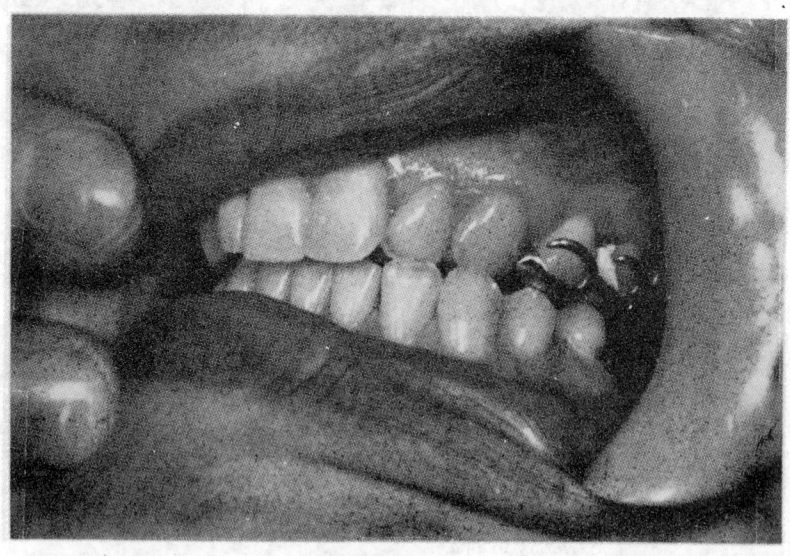

FIG. 508(c).

articulation. The mandible articulates with the skull through the two temporo-mandibular joints and also through the occlusal surfaces of all the teeth. For efficient and comfortable function therefore these three articulations must be in harmony. In addition the muscles controlling the mandible develop a pattern of movement which also harmonizes with the movement of these three surfaces. If one of these articulations fails to fit in functionally with the others then a condition of stress will develop which may produce symptoms of dysfunction and pain. So far as the treatment of these conditions is related to overlays, we are concerned here only with the disharmony of the occlusion and articulation of the teeth in relation to the other articulations. The position of the mandible when the teeth are in contact is determined by the interdigitation of the cusps which act as inclined planes and which under the influence of the powerful muscles of mastication seat the mandible in a definite relationship to the skull on each closure.

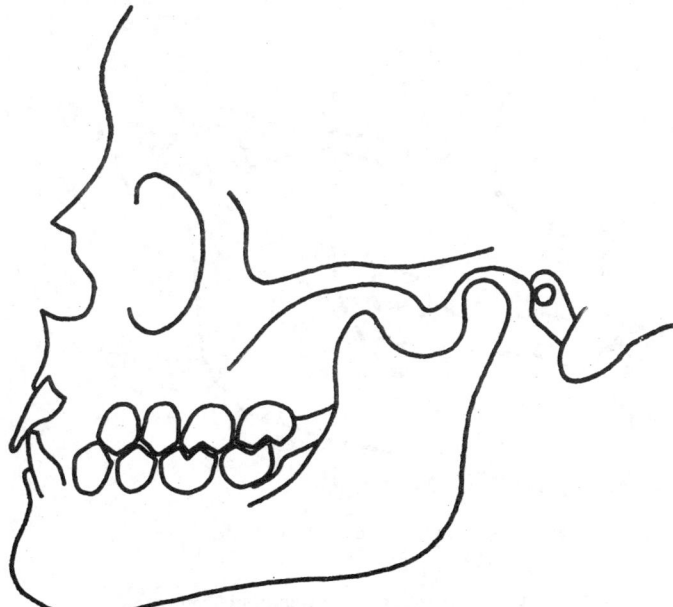

FIG. 509(a). – Anterior teeth and cheek teeth in occlusion; note relationship of condyle to glenoid fossa.

If this position of the mandible is seriously out of harmony with the normal positions which the temporo-mandibular joints and muscles assume, then the joints and muscles will be forced to take up strained positions, and dysfunction of either or both may supervene.

The commonest example of this condition occurs when one or both condyles are forced to retrude further into the glenoid fossae than the normal laxity of the joint structures will allow. Such a condition may develop as a result of the loss of the support of the posterior teeth as illustrated (fig. 509). In figure 509(a) the relationship of the articulating surfaces is illustrated before any teeth were lost. The premolars and first molars are then extracted and as a result of the extra stress induced in them and their lack of support, the last molar teeth tilt. This results in the lower incisors sliding upwards and backwards

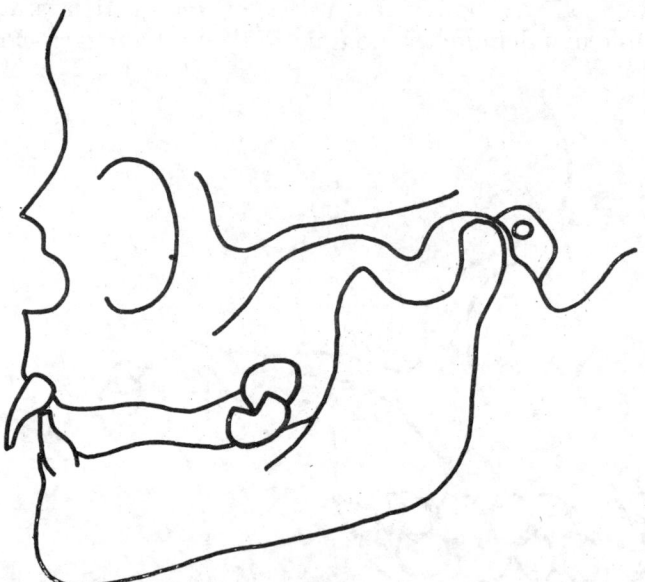

FIG. 509(b). – |456 have been extracted and |7 have tilted.
|456 |7
The palatal surfaces of the upper front teeth have acted as
an inclined plane up which the lower front teeth are drawn
as the teeth occlude, forcing the mandible backwards.
Note the relationship of the condyle to the glenoid fossa and
compare with (a).

along the inclined palatal surfaces of the upper incisors each time the teeth are occluded. This means that part of the power of the muscles of mastication is directed to driving the mandible, and consequently the condyles, upwards and backwards, and therefore on closure the mandible assumes a more retruded position than the temporo-mandibular joints can accommodate. In a majority of cases this condition never develops because the attachments of the upper and lower incisors alter under the extra load applied to them, allowing the upper incisors to tilt forwards and the lowers lingually. If the pressure of the muscles of the lips and tongue is great or the attachments of these teeth is extremely firm however such tilting may not occur, and it is in these cases that symptoms of temporo-mandibular joint derangement or muscular strain may develop. The insertion of a partial denture with an overlay in such cases is aimed at restoring the occlusal relationship of the mandible with the maxilla to the original position, and allowing the condyles to assume their normal relationship to the glenoid fossae.

A similar condition of disharmony can develop without the prior extraction of teeth as illustrated in fig. 510. In fig. 510(a) is illustrated the relationship of the condyles to the glenoid fossae when the mandible is in the relaxed position. From this position to closure of teeth in the position of centric occlusion, a pure hinge movement of the condyles takes place, and when this happens in the type of case illustrated the teeth do not interdigitate (see fig. 510(b)). When the power of the muscles is increased the inclined planes of the teeth act as wedges, and the lower cusps slide up the upper cusps forcing the mandible to assume a retruded position, and driving the heads of the condyles backwards in the glenoid fossae.

As described in the previous example, the teeth usually adjust their positions, by moving, to fit into the joint and muscle position of the mandible, but in some instances the power of the muscles surrounding the teeth is so great or their attachment to the jaw so rigid that no adjustment is made. It is in these cases that the reshaping of the occlusal surfaces by means of an overlay to fit into the temporo-mandibular joint and muscle position of

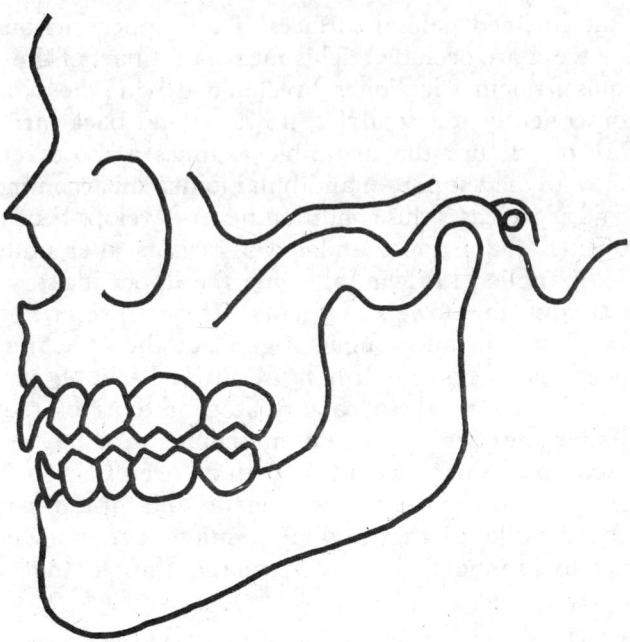

FIG. 510.

(a) A case with an abnormal occlusion with the mandible
  in the relaxed position. Note the relationship of the
  head of the condyle to the glenoid fossa is normal.

(b) An enlarged view of the relationship of the teeth on initial
  contact. As the muscles apply power the lower teeth and
  the mandible will be drawn in the direction of the arrows
  guided by the incline of the cusps and the head of the
  condyle will take up the relationship to the glenoid
  fossa shown in (c) when the teeth are fully interdigitated.

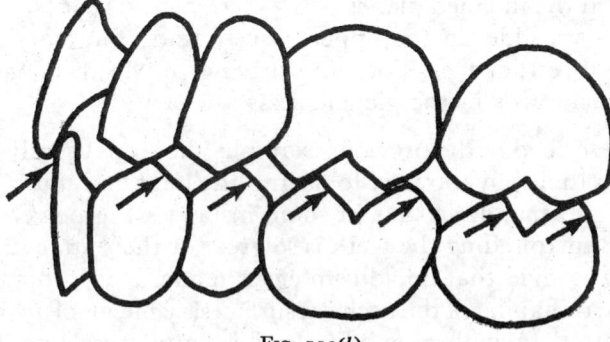

FIG. 510(b).

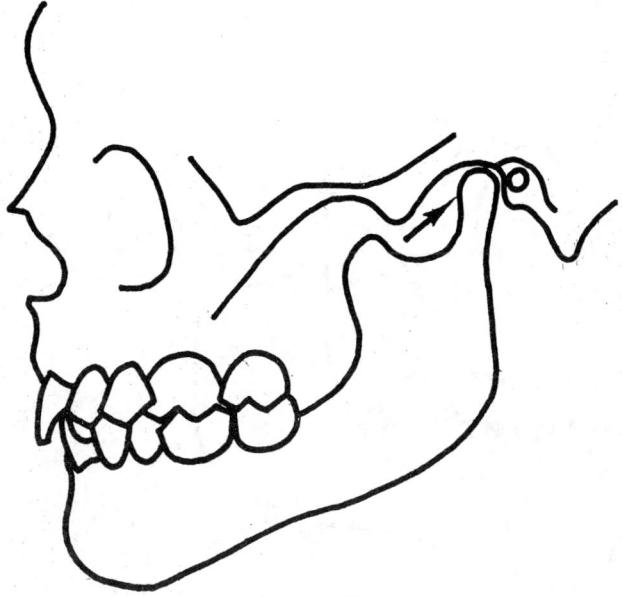

FIG. 510(*c*).

the mandible is of value. Fig. 511 shows how this is effected. Although the above explanation sounds simple and convincing, it leaves a lot unexplained in relation to cases presenting temporo-mandibular joint and muscle symptoms, many of which appear to have no simple explanation. Sush symptoms are becoming increasingly common among young people in the age group of 17 to 25 years, especially females. Many of these cases would appear to be the result of general tension which has centred itself in the masticatory muscles, especially the masseters, and overlay dentures should never be prescribed for cases of temporo-mandibular joint arthrosis unless definite evidence of occlusal disharmony can be demonstrated. The method of assessing the presence of occlusal disharmony is by means of an occlusal analysis. This is carried out in identically the same manner as a check record for full dentures (*see* Chapter XIII) with the difference that models of the patient's natural dentition are used instead of the artificial dentures.

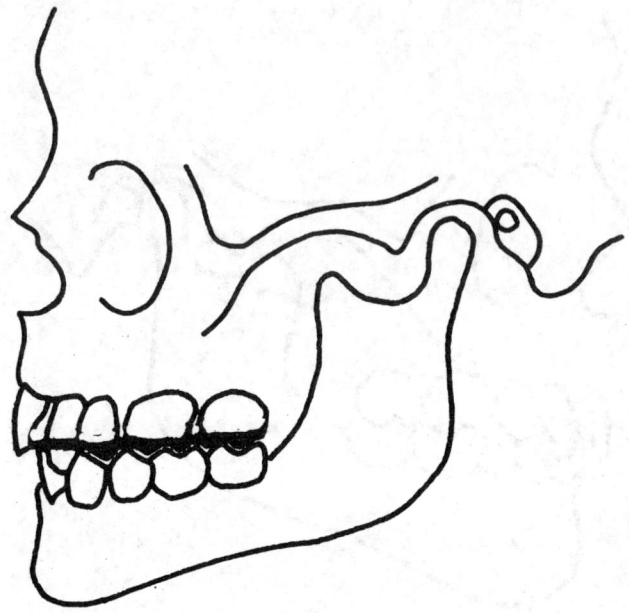

Fig. 511. – An overlay will counteract the backward displacement of the mandible illustrated in fig. 510 by shaping the occlusal surfaces of the upper teeth so that they articulate with the lowers when the mandible and the head of the condyle are in their correct positions.

The Occlusal Analysis

A face-bow reading is taken to enable the upper model to be mounted on the articulator in the correct relationship to the glenoid fossæ. A check record of soft wax is taken with the patient completely relaxed and the teeth closed into but not through the soft wax template. The rationale behind this is that when the mandible is closed from the position in which it is held by the relaxed muscles into the wax, the mandible is following the path which the muscles and the temporo-mandibular joints wish it to take. As it is not closed completely through the wax the cusps of the opposing teeth do not come into contact, and therefore no cusp guidance occurs to divert the mandible from the muscle and joint path of closure. If now, using this wax template, the lower model is articulated to the upper model which has already been mounted by means of the faces bow, and the wax template removed, the models can be closed through the two or three millimetres which separate the occlusal surfaces of the teeth with fair assurance that they are following the same path that the patient's mandible would follow as guided by the joints and muscles. This is because the last few millimetres of closure of the mandible is a hinge movement with the condyles acting as the centres of rotation. When the teeth are occluded on the articulator, it can be observed whether or not they interdigitate correctly, or meet in such a manner that a major shift of the mandible is necessary to effect interdigitation. An occlusal analysis of this type is shown in fig. 512.

In a case such as this an overlay would be constructed to reshape the occlusal surfaces in harmony with the joint and

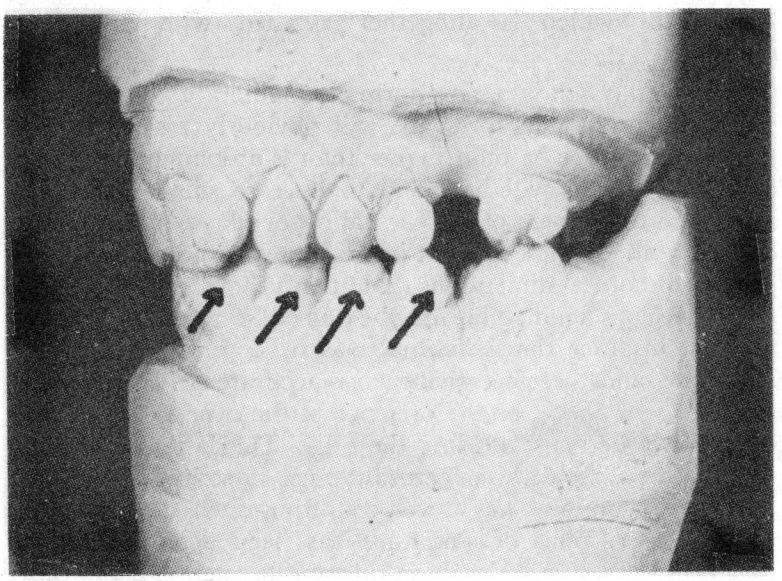

FIG. 512. – Models have been mounted on an anatomical articulator by means of a check record and face bow and closed into the position of tooth contact. It can be seen that when full closure occurs the mesial inclines of the cusps of the lower teeth will force the mandible to retrude as indicated by the arrows. An overlay can prevent this tendency to backward displacement.

muscle path of closure of the mandible and thus prevent the cuspal guidance of the teeth forcing the mandible to assume a strained position.

General Remarks in Relation to Overlays

(1) Overlays should normally be constructed to fit over the upper teeth. The reason for this is that by carrying an acrylic platform behind the upper incisors a surface is presented with which the tips of the lower incisors can occlude, and this prevents any possibility of their over eruption (*see* fig. 508(*b*)). The contact of the acrylic with the palatal surfaces of the upper incisors also prevents their over eruption.

If the overlay is constructed over the lower teeth, in order to prevent over eruption, it is necessary to carry the acrylic over the incisal edges of these teeth, and this produces an unsightly appearance which is altogether avoided with an upper overlay.

(2) Overlays should not normally obliterate the free-way space, although their presence will obviously reduce it, and they should never be built higher than is absolutely necessary. Some individuals will be found to have so small a free-way space that the fitment of even a shallow overlay will completely obliterate it. In these cases it is sometimes found on fitting an overlay of normal dimensions that after a short time a free-way space develops again. This may be due either to the fact that in the first instance the individual was never fully relaxing the mandible, and therefore giving an inaccurate recording of the true free-way space, or the presence of the overlay has caused the teeth to be depressed into the ridge. This latter occurrence the authors view with concern although in some instances no untoward symptoms has developed from such a happening. In some cases relief of symptoms has been achieved by the use of the overlay sufficiently to warrant its retention.

(3) In a case in which it is considered that an overlay might be a suitable form of treatment, the first appliance should be constructed in acrylic resin. Such an appliance might be termed a diagnostic appliance. If after the initial period required for getting used to it, it is worn by the patient with comfort and

abatement of the symptom for the cure of which it was fitted, then it can be assumed that it is a suitable form of treatment, and can be replaced in due course by a metal overlay. The metal appliance is more robust and long-lasting than the acrylic one, as the latter tends after a few months to wear and disintegrate.

If on the other hand no improvement of symptoms occur after a few weeks wear then the acrylic appliance may be discarded and no great loss of time or effort will have occurred.

(4) It is important that overlays and the teeth under them are kept scrupulously clean by the wearer. If they are not then caries is likely to occur.

CHAPTER XXVIII

THE CLEFT PALATE FROM THE PROSTHETIC ASPECT

Definition

A cleft palate may be defined as a lack of continuity of the palate.

It may be congenital i.e. the individual is born with the disability or it may be acquired as a result of injury or disease (frequently a carcinoma spreading from the maxillary antrum). This latter type of deformity is better referred to as a perforation of the palate rather than a cleft and will be dealt with separately.

Development

For full details of the development of cleft palate the reader is referred to the appropriate text; briefly the salient details are as follows:

The Lip. – The upper lip does not develop as a complete entity but is formed by the coalescence of the premaxillary and maxillary growth centres on either side to produce the complete lip.

Fusion of the sections of the lip developing from each growth centre commences around each nostril floor and spreads downwards towards the lower border of the lip uniting the premaxillary and maxillary processes on each side. Failure of this union will result in a cleft or hare-lip which, depending on the degree of failure of union, may vary from a notch in the lower border of the lip on one side to a complete bilateral cleft of the lip with the prolabium (i.e. the middle segment of the lip) only attached loosely to the nasal septum, the cleft extending up into each nostril (*see* fig. 513).

The Palate. – The palate is developed from the maxillary and premaxillary growth centres, union of the three segments commencing at the region of the nasal floor represented in full

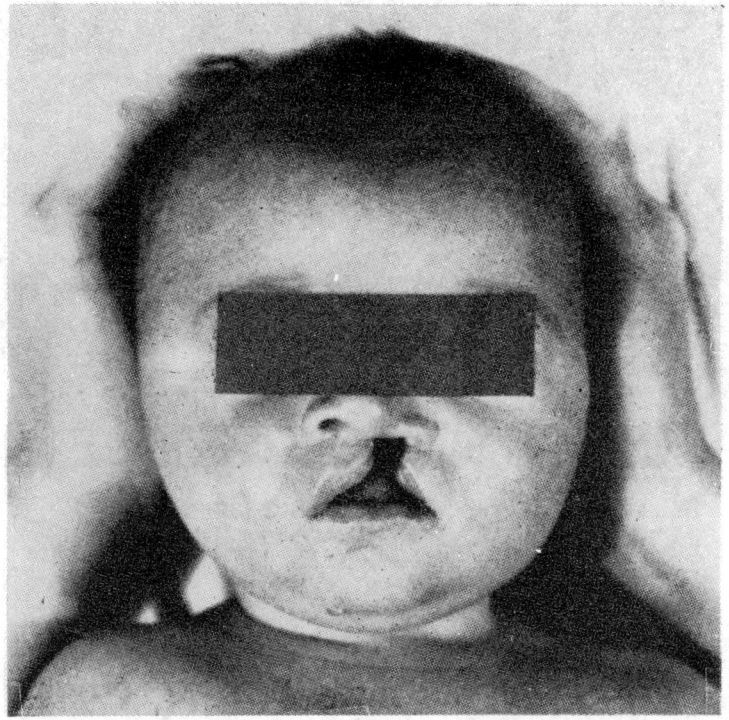

FIG. 513. – A unilateral hare lip.
(Photograph by kind permission of Mr. M. A. Kettle.)

development by the incisive foramen. Union from this point proceeds backwards until both the hard and soft palates and uvula have united, and forwards along the line of the future maxillary premaxillary sutures eventually uniting with the developing lip on either side.

Failure of union at any stage will result in a cleft palate (see fig. 514) which may be pre-alveolar i.e. a hare-lip; post-alveolar i.e. a cleft palate varying from a bifid uvula to a complete failure of union between the two halves of the soft and hard palates up to but behind the incisive foramen, or alveolar which is a cleft palate involving the soft and hard palates and dividing the alveolar process in the region of the lateral incisor

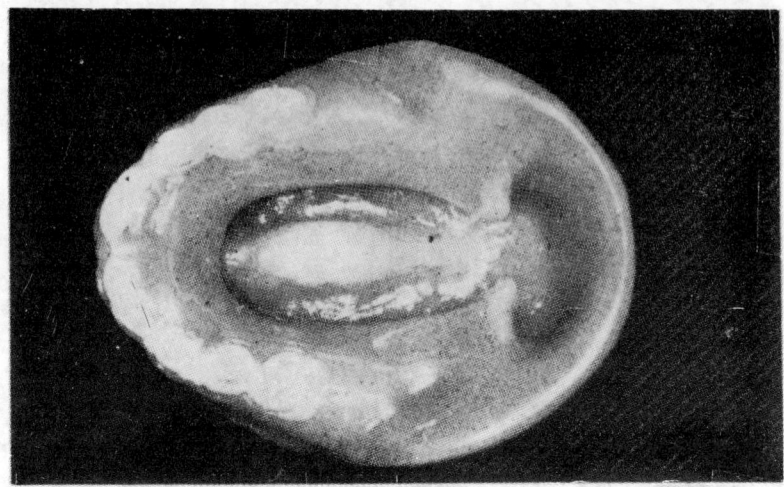

FIG. 514.
(a) Post alveolar or Veau Class I cleft of palate.
(Photograph by kind permission of Professor Malcolm Gibson.)

(b) Alveolar cleft or Veau Class III.

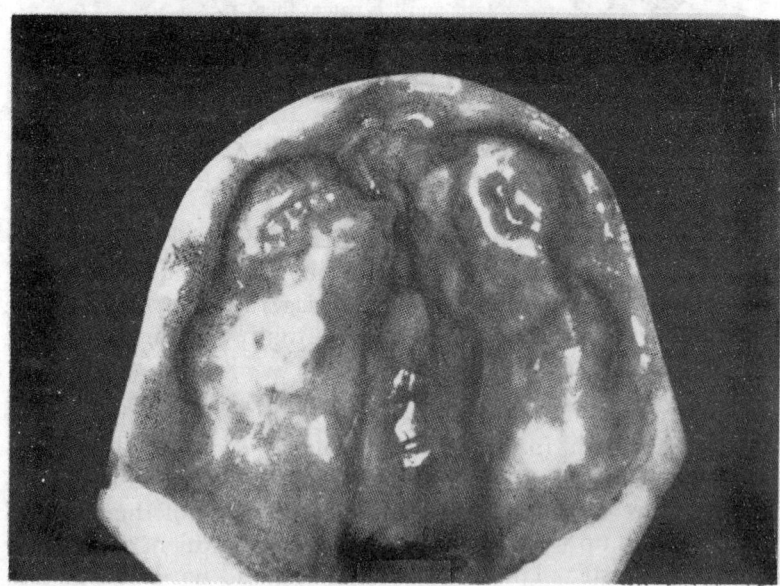

FIG. 514(b).

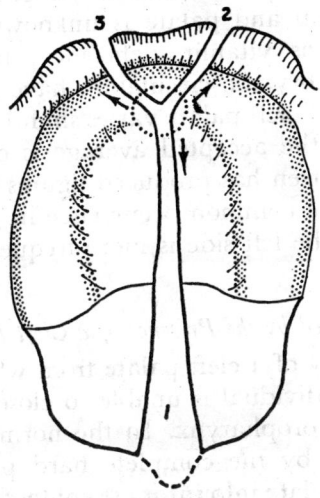

FIG. 515. – Dotted circle indicates area of initial union of segments forming palate and lip; union then proceeds in directions of arrows. If no union occurs and 1, 2 and 3 are patent a bilateral hare lip with a complete alveolar cleft results. If 2 and 3 unite and 1 is patent then a post alveolar cleft results. Union may proceed part way along 1 and then stop.

tooth, continuing into a cleft lip on one or both sides (*see* fig. 515).

Classification of Cleft Palates

A more detailed classification of cleft palates and one that is generally accepted is that of the famous French plastic surgeon, Victor Veau, which is as follows:

Class I.   Clefts involving soft palate only.

Class II.   Clefts involving soft and hard palates up to incisive foramen.

Class III.   Cleft of soft and hard palates, right forwards through alveolar ridge and continues into lip on one side.

Class IV.   Same as Class III only associated with bilateral hare-lip.

The cause of failure of union of the growth centres which produces a cleft lip and palate is unknown, although many suggestions such as vitamin deficiency, malnutrition, deficiencies in the embryonic circulation have been advanced.

The incidence of cleft palate varies slightly in different areas of the world but the accepted average is one in a thousand births. Fogh Andersen has produced figures showing that cleft palates are of more common occurrence in girls and cleft lips in boys and that the left side is more frequently affected than the right.

Disabilities Occasioned by the Presence of a Cleft Palate

The basic disability of a cleft palate from which all the others stem is that the individual is unable to close at will the nasopharynx from the oropharynx. In the normal individual this closure is effected by the complete hard palate and by the raising of the soft palate into intimate contact with the posterior and lateral pharyngeal walls (*see* fig. 516). This airtight

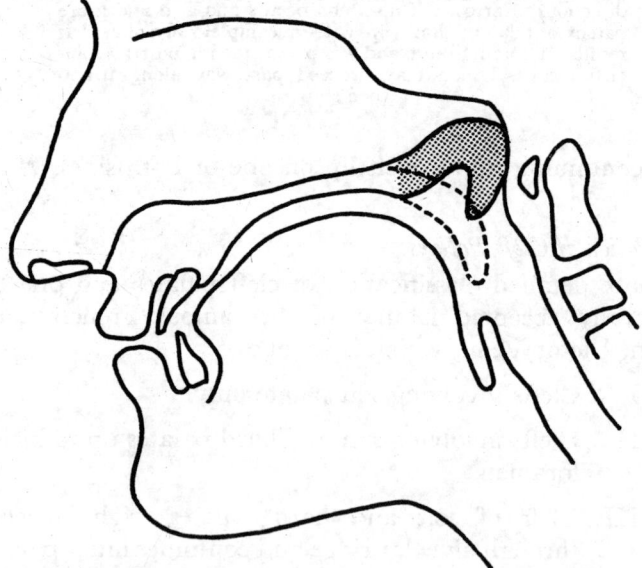

FIG. 516. – Dotted line indicates relaxed position of soft palate. Continuous line indicates position of raised soft palate in contact with pharynx. Note that it is above anterior arch of atlas.

separation of the two cavities is essential to the functions of normal swallowing and speech.

The Action of Swallowing

In swallowing, the food bolus or liquid mass is held in the depressed centre of the tongue the sides of which are pressed hard against the lateral aspects of the hard palate. Peristaltic-like waves then travel along the tongue from before backwards and propel the food or liquid towards the pharynx. The soft palate which is already raised into contact with the walls of the pharynx prevents its escape into the nose and directs it towards the oesophagus; the pharyngeal walls contracting to propel it on its way.

The Problem of Suckling an Infant when the Palate is Cleft

If both the hard and soft palates are cleft the natural process of swallowing is impossible and the first problem facing those nursing a child born with a cleft palate is concerned with its feeding.

A normal child when suckling takes the nipple and part of the breast into the mouth, the nipple resting on the back of the tongue. The alveolar ridges acting with a chewing action express the milk which is deposited on to the tongue and then swallowed. With breast feeding very little, if any, sucking which requires a negative pressure in the mouth is used. With bottle feeding, however, a sucking action is frequently necessary because the design of many artificial teats make it difficult for the action of the ridges alone to express the milk. To produce a negative pressure in the mouth requires a complete soft palate in intimate contact with the walls of the pharynx otherwise air will enter the mouth through the back of the nose.

The Action of Swallowing when the Palate is Cleft

In spite of the problems which face the infant with a cleft palate, in most cases it adapts itself to spoon feeding and sometimes to suckling if the head is turned on one side so that the milk may be swallowed between the tongue and the side of the palate. In the case of a very extensive cleft, however, this is impossible and it may be necessary to construct an acrylic palate to enable the child to swallow.

The Construction of an Acrylic Palate

A composition impression is taken of the infant's upper jaw. This can be accomplished most easily if the child is held on the nurse's knees with its head towards the operator, who himself is sitting down.

To the model, cast from this impression, a simple wax palate is adapted extending to the sulci and two long pieces of stainless steel wire, 2 mm. in diameter, are waxed in place so that they will issue forwards at about the positions of the corners of the mouth after the palate has been processed in acrylic and is in place in the mouth.

The wire extensions are then bent to follow closely the external contours of the cheeks and by means of a skull cap or bonnet support, the appliance is held in place, while the child is feeding.

If surgical closure of the cleft is unsuccessful or no prosthetic treatment is given, as the child grows it adapts iself to swallowing along the side of the tongue using the posterior third thereof to close the cleft in the soft palate, and soon becomes so adept at swallowing in this way, that little if any food or liquid escapes into the nose.

The Technique of Normal Speech

The initial sound of speech is produced in the larynx and travels as a vibrating airstream either through the mouth where it is modulated into articulate sounds by the tongue, palate, lips and teeth, or through the nose where the nasal cavities and associated sinuses produce a nasal resonance.

The production of the correct sound depends in all cases on rapid and accurate positioning of the soft palate.

When speaking, all sounds except for those of m, n and ng, the soft palate is raised preventing all nasal escape of air which is thus wholly directed through the mouth where it is modulated in one of three ways. For the vowel sounds the air stream escapes continually through the mouth the shape of which is altered for the various vowels by raising or lowering the tongue and by altering the shape of the exit through the lips.

The oral consonants are of two kinds – the stopped consonants and the frictives. The sounds of the stopped consonants are produced by first of all stopping the air stream momentarily and then allowing it to escape through a cavity shaped to produce the sound in question.

A few examples will make this clear.

B and P sounds (labials). – The air stream is stopped momentarily by closure of the lips and then released explosively when the lips are suddenly parted (*see* figs. 517 and 518).

T and D sounds (linguo-dentals). – The stop is made for these sounds by the tip of the tongue being pressed against the palatal surfaces of the upper front teeth.

G and K sounds (linguo-palatals). – In these sounds the momentary stop is made by the back of the tongue being pressed hard against the hard palate (*see* fig. 519(*a*)).

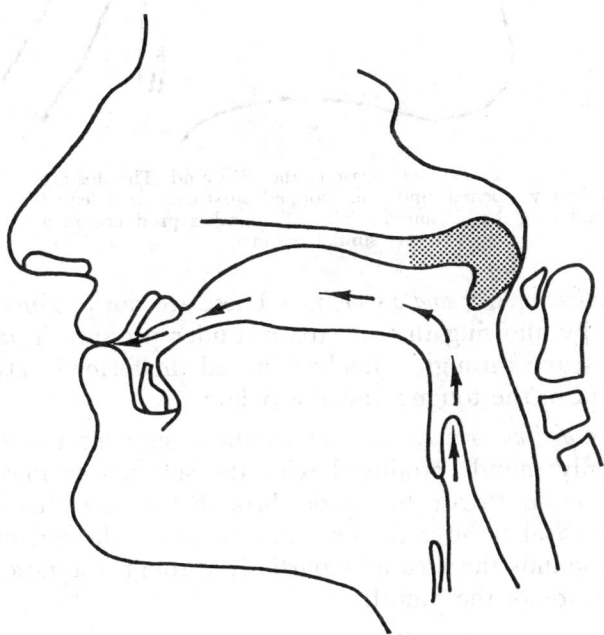

FIG. 517. – The first phase of the 'B' sound. The initial sound is produced in the larynx and travels upwards on the airstream being directed into the mouth by the raised soft palate. The lips are closed and therefore the airstream is stopped when it reaches them and is held there under pressure.

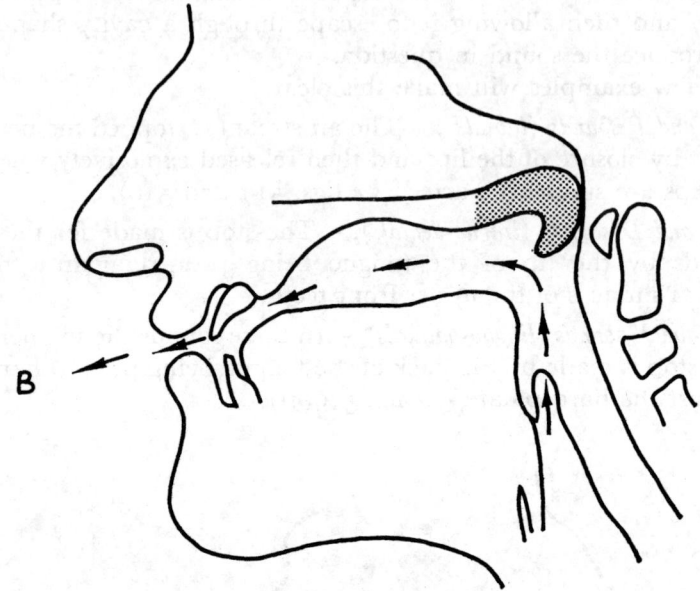

FIG. 518. – The second phase of the 'B' sound. The lips are suddenly opened and the stopped airstream is released producing the 'B' sound. The 'P' sound is produced in a very similar manner.

The frictives or s, z and c sounds. – These are not produced by stops but by allowing the air stream under pressure from the lungs to escape through a finely adjusted slit formed between the dorsum of the tongue and the palate.

The m, n and ng sounds. – These are the nasal consonants and are the only sounds produced with the soft palate lowered, allowing the air stream to escape through the nose. In the m sound the nasal route is the only one taken by the air, in the n and ng sounds the escape is partially through the nose and partially through the mouth.

Speech Faults when the Palate is Cleft

It will be appreciated from the foregoing that the production of all oral sounds requires the airstream to be under some degree of pressure and this can only be maintained and the airstream correctly directed through the cavities of the mouth if

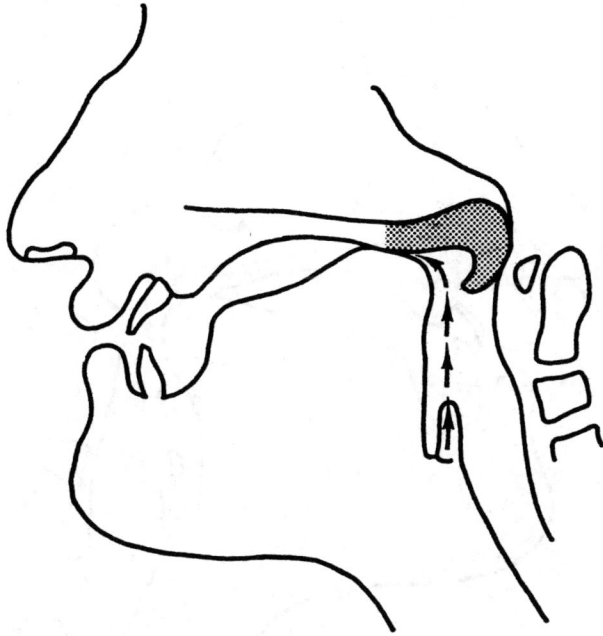

Fig. 519(*a*). – Illustrating how the 'stop' is made with tongue and palate for the 'G' sound.

the soft palate and pharyngeal walls are producing an airtight seal to nasal escape. In the individual with a cleft palate this is not possible and the airstream escapes through the nose. In an attempt to prevent this the back of the tongue is thrust into the cleft and if the treatment of the cleft either by surgical or prosthetic means is delayed much after the second year (which is the age when rapid speech development occurs) this tongue habit becomes well established and even after treatment has been given makes correct speech difficult, because as has already been observed the tongue is a potent factor in the shaping of the modulating cavities and its free play especially forwards is vital to good speech (*see* fig. 519(*b*)).

The Effect of a Cleft on Appearance

The effect of a cleft on the appearance of an individual will depend on whether the lip is cleft as well as the palate.

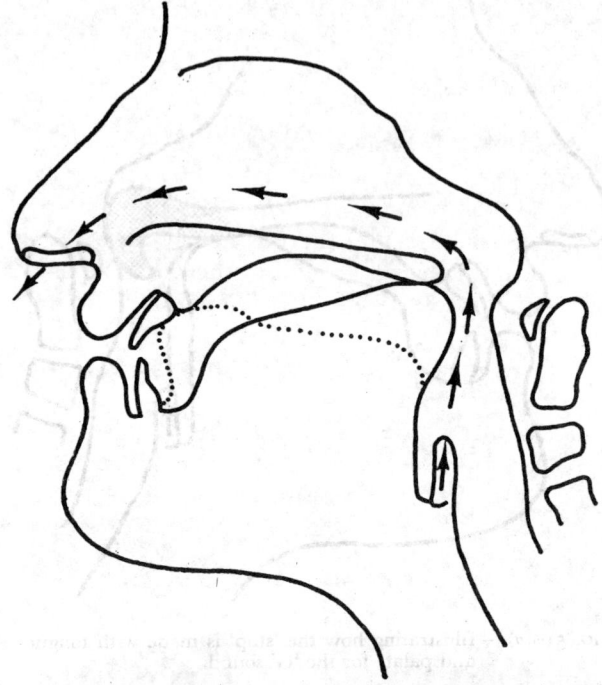

FIG. 519(*b*). – Dotted line shows how the tongue and upper
teeth should make the 'stop' for the 'T' sound but the palate
is cleft and therefore the vibrating airstream escapes
through the nose: in a vain effort to prevent this escape the
individual with a cleft palate pushes the tongue into the
pharynx (continuous line) and thus develops a major fault
of tongue position and thus of articulation.

(*a*) *When the Lip is Cleft.* – The cleft in the lip may be unilateral or bilateral and the premaxilla may be detached
entirely from the maxilla in bilateral clefts. The cleft of the lip
will involve the alveolar process and in most cases the lateral
incisor tooth will either be missing or deformed.

The cleft in the lip will be repaired surgically usually about
six weeks after birth, and most present day operations result in a
functional lip of good appearance, but a repaired lip will bring
more tension to bear than a normal lip on the anterior maxillary ridges and the teeth as they erupt frequently producing
an occlusal relationship of Angle class III type and if the lateral

incisor is missing a closing of the gap (*see* fig. 520). Orthodontic treatment will be necessary to restore the form of the arch and bring the teeth into correct occlusion with the lowers which will not have suffered any deformity. Thereafter a simple denture will be necessary to maintain the expansion and replace the lateral incisor.

(*b*) *When the Hard Palate is Cleft.* – If the cleft in the hard palate is repaired surgically there is nearly always a reduction in the lateral and forward growth of the maxillae as a result of the tension in the scar tissue of the repair. Orthodontic treatment will reduce this contraction of the arch and in doing so frequently open up parts of the cleft. A denture is necessary to maintain the expansion and cover the open cleft.

Modern atraumatic surgery has reduced the resulting contraction of the arch which formerly occurred but it is essential that orthodontic treatment is instituted early and is maintained. If for some reason no orthodontic treatment is given severe deformity of the maxilla may result. Even severer deformation

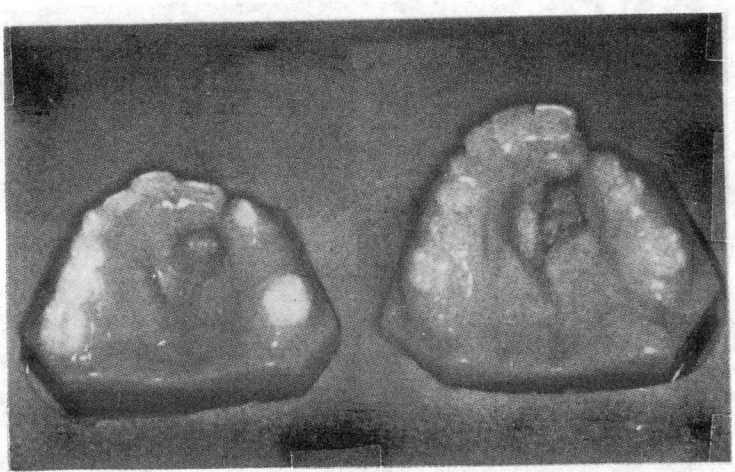

FIG. 520. – (*Left*) Contraction of upper arch following surgery. (*Right*) Orthodontic treatment has restored the shape of the arch but opened up the cleft in the hard palate which can be very simply covered by the denture required to replace |2 which is congenitally missing.

(Photograph by kind permission of Mr. D. F. Glass.)

is seen in older individuals who were operated on by the more traumatic surgical techniques employed earlier in the century. The results of such operations are seen in figs. 521 and 522. The effect of these on the appearance of the individual is marked; the middle third of the face is flattened and contracted (*see* fig. 523). The deformation resulting from uranoplasty (hard palate repair) is made worse if the lip repair was poorly done and has resulted in a tight immobile lip.

The Prosthetic Treatment of Cases with Contracted and Deformed Dental Arches

The treatment of patients with this condition if they are past the age when orthodontic treatment is likely to be effective is to construct a denture which covers the misplaced teeth and set the artificial teeth in a fresh arch corresponding to the position and form of the normal (*see* figs. 524–527). The lower jaw will usually not have suffered any deformation and if the artificial teeth are set to occlude with the lower teeth a very

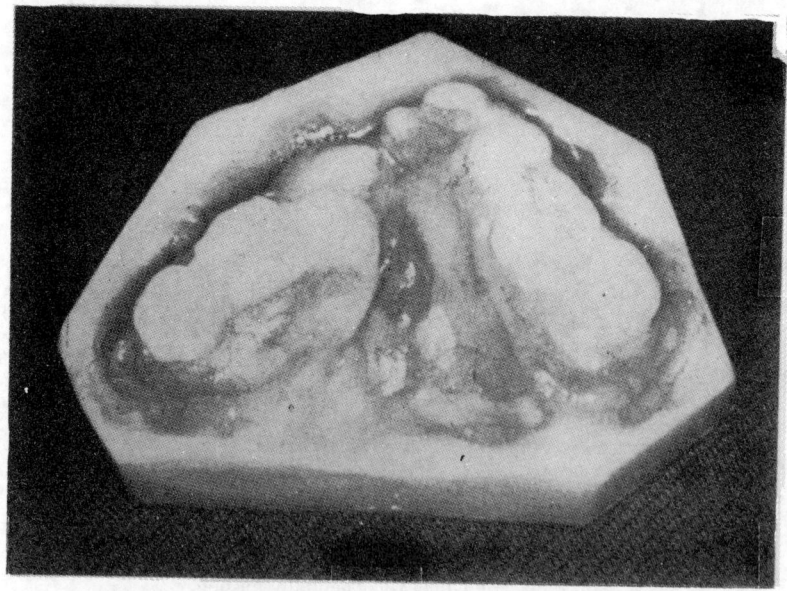

FIG. 521. – Surgical closure of cleft resulting in contraction of arch.

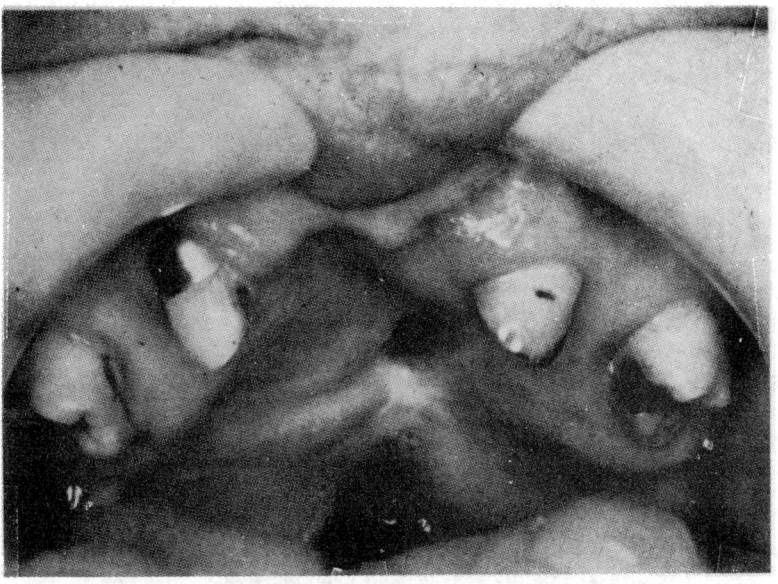

FIG. 522. – Contraction of arch with breakdown of tissue following surgical closure of cleft (patient is too old for orthodontic treatment).

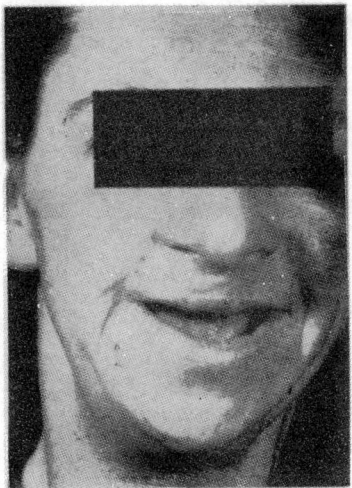

FIG. 523. – Flattening of face and contraction of lips following surgery.

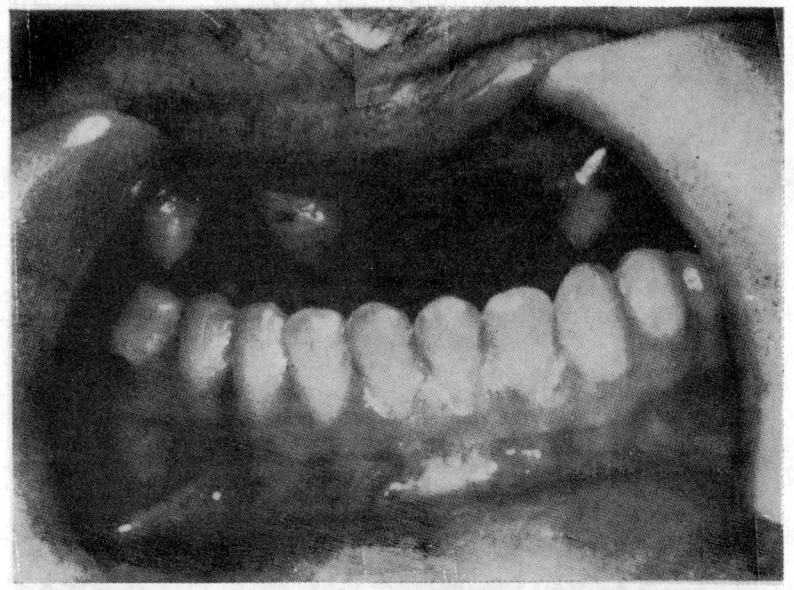

FIG. 524. – Contraction of arch following surgery – contour
of normal arch shown by lower teeth.

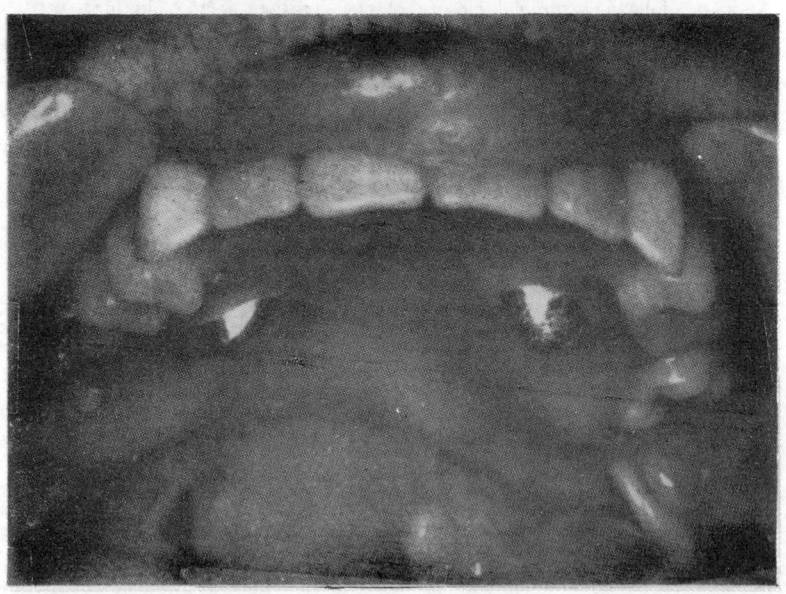

FIG. 525. – Artificial teeth set well forward and 3|3 covered
by denture.

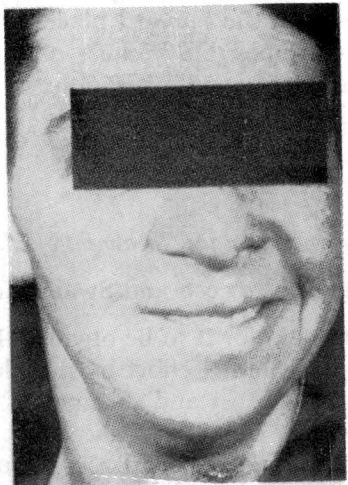

FIG. 526. – Upper lip now supported in more normal position, compare with fig. 523.

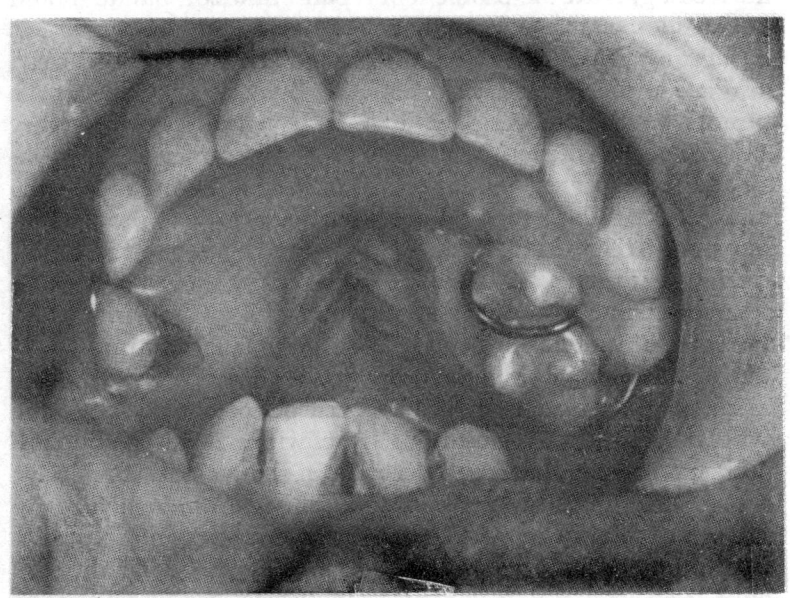

FIG. 527. – Another case of a contracted arch with artificial
teeth set in normal position.

great improvement of the individual's appearance will be effected. In some cases the forward placement of the artificial teeth is difficult or impossible because of the tightness of the lip. In these cases a second operation on the lip may be necessary to relieve the tension before a denture can be constructed.

General Remarks on the Treatment of Cleft Palate

(In Relation to Speech and Swallowing Faults)

Sufficient has been said for it to be obvious that the treatment of cleft palate is a combined effort by the plastic surgeon, the orthodontist, the prosthetist and the speech therapist. Ideally any child born with a cleft palate should be examined by all four specialists in consultation and a combined plan of treatment formulated. The surgeon's main problem will be to repair the lip which he will do at about six weeks after birth if the infant's physical condition allows. Early repair of the lip simplifies feeding. Next the problem of repair of the soft palate should be considered: this is of vital importance because on its success or failure will depend the ability of the child to speak clearly. Surgical repair of the soft palate is obviously superior to the fitting of a prosthesis. This is only true however if surgery can produce a functional soft palate and this will depend on the amount of muscular tissue which is present in the remnants of the soft palate (particularly of the levator muscles). If the cleft is very wide and the muscular remnants poorly developed consideration should be given to abandoning surgery and treating the cleft entirely by fitting a prosthetic obturator. If surgery can only produce a united soft palate which is non-functional the patient is really worse off than if no surgery had been performed, because the problem of fitting an obturator in cases with a repaired and non-functional soft palate is greater than in those cases which have received no surgical treatment. If, in addition, a pharyngoplasty has been performed, the pharyngeal ring mechanisms, on the function of which a successful obturator depends, may have been irreparably damaged. If surgical repair is decided upon this will usually be performed before the end of the second year because it is between the second and third years that the child really commences to talk and if repair is delayed beyond this time faulty habits of speech will have developed which are so difficult to eradicate.

If it is decided that surgery is unlikely to be successful then it is at about two years of age that the first obturator should be fitted. Details of this are given later in the chapter. Finally when the question of the treatment of the lip and soft palate has been decided consideration should be given to the repair of the hard palate. This is the least important problem of all because the cleft in it can be covered so easily and with extremely successful results by means of a simple acrylic or metal palate. If the cleft in the hard palate is at all wide its repair by surgery will almost certainly result in contraction of the dental arch and maxilla and the cleft will be reopened by the subsequent orthodontic treatment.

The Prosthetic Treatment of Soft Palate Clefts

The treatment of clefts in the soft palate is by means of an obturator which means simply something which closes a cavity (Latin, obturare: to close) (see fig. 528). Such an obturator is sometimes called a speech bulb. Its method of function and its form will be fully described later but basically it is a smooth acrylic bulb lying in the plane of maximal pharyngeal contraction so that when the pharynx is relaxed there is a space between it and the bulb allowing free passage of air to and from the nose and when the pharynx is contracted it grips the bulb producing an airtight seal of the nasopharyngeal isthmus (fig. 540).

Types of Obturator

Obturators are of 3 varieties. (a) Fixed pharyngeal (fig. 528); (b) hinged pharyngeal; (c) Meatal.

The fixed variety is an extension of a denture projecting into the pharynx at about the level of the anterior arch of the atlas and so shaped that it can be gripped by the pharyngeal walls. The hinged variety is attached to the posterior border of a denture by a hinge and its lateral borders are shaped so that

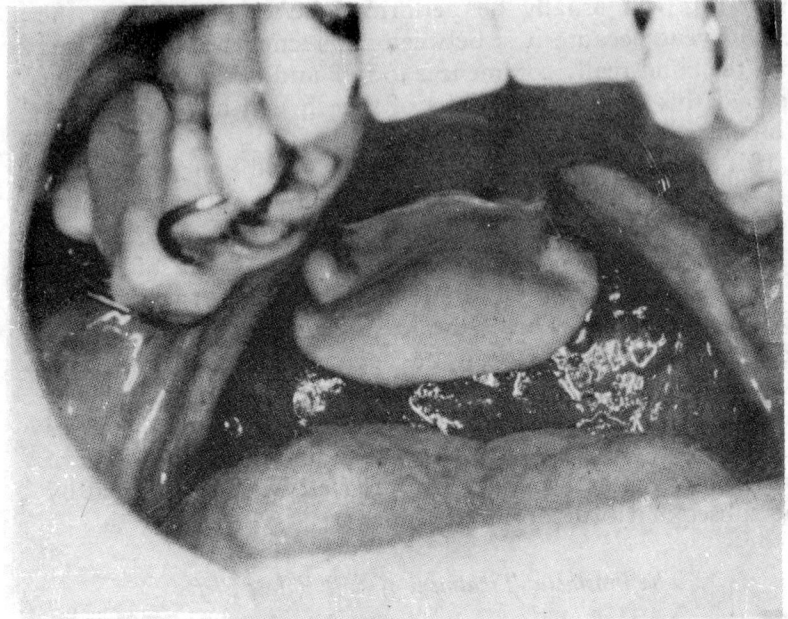

Fig. 528. – A fixed pharyngeal obturator in position in the pharynx.

they may be gripped by the remnants of the soft palate and be raised and lowered with them. The meatal obturator is an extension of the back of a denture upwards at right angles to it so that it occludes the opening of a posterior nares. Present day treatment employs the fixed bulb pharyngeal obturator almost exclusively and this is the only one which will be described. The reasons for this are as follows: the hinged obturator is supposedly designed to function as a substitute soft palate and imitate the movements of the normal soft palate. As will be seen later on this is quite impossible to achieve. The second criticism of the hinged obturator is that the hinge is a source of weakness and frequently gets out of adjustment.

The meatal obturator is only used in cases presenting a very large cleft when no inflammatory swelling of the conchae is present. It is extremely difficult to adjust so that it prevents the nasal escape of air when speaking the oral consonants and yet does not produce hyponasality of the nasal consonants and vowels; also this obturator does not help the patient when swallowing and in the opinion of the authors all that the meatal obturator achieves can be better achieved by the fixed pharyngeal bulb obturator. Before describing the technique, of shaping and constructing a pharyngeal obturator, the following aspects will be discussed. (1) How the normal pharynx and soft palate function in speech and swallowing. (2) How the fixed speech bulb functions. (3) The basic shapes of speech bulbs. These questions will be discussed because a thorough grasp of this information is essential if a speech bulb of an obturator is to be correctly positioned, shaped and adjusted so as to produce the maximum benefit for the patient.

A Brief Outline of the Topographical and Functional Anatomy of the Soft Palate and Pharynx

The soft palate is a curtain of soft tissue attached anteriorly to the posterior border of the hard palate and laterally to the walls of the pharynx. Its posterior border is free and hanging centrally from it is the uvula. The soft palate is composed mainly of extrinsic muscles and covered with mucous membrane cyliated on its nasal surface and squamous on its oral surface.

The muscles which are inserted into the soft palate are paired one entering from each side and consist of the following.

The Tensor Veli Palatini. – These muscles descend from their origins on the base of skull and curving by means of tendons round the hamular processes of the pterygoid plates, fan out into the aponeurosis of the soft palate which they themselves help to form. The function of these muscles is to lower and tense the soft palate from side to side. They are the first to contract in any movement of the palate because they tense the aponeurosis and provide a firm base from which the other muscles can act; they are particularly active in swallowing.

The Levator Veli Palatini Muscles. – These originate from the base of the skull and descending slightly forwards and inwards are inserted into the soft palate over a wide area of the middle third. If the mouth is opened widely when saying 'ah' two dimples can be seen on the oral surface of the soft palate which coincide with the nasal insertions of the levators. The levators raise the soft palate and pull it backwards into contact with the posterior-pharyngeal wall.

The Palato-pharyngeii. – These muscles have two insertions into the soft palate one above and one below the insertion of the levators. They curve laterally and posteriorly into the walls of the pharynx where they spread out descending to their origin from the thyroid cartilage. Covered with mucous membrane this pair of muscles forms the posterior pillars of the fauces. The function of these muscles is to lower the sides of the soft palate and to approximate them. They are particularly active in swallowing.

The Palato-glossus Muscles. – These originate from the sides and base of the tongue and curving outwards and upwards enter the under surface of the soft palate. Covered with mucous membrane they form the anterior pillars of the fauces. They function to both raise the back of the tongue and lower the soft palate and are most active in swallowing.

The Pharynx. – The upper part of the pharynx is formed by the superior constrictor muscle which is slung by its central raphe and pharyngo-basilar fascia from the base of the skull. Its upper border continues downwards and forwards to be attached to the lower part of the internal pterygoid plate. Below this certain specialized fibres are inserted into the aponeurosis of the soft palate and the hamular process. These muscle fibres circle the pharynx to form the palato-pharyngeal sphincter of Whillis. Below this level the superior constrictor muscle is inserted into the pterygo mandibular raphe and finally at its lower border into the mylohyoid ridge with some fibres running inwards to be inserted into the tongue.

The space between the upper border of the superior constrictor and the base of the skull is filled by the pharyngeal fascia. Looked at from above in horizontal section the superior constrictor muscle is roughly pear shaped. Lying in the lateral corners of the pharynx and running downwards from their origin on the mesial plate of the Eustachian tube to mingle with the fibres of the palato-pharyngeus muscle are the salpingo-pharyngeus muscles which, covered with mucous membrane, form the salpingo-pharyngeal folds (figs. 529, 530).

The Action of the Pharynx

The action of the pharynx is complex but basically it contracts from side to side and its posterior surface moves forwards. It is capable of local contractions at various levels, which are mainly used in speech, and also peristaltic type of contractions which travel downwards and which are employed during swallowing. The inward movement of the sides of the pharynx are markedly reinforced by the salpingo-pharyngeus muscles. The function of the soft palate and pharynx must be considered as one because they act in unison to form a combination between a flap valve and a sphincter. The various muscles of the palato-pharyngeal complex act rapidly and accurately together to open and close the oronasal isthmus.

The Action of the Soft Palate and Pharynx in Speech

This has been studied by the methods of direct observation in patients who have had parts of their face removed surgically as treatment for extensive malignancy and also by still and cine radiography using radiopaque media to sharpen the image of the soft tissues.

The Action in Speech. –The tensor muscles contract to tense the aponeurosis to form a firm base from which the other muscles may act. The lateral walls of the pharynx contract and move inwards reinforced by the salpingo-pharyngeus muscles. The levator muscles raise the middle third of the soft palate and bunch it up so that it becomes thicker from above downwards than when relaxed. The posterior third of the soft palate hangs downwards and the uvula curves away from the posterior pharyngeal wall. This position of the palate and pharynx is a preparatory position and when speech commences short rapid movements brought about by the levator muscles close and open the isthmus between the palate and pharynx and raise and lower the palate a limited amount depending on the sound which is being produced. The more explosive the sound the higher the palate rises. The forward movement of

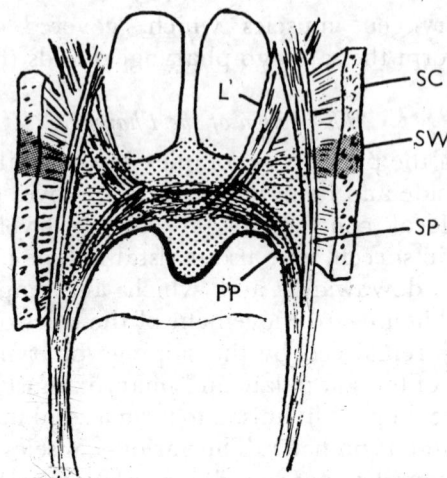

Fig. 529. – Diagrammatic representation of important
   muscles of soft palate and pharynx seen from behind.
SC = Lateral wall of superior constrictor muscle.
SW = Palato-pharyngeal sphincter (sphincter of Whillis).
SP = Salpingo-pharyngeus muscle.
PP = Palato-pharyngeus muscle.
L = Levator muscle.

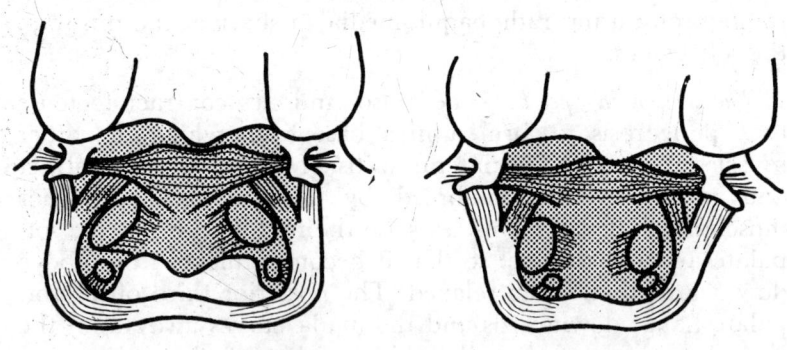

A   B

Fig. 530. – Diagrammatic representation of horizontal section
through palate and pharynx at a level just above the hard
palate showing cut surface of levator and salpingo-pharyngeal
muscles and the palato-pharyngeal sphincter merging with
the tensor muscles and the aponeurosis of the soft palate:
A in the relaxed position.
B, in the closed position.

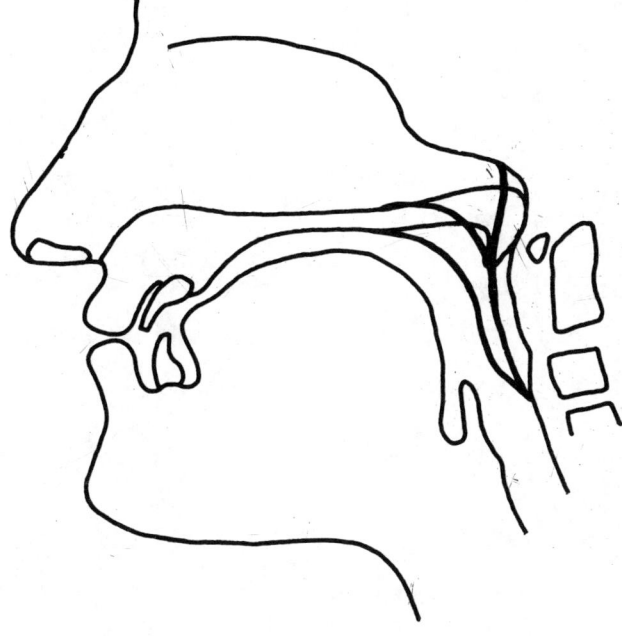

Fig. 531. – Black line illustrates positions of soft palate and posterior pharyngeal wall during speech. Red line illustrates positions of both when swallowing. Note marked forward shift of pharyngeal wall in swallowing position.

the pharynx during speech is small and the area of contact of the palate and pharynx during speech is well above the anterior arch of the atlas i.e. well above the area of the palato-pharyngeal sphincter of Whillis (figs. 518 and 531).

The Action of the Soft Palate and Pharynx in Swallowing

The tensor muscles contract lowering the anterior third of the soft palate so that the palate grips the bolus of food between itself and the tongue. The lateral walls of the pharynx contract and the posterior wall moves forwards. The levator muscles pull the middle third of the palate backwards and the palato-pharyngeus muscles pull the palate downwards and inwards into contact with the posterior pharyngeal wall over a con-siderable area so that frequently the uvula is well below the level of the inferior border of the mandible. The palato-pharyngeal sphincter of Whillis contracts to produce a circular muscular ring at the level of the anterior arch of the atlas which

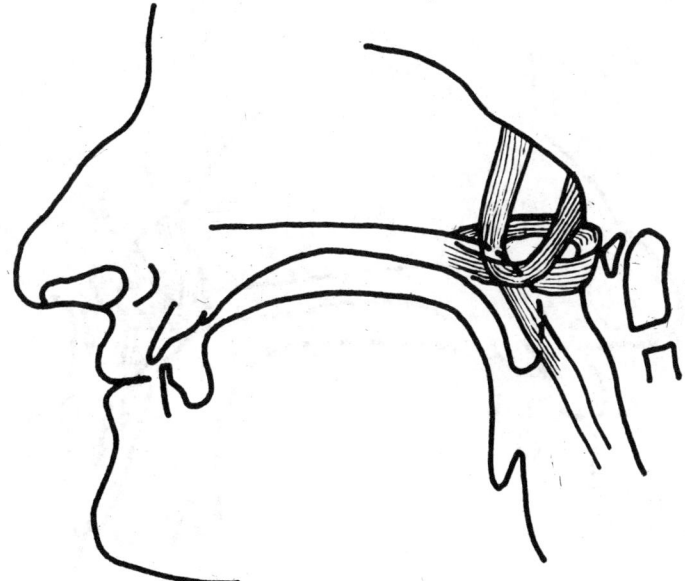

Diagrammatic representation of the action of the levator and palato-pharyngeal muscles and the sphincter when closing the pharynx for swallowing:
Fig. 532. – In the relaxed position.

grips the soft palate with a sphincteric or ring like action (figs. 532 and 533). Waves of contraction then travel down the pharynx from this level. The ring like contraction of the palato-pharyngeal sphincter has been observed for a long time and was described originally by Passavant in 1861, and is now called the bulge of Passavant. For a long time it was considered that the bulge of Passavant was active during speech, remaining raised while speech was in progress and helping to form the seal of the nasopharyngeal isthmus of the soft palate. Recent radiographic observations, however, tend to show that the contact of the soft palate with the pharynx during speech occurs in the normal individual at a higher level than the bulge of Passavant.

The Action of the Palate and Pharynx when the Palate is Cleft

The function of the muscles is similar to the normal but the results are different. The contraction of the tensor muscles,

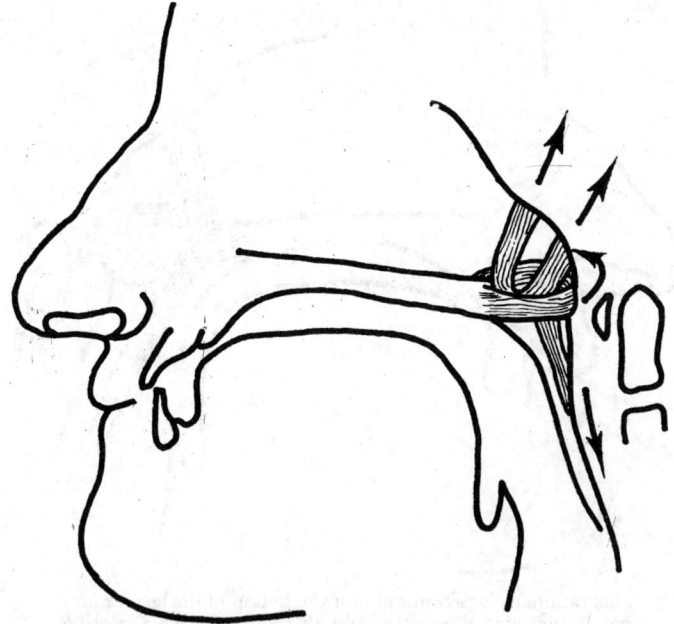

FIG. 533. – Closed. The direction of contraction of the various muscles is indicated by the arrows.

the palato-glossus and palato-pharyngeus muscles tend to draw the two halves of the soft palate away from one another in the areas of their insertions. The contraction of the levators although tending slightly to pull the remnants of the palate away from one another while drawing them upwards and backwards tend by the increase in the bulk of the middle third of the palate, which this contraction produces, to close the cleft to some extent. In an attempt to overcome this disability the palato-pharyngeal sphincter invariably hypertrophies and endeavours to squeeze the muscles of the soft palate together and close the cleft by an increase in its sphincteric grip. In cases of a small cleft this action may be reasonably successful. The other method employed by the individual with the cleft palate to close the gap is to push the dorsum of the tongue into the space and swallow down the sides of the tongue. It is this action and habit which has such a disastrous effect on speech. Another habit which the individual with a cleft palate acquires in an attempt to prevent the nasal escape of air is to contract the nares and in untreated or uncompensated cases of cleft palate this action is most noticeable although its results are quite unsuccessful.

This is the basic muscular pattern therefore into which an obturator has to be fitted and although marked individual variations resulting from the varying size of the cleft and from unsuccessful surgical intervention exist the basic task of the dental surgeon making an obturator is so to shape it and place it so that the muscles of the remnants of the soft palate and pharynx can grip it and thus enable the individual to close off the nasopharynx from the oropharynx at will.

How Can a Fixed Obturator Fit into the Two Different Patterns of Action of the Pharynx in Speech and Swallowing?

Before describing the basic shapes of obturators one other fact must be discussed which will have become apparent from the foregoing discussions of the action of the palato-pharyngeal complex, i.e. the problem of how a fixed obturator can fit the cleft in both the functions of speaking and swallowing when the shape and action of the pharynx differs so much in these two actions. The answer to this problem was perhaps first given by John FitzGibbons who himself suffered from a cleft palate and wore an obturator. He says in relation to the function of an obturator:

> 'The patient must learn new speech habits . . . the gripping of the bulb as in the act of swallowing is the basic principle which must be mastered
>
> and
>
> The action in producing the palatal consonants, particularly the sonants is horizontal instead of vertical and involves the gripping of the bulb as in swallowing.'
>
> (JOHN FITZGIBBONS,
> 'Dental Items of Interest,' 1931.)

The fact that the method by which an individual uses an obturator is entirely by gripping it with his ring or sphincter mechanism and squeezing the remnants of the soft palate against it means therefore that the plane of location of the obturator must be in the plane of action of the palato-pharyngeal sphincter or bulge of Passavant. In practice an obturator is shaped by luting a piece of softened gutta-percha to a wire loop or tail piece extending from the posterior border of the denture along the midline of the cleft into the pharynx. The gutta-percha is then shaped by the muscles as they function. Details of this technique are given later in the chapter

The Horizontal Plane of Location of the Obturator

The following figures show clearly the plane in which the obturator must be placed in relation to the enveloping muscles, and its shape resulting from their actions. Fig. 534 shows the relaxed pharynx of an individual with a repaired cleft of the hard palate and an unrepaired one of the soft palate. The posterior and lateral walls of the pharynx are smooth and the cleft is wide. Fig. 535 shows the same pharynx with the muscles contracted. The sphincter of Whillis can be seen clearly producing the bulge of Passavant on the posterior wall of the pharynx and it can be observed running laterally outside the salpingo-pharyngeal muscles which can be seen as raised vertical ridges in the corners of the pharynx. It then disappears from view laterally to the remnants of the soft palate containing the levator muscles. Fig. 536 shows a model taken from an

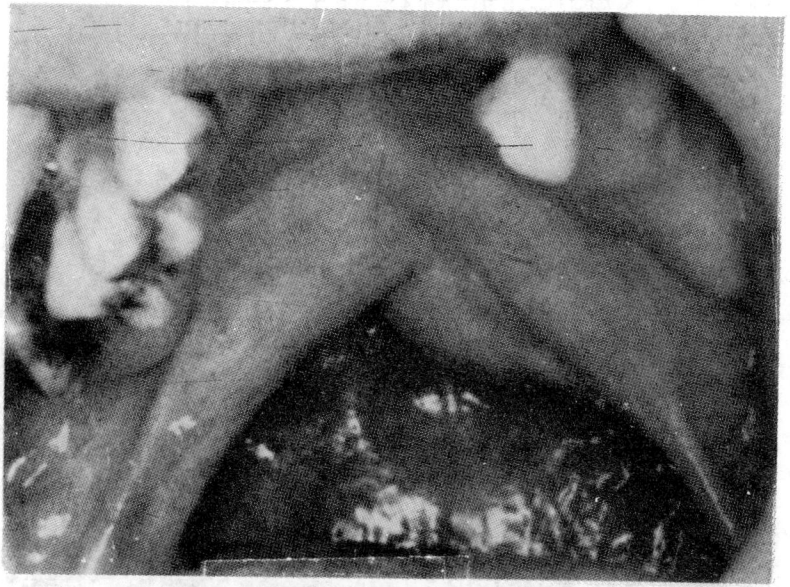

Fig. 534. – Relaxed pharynx.

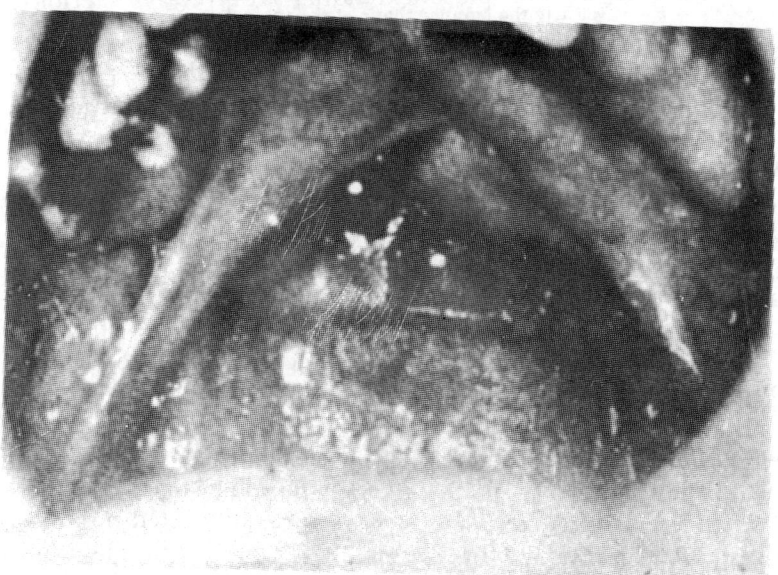

Fig. 535. – Sphincter of Whillis contracted raising bulge of Passavant – note how it circles the pharynx and disappears behind the salpingo-pharyngeal muscles in the lateral corners of the pharynx.

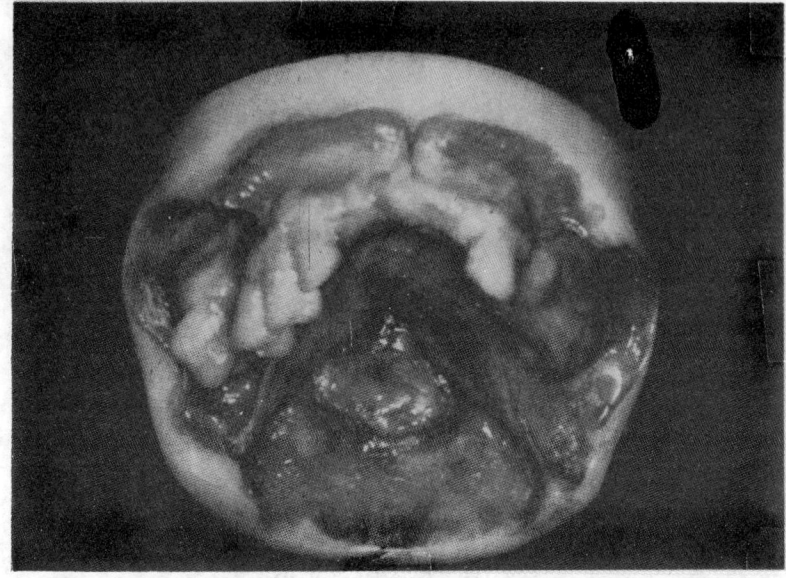

FIG. 536. – Model of same case as 534 and 535 showing more
clearly the circular shape of the sphincter.

alginate impression of the same individual with the pharynx
contracted. The ring mechanism producing a contraction
circling the pharynx can be clearly observed. Fig. 537 is a
sagittal section of this model showing the sphincter of Whillis
from the side and if this is compared with fig. 538 which is a
diagram of the location of the palato-pharyngeal sphincter it
will be observed that the position of the two coincide. Fig. 539
is a photograph of a dissection in the sagittal plane showing
the soft palate and the levator muscles and it will be observed
from fig. 538 which clarifies the dissection how the palato-
pharyngeal sphincter encircles the levator muscles and as
the former contract will squeeze the latter inwards. Fig. 540
shows in horizontal section at the level of the hard palate the
relationship of the levator and salpingo-pharyngeal muscles
and the sphincter in both the relaxed and contracted positions
when an unrepaired cleft is present and illustrates how an
obturator positioned in the plane of the palato-pharyngeal
sphincter will be related to these structures both when relaxed

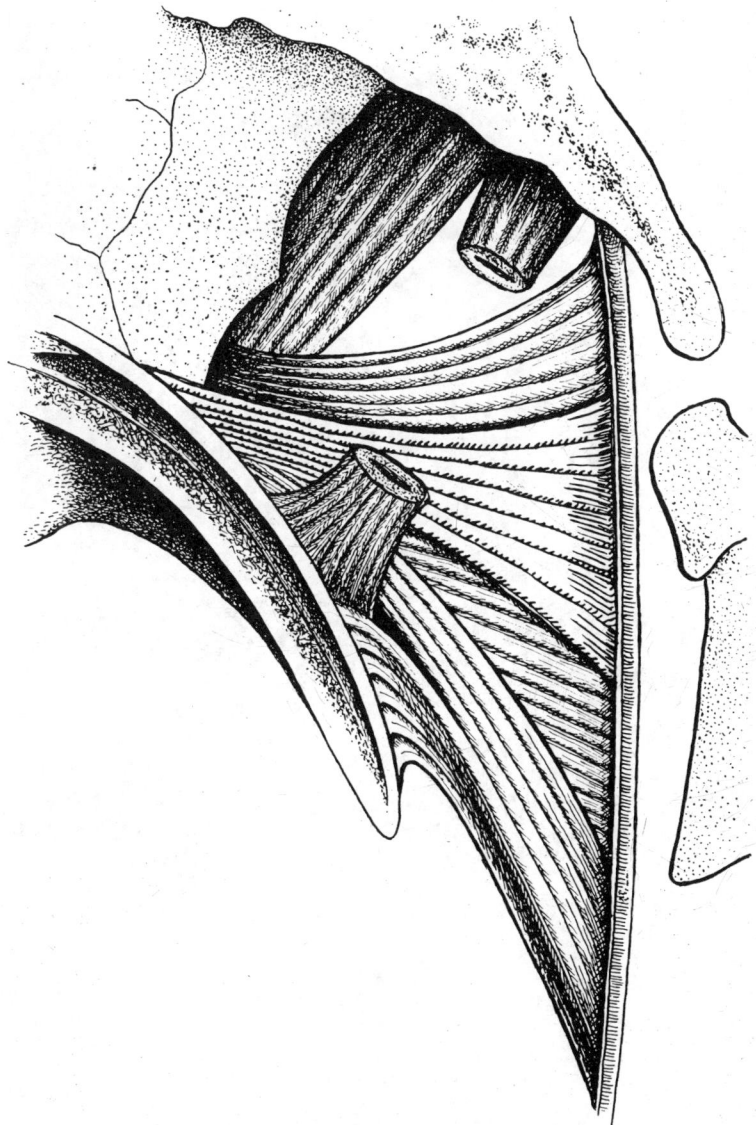

FIG. 538. – Illustrating muscular layer of superior constrictor muscle which acts as the sphincter and produces the bulge of Passavant (partly after an illustration by Whillis).

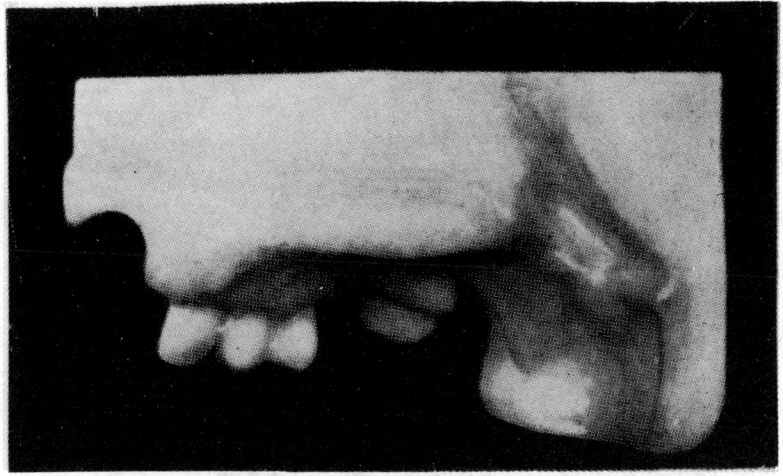

FIG. 537. – Sagittal section of model shown in fig. 536
illustrating how sphincter runs round lateral wall of pharynx
and gains attachment from the palate. Note also bulge of
salpingo-pharyngeus muscle; compare with fig. 538.

and when contracted. It will be observed that in the first
diagram there is a space between the obturator and its related
structures which allows air to pass freely to and from the nose,
whereas in the second diagram the surrounding musculature
grips the periphery of the obturator firmly, producing an
efficient seal of the oronasal isthmus.

The Basic Horizontal Shapes of Obturators[1]

It will be observed that the obturator illustrated in fig. 540 is
T shaped and this is because the remnants of the soft palate are
well developed and their contained levator muscles, being bulky
when squeezed inwards by the palato-pharyngeal sphincter,
produce a neck between the posterior border of the denture
and the pharyngeal section of the obturator. The width and
anteroposterior dimension of the obturator will vary from
patient to patient depending on the size of the pharynx and
the degree of hypertrophy of the palato-pharyngeal sphincter.
In some cases two small horn like processes develop on the
obturator as it is shaped. These result from the extension of

[1]The substance of this section first appeared in an article by one of us in the
Annals of the R.C.S. England (1959) **25**, 245.

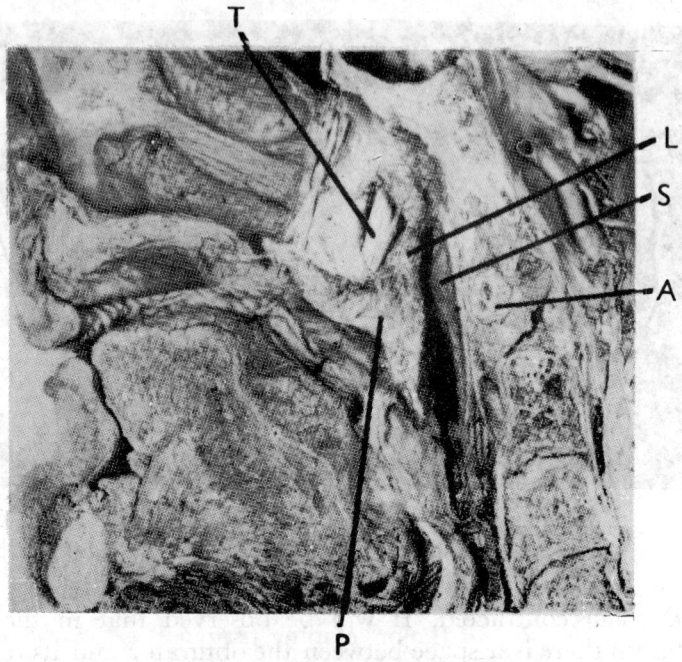

Fig. 539. – Photograph of sagittal section through palate
and pharynx:
P = soft palate.
L = Levator muscle.
T = Tensor muscle.
A = Anterior arch of atlas.
S = Tissues forming sphincter.
(Photograph by kind permission of Professor A. Nicol.)

the obturator into the lateral pharyngeal recess which in
some patients appears to be inactive. The inactivity is probably due to the weakness of the salpingo-pharyngeal muscles
which normally closes this area of the pharynx and it is
probable that closure of the pharynx will be quite effective
without them. In the first instance the obturator should always
be tried without these processes, only replacing them if a
serious air leak is experienced. These horns will also develop if
the obturator is carried in error too high into the pharynx
laterally and enters the sinus of Morgagni. This outline of the
horizontal form of an obturator may be considered as the
basic type and is designated group (a). There are, however,

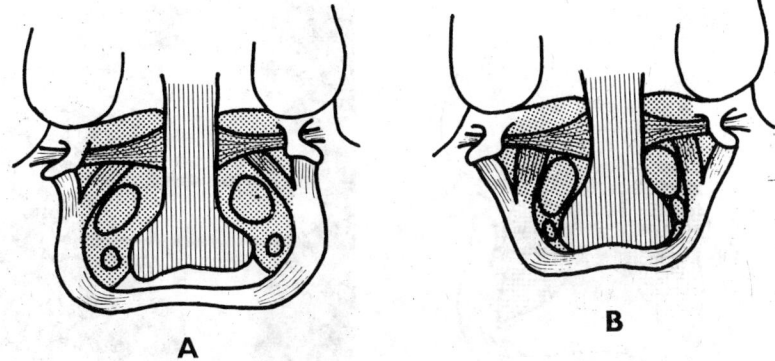

Fig. 540. – A horizontal section through the pharynx and
palate at the level of the hard palate.
A, The obturator in position with the remnants of the soft
palate and pharynx relaxed. Note space for air to pass
from nasopharynx to oropharynx.
B, Palatal remnants and pharynx constricted tightly round
obturator sealing off nasopharynx from oropharynx.

three other modifications of this basic shape depending on the
form and activity of the enveloping tissues.

These modifications are: (b) Those which develop when the
soft palatal remnants are small and inactive. This group also
includes those cases where surgical intervention has been quite
unsuccessful and resulted in deformed and scarred remnants
which are partially or completely bound to the lateral
pharyngeal walls by scar tissue and are partially or completely
immobile (such conditions are found in older patients who were
operated on before the present advances in surgical technique).
(c) Those cases in which a good union of the soft palatal remnants have been achieved but where the resultant palate is too
short or insufficiently functional to close the oro nasal isthmus
completely. (d) Those cases which have been treated surgically
by the Gillies-Fry type of operation in which the united soft
palate is functional posteriorly at the expense of a palatal cleft
between the posterior border of the hard palate and the
anterior border of the united soft palate. The modification in
the horizontal form of the obturator which develops in group
(b) is entirely the result of the inactivity or smallness of the
levator muscles which therefore do not produce the neck.

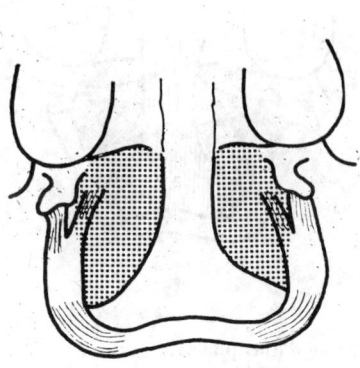
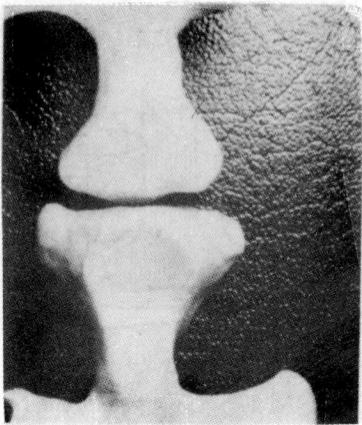

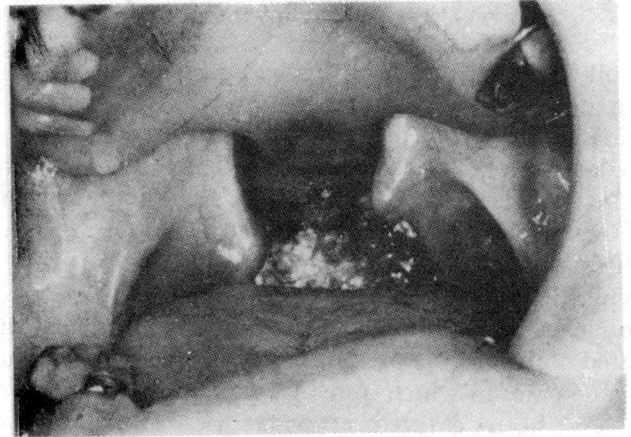

FIG. 541(a).

The illustrations on pages 738 to 743 show the four main variations of cleft which may require prosthetic assistance.

FIG. 541(a). The lower photograph shows a completely untouched post alveolar cleft with an obturator in place. Note the manner in which the soft palate remnants hang down.

The upper photograph illustrates two typical T-shaped obturators made for treating such a cleft, and the line diagram shows the general shape of this class of obturator.

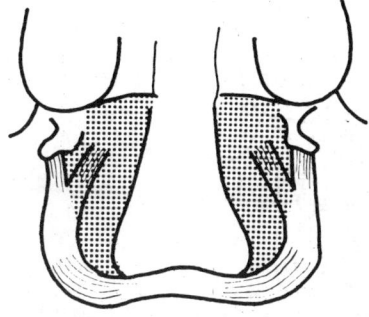
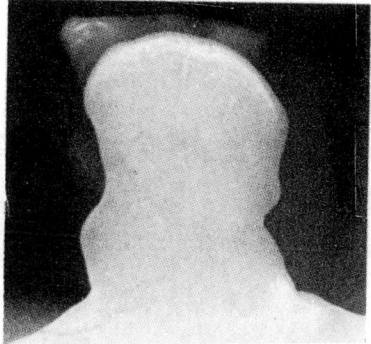

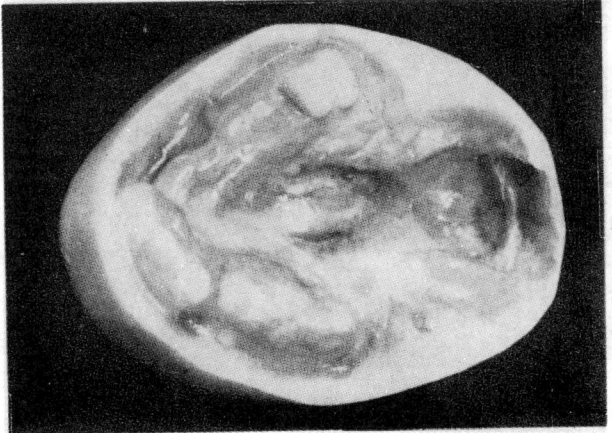

FIG. 541(*b*).

FIG. 541(*b*). The lower photograph shows a cleft which has had surgical treatment which has only been partially successful and the soft palate remnants are fibrosed and inactive. The upper photograph shows the pear shaped type of obturator which is usually suitable for closing such a cleft and the line diagram shows the general shape of this type of obturator.

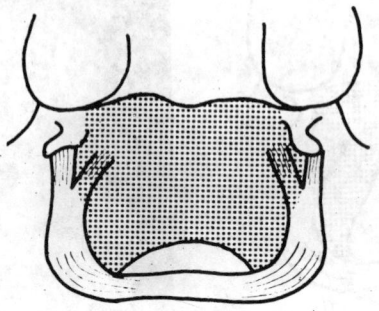

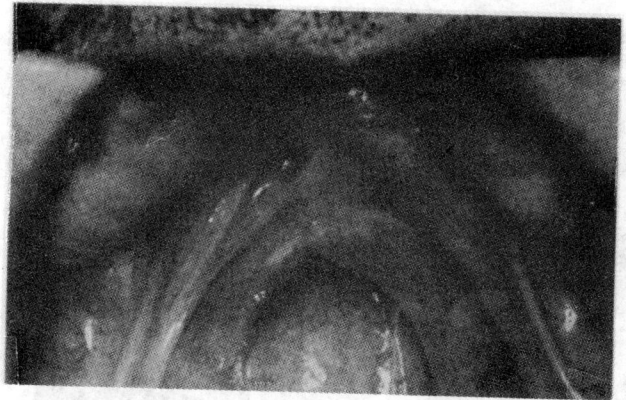

Fig. 541 (c).

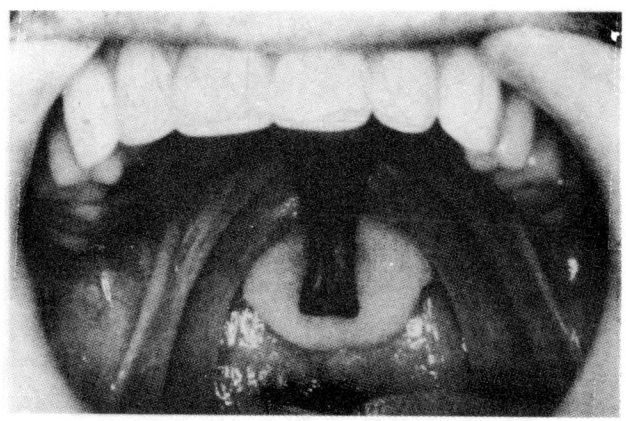

FIG. 541 (c).

FIG. 541 (c). The photograph on page 740 shows a cleft in which the soft palate has apparently been successfully united surgically. The palate however is too short to make contact with the posterior pharyngeal wall.

The photograph on page 741 shows an obturator for this type of case, united to the denture across the soft palate by a tailpiece. The line diagram shows the general shape of this type of obturator.

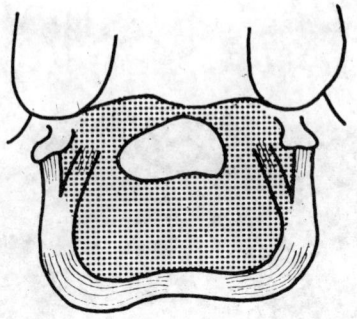

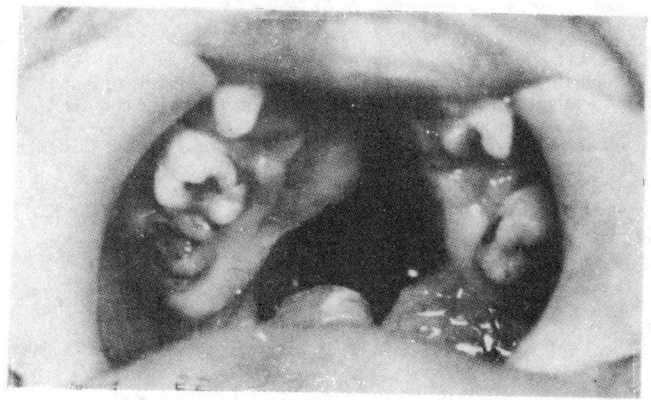

FIG. 541 (d).

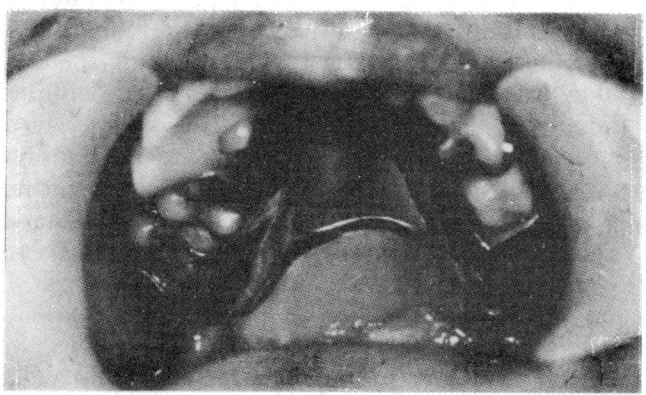

FIG. 541(*d*).

FIG. 541(*d*). The photograph on page 742 shows the post-operative appearance of a cleft palate which has been treated surgically by the Gillies-Fry operation which aims to produce a united functional soft palate distally but leaves a fenestration in the palate anteriorly where it is simpler to close with an obturator.

The photograph on page 743 shows the anterior fenestration closed with an obturator and the line diagram illustrates the general shape of this type of obturator.

Such obturators have a horizontal form which is pear shaped or circular (*see* figs. 541, 542 and 543 for all these types). Obturators in Group (*c*) differ from the preceding types mainly by the fact that the neck section joining the obturator to the denture does not function as part of the obturator by occluding the palatal section of the cleft but merely acts as a bridge to unite the pharyngeal section to the denture. The pharyngeal bulb of the obturators in this class are moulded by the pharynx and sphincter of Whillis on their posterior and lateral surfaces in the same way as the other classes but the anterior surface of the bulb is moulded by the posterior border of the united soft palate and the degree of moulding will depend on the degree of activity of the muscles of the palate. The general form of such obturators is that of a flattened elipse which varies in size depending on the degree of failure of the soft palate to close with the pharyngeal walls. Group (*d*) obturators occluding clefts resulting from Gillies-Fry operations

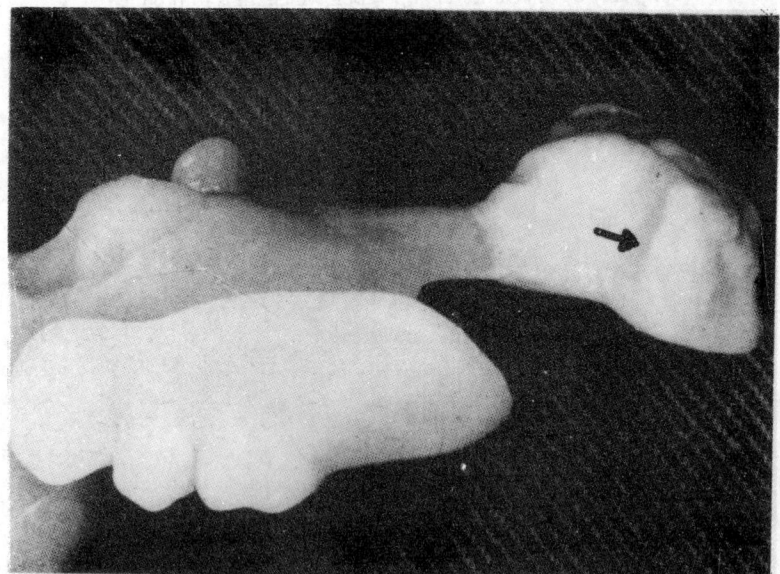

Fig. 542. – Lateral views of speech bulb. Arrow points to:
(*a*) Levator groove.

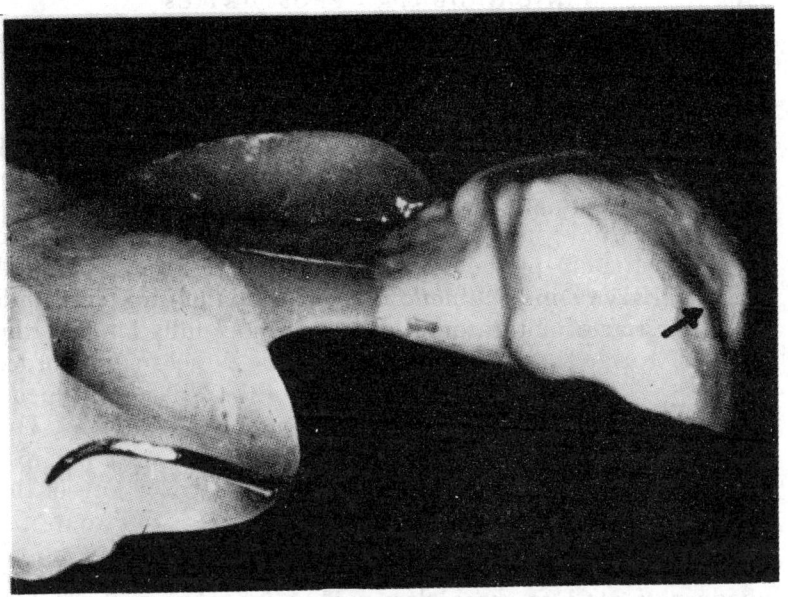

FIG. 542.
(b) Salpingo-pharyngeus groove.

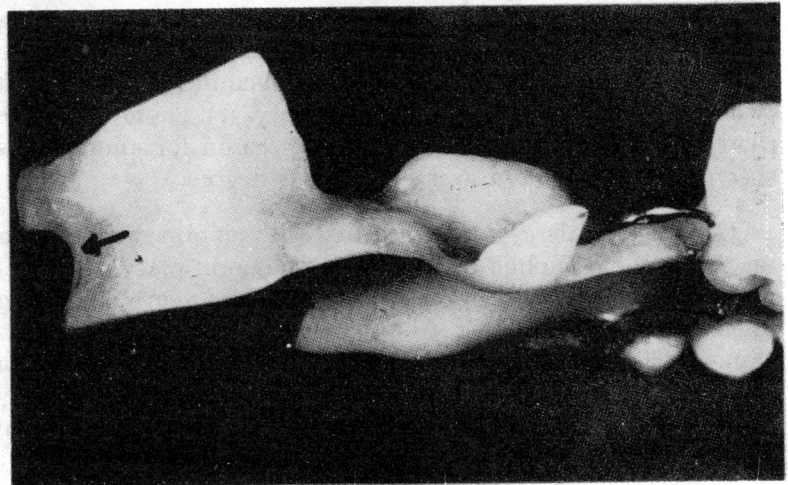

FIG. 543. – Palato-pharyngeal sphincter (bulge of Passavant)
groove.
Note the grooves made by these muscles illustrated in figs.
542(a and b) and 543 are not always as well marked as illustrated nor are they always all present on the same obturator.
The presence and depth of the grooves depends on the
development and activity of the muscles in each case.

are mainly static bungs and not moulded bv any muscle action at all except perhaps to a limited amount on their posterior border by the slight rise and fall of the anterior border of the repaired soft palate as its posterior section functions to close the oral nasal isthmus. A typical obturator used to close the residual cleft of the Gillies-Fry operation is shown in fig. 541(d).

The Sagittal Form of Obturators. – The shape of the upper and lower surfaces of obturators is discussed more fully later in the chapter.

Factors to be Taken into Consideration Before Deciding Whether to Fit an Obturator or Not

For the purpose of making such a decision it is convenient to divide patients into three classes, viz.: (a) those not suitable for surgical closure of the soft palate (b) those who have grown up without any surgical treatment either because they were born before the widespread application of surgery using modern techniques or because of the failure of their parents to take advantage on their behalf of the facilities available, but whose soft palates are suitable for surgery. (c) Those who have had surgical treatment which for one reason for another has been unsuccessful to a greater or lesser degree.

Group (a) patients should be fitted with an obturator as soon as they are old enough to allow it to remain in place. This will be in most cases between the second and third year. The fitting of an obturator should not be delayed later than this and its fitment, if possible, should be earlier otherwise bad habits of speech will be developed. Group (b) patients require very careful consideration because there are three possibilities open to them and it is important that the correct one be selected.

The first possibility is that no treatment at all be given. Some individuals who have reached maturity with no treatment for their cleft have adapted to the disability remarkably well.

They can swallow liquids and solids competently with no nasal escape and their speech, although exhibiting marked hypernasality, is sufficiently intelligible for them to be understood. Others however suffer from such degradation of speech that they are quite unintelligible. The possible lines of treatment for these individuals is (1) the fitting of a denture carrying an obturator and the second is a surgical repair of the cleft, both aimed primarily at improving speech. The success of either line of treatment will depend on: (a) the intelligence of the individual and their desire to improve their speech because in adult life improvement of speech demands the eradication of deeply ingrained faulty habits of articulation and improvement will require years of training by a competent speech therapist and continual perseverance by the individual. (b) Acuity of hearing because the individual will hear his own voice as if it is producing the same sounds that people with normal voices make, and accurate listening is necessary if he is to appreciate his own faults and learn to correct them.

Two further requirements are necessary before surgical treatment is considered, the first is that sufficient muscular tissue is present in the remnants of the soft palatal to ensure that the palate is functional when repaired and the second is that the individual is prepared to face a major operation after having managed with the disability for so long. All these aspects should be considered by the dental surgeon and then explained to the patient and only if he shows a marked keenness for surgery should he be referred to a plastic surgeon for an opinion and possible treatment. The opinion of an Ear, Nose and Throat Surgeon and speech therapist should be sought when assessing the possibility of improved speech with either line of treatment.

Generally for patients of this class the ideal treatment is the fitting of an obturator which, if after due trial confers no advantage, can be discarded and the individual will have been put to little discomfort. In most cases, however, if speech training is given, the improvement with an obturator is sufficient for the patient to continue to wear the appliance with benefit and in some cases the improvement is outstanding.

Perhaps the most difficult class of case in which to make a decision as to whether the fitting of an obturator will confer benefit is the one where surgery has produced a united soft palate but without any marked improvement of speech. In these cases a diagnosis must be made as to the cause of failure. It may be due to faults of articulation which the individual has been unable to eradicate either because of lack of perseverance or of desire to improve or because of dullness of hearing or lack of intelligence. It may on the other hand be due to failure of function of the united palate which, although it appears from examination through the mouth to be long enough and sufficiently functional to occlude the nasopharyngeal isthmus, is in fact neither of these. Examination of palato-pharyngeal contact by observation through the mouth is misleading because the main area of contact of the palate with the pharynx is in the middle third of the palate which is bunched up by the action of the levators and this cannot be seen by observations through the mouth. A palate which appears long enough may in fact entirely lack this bunching up action. Another test of palato-pharyngeal closure, which in many cases is valueless is the blowing up of a balloon or manometer because frequently an individual with palatal insufficiency or even a patent cleft can produce quite impressive rise of mercury by filling the cleft or pushing the short palate up with the back of the tongue. The two tests which are valuable however are (1) the snoring test and (2) a lateral X-ray.

Snoring results from drawing air in through the nose and by its passage to the lungs forcefully separating the raised soft palate from the pharyngeal wall. The air passes in a series of short puffs causing the soft palate to vibrate producing the snoring sound. If the soft palate is incapable of making firm contact with the pharynx snoring is impossible.

A lateral X-ray is taken after several drops of barium solution have been introduced into each nostril while the individual is lying down and the head gently moved from side to side to spread the barium over the palate and pharynx. The exposure should be made while the patient is making the action of sounding a prolonged 'P' but without actually parting the lips.

This will cause the soft palate to rise to its high level if it is capable of so doing. Several X-rays may be needed to produce convincing evidence of palatal position and function. Such X-rays frequently reveal what appears from oral examination to be an adequate palate, to be merely a thin sheet of soft tissue completely out of contact with the posterior pharyngeal wall. At other times, it reveals a fully functional and competent palate.

In the former case an obturator shaped and placed to occlude the space which exists between the repaired soft palate and the pharynx is justified and frequently produces excellent results. Such an obturator is attached to the supporting denture by a tailpiece which crosses the united soft palate (*see* fig. 542). Details of this are given later in the chapter.

The Clinical Technique for Producing an Obturator

There are some differences in the technique for making an obturator for those cases where the cleft is patent along the length of the soft palate or hard and soft palates and those where surgery has produced a united but incompetent soft palate. The differences in technique only apply up to the point of commencing to trim the speech bulb, thereafter they are similar and therefore up to this point they will be described separately.

The Technique for an Unrepaired Cleft of the Hard and Soft Palates

A composition impression is taken in a stock tray and there is no need to extend this impression much beyond the posterior border of the hard palate as nothing is to be gained at this stage by trying to obtain a comprehensive impression of the remnants of the soft palate and the pharynx.[1] In cases with unrepaired clefts involving both the hard and soft palates the composition will of its own accord flow upwards into the cleft in the hard palate.

On the model cast from this impression a special tray is constructed of base plate tray material which straddles the

[1]At the end of this chapter details are given of the technique of taking a comprehensive impression of the pharyngeal structures if such an impression is required for record purposes.

cleft in the hard palate and is not contoured into it. In this tray an alginate impression is taken (*see* fig. 544): normally no impression material is placed in the cleft, because, if an adequate amount is put on the tray, sufficient flows into the cleft to give a satisfactory impression and if too much material is present it may flow excessively on to the nasal side of the cleft of the hard palate and when the tray is removed the material will tear, leaving the nasal section of the impression *in situ*. If this does happen, in most cases it can be retrieved by inserting a probe deeply into the remnant of the impression and sliding it back towards the soft palatal cleft where it can be brought downwards into the mouth. Sometimes, however, the nasal section becomes locked into place by the turbinate bones and then has to be removed piecemeal which can be a trying proceeding for both the patient and the operator and as nothing is gained by obtaining an excessive impression of the nasal cavities it is wisest to limit the impression material in this region. In wide clefts no problems are usually encountered with excess material, but in

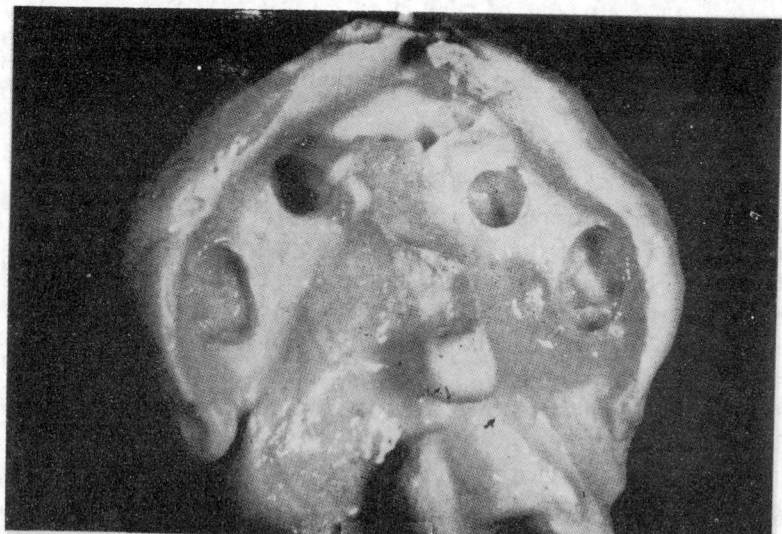

Fig. 544. – Alginate impression of the mouth of an individual with a cleft palate.

narrow ones or those where a surgical union has broken
down, leaving a hole or series of holes in the palate (*see* fig. 522)
it is wise to pack these with vaseline gauze prior to taking the
impression, for if alginate material does flow into the nose
through a small defect, serious difficulty may be experienced
in its removal.

The working model cast from the alginate impression is
surveyed in the normal way and the cleft in the hard palate
filled in with plaster of Paris so as to reproduce the contour of
a normal palate and on this prepared model a record block is
constructed. The records are then taken in the usual manner
and if the case is one where a reconstruction of the appearance
is to be undertaken, the record block is built up and contoured
with wax, to which trial teeth may be attached if necessary,
until a pleasing fullness of the lips has been obtained.

On the articulated models the artificial teeth are set in
positions demanded by appearance and occlusion.

At the try-in the usual points are checked and a wire loop
made of German silver of dental wire gauge 2, is bent to
shape and attached with sticky wax to the base of the trial
denture. This loop should lie along the centre of the cleft of
the soft palate, completely out of contact with its remnants
or with the posterior pharyngeal wall when a prolonged 'Ah'
is sounded and its plane should be slightly above that to which
the soft palate remnants rise when the 'Ah' sound is made
(*see* fig. 545). It should be adjusted by bending and altering
its position in the wax until it satisfies these requirements.
If the loop is made of German silver wire it is more easily
adjusted than if made of stainless steel. When the trial denture
is satisfactory it is returned to the model and plaster is flowed
around the wire loop to hold it in position and the case processed and finished. The denture is now ready for the trimming
of the speech bulb.

In those cases where difficulty with regard to the wearing of
the denture is anticipated it is sometimes desirable to leave the
wire loop off the denture altogether allowing the patient to
wear the denture by itself for a week or two until it is quite
comfortable. The wire loop may then be added to the denture

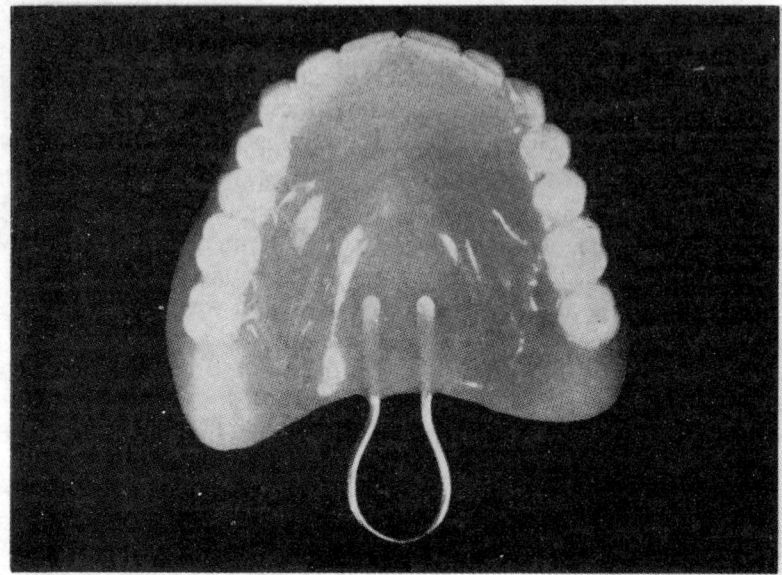

FIG. 545. – Denture carrying wire loop.

with cold cure resin so as not to induce extra strains in the acrylic by a second processing.

A Technique for Repaired but Incompetent Soft Palates

After the denture has been completed and fitted, a tailpiece must be made and positioned so that when attached to the back edge of the denture it crosses the united soft palate at a level just below that which the latter assumes when fully relaxed. If the tailpiece is at a higher level when the soft palate relaxes it will rest on the tailpiece, which, being narrow, will cause discomfort and pressure sores. If on the other hand the plane of the tailpiece is much below that assumed by the relaxed soft palate, then it will cause discomfort by obstructing the movements of the tongue.

The technique of locating the plane of the tailpiece is as follows: to the back edge of the denture a piece of pink baseplate wax is luted with sticky wax, this wax should be about $\frac{3}{8}$ in. wide and long enough to cross the soft palate into the pharynx. The denture carrying the wax is then inserted into the

mouth and the patient asked to relax and breathe through the
nose. If left in place for a few minutes the wax will be moulded
by the relaxed soft palate above and the tongue below to conform to the plane and contour of the relaxed palate. The denture is carefully removed and the wax chilled thoroughly. The
denture is then replaced into the mouth and a check made of
the plane of the wax in relation to the relaxed soft palate
when observed with the mouth open. To do this the patient is
asked to open the mouth, to relax fully and breathe through the
nose; if there is any appearance of the wax supporting the soft
palate the shaping technique as previously described should be
repeated. When the plane and contour of the wax is satisfactory, a plaster model is cast under the palatal side of the wax
and extending sufficiently far under the denture to enable it
to be located. When the plaster is set, and this will only take a
few minutes if an accelerator is used, the wax is removed, the
plaster painted with cold mould seal and a thin mix of cold
cure resin is run on to the plaster in place of the wax and
carried on to the back of the denture which has been roughened
sufficiently to ensure a firm union. When the cold cure resin
has hardened it is trimmed and rough polished and tried in the
mouth to ensure it is in the same relation to the soft palate
as was its wax precursor. The pharyngeal end of the cold
cure tailpiece is then grooved and holes are bored in it and
a piece of gutta-percha, softened in boiling water, is firmly
secured to the tailpiece and roughly shaped into a flattened
ellipse, with its long axis lying laterally. The denture carrying
this tailpiece and gutta-percha is then inserted into the mouth
and the gutta-percha gently pressed upwards, behind the
soft palate, into the region of the nasopharynx and the patient
requested to swallow, say 'Ah' and move the head from side to
side. A drink of warm water or preferably hot tea will facilitate
swallowing. This action will bring the muscular pressure of
the posterior and the lateral walls of the pharynx and the
posterior border of the soft palate to bear on the softened gutta-
percha and shape it to conform to the space which exists in the
nasopharyngeal isthmus due to the incompetence of the soft
palate (*see* fig. 546). The denture is then removed and the gutta-
percha inspected; it will probably have increased in dimension

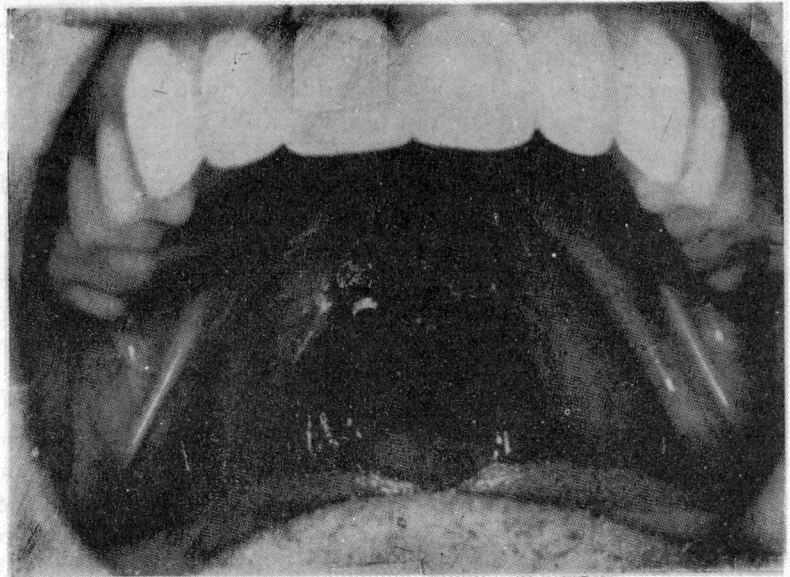

Fig. 546. – Cold cure acrylic 'bridge' crossing soft palate with gutta-percha attached to it being moulded into the incompetent area of the united palate.

from top to bottom and become flattened anteroposteriorly and show evidence of moulding, and its periphery, where the gutta-percha has been squeezed into the nasopharynx, should be trimmed slightly with a very hot wax knife which will cut the gutta-percha easily without dragging. The gutta-percha should then be dipped into very hot water, tested for temperature on the back of the hand, because gutta-percha, being a very poor thermal conductor, holds its heat and, when cool enough, inserted into the mouth and the trimming routine repeated. In order to check that the gutta-percha has been moulded by the delicate tissues of the palate instead of distorting them, some zinc oxide starch and lanoline paste is applied to the dried palatal surface of the acrylic tailpiece and the anterior surface of the gutta-percha and the whole reinserted and the trimming routine repeated. On removal, a completely unbroken film of white paste with clear-cut evidence of tissue moulding should be evident. If the black gutta-percha or

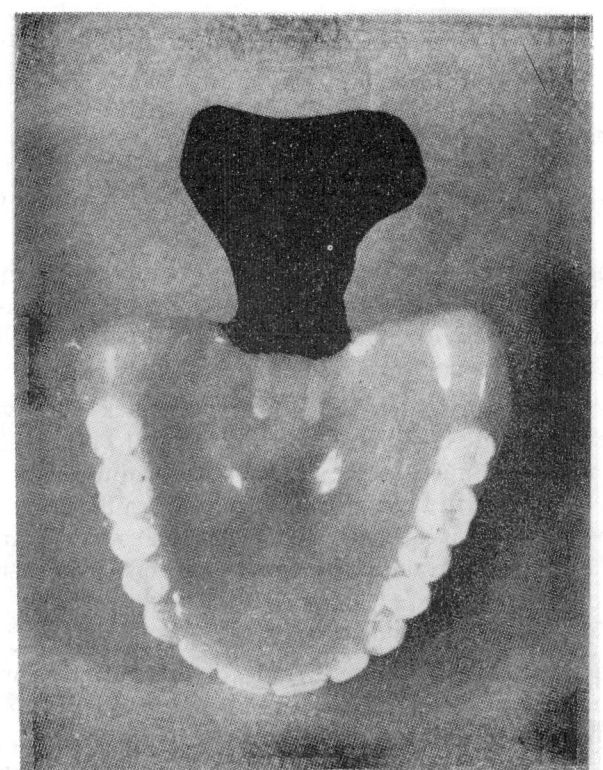

FIG. 547(b).

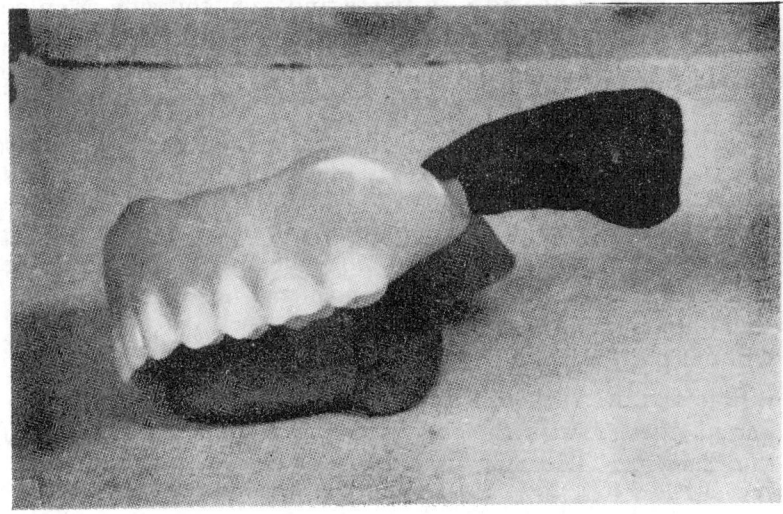

FIG. 547(c).

piece if desired, but it is more bulky than a well-contoured chrome cobalt tailpiece. The assembly is now ready for the final trimming of the speech bulb.

The Trimming and Shaping of the Speech Bulb for Dentures Carrying a Wire Loop or a Tailpiece

In both the case of the patent cleft and the repaired but incompetent palate, the speech bulb is formed in gutta-percha and fully adjusted to fit the movements of the pharynx and palatal remnants before being processed in acrylic.

The type of gutta-percha used is the black variety which has the advantage of remaining soft enough to be moulded by the pharyngeal musculature for about 5 minutes after each heating, while at the same time remaining sufficiently viscous to support its own weight. It is therefore deformed by muscular pressure and then retains the shape impressed on it by that pressure.

Gutta-percha is supplied in sheets about ⅛ in. thick and about a third of a sheet is sufficient for the construction of the average speech bulb. This amount is placed in boiling water; it can be dropped in a sterilizer for convenience. After three to four minutes it will be quite soft and it is then removed from the boiling water, dried in a napkin, rolled into a ball, one side of which is heated in a flame and then this side adapted to the wire loop or the tailpiece of the denture. The dry heat will make the gutta-percha sticky and it will adhere firmly to the support. The ball of gutta-percha is then roughly adapted with the fingers to conform to the shape of the deficiency as it appears on the master model, that is T-shaped, pear-shaped or a flattened ellipse (*see* pages 738 *et seq.*). By this time the gutta-percha should have cooled sufficiently to be tolerable to the tissues, but before inserting it into the mouth it should be tested on the back of the hand and if too hot held under the cold tap for a few seconds: such cooling, unless protracted, will not reduce its ability to flow.

The denture is then inserted into the mouth and the gutta-percha pressed with the fingers upwards and backwards into the pharynx. The patient should be given a cup of hot tea to

drink; the heat of the tea will tend to maintain the ability of
the gutta-percha to flow. The swallowing action thus initiated
will cause the palato-pharyngeal sphincter to contract and the
muscles of the soft palate to function and they will commence
to mould the gutta-percha so that it fills the space occupied by
the cleft and adapts itself at its periphery to the form of the
functioning muscles. After several sips of tea the denture is
removed and the gutta-percha inspected. A limited change
will have taken place in its shape and it should show evidence
of having been moulded: the posterior border should show a
tendency to be flattened, the lateral corners a tendency to
roundness and, in the case of a T-shaped cleft, the lateral surfaces a tendency to narrowing. The pear-shaped clefts will
produce less or no narrowing at all, but show evidence of a
side to side flattening while the repaired soft palate type will
show evidence on its anterior surface of moulding by the
posterior border of the unrepaired palate. If the amount
of gutta-percha is excessive, the excess will have been forced
mostly up into the nasopharynx but a little may have escaped
downwards, between the back of the tongue and the posterior
pharyngeal wall. If insufficient gutta-percha was present to
fill the cleft, none will have been forced into the nasopharynx
and some of its surfaces will show no evidence of moulding.
The moulded surfaces will develop a matt appearance and
those not moulded will still retain some of the shiny appearance of the gutta-percha as originally inserted. Where evidence of excess gutta-percha is present it should be removed
with a very hot wax knife which will cut it easily and cleanly
without dragging. Where a deficiency appears more soft gutta-
percha should be added by drying and flaming both the
surfaces to be united. After these adjustments the gutta-percha
bulb should be dipped in very hot water for about a minute
and after testing for temperature reinserted in the mouth and
more tea drunk. This routine should be carried out several
times and on each removal further evidence of moulding or
lack of it will be evident with its need for removal or addition
of gutta-percha (see fig. 547).

When swallowing has impressed on the gutta-percha a
definite form, movements of the head should be instituted

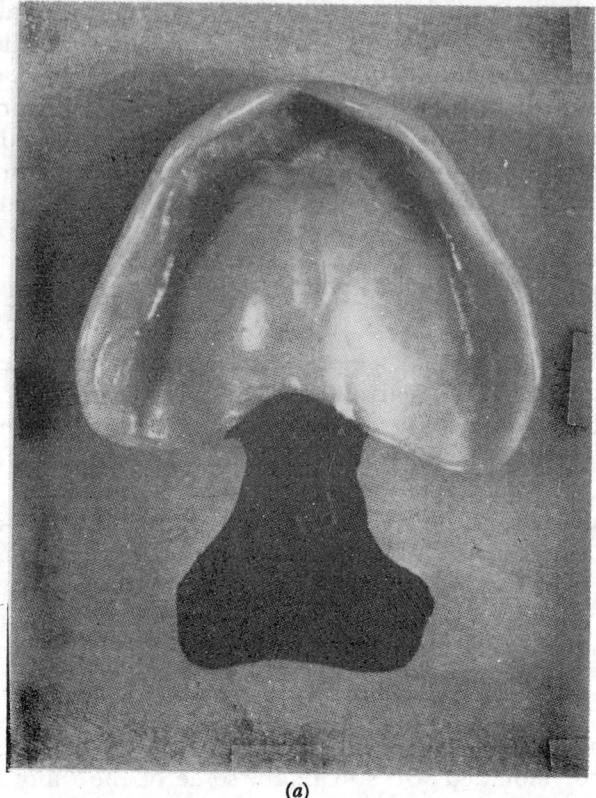

(a)

Fig. 547. – Speech bulb in process of being moulded in gutta-percha looked at from (*a*) Top, (*b*) Bottom, (*c*) Side.

because these have an effect on the shape of the pharynx and if the gutta-percha is not moulded to accommodate them the finished speech bulb will cause pressure with ultimate ulceration when such movements are made. The patient is therefore requested to bend the head forward and then move it from side to side. These actions should be performed several times. Next the action of speaking should be induced to mould the gutta-percha and the patient should be asked to say some of the plosive consonants, which produce the greatest action of the pharynx and palate, as forcefully as possible. The sounds themselves and words containing them should be spoken, such

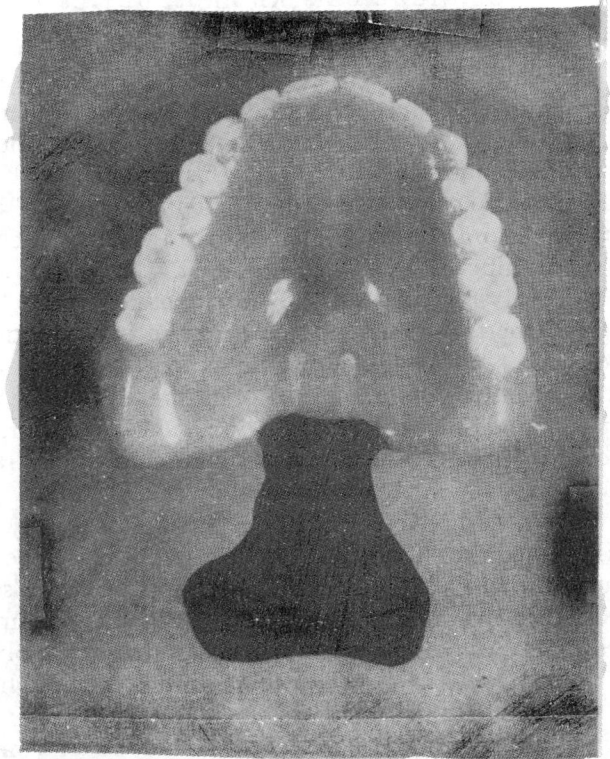

FIG. 547(b).

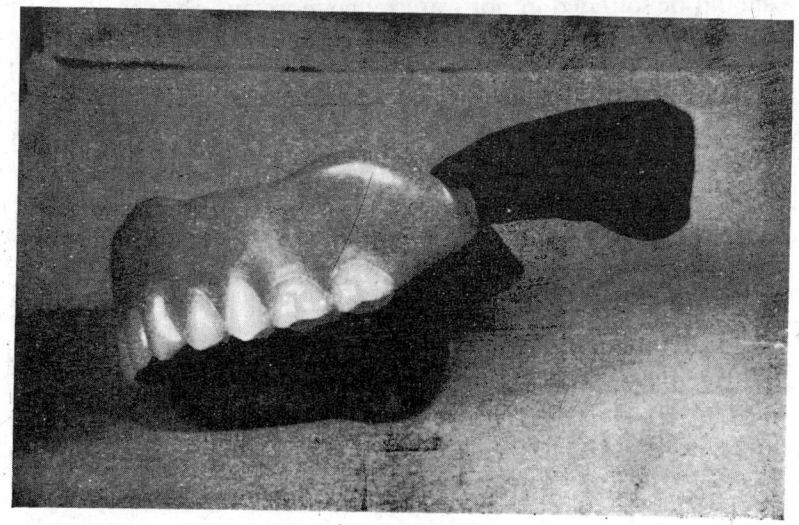

FIG. 547(c).

as 'P' and 'pa', 'B' and 'bar', 'C' and 'car', 'G' and 'gar'. By this time the gutta-percha bulb will have developed a very definite form around its periphery, but its superior and inferior surfaces and its thickness will be variable. These should now be adjusted and to do this the bulge of Passavant should be evoked by asking the patient to say 'Ah' with the mouth open and the bulge painted with a little zinc oxide in olive oil of sufficient viscosity not to run. The dentures should then be gently replaced and the patient asked to say 'Ah' and swallow. When the denture is removed the area of action of the bulge of Passavant will be visible as a white smudge on the back of the gutta-percha and the bung should then be trimmed superiorly and inferiorly so that it is ⅛ in. above the highest plane and ₁₆ in. below the lowest plane of travel of the bulge of Passavant.

The form of the inferior surface should be gently concave looking downwards because this shape will allow the greatest amount of room for the dorsum of the tongue and also deflect the airstream from the larynx into the mouth. The upper surface should curve as steeply as possible towards the pharynx so that nasal secretions can flow backwards towards the throat (*see* fig. 547).

By now the gutta-percha bulb should be of comfortable proportions and the patient should be tolerating it easily. It should be softened in hot water once more and then the patient dismissed to wear it for twenty-four hours or so with the warning that it may feel strange to begin with but that he will soon become used to it.

When the patient returns it will be found in most cases that the bulb has undergone further considerable moulding, especially in the areas within the grasp of the palato-pharyngeal sphincter and, in the case of T-shaped bulbs, in the region of the levator muscles. Excess gutta-percha which has been squeezed upwards and downwards by this action should be trimmed away and the patient should then be questioned regarding the 'feel' of the speech bulb. Such questions as 'does it make the throat sore', 'does it help or impede swallowing', 'does it impede nasal breathing' are asked. If a complaint of soreness is made the whole bulb should be coated with a paste made of zinc oxide and starch mixed with lanoline and the patient given more tea to drink. Hard pressure spots will then be revealed as areas where the white paste is completely thinned by the pressure of the enveloping muscles and the black gutta-percha will show through. These areas should be trimmed with a hot wax knife and more paste applied to check whether or not the over-extension has been reduced. This should be continued until the black gutta-percha remains covered by the white paste. If swallowing becomes more difficult with the bulb in place it may be due to the fact that the inferior surface of the bulb is too concave and part of the food bolus lodges in it. A flattening of the concavity should be effected. In most cases where nasal breathing is impeded it will be found by the white paste test that the whole bulb is over size so that the tissues are unable to relax away from it and produce a breathing space around it. In these cases the whole bulb should be re-softened and the whole cycle of trimming movements vigorously and persistently repeated. If any doubt exists in the operator's mind that the bulb is not fully or correctly adapted it should be wiped clear of white paste and fully re-softened and the patient dismissed for another twenty-four hours.

When the bulb appears to have reached a final shape it should be coated all over including the upper and lower surfaces with white lanoline paste and subjected to the trimming movements of swallowing, speaking, and head movement (*see* figs. 548, 549, 550). It should then be removed from the mouth, care being taken not to distort the paste and on inspection it will be observed that the tissues have moulded the paste into a form perfectly adapted to their movements. Provided no hard areas of gutta-percha are visible through the paste the whole should be invested in plaster of Paris, the gutta-percha and paste removed and the resulting cavity filled with wax and processed in acrylic resin.

If the denture is well retained and the speech bulb is not too large the latter can be made of solid acrylic. If, however, the denture is poorly retained due to there being only a few natural teeth present in the upper jaw or if it is a full upper denture, or if the speech bulb is large, then to reduce

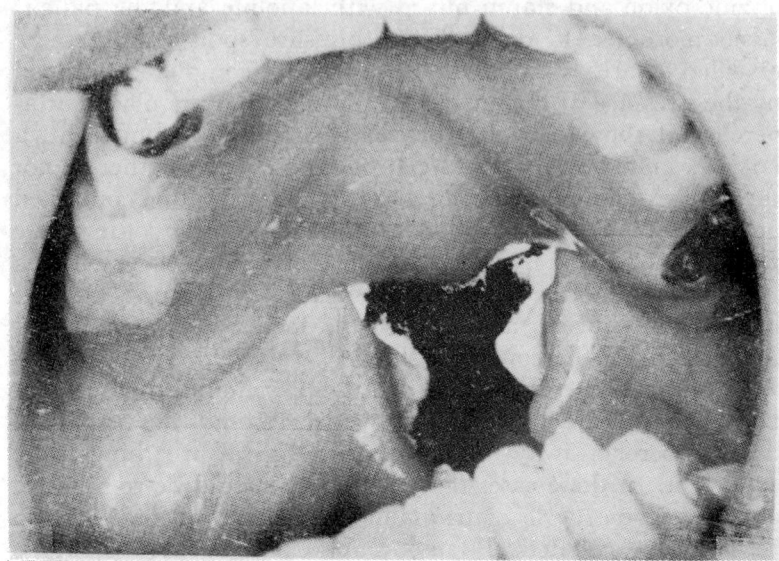

FIG. 548. – Speech bulb made of gutta-percha covered with zinc oxide paste, for final detailed trimming, in place.

the weight of the appliance the speech bulb can be made hollow (*see* fig. 551).

The Technique for Taking a Comprehensive Impression of a Cleft

A preliminary impression is taken in composition in a suitable stock tray. The tray is loaded with an excess of composition and introduced into the mouth in the normal manner raising the front of the tray in place first. Due to the presence of the excess impression material as the back of the tray is raised the composition will flow backwards and due to its own weight tend to drop on to the tongue. At this stage a finger should be introduced into the mouth and the composition gently pushed backwards and upwards into the cleft of the soft palate and against the posterior pharyngeal wall. The patient should be requested to breathe through the mouth as nasal breathing will, of course, be impossible. When the composition is in place the patient should be encouraged to raise the remnants of the palate and contract the pharynx by saying 'Ah'. The tray should be removed carefully before the compound has

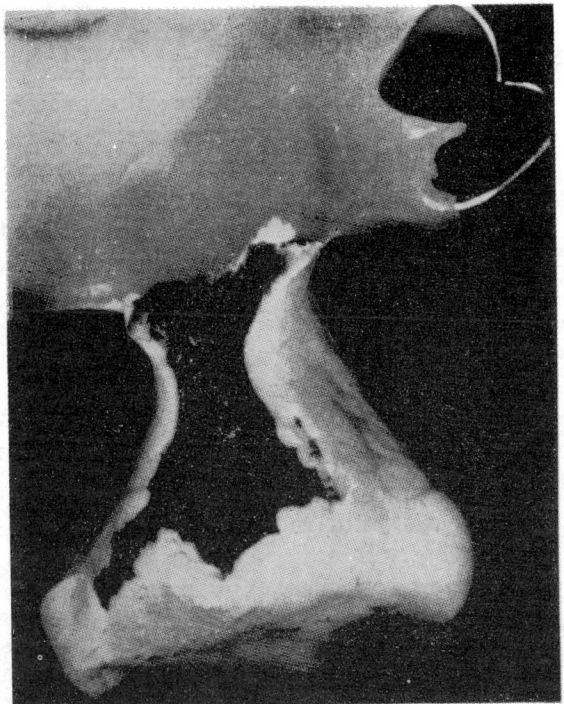

FIG. 549. – Speech bulb shown in fig. 548 after trimming. Note the 'waist' area trimmed by the palatal remnants and the distal area trimmed by the posterior wall of the pharynx.

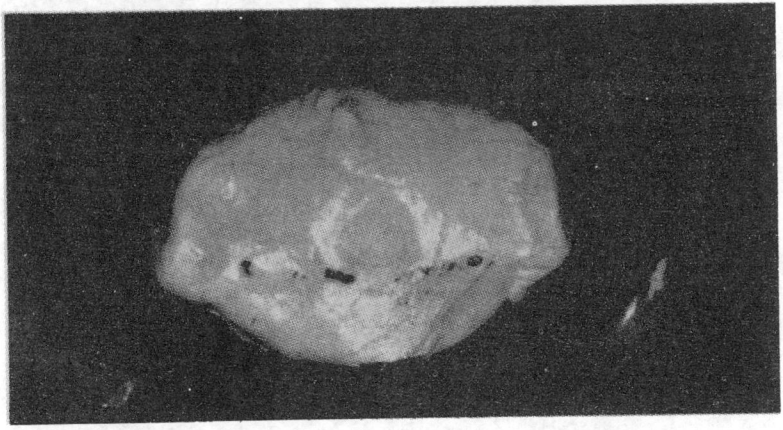

FIG. 550. – Speech bulb shown in figs. 548 and 549 looked at from the back showing in greater detail the effects of the pharyngeal trimming. Note the hollow in the centre made by the tissues overlaying the anterior arch of the atlas (*see* fig. 438(*b*)) and the lateral grooves made by the salpingo-pharyngeal muscles. The pencil line indicates a groove made by the sphincter muscle.

hardened fully and then immediately chilled. The large majority of patients with cleft palates exhibit marked insensitivity of the palatal and pharyngeal regions to contact stimuli and are usually quite unembarrassed by the presence of a large mass of composition in the pharynx. A few individuals, however, do exhibit retching. In some of these the sucking of a benzocaine tablet will enable a comprehensive impression to be obtained, but in a few cases such an impression is impossible. In these individuals the operator should be content with obtaining an impression up to the normal limits usually secured for making a denture and not attempt an impression or the pharynx. Although a comprehensive impression is valuable when constructing an obturator its absence does not make its construction impossible.

On the model cast from the preliminary composition impression, a special tray is constructed of base-plate tray compound over a generous spacer. It is extended to the normal outline in its normal part and merely straddles the cleft in the hard palate, if one exists, and is not pushed up into it. The

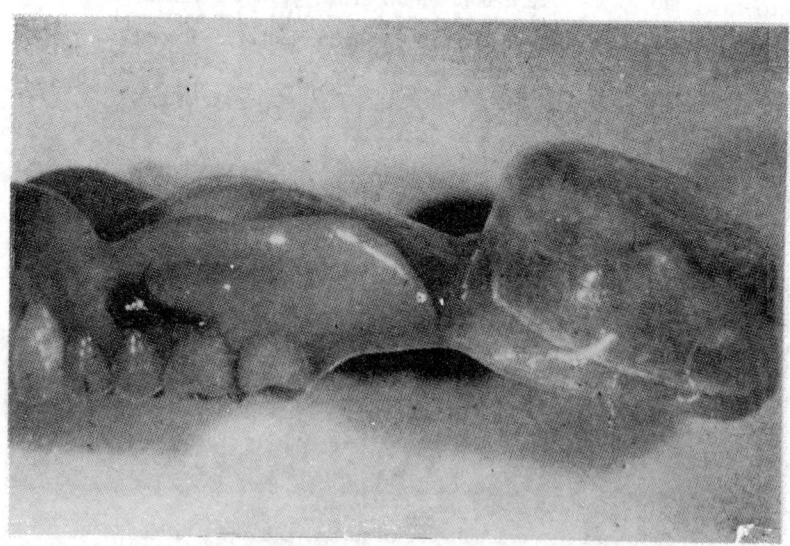

FIG. 551. – Hollow bulb obturator to reduce weight.

extent of the pharyngeal part of the tray should be to within
⅟₁₆ in. of the pharyngeal walls all round.

In this tray an alginate impression is taken. The alginate
material is spread evenly over the tray and then introduced
into the mouth, raising the front of the tray first and then the
back of the tray is gradually brought into position with a
gentle wriggling motion which spreads the impression material
out and allows it to flow gently up into the cleft. When the tray
is in place, the patient is requested to say 'Ah' once or twice
and to contract the pharyngeal walls. Normally no impression
material is placed in the cleft, because, if an adequate amount is
put on the tray, sufficient flows into the cleft to give a satisfactory impression and if too much material is present it may
flow excessively on to the nasal side of the cleft of the hard
palate and when the tray is removed the material will tear,
leaving the nasal section of the impression *in situ*. If the tray is
correctly extended and correctly positioned no problem is
usually experienced with impression material flowing towards
the throat, because any excess can escape more easily into the
nasopharynx. If some material does commence to flow down
towards the throat, however, it can be retrieved easily by a
long, flat, wooden spatula which should always be at hand.
A simple way of reducing this problem is to mix the alginate
material for a cleft impression with a few drops of water less
than the normal, and this will increase the viscosity of the
material sufficiently to limit its tendency to drip. If when the
alginate impression is in place, the patient commences to retch,
he should be reassured in the normal manner and under no
circumstances should the impression be removed before it is
set. Even if the patient vomits, provided that a bowl is placed
under his chin he will come to no real harm. It is wise,
however, to limit the alginate impression to the oral cavity in
patients who showed any tendency to retch when the composition impression was being taken. A model is cast in the
alginate impression and immediately duplicated so that a
record and reference model is available.

After-care of Patients with Obturators

It will take a little while for an individual to adapt himself to wearing an obturator and he must be encouraged to learn to grip the bulb when speaking as in the act of swallowing.

The only improvement in the voice to be anticipated when the obturator is fitted is in the tone: the deeply ingrained faults of articulation will only be rectified by speech training given by an experienced speech therapist, to whom the patient should be referred when the obturator has been fitted. Close co-operation with the speech therapist will ensure any adjustment in the shape of the speech bulb which may be necessary as progress in voice production is made.

CHAPTER XXIX

SURGICAL PROSTHESES

The replacement of tissue lost from the mouth or face as the result of trauma (such as road accidents and war wounds) or surgery for the removal of malignant growths all comes within the province of prosthetic dentistry and the following section gives information on some of the commoner types of appliance needed for the treatment of these conditions.

Obturators for Intra-oral Loss of Tissue by Surgery

The commonest cause of tissue loss results from the removal of growths in the maxillary antrum. Such growths frequently involve the alveolar process and part of the palate and the

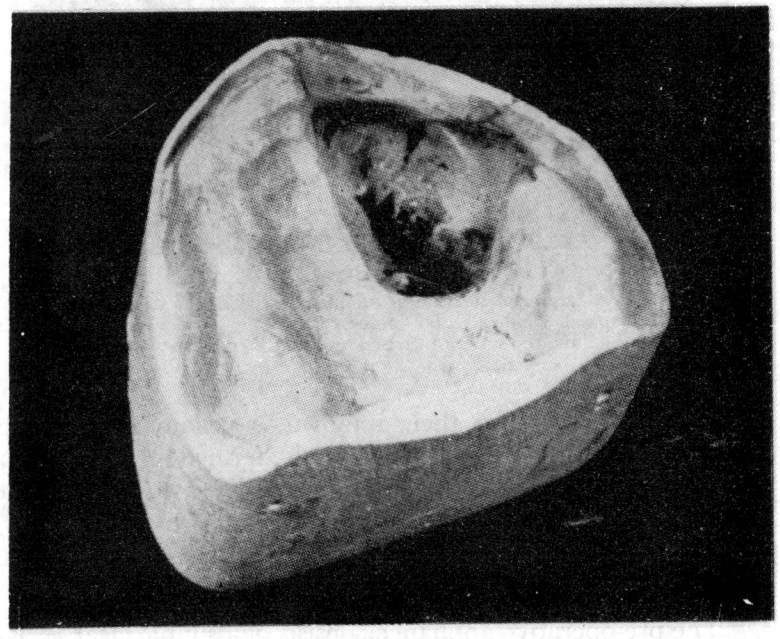

Fig. 552.
(a) Model of a medium-sized palatal fenestration.

767

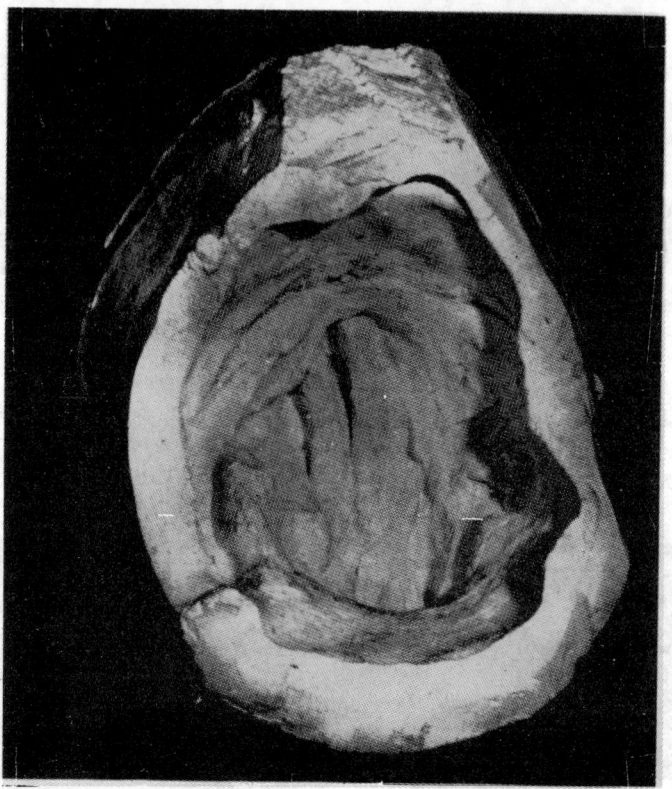

FIG. 552.
(b) A large fenestration involving the whole of the hard palate and alveolar process. Anterior border of soft palate, the superior turbinates and the maxillary antrum can be seen.

surgical approach for their removal is usually through the mouth, leaving post operatively a hole, termed a 'fenestration', varying from the size of a penny to complete loss of palate and alveolar process (*see* fig. 552).

The prosthetic treatment for these conditions demands a pre-operative and post-operative appliance.

The pre-operative appliance consists of a simple clear acrylic palate made to an impression of the upper jaw taken pre-operatively (*see* fig. 553). Immediately after operation the

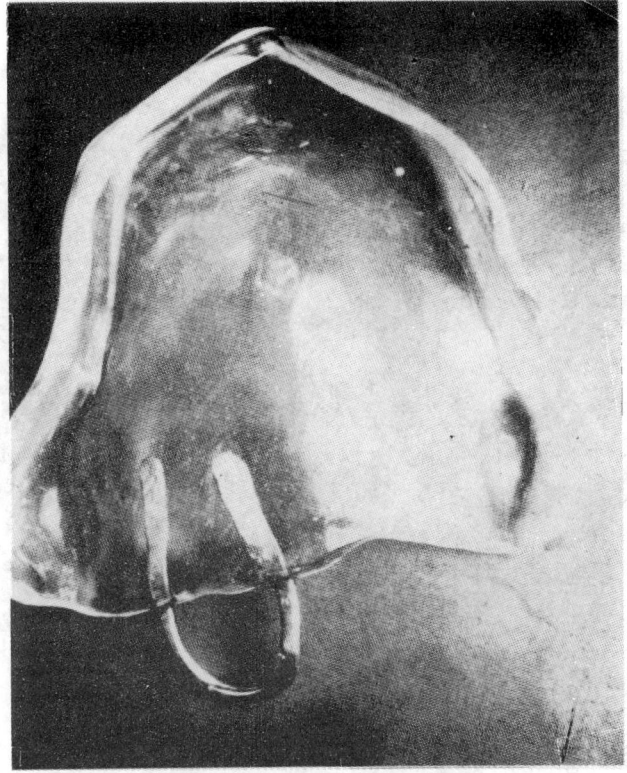

FIG. 553. – Pre-operative palates for fenestration cases.
(a) With a wire loop to carry gutta-percha.
(b) With Vitallium screws for fixing in the bone of the midline of the palate.
(c) Plate (b) in place in mouth. This type of fixation is only rarely called for when extensive surgery prevents simpler methods of fixation being used.

palate is inserted and held in place by gum tragacanth or, in extreme case, by Vitallium screws placed in the midline of the palate (*see* fig. 553). The purpose of this appliance is to enable the patient to speak, eat and drink normally. As soon as the wound has healed sufficiently and is no longer painful an alginate impression is taken in a special tray, care being taken to ensure that excess alginate does not flow into the nasal cavities and become locked therein so that it remains

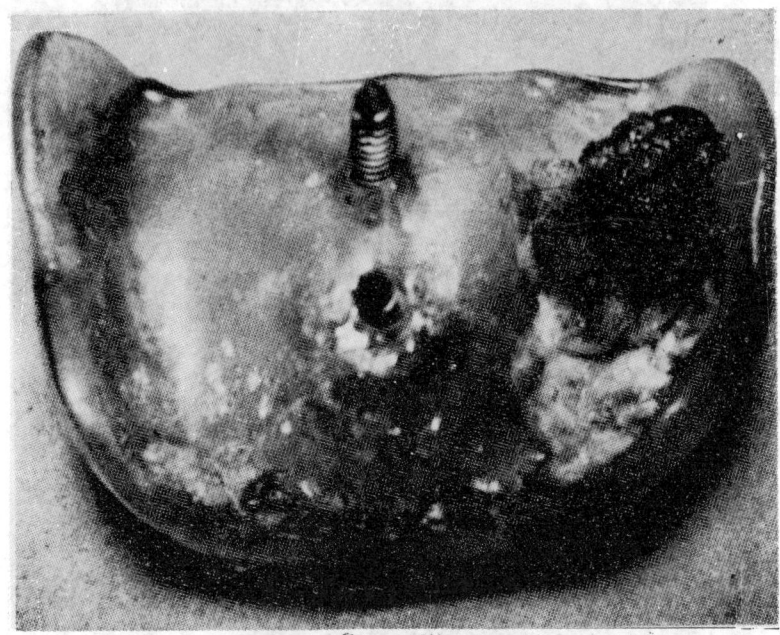

FIG. 553(b).

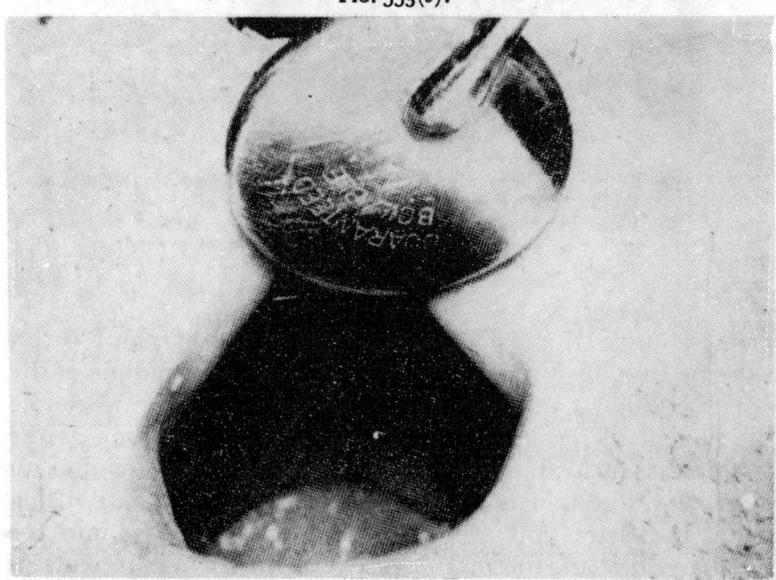

FIG. 553(c).

in place on removal of the main impression (*see* fig. 554). Judgment of the amount of impression material used is the simplest way to ensure this, but Vaseline gauze can be packed into parts of the nasal cavity if necessary.

On the model cast from this impression an acrylic base-plate is constructed to the normal outline of an upper denture and penetrating into the cavity for as short a distance as is necessary to produce a seal. On this base-plate the records and try-in are carried out and then the denture is finished by processing teeth to the base-plate with cold cure resin so as not to warp the base-plate by heat.

The retention of the denture will depend to some extent on the size of the fenestration wound. If this is small the denture can be retained normally by adhesion and peripheral seal, although this latter is naturally reduced, and tongue control.

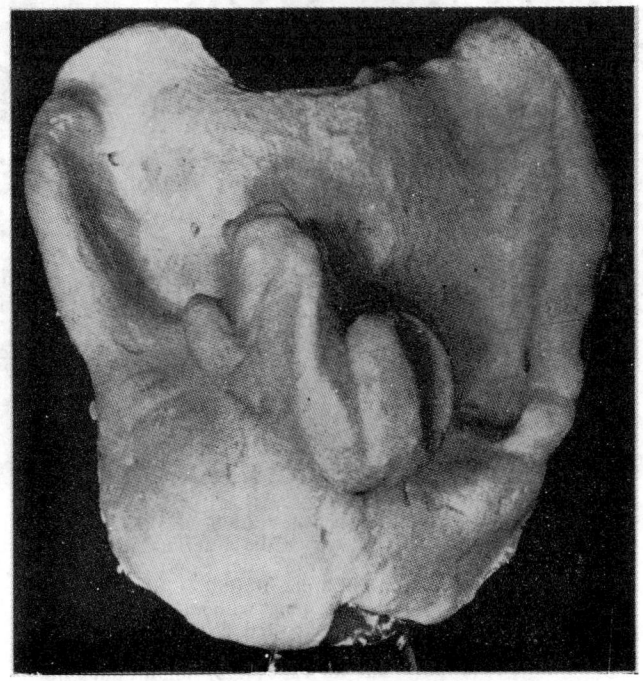

FIG. 554. – An alginate impression for a fenestration case.

In cases presenting a large wound, springs are usually successful.

In cases of extreme loss of tissue, such as shown in fig. 555 where the whole of the palate was removed, the appliance requires to be made hollow to reduce its weight. This is achieved by the use of a plaster and pumice core.

Facial Prostheses

Any part of the face may need to be replaced by a prosthesis, either as a temporary measure prior to plastic surgery or as a permanency.

The technique is briefly as follows: An impression is taken of the area surrounding the missing parts. This may need to be done in plaster, alginate or a combination of the two. If the

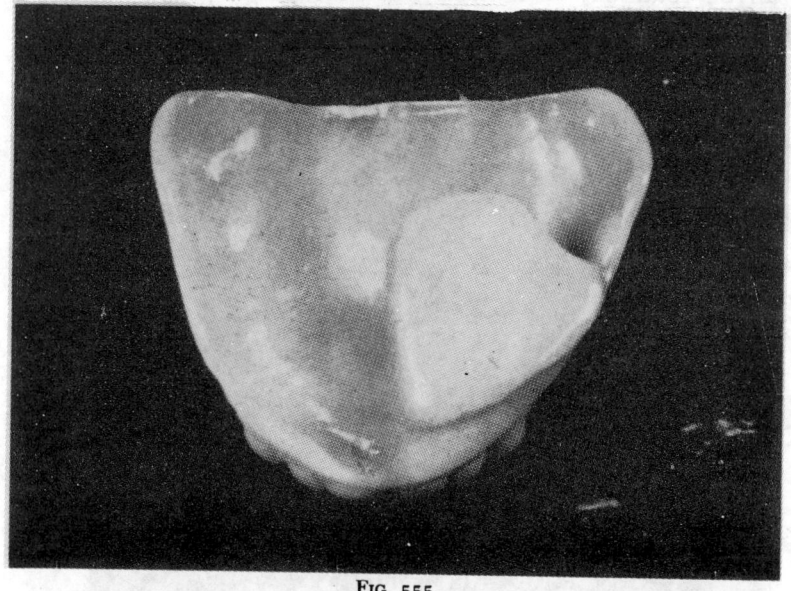

FIG. 555.

(a) A simple denture for a fenestration case with little penetration into the cavity because stability and retention are good; (b) from the side.

(c) A denture with complete penetration into the cavity because stability was very poor without it. This type of obturator must be hollow to reduce weight and have a tube to facilitate nasal breathing.

(d) A large obturator made for case 552(b) hollow and with springs for retention.

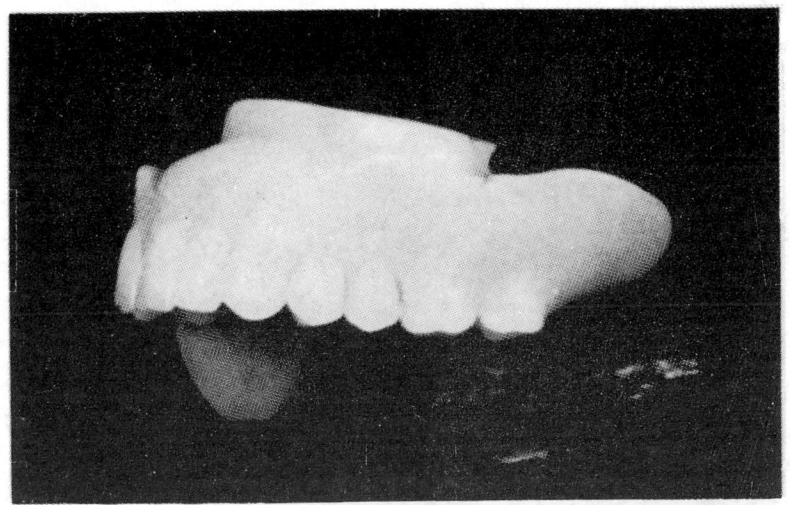

FIG. 555(b).

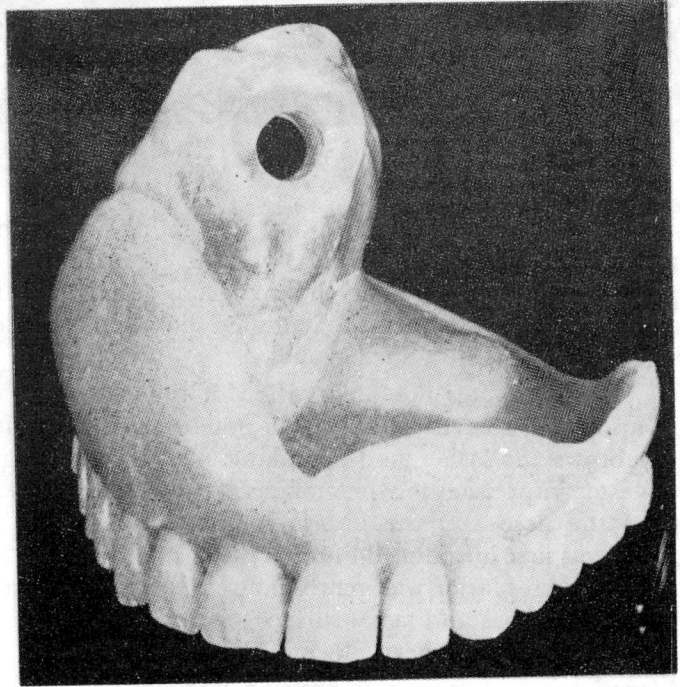

FIG. 555(c).

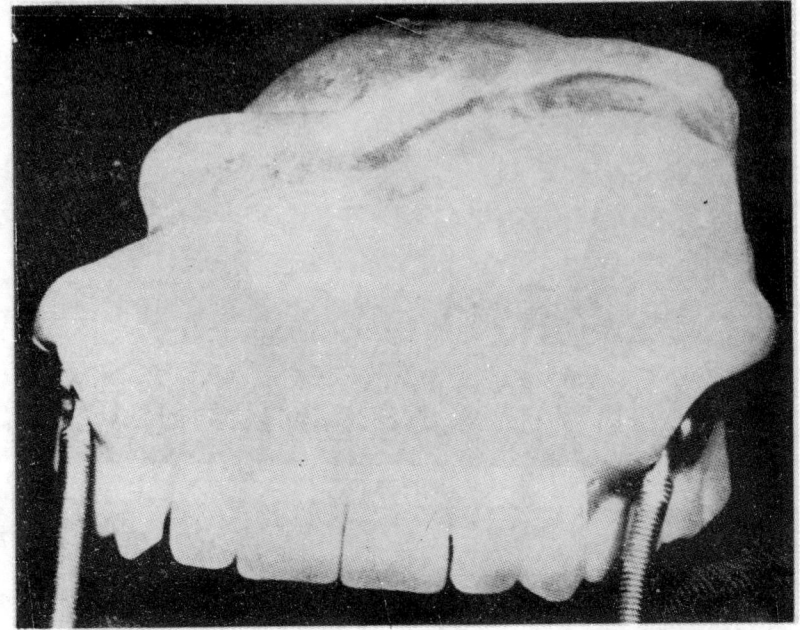

FIG. 555(d).

tissues to be impressed are firm and unyielding or part of the nasal cavities with undercut areas need to be included in the impression, then alginate is the material of choice. If the tissues are soft and mobile then plaster should be employed, for alginate will distort such tissues.

Fig. 556 illustrates the preparation of the patient prior to the impression, so that plaster does not become entangled in the eyebrows and lashes, and the taking of a combined alginate and plaster impression for the making of a prosthesis to replace part of the nose and the upper lip. In the case illustrated alginate was first introduced into the nasal cavities and allowed to set and then plaster was gently poured and shaped over the outside of the nose and facial surfaces with the patient supine. The impression is shown in place in fig. 556.

A model is cast to this impression and on this model the missing parts of the nose and lip are fashioned in plasticine

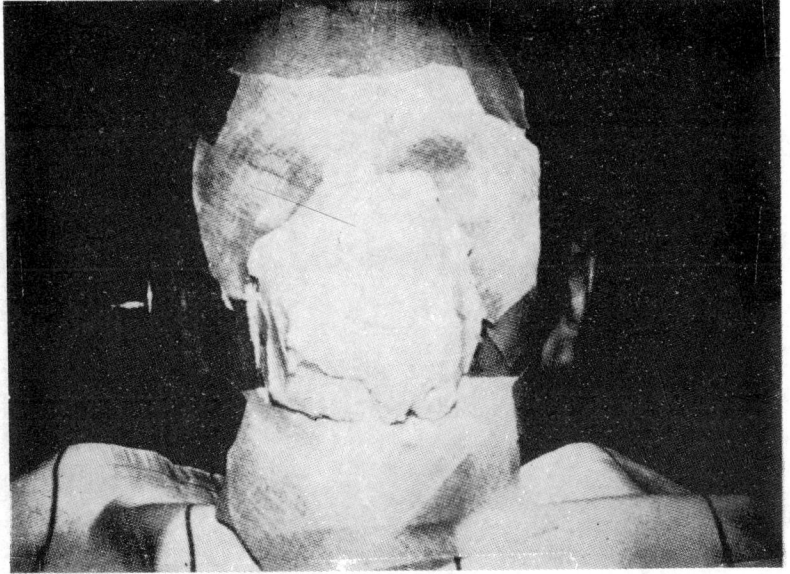

Fig. 556. – Plaster impression being taken for patient
illustrated in fig. 558.

(*see* fig. 557). This model is then duplicated and cast in plaster
and on this plaster model a thin sheet of casting wax is laid and
moulded to reproduce all the contours. The use of negative
cores is sometimes a help in achieving this. This wax template
is then finally fitted to the master model from which the plasticine has been removed and then processed in clear acrylic
resin. This results in a very thin, completely clear, template of
the correct shape of the missing parts. This is tried on the
patient's face and, if acceptable with regard to shape and fit,
is coloured on the under-surface with artists' oil paints. These
can be mixed at the chairside and painted on and removed
until the correct shade and match to the patient's skin is obtained.
The paint is allowed to dry for a few days and then sandwiched
between the original template and a layer of cold cure acrylic
which is painted thinly over the dried paint. This type of
appliance can produce an excellent colour match and is clean,
as it can be washed; it is very light and adequately durable
and simply replaced if the models are kept.

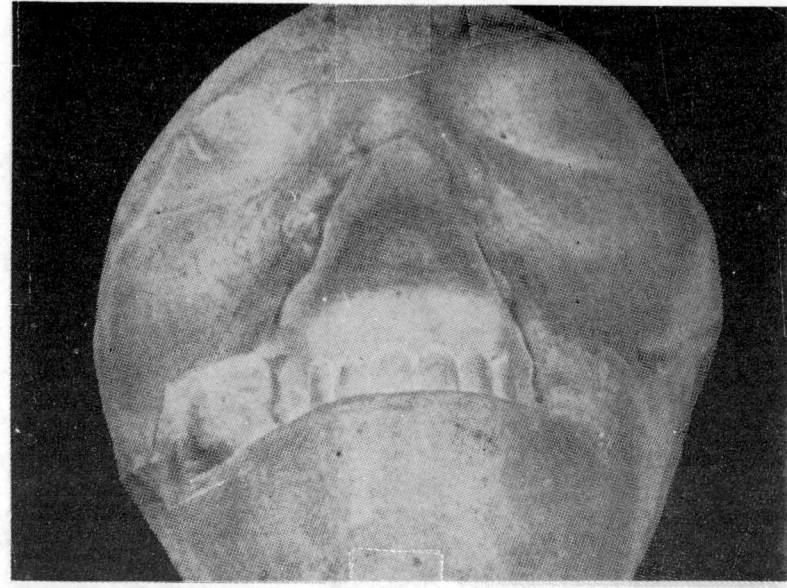

Fig. 557(a). – Model cast from impression of face.

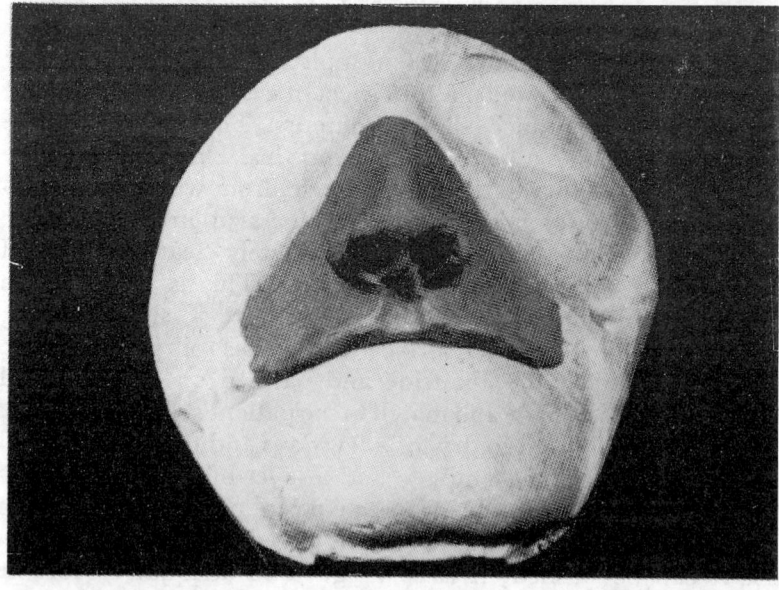

Fig. 557(b). – Plasticine nose and lip in process of being fashioned in this model.

The polyvinyl chloride prostheses, however, have the advantage of resiliency and are frequently preferred by patients for this reason.

Basically, polyvinyl chloride for dental use consists of a mixture of 'Corvic. S.U.' powder sold by I.C.I. together with an equal weight of dibutyl phthalate plasticizer which is then heated in the plaster mould to a temperature of 147° C. This temperature is critical, if only slightly exceeded burning of the final product ensues. To reduce the danger of charring a small quantity (about 10 per cent by volume) of calcium stearate is included in the mixture.

Processed P.V.C. is translucent and human tissue is semi-opaque, therefore a variable quantity of an opacifier is also required and this may be either zinc oxide or titanium oxide powder and the quantity should be varied to suit the part being made.

The colouring of polyvinyl chloride prostheses to match the surrounding tissue is not simple and trial and error, using test pieces of P.V.C., is necessary to achieve a satisfactory result.

Dyes are produced by I.C.I. in the form of powders which may be mixed with the dibutyl phthalate: a selection is as follows:

Lithafor Red A.S.
Waxolene Red O.S.
Waxolene Green G.S.
Waxolene Blue
Lithafor Yellow A.S.
Lithafor Brown A.S.

The dyes should be made up separately in a concentrated solution with dibutyl phthalate and the required number of drops of each put into the clear plasticizers with a pipette before mixing in the powders.

Final colouring of the prostheses may be achieved after processing by reducing excessive colouring by rubbing the surface of the prosthesis with a pad of cotton-wool soaked in acrylic monomer. Extra colouring may then be added by working in various dyes dissolved either in acrylic monomer or dibutyl phthalate on a pad.

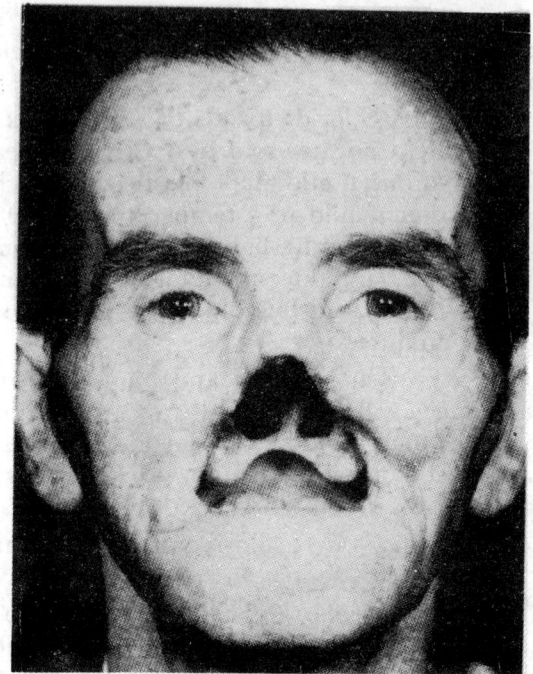

Fig. 558 (*a* and *b*). – Patient who has lost nose and upper lip.

Facial prostheses can, in most instances, be retained by a pair of spectacles (*see* figs. 558 to 561) and if the patient does not need glasses for vision plain lenses are employed.

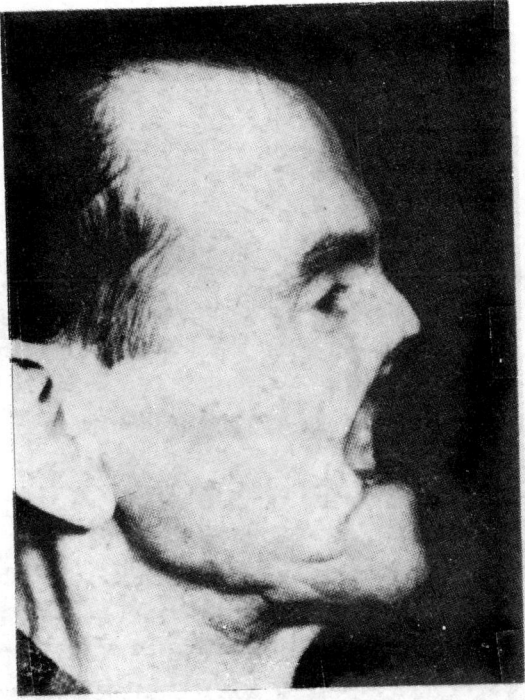

Fig. 558(*b*).

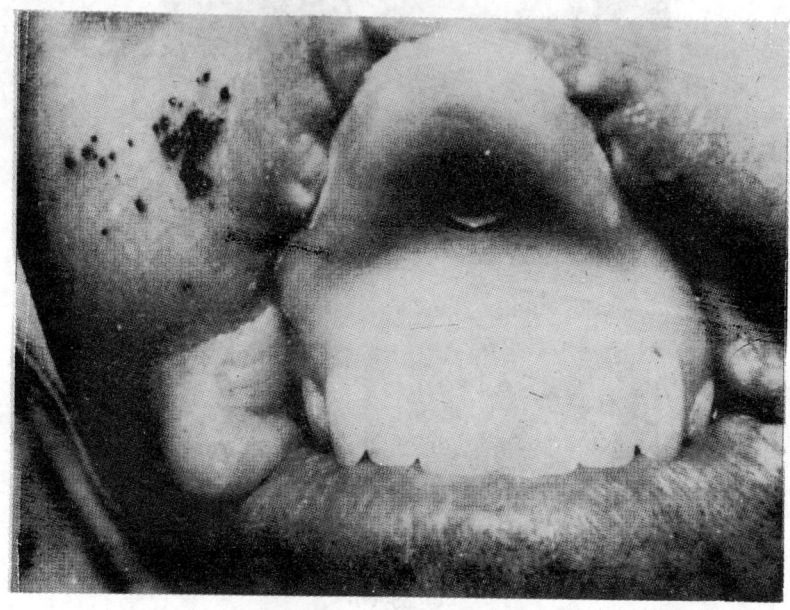

FIG. 559(a). – Denture in place for patient illustrated in fig. 558. Note breathing tube.

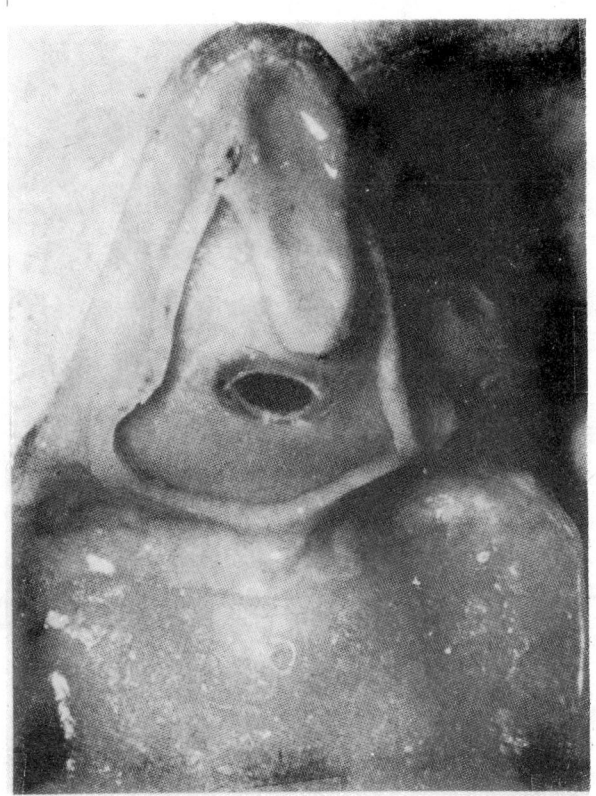

Fig. 559(b).

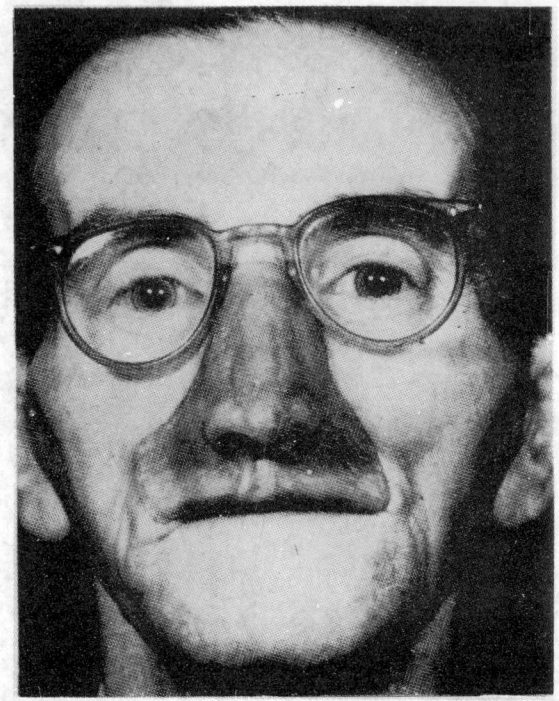

FIG. 560 (*a* and *b*). – Patient illustrated in fig. 558 wearing P.V.C. prosthesis held in place by denture and glasses.

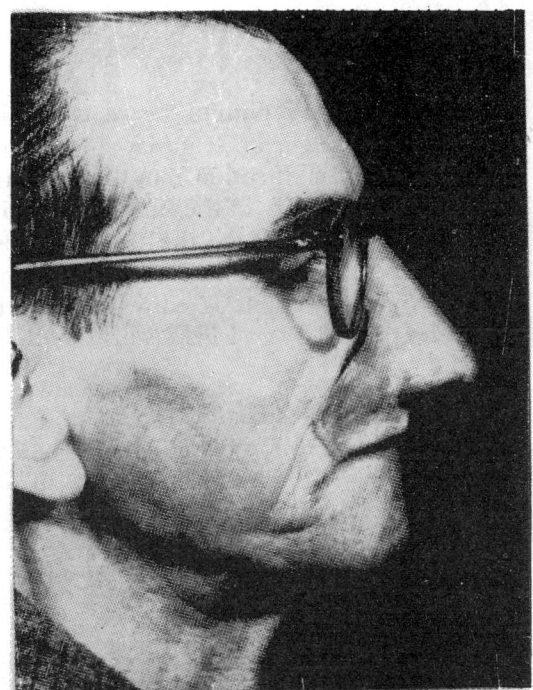

Fig. 560(*b*).

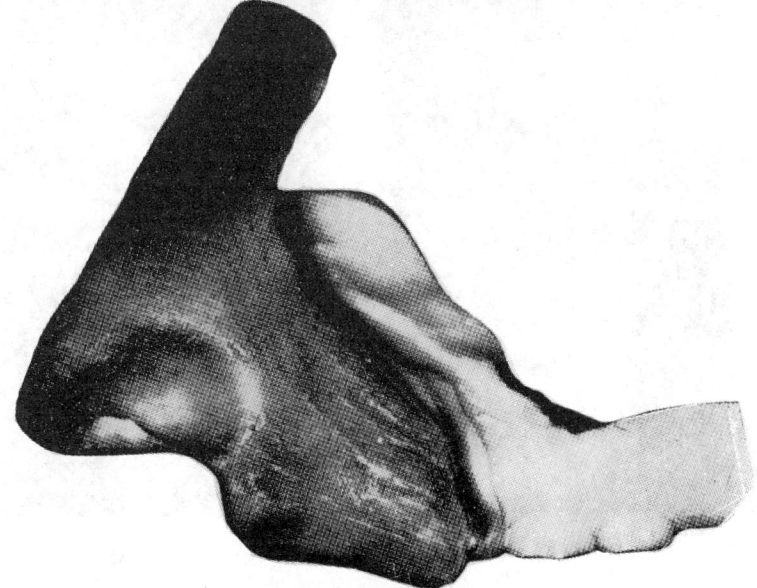

Fig. 561. – Prosthesis attached to denture.

Lip Splints

Paralysis of the seventh cranial nerve is a fairly common occurrence. It may result from trauma, surgery, or sometimes occurs spontaneously. Its duration may be permanent or temporary. It results in flaccidity of the muscles of facial expression on the side affected. Frequently the physician or surgeon in charge of the patient requests the construction of a splint to support the lip. Such a splint is conveniently attached to a denture or, if the patient has all his natural teeth, to an acrylic palate.

The splint is made of cold cure acrylic and attached to a wire loop or to a removable rod and should be adjusted to fit at the corner of the mouth and support the lip in its normal position, that is, level with the opposite functional side (*see* fig. 562).

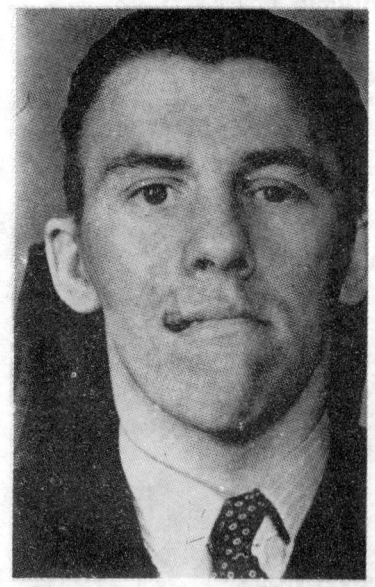 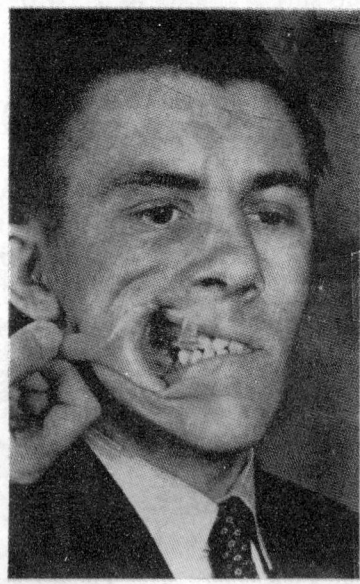

FIG. 562. – A lip splint.

Chapter XXX

IMPLANT DENTURES

Ever since prosthetic dentistry became an entity practitioners have sought for a means of increasing the retention, stability, efficiency and comfort of dentures for those patients presenting grossly absorbed edentulous ridges. The life of such individuals is often made miserable by the continual instability of their dentures or by the pain engendered through pressure on friable mucosa overlying an irregular bone surface or on a mandibular or mental nerve which has come to lie submucously as a result of the excessive absorption of the alveolar ridge.

It has long been obvious that were it possible to anchor a denture in such cases to the bone by means of a metal insert that a great deal could be achieved. Such a metal insert attached to the surface of the bone with abutment posts penetrating the mucous membrane is termed an implant and during the last century many spasmodic attempts have been made with a variety of metals and alloys, employing a large number of techniques, to perfect such implants. Metal teeth with fenestrated roots made of lead, gold, platinum, silver and stainless steel have been inserted into tooth sockets after extraction. All these failed because the implant was rapidly exfoliated.

One of the main reasons for this failure was the electrolytic incompatibility of such metals and alloys with the body tissues. This major disadvantage disappeared with the advent of the chrome cobalt alloys, such alloys being electrolytically inert as discovered by Venable and Stuck (1936). The usefulness of these alloys in surgery and their compatibility with the body tissues was first utilized by the orthopaedic surgeons who used Vitallium as plates and screws for positioning the ends of fractured bones.

About fifteen years ago serious attempts were made by dental surgeons to develop a method for implanting chrome cobalt structures into the jaws which would provide a firm stable base to support dentures in cases presenting major prob- lems of stability or discomfort. The first subperiosteal implant was placed by Dahl of Sweden in 1943 and this was followed by Gershkoff and Goldberg in 1948, and in Great Britain by Mack and Trainin in 1952/53.

From the earliest attempts to the present day there have been many successes and many failures and many techniques have been tried and modified or abandoned. At the present time however as the result of the work of a comparatively small number of pioneers, a technique for making and inserting a chrome cobalt implant has been developed which is sufficiently reliable to employ in those cases in which all other normal methods of providing comfortable and efficient dentures have failed, and the following pages give in outline form the stages of this technique:

The Technique of Making and Fitting a Lower Chrome Cobalt Implant

The normal prosthetic procedure for constructing full upper and lower dentures is carried out until the dentures have reached the 'try-in' stage. At this point the occlusion and appearance of the dentures are carefully checked and if approved the upper denture is finished in the normal way, the lower denture being retained in the waxed up stage. In the laboratory the first molars and the canines are removed from the waxed up lower denture and a sharp instrument is thrust through the wax in approximately the centre of the areas occupied by these teeth until it penetrates the surface of the ridge of the plaster model beneath sufficiently to mark it (*see* fig. 563). These marks on the model locate the positions of the abut- ments of the future implant. A piece of base plate wax is next adapted to the ridge of the model and contoured to the shape of a denture base and then withdrawn and processed in clear acrylic. It is replaced on the model and small holes are drilled through it in the areas marked for the future abutment (*see* fig. 564). The purpose of this acrylic template will become apparent in due course.

Next two special trays are made to fit the model of the lower

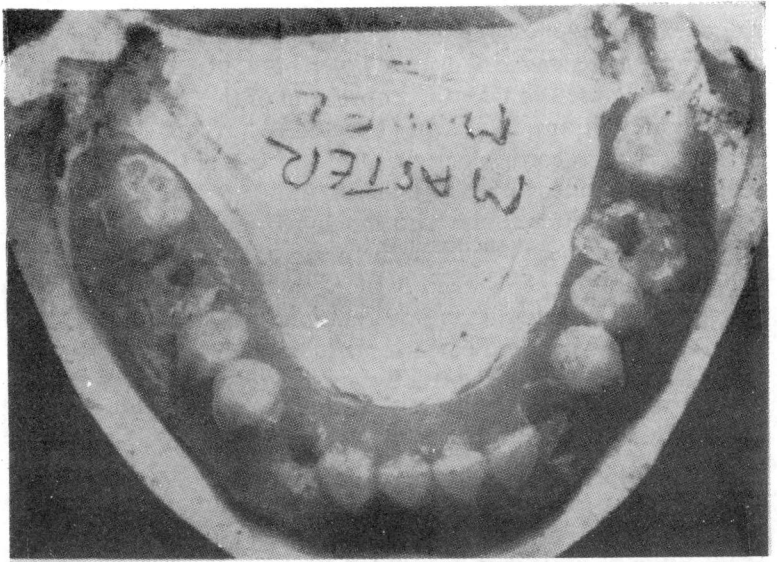

Fig. 563. – Lower denture after 'try-in' with canine and molar teeth removed and holes bored through wax into surface of ridge of model.

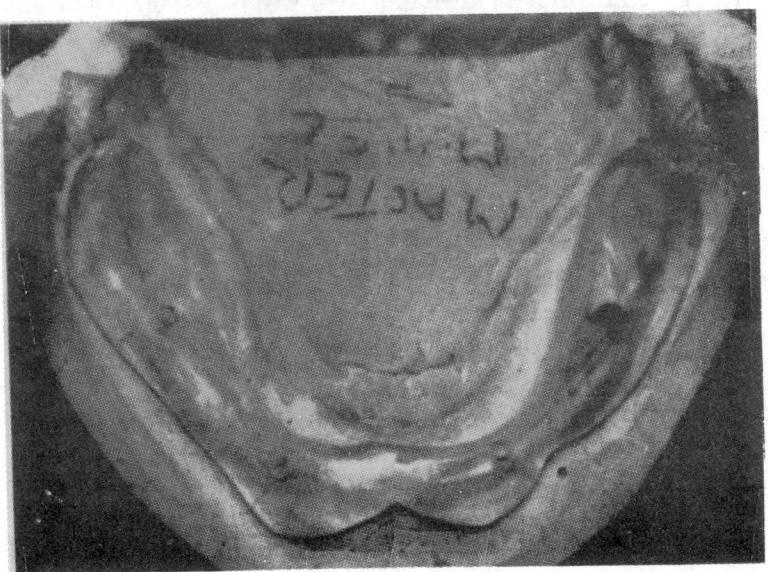

Fig. 564. – Clear acrylic template, fitting lower model, with holes bored.

ridge extending buccally and labially. These trays may be constructed in swaged German silver or light cast tray metal. They will be used to take the impression of the bone when the mucous membrane has been reflected.

An acrylic record block is also constructed to the lower model to occlude with the finished upper denture. Rims are only built in the premolar and molar regions, and wire staples are inserted into the acrylic in the premolar regions to facilitate its manipulation. This record block will be used lined with gutta-percha to record the jaw relationship when the mucous membrane has been reflected so as to enable the models of the bone impression to be correctly articulated in relation to the upper denture.

The Exposure of the Bone and the Taking of the Bone Impression

If an implant is to be successful it must fit the surface of the bone accurately and for this to be possible it must be constructed to an impression of the bone itself, therefore, the fitting of an implant demands two surgical stages. The first consists of the reflection of the mucous membrane followed by the taking of at least two impressions of the surface of the bone, together with the recording of the occlusion, also taken with the record block fitting the bone. The second stage which is usually carried out about three weeks after the first operation consists of the reflection of the mucous membrane and the insertion of the completed implant.

The First Operation

For this the acrylic template, the special trays, the acrylic record block and the finished full upper denture are needed, together with all those surgical instruments usually employed for the reflection of mucous membrane and its stitching together again. In addition some composition, gutta-percha and rubber or silicone base impression material is required.

The patient is pre-medicated and the mandible anaesthetized with double mandibular and long buccal injections. (It is possible to perform this operation under general anaesthesia but a local is preferred because the co-operation of the patient is helpful.)

The clear template is positioned on the surface of the lower ridge and the point of a probe thrust successively through the holes in the template. This action produces four bleeding points corresponding to the location of the future abutment posts. Next the thickness of the mucous membrane at the site of the bleeding points is measured using a probe with a sliding rubber washer on it. A tungsten carbide round bur size No. 3 is now sunk into the bleeding points and shallow pits drilled into the surface of the bony ridge. The purpose of these pits is that they will be recorded in the impression of the bone and thus in the model cast from this impression, and locate clearly the positions of the abutment posts. It is important that a tungsten carbide bur is used because a steel bur might leave small steel particles in the pits in the bone and these could produce an electrolytic action with the implant which might be sufficient to invalidate it.

Next an incision is made on the crest of the ridge commencing at the retromolar pad of one side and passing successively through each bleeding point and finishing at the opposite retromolar pad. Cross incisions are made lingually and buccally in the retromolar pad regions and in the mid-line. The mucoperiosteum is now carefully reflected to expose the mylohyoid ridges, the external oblique ridges, the genioid tubercles and the mental nerves which are carefully identified. As wide a reflection of the mucous membrane as possible is desirable.

The reflection complete, the surface of the exposed bone is examined and any sharp or rough areas smoothed with a bone file (see fig. 565).

Taking the Bone Impression

The next operation is the taking of the bone impression, and on its accuracy success or failure of the implant to a large extent depends. If the substructure of the implant is a close fit over as wide an area of the bone as possible, it will posses an inherent stability which is all important.

To facilitate the insertion of the impression tray the lingual mucoperiosteal flaps are joined with sutures passing under the

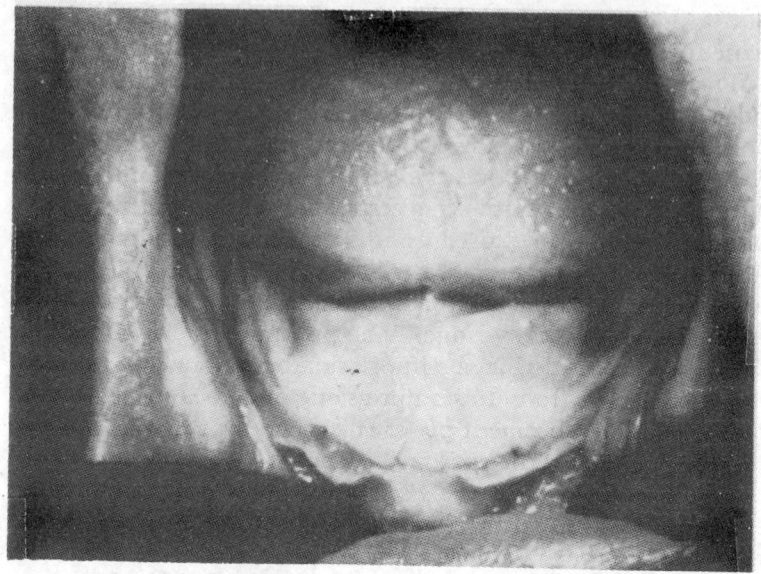

FIG. 565. – Mucous membrane reflected and bone exposed.
Note sharp ledges of bone which were removed prior to
taking impression and holes bored in surface of bone in
$\overline{3|3}$ region.
(Photograph by kind permission of Mr. M. A. Kettle.)

tongue, and when the sutures are looped and pulled tight the
lingual flaps are retracted.

The impression tray is now tried in. Its insertion is simplified
if it is inserted under the buccal flap of one side first, and then
rotated into position while the opposite buccal flap is elevated
out of the way. The front part of the tray being seated finally
while the labial flap is retracted. The tray should cover the
whole of the bony region, and should only be trimmed if too
large. An over extended bone impression is far better than an
under extended one. The tray is withdrawn and loaded with
composition of an even thickness (about ⅛ in.) and reinserted
in the manner previously described for the empty tray. Before
seating the composition fully into place any mucoperiosteal
flaps which have been trapped under its edges must be carefully retracted. When fully in place the composition is chilled

with a jet of sterile iced water. When set hard the composition is removed and inspected. It should show impressions of the mylohyoid ridges, the external oblique ridges, the mental nerves and the genioid tubercles, and should be well extended over the labial surface of the ridge. The surface of the composition is now carefully dried, and then covered with an even thickness of mixed rubber base or silicone impression material and again inserted and held in place until the impression material has fully set. The composition stage can be omitted and the rubber base material used alone if desired. A typical completed bone impression is shown in fig. 566. A second bone impression is then taken. It is essential that two impressions are taken because it is difficult to assess their absolute accuracy and therefore it is a safe precaution to have two implants made, one to each impression. If facilities allow it is wise to have the models cast to these impressions while the occlusal record is being taken and then the models checked visually with the surface of the bone before suturing the flaps together. After

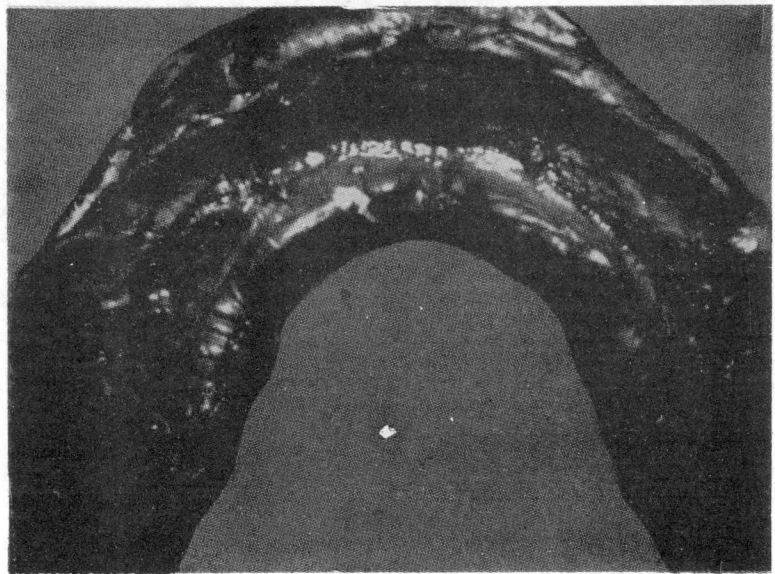

FIG. 566. – Rubber base impression of bone surface.

the impressions have been taken and the wound cleaned of any small pieces of impression material which may have remained in place, the fitting surface of the acrylic record block is lined with softened black gutta-percha, and a little soft wax placed on the occlusal surfaces of the blocks. The gutta-percha is located on the bone surface and the patient instructed to relax and close the softened wax gently against the teeth of the finished upper denture which has previously been inserted (*see* fig. 567). The positioning and stabilizing of the record block is facilitated by inserting the fingers into the wire staples in the pre-molar regions of the block. The final stage of the first operation is the careful approximation of the mucoperiosteal flaps with sutures.

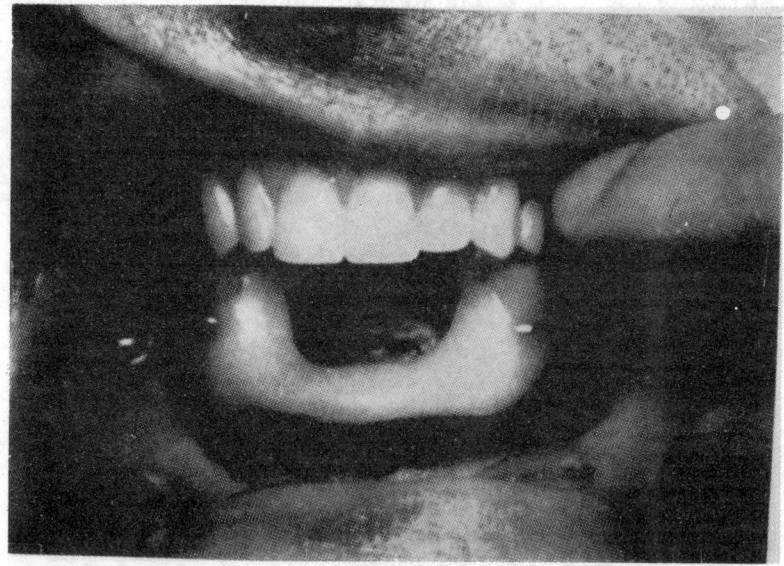

FIG. 567.
(a) Acrylic record block lined with gutta-percha in place on ridge.
(b) Record block out of mouth.
Note wire loops to facilitate holding block in place.

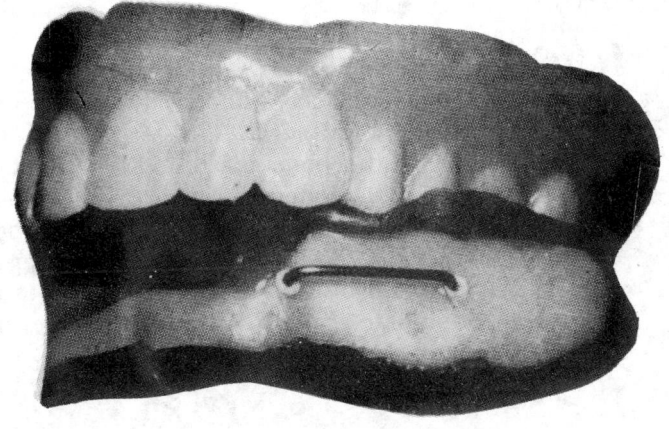

FIG. 567(b).

A Brief Outline of the Laboratory Procedure for Producing an Implant

(1) The model of the bone (fig. 568) is articulated with the upper denture by means of the record block.

(2) The model is duplicated in chrome cobalt investment material.

(3) The substructure of the implant is outlined on this model. The abutment posts are positioned as indicated by the small location pits in the model and the bars of the frame-work are kept as narrow as possible commensurate with strength. The periphery of the frame-work is located on or over the external oblique ridges, and well short of the mylohyoid ridges, because if it protrudes lingually beyond these structures it will ulcerate through the thin lingual mucosa. It is kept well clear of the mental nerves and is carried as deeply as possible down the labial surface of the ridge. The struts joining the abutment posts to the periphery of the framework are kept narrow and the spaces between them wide. Any additional struts required for strengthening the substructure should be as few as possible and little or no metal should be placed in or across the incision line. The proposed outline of a typical implant substructure framework is shown in fig. 569.

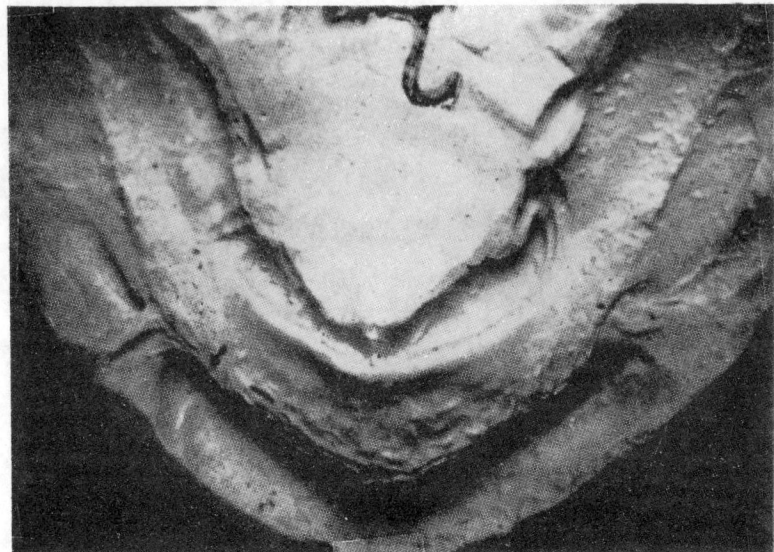

FIG. 568. – Model cast from impression of surface of bone.
Note the neurovascular bundles.

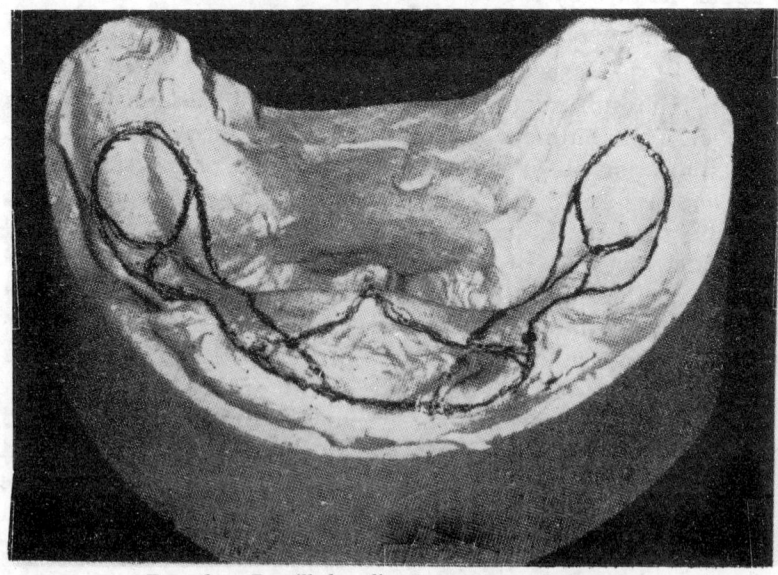

FIG. 569. – Pencilled outline for implant substructure.

(4) The implant is waxed up to the proposed outline (*see* fig. 570). The abutment posts should be shaped as shown in fig. 571 with a neck of $2\frac{1}{2}$ to 3 mm. diameter and of a depth of slightly greater than the thickness of the mucous membrane (when the mucosa is no longer subjected to the pressure of the fitting surface of a denture, its thickness will increase slightly). The height of the abutment posts above the mucous membrane should be such that they will be well short of the occlusal surfaces of the upper teeth. This height can be gauged from the articulated model and upper denture. The diameter of the base of the abutment posts should be about 4 mm. in the canine regions and 6 mm. in the molar regions and each post should have a 5 degree (approx.) taper. The patterns of the posts can be made in either wax or acrylic resin. Casting of the pattern is carried out in the normal manner and care should be taken to use only an alloy which has been proved to be electrolytically compatible with the body tissues.

The cast implant is trimmed and finished, the substructure being left with a sand blast surface, and the abutment posts

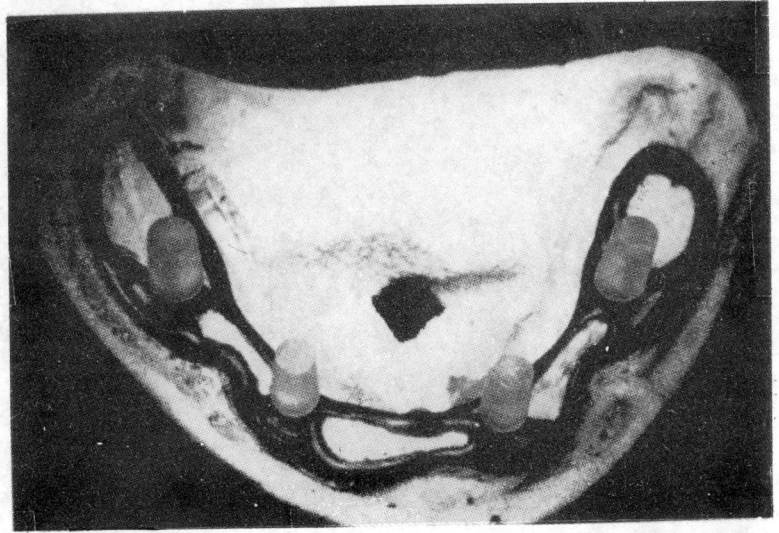

FIG. 570. – Wax pattern for substructure. Posts made of acrylic resin turned on lathe.

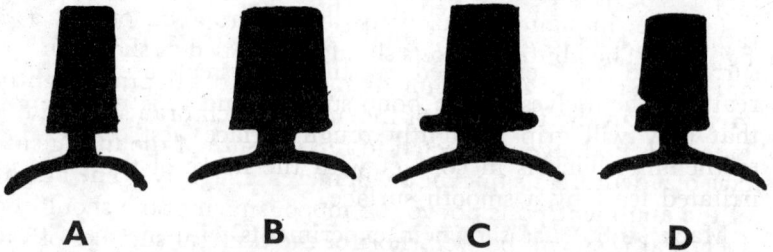

A   B   C   D

Fig. 571. – Silhouettes of shapes of implant posts: all have
approximately a 5 degree taper.
A, Canine post, dimensions are: diameter at base 4 mm.,
diameter of neck joining it with substructure 2½ mm.
B, Molar post, diameter at base 6 mm., diameter of
neck 3 mm.
C, Illustrates an alternative shape to provide a ledge to
support the superstructure and provide extra protection
·for the gingival margin.
D, Illustrates a post with a neck in it to engage a clasp if
required.
The dimensions given are arbitrary; the height of the
neck will be slightly more than the thickness of the mucosa;·
the height of the post will depend on the interalveolar distance.

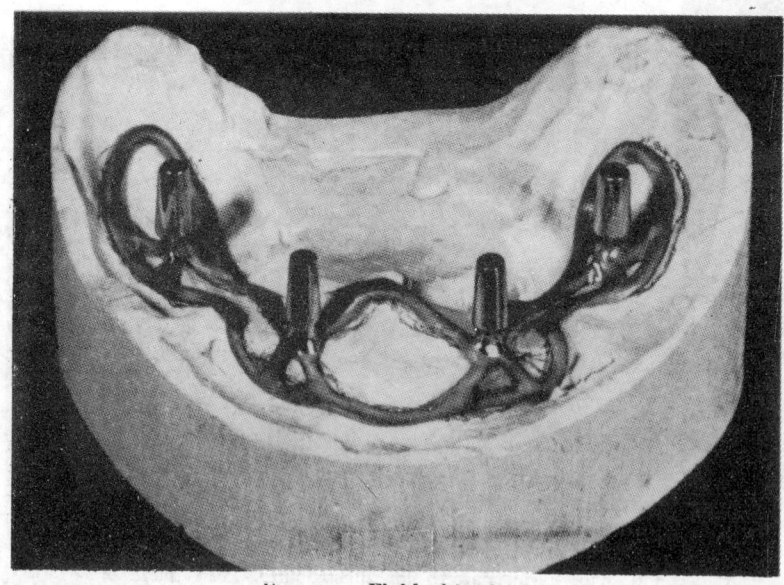

Fig. 572. – Finished implant.

and necks highly polished (*see* figs. 572, 573, 574). The rationale behind this is that the substructure becomes surrounded and embedded in the periosteal fibres which reattach themselves to the bone surface, and it is considered that they will grip a slightly rough surface best, while the epithelium which is in contact with the necks of the posts is irritated least by a smooth surface.

Mack (1960) has shown in experiments with monkeys that it is probable that the whole implant substructure becomes in time surrounded by epithelium and if this indeed proves to be the case it might be better practice to polish highly the whole of the implant.

Before finally finishing and polishing the implant it must be carefully inspected visually for imperfections likely to weaken it, and then X-rayed for evidence of any internal porosity.

(5) The implant is positioned on the model and the sub-

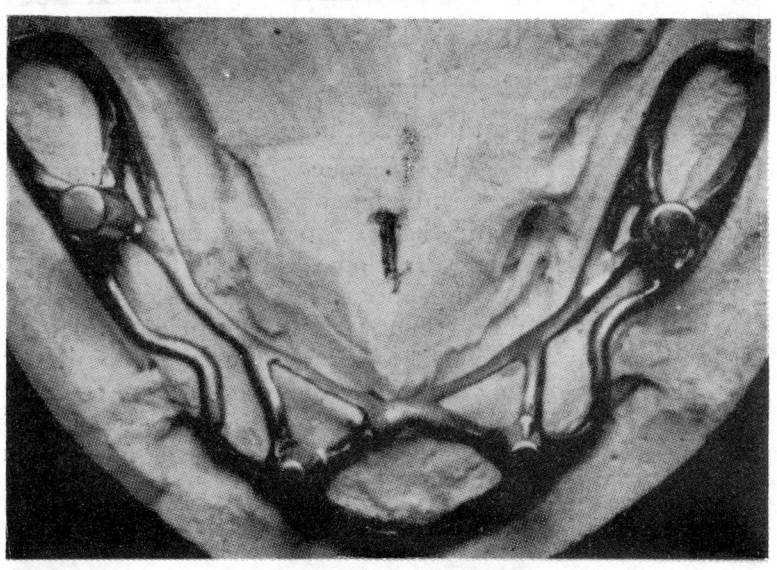

FIG. 573. – Finished implant. Note wide coverage of substructure, area of incision left free from metal, clearance of mental nerves and that the substructure is short of the mylohyoid ridge.

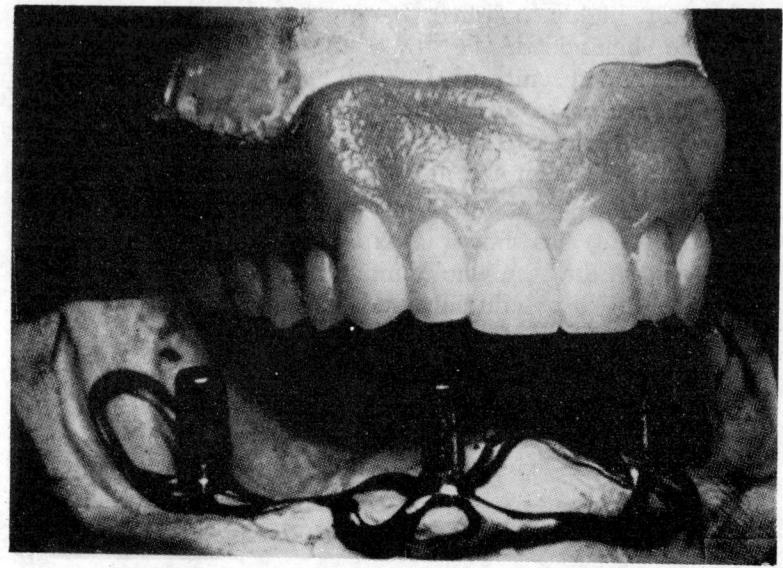

FIG. 574. – Implant on model articulated by means of
records taken at operation. Note clearance between tops of
posts and occlusal surfaces of teeth of upper denture.

structure covered with a thickness of base plate wax of approximately twice the thickness of the mucous membrane. Thimbles
are then waxed to fit the abutment posts and joined by wax
bars. The whole is cast in chrome cobalt and then trimmed to
be a comfortable and inert frictional fit on the four abutment
posts (see fig. 575). This superstructure frame work is an
important part of the implant because it confers additional
rigidity to it by its close fit to the abutments, joining them
by the rigid connecting bars. The connecting bars also ensure
that when the superstructure is processed into the lower
denture that the contraction of the acrylic will not distort
the position of the thimbles and therefore ensures that the
denture will be a stable fit on the abutment posts. Two of
these superstructure castings are required for each implant;
one is processed into the initial denture and one kept for use
with the final denture.

(6) The cast superstructure is seated on the abutment posts

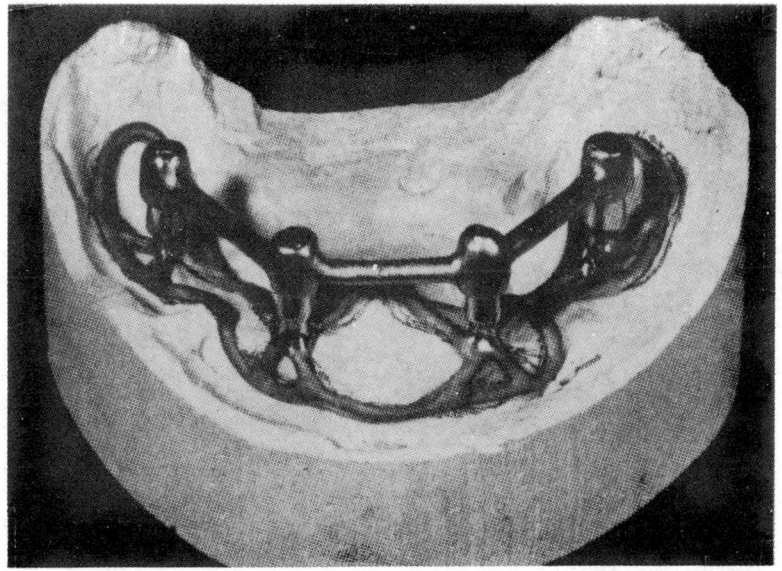

Fig. 575. – Cast superstructure fitted on to posts.

and the initial lower denture is waxed up around it. This denture carries six anterior teeth, but the posterior teeth are represented by blocks built to occlude with the molars and pre-molars of the upper denture (*see* fig. 577). The reason for this is that such a procedure simplifies any occlusal adjustment which may be necessary after the fitting of the implant and the flat surfaces of the lower blocks cause little or no lateral drag to be applied to the implant. Some operators dispense altogether with the initial denture and fit no lower denture until the tissues have healed around the implant. Fitting the denture to the implant as soon as it is placed has two advantages; firstly it covers the wound, protecting it from the inquisitive tongue, and secondly and perhaps more important each time the patient occludes it tends to seat the implant firmly on to the bone surface.

The waxed up initial denture is processed in acrylic and then finally shaped and polished. The shape of an implant supported denture has no relationship to that of a normal lower denture.

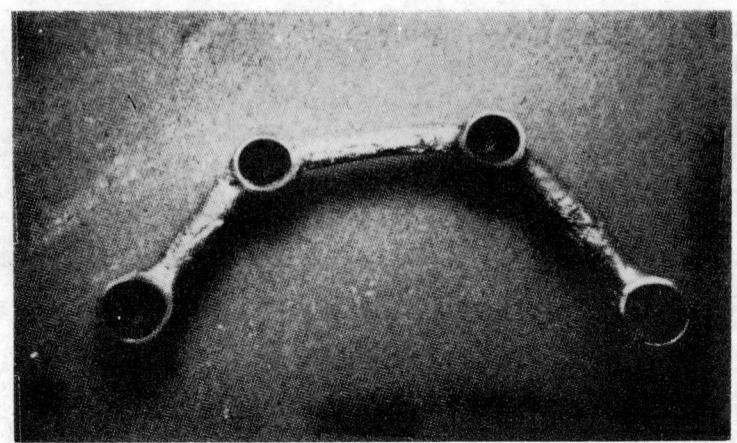

FIG. 576. – Looking into fitting surface of thimbles of superstructure.

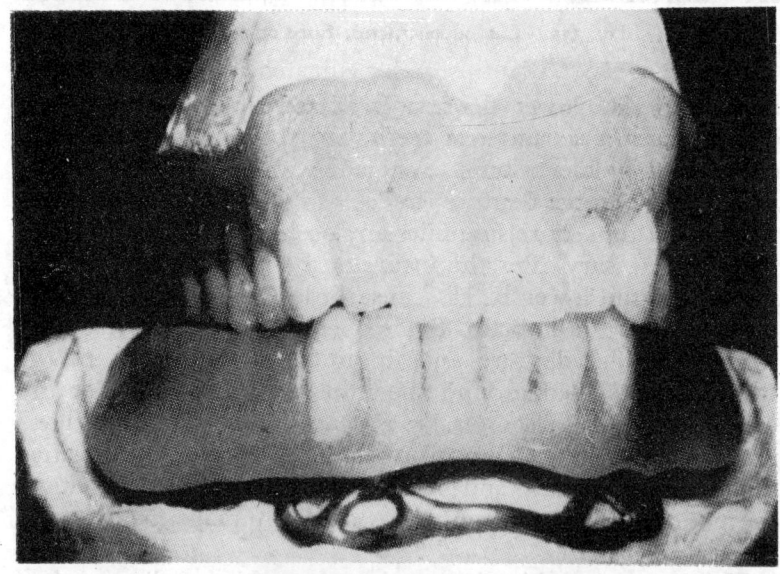

FIG. 577. – The denture fitted at the second operation in place on implant. Note wide clearance between it and substructure to allow for thickness of mucosa.

Firstly its fitting surface must be clear of the mucous membrane by at least one millimetre because it is supported entirely by the abutments, and secondly its bucco-lingual and labio-lingual bulk must be minimal and it must lie as accurately as possible in the volume of the neutral space. This is of vital importance because the success of the implant depends to a large extent on its not being subjected to continuous antero-posterior or lateral forces. Such continuous forces are likely to develop if for instance the denture is shaped so that the lip or the cheek bring a constant pressure to bear on it, not counter balanced by the tongue. Such unbalanced forces will cause the implant to move backwards or sideways with possible loosening of it. If, however, the denture is placed in the neutral zone the forces applied around its periphery will cancel one another out and it will remain in position. The shape of a typical implant supported denture is shown in fig. 578.

THE INSERTION OF THE IMPLANT

This usually takes place about three weeks after the first operation. The patient is pre-medicated and the mandible

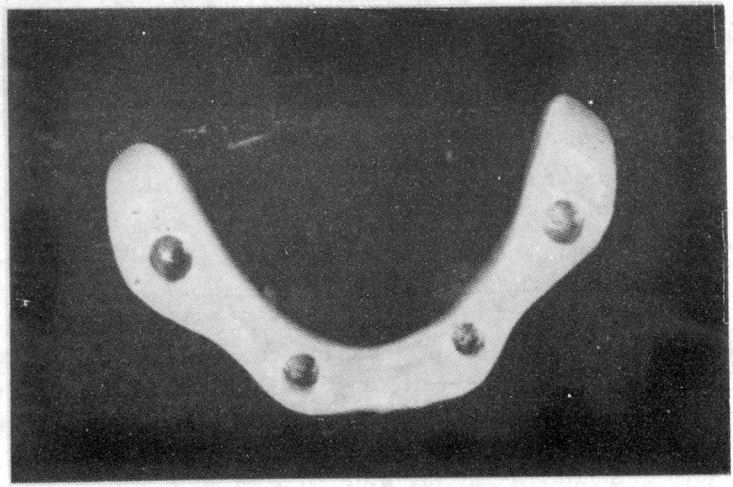

FIG. 578. – An implant supported denture viewed from below. Note narrowness, especially labially and in region of modiolii.

anaesthetized as for the initial operation. The mucous membrane is incised following the line of the original incision which will still be visible. The second incisions posteriorly and in the mid-line are not usually necessary. The mucoperiosteum is reflected but not so widely as previously, and as soon as it has been retracted sufficiently from the bone one of the implants which have been previously degreased in trichlorethylene and sterilized is tried-in. It should fit the bone surface accurately all round the area of the frame work and lie completely inert when pressure is applied to each abutment post successively (*see* fig. 579). If the first implant does not fulfil these require-

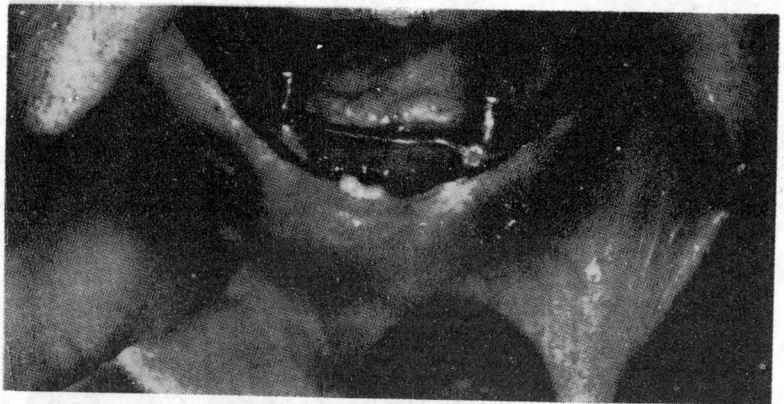

FIG. 579. – Implant in place prior to suturing of mucous membrane.
(Photograph by kind permission of Mr. M. A. Kettle.)

ments in any particular, the second one is tried-in and the more suitable of the two selected for insertion.

Some authorities advocate the initial stabilization of the implant by fixing it to the bone by screws placed one in the molar region on each side, and one in the region of the symphysis. The technique here described does not employ screws, and provided the extension of the implant frame work is adequate and its fit accurate they do not appear to be necessary. When the implant has been positioned, the mucoperiosteum is carefully united with sutures (*see* fig. 580). The

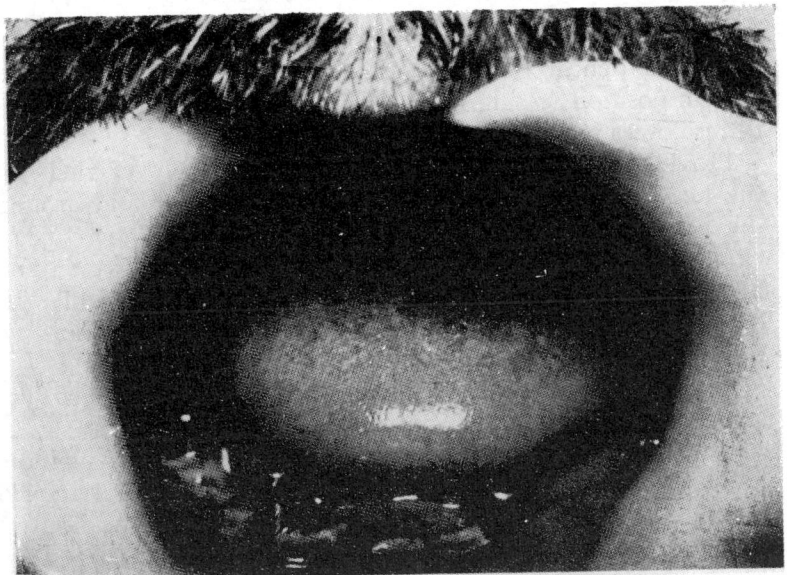

FIG. 580. – Implant in place after forty-eight hours.
(Photograph by kind permission of Mr. M. A. Kettle.)

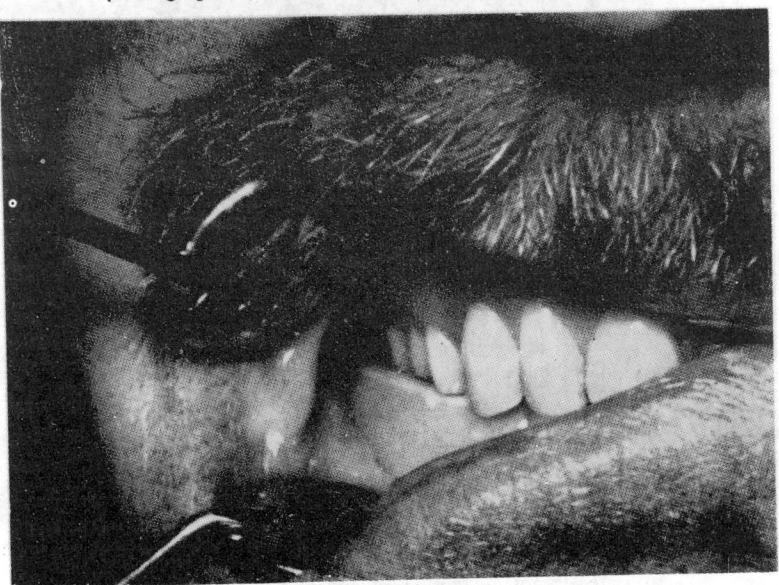

FIG. 581. – First denture in place. Note even occlusal contact
has been obtained by cold cure acrylic on surface of posterior
blocks.

initial denture is then placed in position, and its occlusion with the upper denture carefully adjusted to be quite even in the centric position (*see* fig. 581). This is important for otherwise tilting forces may be applied to the implant.

Provided all the stages have been accurately carried out the healing of the tissues over the substructure and around the abutments should be uneventful (*see* fig. 583). Commonly the wound breaks down in the anterior region and heals slowly by second intention. It is important that while the denture is a firm frictional fit on the abutment posts it is not so tight that undue force is needed to remove it.

As soon as the tissues are completely healed the second or final lower denture should be constructed. The second cast superstructure is seated on the abutment posts and an alginate impression taken around it. When the impression is removed the superstructure will be withdrawn buried in the impres-

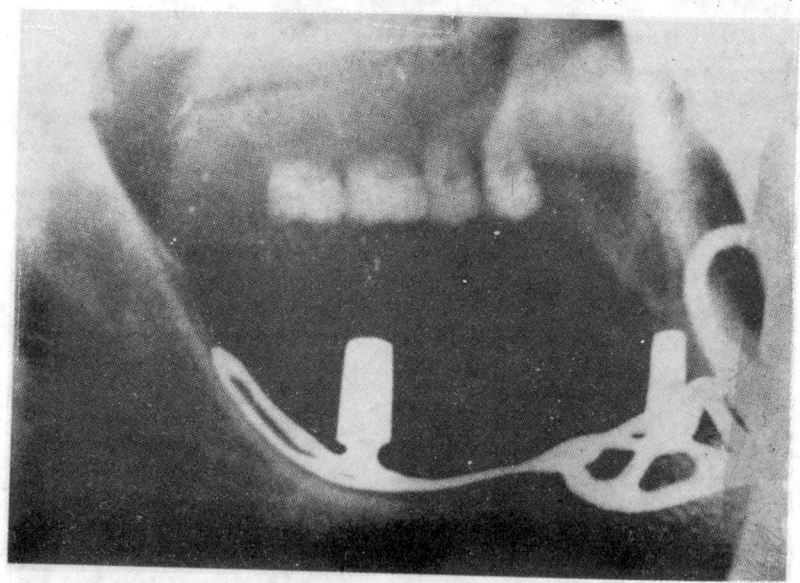

Fig. 582. – X-ray photographs of implants in place.
(a) Lateral; note extension of substructure up ascending ramus and deep extension of framework labially, both designed to resist backward pressures of lower lip.

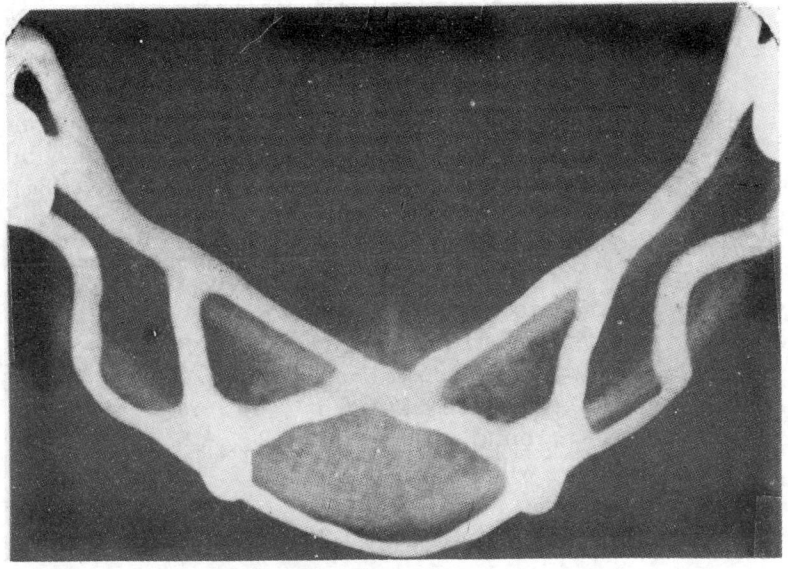

Fig. 582
(b) Occlusal view of same implant.

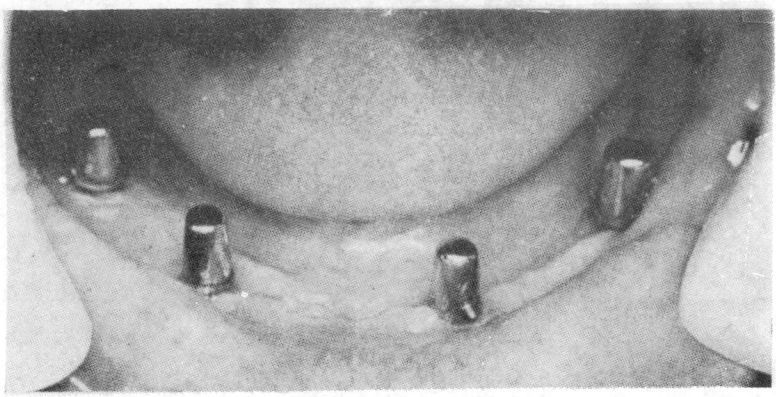

Fig. 583.
(a) A completed implant after three months.

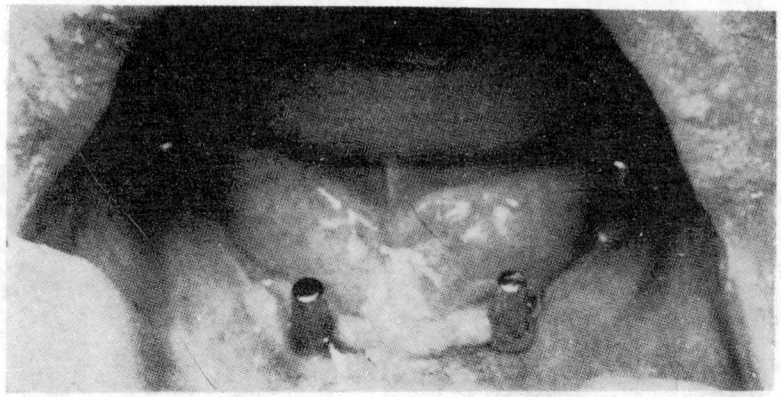

FIG. 583.
(b) A completed implant after nine months.

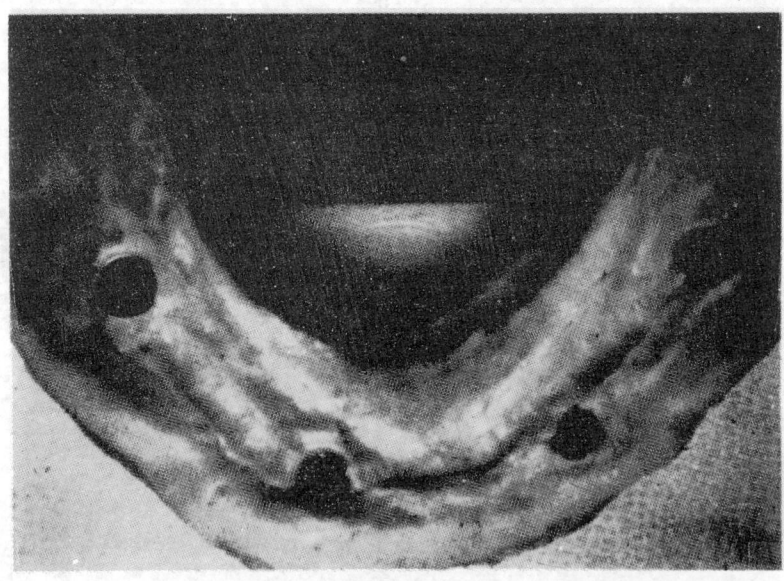

FIG. 584. – Alginate impression for second denture with
second superstructure contained in impression.

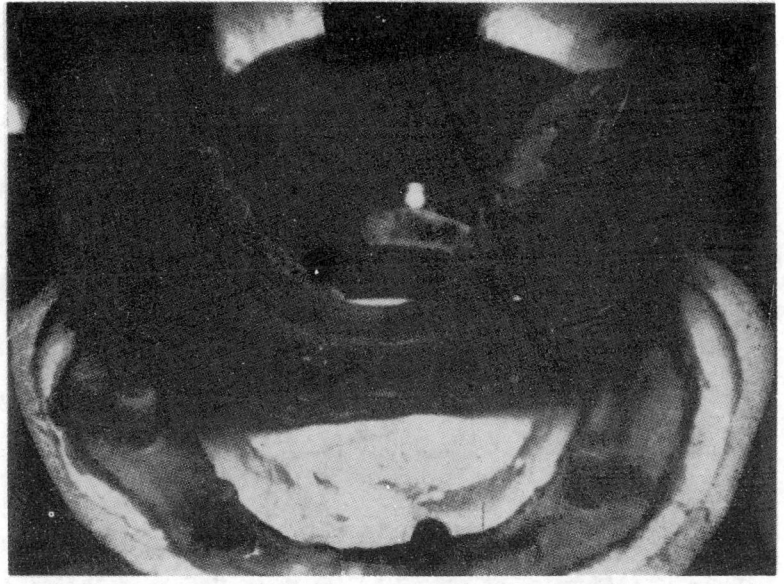

Fig. 585. – Model cast from alginate impression. Posts are cast in cold cure acrylic. Record block is also shown containing second superstructure.

sion (*see* fig. 584). Cold cure acrylic resin is mixed and vibrated into the thimbles of the cast superstructure, and when this is set plaster is cast into the rest of the impression (*see* fig. 585). This technique is employed because if plaster is cast into the thimbles it usually breaks off when an attempt is made to remove the superstructure from the model. The ridge surface of the model is covered with a thickness of base plate wax to act as a separator and prevent the base of the denture touching the mucous membrane.

A record block is then built round the superstructure and the records taken against the upper denture in the normal manner for setting the case on anatomical articulator. From here on the technique is similar for that of a normal denture, except for its shaping which is similar to that of the initial denture (*see* fig. 586). Careful attention must be paid to obtaining a balanced articulation because all unnecessary lateral or antero-posterior drag on the implant must be avoided. When the final

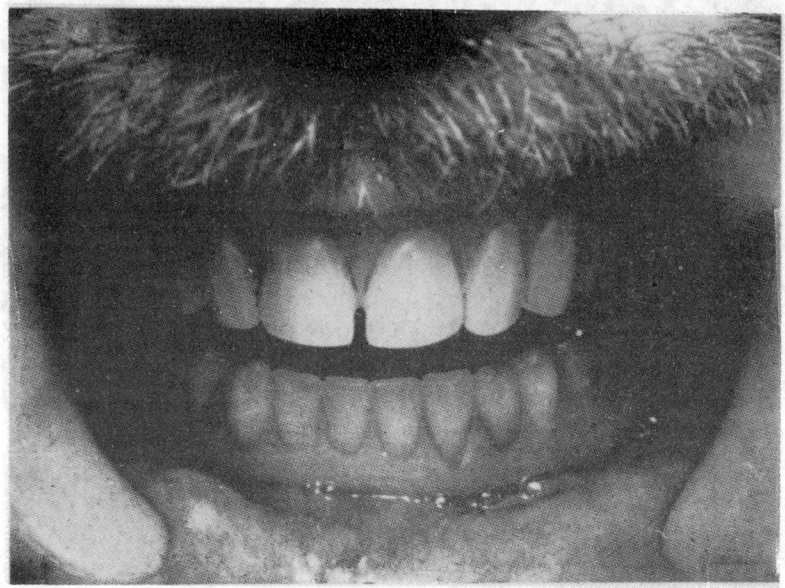

FIG. 586. – Finished second denture in place.

denture is fitted the initial denture is retained because when the second denture needs replacing in due course the cast superstructure buried in the first denture will be needed again.

GENERAL REMARKS IN RELATION TO SUBPERIOSTEAL IMPLANTS

Several thousand implants have been inserted throughout the world during the last ten years. Many of these have been in place and highly successful for five years or more. If an implant is successful the benefit to the patient is most marked. Many implants, however, have been failures; they have become loose and infection has penetrated around the abutment posts, and along the substructure. In many of these the failure is attributed to a failure of one or more of the following important points:

(a) Accurate fit on the surface of the bone.

(b) Correct outline and adequate extension of the substructure frame work.

(*c*) Shape of the denture leading to uneven pressure being applied to it by the surrounding muscles or to uneven occlusion.

(*d*) Careless surgical technique.

(*e*) Inserting an implant in an individual whose health was poor as a result of some systemic disease or whose health has degenerated after the insertion of the implant.

In some cases although the general healing of the tissues over the sub-structure frame work has been good, in some areas the tissues have failed to cover the metal. In some of these cases a *status quo* has developed and the implant has remained in place, in others it has had to be removed. An implant is held in place by the periosteal fibres re-attaching themselves to the surface of the bone around the frame work of the substructure and binding it firmly in place. In a well fitting properly extended implant the firmness of this retention is very great.

Why infection does not penetrate between the abutment posts and the mucous membrane is not fully understood. A gingival margin similar in many respects to the gingival margin surrounding a natural tooth develops, and it is also thought that there is a current of tissue fluid sweeping up from the substructure of implant around the false gingival margins which prevents the ingress of infection. A great deal of experiment and research is needed before implants are completely understood and evaluated. There is no doubt however, that in successful implants these false gingival margins appear to be perfectly healthy.

Bibliography

BOOKS

ANDERSON, J. N. Applied Dental Materials. Blackwell Scientific Publication, Oxford.

BRASIER, S. Maxillo-facial Laboratory Technique and Facial Prostheses. H. Kimpton, London.

BRENNER, M. D. K. The Story of Dentistry. Dental Items of Interest Publishing Co.

CRADDOCK, F. W. Prosthetic Dentistry. A Clinical Outline. Henry Kimpton, London.

DORRANCE, G. N. Operative Story of the Cleft Palate. W. B. Saunders, Philadelphia and London.

FISH, E. W. Principles of Full Denture Prosthesis. 4th ed. revised. Staples Press Limited, London.

FOCH-ANDERSON. Inheritance of Hare Lip and Cleft Palate. Arnold Busck.

FRAHM, F. W. The Principles and Techniques of Full Denture Construction. Dental Items of Interest Publishing Co., Brooklyn, New York; Henry Kimpton, London.

GERSHKOFF, A. and GOLDBERG, N. I. Implant Dentures. Pitman, London.

HOLDSWORTH, W. J. Cleft Lip and Palate. William Heinemann Medical Books Ltd.

KENNEDY, E. Partial Denture Construction. Dental Items of Interest Publishing Co., Brooklyn, New York; Henry Kimpton, London.

LANDA, J. S. Practical Full Denture Prosthesis. Dental Items of Interest Publishing Co., Brooklyn, New York; Henry Kimpton, London.

LINDSAY, LILIAN. Short History of Dentistry. John Bale, Sons and Danielsson Ltd.

MILLER, R. G. Synopsis of Full and Partial Dentures. Henry Kimpton, London.

MORLEY, M. E. Cleft Palate and Speech. 4th ed. Livingstone, Edinburgh.

OSBORNE, JOHN. Dental Mechanics for Students. Staples Press Limited, London.

OSBORNE, J., and LAMMIE, G. A. Partial Dentures. Blackwell Scientific Publications, Oxford.

PEYTON, F. A. Restorative Dental Materials. C. V. Mosby Co. Ltd.
PRINZ, HERMAN. Dental Chronology. H. Kimpton, London.
SCHLOSSER, R. O. Complete Denture Prosthesis. W. B. Saunders, Philadelphia.
SICHER, H. Oral Anatomy. H. Kimpton, London.
SKINNER, E. W. Science of Dental Materials. W. B. Saunders & Co.
SWENSON, M. G. Complete Dentures. 2nd ed. C. V. Mosby Co., and Henry Kimpton, London.
TUCKFIELD, W. J. Full Denture Technique. Ramsay Ware Publishing Pty., Melbourne, Australia.

PERIODICALS

Aesthetics and Appearance

ASPIN, M. E., TOMLIN, H. R., and OSBORNE, J. (1960) Brit. Dent. J., **109** 271–274.
CLARK, E. B. (1947) Selection of tooth colour for the edentulous patient, J.A.D.A., **35**, 787–793.
FRUSH, J. P., and FISHER, R. D. (1955) J.P.D., **5**, 586–595.
——— (1956) J.P.D., **6**, 160–172.
——— (1956) J.P.D., **6**, 441–449.
——— (1957) J.P.D., **7**, 5–13.
——— (1958) J.P.D., **8**, 558–581.
——— (1959) J.P.D., **9**, 914–921.
FURNAS, I. L. (1936) Esthetics in full denture construction, J.A.D.A. **23**, 3–13.
HARDY, I. R. (1939) Ways and means of avoiding obvious artificiality, J.A.D.A., **26**, 1289–1291.
MENDELSOHN, W. A. (1938) Light as related to matching shades of, teeth, Dental Digest, **44**, 12–14.
POUND, E. (1951) J.P.D., **1**, 98–111.
——— (1954) J.P.D., **4**, 6–16.
YOUNG, H. A. (1954) J.P.D., **4**, 748–760.
——— (1956) J.P.D., **6**, 748—755.
WARBURTON, W. L. (1946) Pre-extraction records, Dental Survey, **22**, 2069–2073.

Alveolectomy

BOWDEN, A. C. (1943) Indications for alveolectomy and the technique of the operation, D. Gazette, **9**, 289–293.
CASH, H. R. (1944) Surgical treatment of abnormal soft tissue ridge attachment, Australian J. D., **48**, 141–143.
FLEMING, W. E. (1944) Surgical preparation of the mouth for prostheses, Australian J. D., **48**, 197–199.

Articulation

CRADDOCK, F. W. (1949) Accuracy and practical value of records of condylar path inclinations, *J.A.D.A.*, **38**, 697–710.

FRIEDMAN, S. (1947) Occlusal harmony in complete artificial dentures, *J.A.D.A.*, **35**, 873–875.

LINDBLOM, GOSTA (1949) Term 'Balanced articulation', its origin, development and present significance in modern odontology, *D. Record*, **69**, 304–312.

THOMPSON, J. R. (1946) Rest position of the mandible and its significance of dental science, *J.A.D.A.*, **33**, 151–180

Bases

LEADER, S. A. (1952) Laminated acrylic dentures, *Brit. dent. J.*, **93**, 179–182.

OSBORNE, JOHN (1952) The use of self-curing resins in prosthetic dentistry, *Brit. Dent. J.*, **93**, 309–312.

—— (1953) Some observations concerning chrome cobalt denture bases, *Brit. Dent. J.*, **94**, 55–67.

Cleft Palate

CALNAN, J. S. (1953) *J. Plastic Surg.*, **5**, 286.

FITZGIBBONS, J. S. (1931) *Dental Items of Interest*, **53**, 737.

LIDDELOW, K. P. (1959) *Annals Roy. Coll. Surg.*, **25**, 246.

MALSON, T. S. (1957) Non obstructing prosthetic speech aid during growth and orthodontic treatment, *J. Pros. Dent.*, **7**, 403–415.

NOBISTROM, P. H., and ANDERSON, B. D. (1959) *Oral Surg.*, **12**, 142.

RAMSEY, G. H., WATSON, J. S., *et al.* (1955) Cinefluorographic analysis of the mechanism of swallowing, *J. Radio.*, **64**, 498.

ROSEN, M. S., and BZOCH, K. R. (1957) *J. Amer. Dent. Ass.*, **57**, 203.

TOWNSHEND, R. H. (1940) The formation of Passevant's bar. *Journ. Laryng. & Otol.*, **55**, 154.

WARDILL, W. E. M. (1930) *Dental Record*, **50**, 547.

WHILLIS, J. (1930) A note on the muscles of the palate and the Inferior Constrictor, *Journ. Anat.*, **65**, 92–95.

Dentures

FLETCHER, L. S. (1947) Fundamental principles of full denture construction, *D. Survey*, **23**, 1765–1769.

MATTHEWS, E. (1944) New approach to full denture construction, *Brit. Dent. J.*, **76**, 262–268.

—— (1945) Some common causes of failure in dentures, *D. Gazette*, **11**, 258–259.

—— (1942) Stabilisation of lower dentures, *D. Gazette*, **8**, 315–316.

TIGHE, J. C. (1949) Construction of full dentures, *J.A.D.A.*, **39**, 703–708.

Impressions

ALBINSON, R. N. (1948) What is mucostatics? *D. Survey*, **24**, 967–970

CHICK, A. O., and PEACOCK, J. N. (1945) Notes on prosthetic procedures, *Brit. Dent. J.*, **79**, 243–249.

—— (1946) *Brit. Dent. J.*, **80**, 23.

CHRISTY, R. L. (1943) Impression technique for flabby ridge. Need for surgery eliminated, *D. Survey*, **19**, 44–46.

GLUPKER, H. (1942) Complete denture impression materials, their application and manipulation, *J.A.D.A.*, **29**, 2216–2220.

HURST, W. W. (1946) Importance of a thorough mouth examination as related to the selection of suitable impression methods for edentulous cases, *Pennsylvania D. J.*, **13**, 179–187.

JØRGENSEN, K. D. (1956) Thiokol as a dental impression material, *Acta Odont. Scand.*, **14**, 313–334.

KILE, C. S. (1942) Muscle trimming the hamular notch and soft palate area to get perfect upper impressions, *D. Survey*, **18**, 1632–1634.

KINGHORN, A., and ALLEN, D. N. (1957) Inlay production from rubber base impressions, *Brit. Dent. J.*, **103**, 1–6.

KNAPP, K. W. (1948) Hydrocolloid impressions after ten years, *New York D. J.*, **14**, 249–253.

MACK, A. O. (1950) Closed mouth impression technique for full denture construction, *Brit. Dent. J.*, **89**, 104–105.

MORANGE, R. M. (1948) Fournet-Tuller technique for lower dentures, *D. Digest*, **54**, 406–409.

PRYOR, W. J. (1948) Evaluation of several full denture impression techniques, *J.A.D.A.*, **37**, 159–167.

SKINNER, E. W. (1946) Dimensional stability of alginate impression material, *J.A.D.A.*, **33**, 1253–1260.

SPICER, G. H. (1953) Impressions of ridges with hyperplastic tissue, *J. Pros. Dent.*, **3**, 163.

TOMLIN, H. R., and OSBORNE, J. (1958) Some observations on silicone impression materials, *Brit. Dent. J.*, **104**, 407–412.

TUCKFIELD, W. J. (1947) Relative importance of impressions in full denture construction, *Austr. D.J.*, **51**, 361–365.
—— (1950) Review of impression techniques in full denture prosthesis, *Internat. Dent. J.*, **1**, 112.

Immediate Dentures

ALLEN, A. G. (1952) Immediate dentures, *Brit. Dent. J.*, **92**, 212–215

COBLE, L. G. (1946) Immediate denture technique, *D. Survey*, **22**, 1870–1873.

DAWBORN, R. K. (1948) Immediate denture service, gum faced technique, with partial alveolectomy, *Aus. Dental Congress*, 11*th Proceedings*, pp. 152–161.

GIELER, C. W. (1947) Immediate denture prostheses, tooth arrangement and aesthetics, *J.A.D.A.*, **35**, 185–191.

KEENEY, B. L. (1948) One day immediate denture service, *D. Survey* **24**, 1745–1747.

OSBORNE, JOHN (1945) Immediate restorations, *D. Gazette*, **11**, 300–304.

SCHLOSSER, R. O. (1946) Rational clinical procedure in complete immediate denture prosthesis, *J. South California Dental Ass.*, **13**, 13–17.
—— (1948) Advantages of conservative procedure in complete immediate denture prosthesis, *J. Canadian Dental Ass.*, **14**, 611–616.

SWENSON, M. G. (1939) Immediate denture service, *J.A.D.A.*, **26** 719–730.

Implant Dentures

DAHL, G. S. A. (1943) *Odontol. Tidsk.*, **51**, 440.

MACK, A. O. (1955) *Brit. Dent. J.*, **99**, 287.
—— (1960) *Brit. Dent. J.*, **108**, 127.

TRAININ, B. (1954) *Brit. Dent. J.*, **96**, 224.
—— (1954) *Brit. Dent. J.*, **102**, 389.

VENABLE, C. S., STUCK, W. G., and BEACH, A. (1937) *Ann. Surg.*, **105**, 917.

Mandible

CHICK, A. O. (1949) Forward movement of the mandible during bite closure and its relation to excessive alveolar resorption in edentulous cases, *Brit. Dent. J.*, **87**, 243–246.

KURTH, L. E. (1949) Physiology of mandibular movements related to prosthodontia, *New York D.J.*, **15**, 323–329.

—— (1942) Mandibular movements in mastication, *J.A.D.A.*, **29**, 1769–1790.

PENDLETON, E. C. (1942) Minute anatomy of the lower jaw in relation to the denture problem, *J.A.D.A.*, **29**, 719–736.

THOMPSON, J. R., and BRODIE, A. G. (1942) Factors in the position of the mandible, *J.A.D.A.*, **29**, 925–941.

Occlusion

CASON, W. H. (1947) Securing centric relation, *D. Survey*, **23**, 631–635.

HOLIC, R. (1948) Centric registration in full denture construction, *J.A.D.A.*, **36**, 296–301.

MCGEE, G. F. (1947) Use of facial measurements in determining vertical dimension, *J.A.D.A.*, **35**, 342–350.

OSBORNE, JOHN (1949) Recording centric occlusion for edentulous cases, *D. Record*, **69**, 6–12.

SCHWEITZER, J. M. (1942) Vertical dimension, *J.A.D.A.*, **29**, 419–422.

SICHER, H. (1948) Temporomandibular articulation in mandibular overclosure, *J.A.D.A.*, **36**, 131–139.

Overlay Dentures

BRILL, NIELS, et al. (1959) *Brit. Dent. J.*, **106**, 2.

HANKEY, G. T. (1954) *Brit. Dent. J.*, **97**, 249.

LAMMIE, G. A. et al. (1956) *Brit. Dent. J.*, **100**, 33.

LINDBLOM, GÖSTA (1954) *J. Amer. Dent. Ass.*, **48**, 620.

POSSELT, U. (1959) *Dent. Pract.*, **9**, 255.

—— (1959) *Paradontologie*, **1**, 3.

REES, L. A. (1954) *Brit. Dent. J.*, **96**, 125.

SICHER, H. (1954) *J. Amer. Dent. Ass.*, **48**, 620.

WILSON, H. E. (1957) *Dent. Pract.*, **7**, 218.

Partial Dentures

ANDERSON, J. N., and LAMMIE, G. A. (1952) A clinical survey of partial dentures, *Brit. Dent. J.*, **92**, 59–67.

CRADDOCK, F. W. (1946) Labial bar partial denture, *New Zealand D.J.*, **42**, 67.

MATTHEWS, E. (1952) The partial denture problem, *Brit. Dent. J.*, **92**, 173–179.

—— (1948) Clasp design in partial dentures, *Brit. Dent. J.*, **85**, 152–158.

SCHMIDT, A. H. (1947) Partial dentures; planning and designing, *J.A.D.A.*, **35**, 562–569.

SMITH, E. S. (1949) Importance of evaluating mouth conditions preparatory to the construction of partial dentures, *J.A.D.A.*, **39**, 693–702.

WATT, D. M., MACGREGOR, A. R., *et al.* (1958) A preliminary investigation of the support of partial dentures and its relationship to vertical load, *Dent. Pract.*, **9**, 2.

Perfecting Occlusion and Articulation

COBLE, L. G. C. (1958) *New York Journal of Dentistry*, **28**, 306–307.

CRADDOCK, F. W. (1949) *J.A.D.A.*, **38**, 697.

GRAHAM, C. H. (1953) *The Australian Journal of Dentistry*, **59**, 100–110.

KROGH-POULSEN, W. (1958) *Internat. D.J.*, **8**, 374–376

LINDBLOM, G. (1949) *Dental Record*, **69**, 304–311

SCHUYLER, C. H. (1935) *J.A.D.A.*, **22**, 1193.

SICHER, H. (1956) *J.P.D.*, **6**, 616–620.

Relining

ARONSON, H. L. (1942) Simple method of relining metal partials, *D. Digest*, **48**, 380.

CHICK, A. O., and PEACOCK, J. N. (1946) Relining technique for full upper dentures, *Brit. Dent. J.*, **80**, 120.

CRAIG, W. E. (1943) Relining an upper denture. *Oral Hygiene*, **33**, 798–799.

LEVY, CLEMENT (1944) Denture rebase with acrylic resin. Cured at mouth temperature, *Brit. Dent. J.*, **76**, 305–306.

—— (1946) Denture relining and acrylic burns, *S. Africa D.J.*, **20**, 195–197.

OSBORNE, JOHN (1952) Relining and rebasing, *Brit. Dent. J.*, **92**, 149–153.

Stability

MATTHEWS, E. (1942) Stabilisation of lower dentures, *D. Gazette*, **8**, 315–316.

RAYBIN, N. H. (1949) Analysis of the unstable and ill-fitting artificial denture, *J.A.D.A.*, **39**, 177–184.

Stomatitis

CAHN, L. R. (1949) Denture sore mouth, *New York D.J.*, **15**, 158–160.

HEAVENOR, R. G. M. (1943) Acute stomatitis caused by ill-fitting dentures, *Brit. Dent. J.*, **74**, 319–320.

LYON, D. G., and CHICK, A. O. (1957) Denture sore mouth and angular cheilitis, *Dent. Pract.*, **7**, 212–217.

Teeth

ANDERSON, B. G. (1947) Functions of the teeth, *Ann. Den.*, **5**, 103–107.

MATTHEWS, E. (1949) Tooth placement in full denture construction, *Dental Record*, **69**, 13–17.

Tongue

FISH, E. W. (1947) Tongue space in full denture construction, *Brit. Dent. J.*, **83**, 137–142.

LANDA, J. S. (1945) Practical full denture prosthesis, *D. Items of Interest*, **67**, 470–478.

Index